MAMMALIAN
PHYSIOLOGY

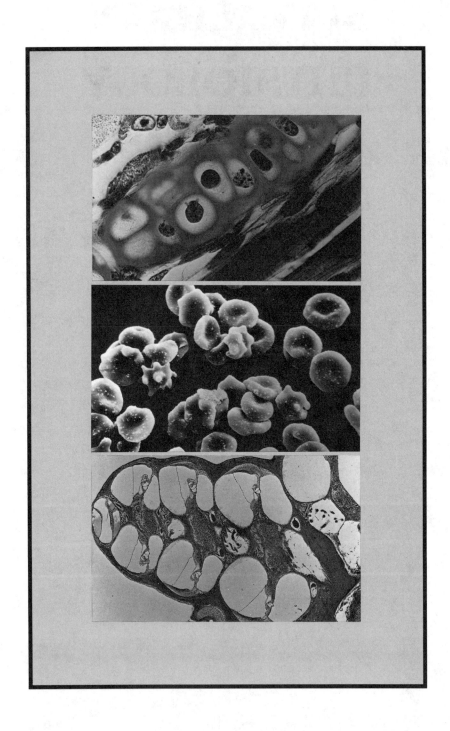

MAMMALIAN

PHYSIOLOGY

J. Homer Ferguson
formerly
University of Idaho

Charles E. Merrill Publishing Company
A Bell & Howell Company
Columbus   Toronto   London   Sydney

To my wife
Carolyn Hawley Ferguson
To my aunt
Agnes Henson Bynum
And to the memory of my parents
Mr. and Mrs. Morgan Ferguson

Published by Charles E. Merrill Publishing Company
A Bell & Howell Company
Columbus, Ohio   43216

This book was set in Zapf Book Light
Production Coordinator: Mary Henkener
Text Designer: Cynthia Brunk
Cover Designer: Cathy Watterson
Original biological art: Ron McLean
Line art: Steve Botts

Library of Congress Catalog Card Number: 84–62174
International Standard Book Number: 0–675–20384–8
Printed in the United States of America
1 2 3 4 5 6 7 8 9 90 89 88 87 86 85

Cover photos © Manfred Kage, Peter Arnold, Inc. *Top,*
muscle-cartilage-connective tissue; *center,* healthy red
blood cells of rat; *bottom,* cochlea of ear of guinea pig.

CONTENTS

CONTENTS

19 The Physiology of Some Specialized Mammalian Adaptations   457

PREFACE

In this text I have attempted to introduce the student to a wide variety of physiological adaptations that enable mammals to inhabit the many habitats available to them. The organ systems concept is utilized here since this more nearly fills the need of the biology or zoology student at the undergraduate level. Comparative aspects of mammalian adaptations have been included wherever possible but this is by no means an exhaustive treatise of the comparative physiology of mammals. It is hoped that this text will be used in organ systems physiology courses that are not devoted exclusively to human or medical physiology.

The major intent is to round out the background of undergraduates in zoology and to prepare them for advanced studies in basic or applied physiology. This text is also intended to provide a physiological foundation which many students in applied areas of zoology such as game and wildlife management must rely upon as they follow careers aligned with ecology and natural history.

In some cases it has not been possible to cover the material in depth from a comparative approach since the majority of the literature in specific areas is developed from human-oriented research. However, in as many instances as possible, hiatuses in the literature are pointed out and the student is encouraged to pursue these areas as his or her own interest dictates. This book is not intended to be an ending or resource in itself, but should be a beginning where the pathways of endeavor into the study of physiology may be discovered.

I wish to express my appreciation to my wife, Carolyn Hawley Ferguson, for typing this manuscript and for devoting countless hours to proofreading as well as other valuable aspects of preparation. Christopher J. Gordon extended his encouragement and suggestions throughout the writing and preparation of this book. To him I owe special thanks for his assistance and participation in many writing as well as research efforts over the past ten years. I would also like to thank Robert Lakemacher of Charles E. Merrill Publishing Company for his patience and encouragement throughout the preparation of this text. Mary Henkener, Linda

Thornhill, and Linda Bayma also of Merrill devoted many hours to manuscript preparation and final editing. The help and suggestions from the reviewers are gratefully acknowledged. Their expertise and knowledge were a tremendous resource. I would especially like to thank Richard V. Andrews of Creighton University for his critical review in this process.

During the course of writing this text I was granted a sabbatical leave by the University of Idaho. I owe sincere appreciation to the chairman of that committee, Philip Deutchman, and the other members of the commit-

tee who made the final efforts in the preparation of this book possible.

Dr. G. Edgar Folk provided me with an environment for research at the University of Iowa and introduced me to arctic Alaska. I am grateful for his warm generosity and assistance. Finally, I would like to take this opportunity to express my gratitude to Dr. Charles H. Lower of the University of Arizona for his constant devotion to his students and for his persistent demands for excellence both in research and teaching.

J. H. Ferguson

1

INTRODUCTION

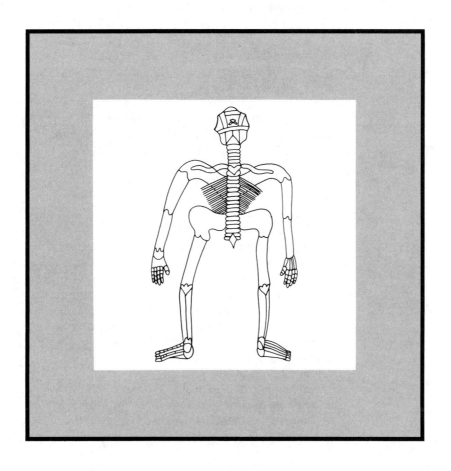

Physiology *is the study of function in the living organism; by its very nature it is closely associated with anatomy, or the study of structure. To understand function, structure must first be known. Early physiology was usually an interpretation of function based upon current knowledge of the structure of an organism. Aristotle's use of the term physiology encompassed all knowledge about nature, without restriction to living systems. In general, the term was unknown to most people and crept into the language very slowly. Galen of Pergamum (130?–?201), one of the most famous physicians of antiquity, used the term physiology to designate a branch of medicine alongside etiology, pathology, hygiene, and therapeutics. The term* physiologia *was first used by Jean Fernel (1497–1558) in his* Universa medicina *and gradually gained medical usage as a term describing functions that were distinct from basic anatomy. In the 18th century, Hermann Boerhaave (1668–1738) described physiology as the science concerned with the vital and organic functions. In 1708, Boerhaave published a series of lectures given at Leyden, the Netherlands, which dealt in part with "physiologia." A German translation of Boerhaave's work was published in 1754 entitled* Hermann Boerhaave's Physiology. *The subject of physiology was elevated to a position of independence in science by two publications,* Primae linea physiologiae *(1747) and the eight-volume* Elementa physiologiae corporis humani *(1757–1766), both by the Swiss Albrecht von Haller (1708–1777).*

Today there are many well-delineated areas within the field of physiology that deal with specific aspects of a very large and growing science, including cell physiology, comparative physiology, and medical physiology. In those and other areas literally thousands of scientists are involved in teaching and research. Medical physiology encompasses the basics of physiology because it concerns the function of organ systems in the human species, which was perhaps the first mammal to be studied from a physiological perspective. In mammalian physiology examples are cited from other species as well, thus covering aspects of function foreign to humans but quite characteristic of other mammals. The mammalian physiologist must never lose sight of the whole organism and its natural position in the environment. In that sense, mammalian physiology comprises environmental physiology as well as the comparative physiology both of mammals and of nonmammalian vertebrates.

The modern physiologist is concerned with how biological systems are designed and how they are controlled within the organism in the context of the environment. Two principles have utmost importance here: homeostasis *and* feedback regulation. *Homeostasis, a term proposed by American physiologist Walter Cannon (1871–1945), is the result of a group of regulating mechanisms that act to maintain the steady state of the organism in relation to its environment. Homeostasis, which is relevant to all aspects of mammalian physiology, is essential for maintainance of the so-called normal condition. Body temperature, blood calcium levels, and blood glucose levels, to name a few examples, must be maintained at steady states by homeostatic mechanisms. The most plausible and well-documented regulatory system in maintaining homeostasis is feedback regulation, a model of which appears in Figure 1–1. As an example, consider the homeostatic mechanism of body temperature maintenance in a relatively cold environment. The* sensor *represents temperature receptors in the skin and elsewhere in the body, the* control apparatus *represents the hypothalamus, and the* effector *represents metabolic tissue that produces heat. If heat is built up in the tissue as a result of metabolism, the receptors become warmed and the rate of internal heat production is reduced. Such feedback regulation is essential to numerous processes.*

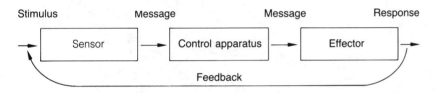

FIGURE 1–1
Simple model of feedback regulation

HISTORY OF PHYSIOLOGY

The history of physiology is rich and cannot be comprehensively covered here. Rather, the intent in this section is to demonstrate that our present knowledge is an accumulation resulting from the hard work of numerous philosophers and researchers over the past two millennia and more.

The study of physiology began in antiquity, almost simultaneously with the study of medicine. Some ancient theories long defended with almost religious fervor now appear ludicrous. But those theories were very important because many of them provided the hypotheses that allowed scientists to progress to the present level of thinking. Among the early Greek philosophers three

stand out as precursors to the present science of physiology. Hippocrates (460?–?377 B.C.), who lived on the island of Cos in the Aegean Sea, is considered the father of Western medicine. His major contribution to physiology is the so-called *Corpus Hippocraticum*, which was compiled in the 4th century B.C. The *Corpus* comprises many essays on cures and treatments of the time, only a few of which were actually written by Hippocrates himself. Aristotle (384–322 B.C.), probably the most famous and perhaps the greatest contributor to physiological thought of antiquity, wrote several important biological works expressing his ideas on physiology and medicine. His contributions remained the most accurate characterizations of physiological thought for many years. During the second century of the Christian era, the physician Galen rose to such heights and dominance in the field of medicine and physiology that for centuries none dared contradict his theories. Many important scholars of the Middle Ages are known to have suppressed knowledge simply because to have disagreed with the writings of Galen would have been considered heresy.

Physiology was in great turmoil during the 16th and 17th centuries. Traditional theories, such as those of Galen, gained opposition, and the reformation movement in physiology began. During that period one of the best

and well-documented treatises on anatomy, *De humani corporis fabrica*, was written by the Flemish physician and anatomist Andreas Vesalius (1514–1564). The reader might appreciate more thoroughly the work of Vesalius by comparing the diagrams in Figure 1–2. Also during that period, the Swiss scientist Paracelsus (Theophrastus von Hohenheim) (1493–1541) paved the way for the development of modern physiology through his statements on the vital actions of chemicals and their roles in the living animal.

During the 17th century, William Harvey (1578–1657) discovered the circulation of

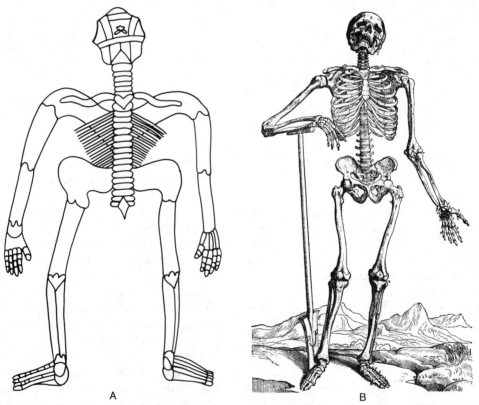

A   B

FIGURE 1–2
Depiction of the human skeletons from (A) the 14th century and (B) Andreas Vesalius's *De humani corporis fabrica* (1543)

blood, an essential concept for the discovery of the majority of the systemic functions which followed. Of primary importance was that observations and various data left no doubt that Harvey's views on blood circulation were correct. Anything short of outstanding evidence would have immediately been branded as heresy, since his discovery differed substantially in principle from the teachings of Galen. Also during that century, Giovanni A. Borelli (1608–1679) began applying mathematical analysis to muscular force and action. Respiratory physiology gained widespread interest, and it was shown experimentally that animals required an airborne substance for life. The respiratory experiments of John Mayow (1640–1679) proved that metabolism, respiration, and oxidation of metals are phenomena that require the presence of oxygen.

The 18th century saw the measurement of blood pressure by the Reverend Stephen Hales (1677–1761). His work paved the way for the calculation of cardiac output as well as for the calculation of other circulatory phenomena by the Swiss physician Daniel Bernoulli (1700–1782). During the latter part of the 18th century, the digestive process was established as a chemical phenomenon by the great Italian naturalist Lazzaro Spallanzani (1729–1799), who demonstrated the chemical nature of the digestive juices using himself as a guinea pig. Spallanzani, with remarkable fortitude, swallowed linen bags filled with food and regurgitated them at intervals in order to inspect the digestion of their contents. Despite Spallanzani's heroics, well-known scientists such as John Hunter (1628–1693) asserted that the Italian's experimental results were invalid. Hunter, a so-called vitalist, believed that digested materials were transformed into animal tissue by some "vital" occurrence. During that period

the central nervous system was studied extensively. Alexander Stuart studied spinal reflexes in frogs and from his research developed the concept of the central nervous system. Publications by G. Prochaska (1749–1820) later outlined the basic ingredients of the reflex mechanism. One of the most significant discoveries during the latter part of the 18th century involved the electrical nature of nerves. Luigi Galvani (1737–1798), a native of Bologna, demonstrated that electrical stimulation of nerves in frogs resulted in muscular contraction. Also in the late 18th century, Antoine L. Lavoisier (1743–1794) recognized the processes of metabolism and oxidation and demonstrated that metabolism produced heat not unlike that produced by burning. Lavoisier fell to the guillotine in 1794 after the revolutionary tribunal concluded, "Nous n'avons plus besoin des savants" (we no longer have need of wise men). It is unfortunate that "savants" were no longer needed: persons of his insight are as rare as perfection itself, and other scientists of his caliber were not to emerge for decades.

The 19th century saw the likes of Claude Bernard (1813–1878), Francois Magendie (1783–1855), and Johannes E. Purkinje (1787–1869), all of whom were outstanding scientists, dedicated to experimentation and observation as methods of obtaining scientific truth. Bernard described the "milieu interieur" (interior environment), thus paving the way for physiologists such as Walter Cannon and others in the study of homeostasis. Magendie made numerous scientific contributions, such as describing the mechanism of absorption, the function of the dorsal root nerves, and the localization of drug action. Purkinje is widely recognized for his achievements in both embryology and physiology. He studied epithelial tissue and, among other things, classified fingerprints.

The so-called Romantic interlude, which occurred in the 19th century, was largely the product of the German philosopher Friedrich W. J. von Schelling (1775–1854). Largely owing to Schelling, physiological theory was derived philosophically, and experimentation was given only casual consideration. In the United States, the first physiological laboratory was opened at Harvard Medical School in 1871 by Henry Bowditch (1840–1911). The American Physiological Society was founded on December 30, 1887, in New York. The society initially had twenty-eight members, and Bowditch was elected its first president. In 1938 there were less than 700 members; today there are several thousand members, and the society is divided into units dedicated to the study of specific areas within the field of physiology.

The 20th century brought to light such scientists as Ernest H. Starling (1866–1927) and William Bayliss (1860–1924), who together discovered the existence of blood-borne messengers, later given the name hormones by Starling. Many landmark contributions in the 20th century involve the work of Elmer V. McCollum (1879–1967), who described the nature and function of vitamin A; Otto Warburg (1883–1970), who pioneered metabolic research; and Ivan Pavlov (1849–1936), who discovered the process of conditioning reflexes.

The list of landmark contributions, many of which will be noted later, is lengthy. As knowledge of physiology has increased, the number of physiologists has also increased, and it would be extremely difficult to provide a chronology of significant contributions of the past fifty years. In order to abbreviate an otherwise lengthy discussion of the major developments in modern physiology, a number of important contributors and their contributions have been listed in Table 1–1.

EXPERIMENTAL DESIGN

One could hardly express the difficulties confronted in all good physiological research better than Johannes P. Müller, who in 1792 said:

> An observation should be carried out in a plain, candid and industrious manner without preconceived opinions. . . . But nothing is more difficult than the correct interpretation of nature, nothing tougher than to plan a truly valid experiment. We consider it the foremost objective of contemporary physiology to show and clearly grasp these obstacles. . . . Abstract thought about nature is not the proper area for physiological endeavor, since the physiologist must experience nature in order to develop thoughts about her. (Rothschuh 1973, p. 197)

In those sentences Müller conveyed several thoughts on the philosophy and mechanics of physiological research that are particularly germane. He expressed the need for the physiologist to "experience nature." No one can design a proper experiment without a fundamental knowledge of the natural situation which initiates the questions, "How does it work?" and "What is its mechanism?" How can a truly valid experiment be designed? Frequently, one is intrigued by elaborate apparatuses, conceiving experiments that require expensive equipment but achieve little in the way of data. Many landmark studies in physiology have been conducted with a modicum of equipment, and many excellent experiments have been conducted with equipment designed and constructed by the investigator. When an experiment is properly designed, bias is eliminated, the data are clear, and the results can be expressed plainly and concisely.

A systematic approach to scientific experimentation demands an *experimental design*.

Name	Date*	Contribution
C. Bohr	1886	Effect of carbon dioxide tension on hemoglobin
W. H. Nernst	1889	Related cell potential to ion distribution
I. Pavlov	1897	Process of conditioning of reflexes
K. Landsteiner	1900	Blood physiology and blood types
C. S. Sherrington	1906	Reflex control by means of the central nervous system
E. V. McCollum	1912	Discovery of vitamin A
K. Lucas	1917	"All or none law" of nerves
A. Krogh	1919	Capillary circulation and regulation
A. V. Hill	1922	Energy relations during muscle contraction
A. N. Richards	1924	Renal filtration
O. Warburg	1931	Metabolic processes
W. Cannon	1933	Physiology of the autonomic nervous system
R. Schoenheimer	1935	Use of isotopes in metabolic studies
F. G. Benedict	1938	Animal metabolism
H. Selye	1941	General Adaptation Syndrome
A. L. Hodgkin and A. F. Huxley	1945	Nerve action
G. W. Harris	1945	Secretion of releasing hormones
H. Smith	1950	Renal physiology
P. F. Scholander	1955	Countercurrent exchange, thermoregulation
H. E. and A. F. Huxley	1957	Muscle contraction
L. Irving	1957	Adaptation to cold
J. Olds	1960	Behavior control
G. von Békésy	1961	Mechanism of sound reception
J. C. Eccles	1963	Mechanism of synaptic activity

TABLE 1–1
Recent contributions instrumental in developing an understanding of particular areas of physiology

*Dates are approximate and do not necessarily represent dates of publication

A well-designed experiment should leave no doubt in the mind of the investigator as to the nature of the data, the method of analysis, the absence of redundancy, and the possible significance of the results. If one designs an experiment carefully, there should be little additional effort necessary when the time arrives for preparation of a manuscript.

After the experimental design has been worked out with care and consideration, an experiment should be easily conducted and should yield fruitful results, barring technical difficulties. The data, analyzed in a prescribed way, should fit a prescribed pattern. From that material, the investigator can readily draw necessary conclusions and explain his or her results in terms of previously published material.

An experimental design could be constructed as follows, though this is by no means the only way of developing such a design.

Introduction

This section of an experimental design should include a description of experiments which have bearing on the research at hand, and it should give the reader an idea of the scope of the problem to be addressed. The hypothesis to be tested should be stated in this section. The last sentence of the introduction should define the problem and state the purpose of the experiment.

Materials and Methods (Experimental Protocol)

In this section, techniques, both established and improvised, should be described in detail. The equipment should be described along with the role fulfilled by each item. The form in which the data will be obtained (i.e., millimeters of oxygen per work load, water loss per gram salt intake, etc.) should be specified. The nature of the data should be clearly described; the data should be amenable to an accepted mode of statistical analysis. All statistical steps and techniques should be outlined, unless a well-known standard such as chi-square, Student's *t*, or regression is used. The better-known statistical procedures need only be referred to by name.

Every experiment should have adequate *controls.* In other words, the experimental

treatment should be duplicated in a second group of animals—the *control group*—as closely as possible but with the omission of the final experimental step. For instance, an experiment is conducted to determine the effects of insulin on blood sugar levels, and the technique requires that fasted animals be injected with insulin dissolved in physiological saline at 8:00 A.M. A second group should be treated similarly but injected with physiological saline free of insulin, also at 8:00 A.M. The importance of a control cannot be overemphasized. Without adequate controls, data are not clear and cannot be relied upon.

Results

In a well-designed experiment one should be able to anticipate the type of results to be obtained. For example, the data might be expressed in terms of metabolism, force, temperature, and so on, or as a function of time or some other dependent variable. If proper judgment is used, the investigator should be able to anticipate several possible results and show how they will support the hypothesis and purpose of the experiment, which were stated in the introduction.

Discussion

The relevance of the experiment or group of experiments should be explained in terms of existing data or knowledge in the area. The pertinence of the results of the experiment in explaining a previous problem or problems should be clearly delineated.

Literature Cited

This section of the experimental design should only include the published papers cited in the text of the design. This should not be a reading list for interested observers.

Note that this example of an experimental design is also the basic form of most manuscripts submitted for publication: the similarity is not fortuitous but represents a planned approach. If the design of an experiment is placed in that form, not only are the investigator's thoughts organized, but the experiment when finished is also decidedly close to final manuscript form. It may need only a modicum of preparation to bring it into acceptable journal style.

Publication is central to all scientific progress. Without publication as a record, scientists would periodically be forced to redis-

TABLE 1–2
Some of the more common subdivisions of the class Mammalia

Classification	Common Name
Subclass Prototheria	
Order Monotremata	Duckbill platypuses, spiny anteaters (echidnas)
Subclass Theria	
Infraclass Metatheria	
Order Marsupialia	Opossums, koalas, kangaroos, wombats
Infraclass Eutheria	
Order Insectivora	Moles, shrews
Order Dermoptera	Flying lemurs
Order Chiroptera	Bats
Order Primates	Lemurs, New and Old World Monkeys, humans
Order Edentata	Anteaters, sloths, armadillos
Order Pholidota	Scaly anteaters
Order Lagomorpha	Pikas, rabbits, hares
Order Rodentia	Beavers, squirrels, mice, rats
Order Mysticeti	Right whales, gray whales, rorquals
Order Odontoceti	Dolphins, porpoises, sperm whales, norwhals
Order Carnivora	Dogs (Canidae), Cats (Felidae), Bears (Ursidae), Racoons (Procyonidae), Skunks, weasels, badgers, wolverines, otters (Mustelidae)
Order Tubulidentata	Aardvarks
Order Proboscidea	Elephants
Order Hyracoidea	Hyraxes
Order Sirenia	Dugongs, sea cows, manatees
Order Perissodactyla	Horses, rhinoceri
Order Artiodactyla	Swine, camels, hippopotami, deer, giraffe, sheep, cattle, pronghorn

cover all the information accumulated over time. Heraclitus once said that one cannot step into the same stream twice: perhaps, but without a written history of physiology an attempt would have to be made to do just that.

The purpose and importance of research has been stated in many ways, sometimes quite eloquently, by any number of outstanding researchers. But the statement by Ida Henrietta Hyde, the first woman member of the American Physiological Society, is perhaps the most clear and expressive: "All research requires patience and inspiration, and the results in themselves are difficult to estimate. They lead to other problems, and may inspire others to new ideas."

MAMMALS

The Class Mammalia comprises a very broad group, consisting of many orders and families (Table 1–2). In many cases the adaptations seen in the nonhuman species of this class are truly awe inspiring. The mechanisms that enable them to exist in a habitat quite different from ours require considerable insight and research to be clearly understood.

In addition to their unique adaptations to specific habitats, all mammals exhibit overriding physiological similarities. For instance, even though seals' well-developed circulatory adaptations to diving are not comparable to many terrestrial mammals, their circulatory system relates generally in principle to that of all mammals. More similarities include live birth (except for certain monotremes), suckling their young, and employing internal production of heat in thermoregulation. These likenesses are remarkable, but it is the differences in physiological mechanisms that make this class so interesting.

SUMMARY

Physiology is the study of function in the living organism. It demands a knowledge of anatomy, physics, chemistry and mathematics to achieve its maximum expression. As a branch of science, its roots are founded in antiquity; as new problems are solved, new questions arise. There are more physiologists alive today than ever before, and solutions to new problems are proceeding at an ever-increasing rate.

The most commendable aspects of the study of physiology are research, or the discovery of knowledge and its publication, and teaching, or the dissemination of knowledge. The objectives of physiology are the measurement of function and the understanding of the mechanisms by which organisms exist.

2

A REVIEW OF
BASIC CHEMICAL AND
CELLULAR CONCEPTS

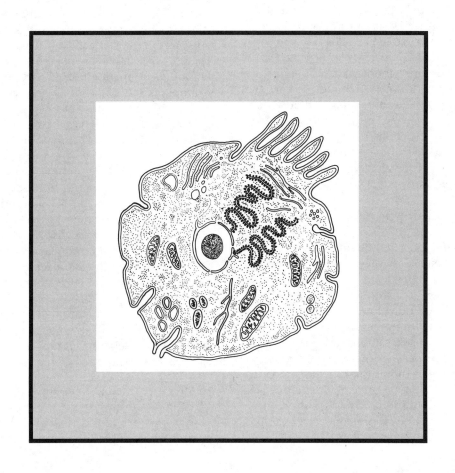

*L*iving organisms are composed of specific chemicals which are arranged in organized fashion. Basic principles can be applied to the role of chemicals in the cell and the organism. The function of an organ or even an organism in its relationship to its environment is controlled through these chemicals and the physical elements which affect them.

CHEMICAL PRINCIPLES

Compounds found in living systems are generally of two types: *organic* and *inorganic*. Organic compounds are molecules which contain carbon, and usually oxygen and hydrogen as well. The organic compounds found in living systems are usually rather large and are held together almost entirely by covalent bonds. The principal organic compounds found in living cells are *carbohydrates*, *lipids*, *nucleic acids*, and *proteins* (including enzymes). Inorganic compounds, on the other hand, do not contain carbon and are not of organic origin. That is, they are not derived from living cells. Inorganic compounds are generally rather small and are held together by ionic bonds. Inorganic compounds found in living cells include *water*, *acids*, *bases*, and *salts.*

Organic Compounds

Carbohydrates Carbohydrates, such as sugars and starches, play a number of important roles in the living system. There are three classes of carbohydrates, defined by the number of individual sugar units present: *monosaccharides* (one simple sugar molecule), *disaccharides* (two simple sugar units), and *polysaccharides* (more than two sugar units). These compounds provide energy by their *catabolism*, or breakdown in the cell. They are also important for the production of other cellular components. For example, deoxyribose, a pentose or five-carbon sugar,

is the structural backbone of deoxyribonucleic acid (DNA). Examples of carbohydrates are shown in Figure 2–1.

Lipids Lipids are organic compounds that are water insoluble but are soluble in solvents such as ether, alcohol, and chloroform. These molecules are important to the structure of such cellular membranes as the plasma membrane and those membranes surrounding cell organelles. They also serve as a storage form of metabolic fuel. Lipids contain carbon, hydrogen, and oxygen. An example of a lipid is shown in Figure 2–1.

There are a number of types of lipids. *Triglycerides*, found in fatty tissues, are composed of glycerol and three fatty acid molecules. They function in the insulation of the body and as energy sources. *Phospholipids* are found in membranes and also found in high concentrations in brain and other nerve tissues. *Steroids* include cholesterol (a constituent of all animal cells, blood, and nervous tissue), sex hormones (estrogens and androgens), bile salts (important in the emulsification of fats for digestion), vitamin D (necessary for proper bone growth and development), the cytochromes (important for energy production), and various other lipid substances, such as vitamins E and K and the prostaglandins.

Proteins Proteins, another group of organic compounds, are composed of building blocks called *amino acids*, which are connected through peptide bonds. The order in

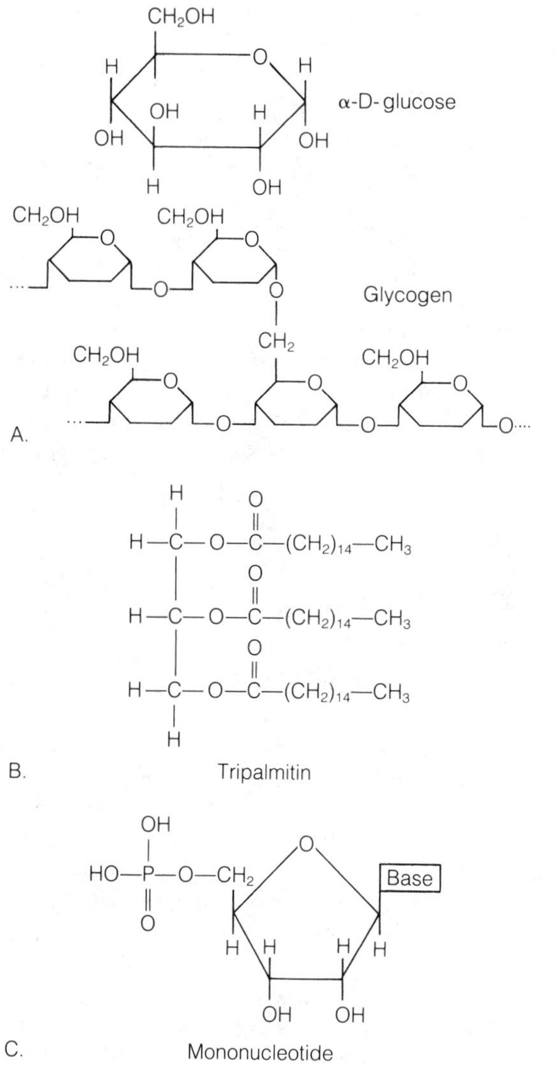

CH₂OH

α-D-glucose

Glycogen

A.

B.   Tripalmitin

C.   Mononucleotide

FIGURE 2–1
Examples of organic compounds: (A) carbohydrates—
glucose (monosaccharide) and glycogen (polysaccharide; (B) lipid—tripalmitin (composed of glycerol and
three molecules of the triglyceride palmitic acid); (C) nucleotide—the building block of nucleic acids

which these amino acids occur is specific to each protein molecule. Each amino acid is composed of carbon, hydrogen, oxygen, and nitrogen. Proteins may be grouped according to the function. For instance, *enzymes* are catalytic molecules functioning in the control of biological reactions within the cell. Another group of proteins constitute the structural elements of the body, such as collagen in connective tissue and keratin in hair and fingernails. *Hormones*, such as insulin, comprise a third class of proteins. *Plasma proteins*, such as gamma globulin, serve as antibodies in the immune system. *Contractile proteins*, such as actin and myosin, are found in muscle cells and allow the muscle fibers to contract.

Nucleic acids Nucleic acids, a fundamental component of chromosomes, are composed of a number of building blocks called *nucleotides*. Nucleotides are in turn composed of a five-carbon sugar (either ribose or deoxyribose), phosphoric acid, and one of five nitrogenous bases (thymine, cytosine, guanine, adenine, and uracil). Each of those bases contains carbon, hydrogen, oxygen, and nitrogen. An example of a nucleotide is shown in Figure 2–1. Both the type of sugar and the type of base vary with the type of nucleic acid in question. *Deoxyribonucleic acid (DNA)* contains the sugar deoxyribose and any of the first four bases listed. *Ribonucleic acid (RNA)* contains the sugar ribose and any of the last four bases listed. Those nucleotides are covalently bonded to form long chains. In the cell nucleus of vertebrates, DNA is a double stranded helix and thus in form resembles a twisted ladder. The nucleotides of DNA provide the genes of the cell. Ribonucleic acid, found in the nucleus as well as in the cytoplasm, is essential in the synthesis of proteins.

Inorganic Compounds

Water Water, the most important inorganic compound in the living body, is the most abundant material in living tissues. It has been called the universal solvent because of its unique properties. Its presence is essential in certain chemical reactions, such as hydrolysis and oxidation reactions. Water is a *thermostabilizer* in that it has a high heat of vaporization (approximately 580 cals/g). That is, it takes a large amount of heat to increase water's temperature sufficiently to change from a liquid to a gas. Water also has a high heat of fusion. In other words, more heat is required to change water from a solid to a liquid than is required for most other substances. A third reason why water is a good thermostabilizer is its high *specific heat* (approximately 1.0 cal/g/C), or that amount of heat necessary to raise the temperature of one gram of that substance one degree centigrade.

Acids, bases, and salts Acids, bases, and salts are other classes of inorganic compounds important to living systems, and for simplicity's sake are grouped together here. An acid is a substance which gives up hydrogen ions (hydrogen atoms or protons) in solution. A base is a substance which yields hydroxyl ions in solution and which can react with an acid to form a salt and water. A salt then is defined as the substance resulting from the combination of an acid and a base. When put into solution, any compound of the three categories of inorganic compounds dissociates, or *ionizes*. An acid forms hydrogen ions and anions, a base forms hydroxyl ions and cations, and a salt forms anions and cations, the specific nature of which is dependent upon the type of salt. In extracellular fluids sodium and chloride ions predominate, whereas in the intracellular environment potassium and phosphate ions predominate.

In order for life to be sustained there must be a constant balance between the amount of acids and bases in the living system. The more hydrogen ions present the more acidic a solution is; conversely, the more hydroxyl ions present the more basic the solution. The correct acidity of a system is maintained by a *buffer system*. A buffer system reacts with strong acids and bases and converts them to weaker species. An example of such a system in mammals is the carbonate-bicarbonate buffer system found in cells, blood plasma, and other body fluids (see chapter 15, Respiration).

THE CELL AND ITS FUNCTION

The cell is the basic structural unit in living organisms, and within each cell can be found all of the mechanisms necessary to sustain life. The *eucaryotic cell*, a cell that has a discrete nucleus separated from the cytoplasm by a nuclear membrane, is found in all higher plants and animals (see Figure 2–2). The cell is enveloped by a *plasma membrane*, or *cell membrane*, which maintains the cell as a distinct unit separate from the surrounding environment. The *cytoplasm* is the fluid matrix found within the plasma membrane. It is the cytoplasm that contains the various cellular organelles and inclusions which constitute the remainder of the cell.

Plasma membrane The plasma membrane, complex in structure, is approximately 80 angstroms thick and is composed of a protein-containing phospholipid bilayer (see Figure 2–3). The phospholipids are arranged so that the hydrophobic (water fearing) ends of the molecules are drawn to the inside of the bilipid layer, thus exposing the hydro-

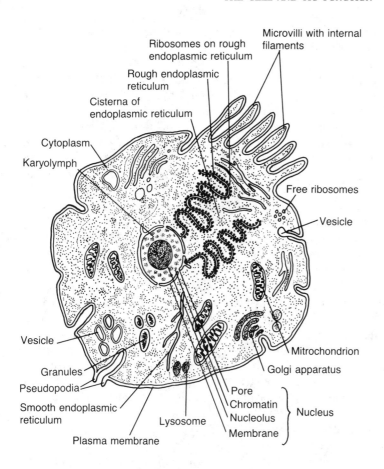

FIGURE 2–2
A generalized eucaryotic cell

Microvilli with internal filaments

Ribosomes on rough endoplasmic reticulum

Rough endoplasmic reticulum

Cisterna of endoplasmic reticulum

Cytoplasm

Karyolymph

Free ribosomes

Vesicle

Vesicle

Granules

Pseudopodia

Smooth endoplasmic reticulum

Lysosome

Plasma membrane

Mitrochondrion

Golgi apparatus

Pore
Chromatin
Nucleolus
Membrane
} Nucleus

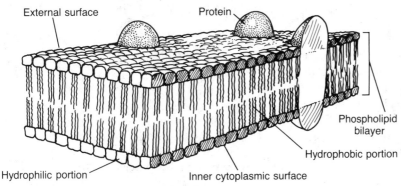

FIGURE 2–3
The plasma or cell membrane is composed of a protein-containing phospholipid bilayer. Hydrophobic portions of the lipid molecules are directed inward. The randomly dispersed protein units form a mosaic.

External surface

Protein

Phospholipid bilayer

Hydrophobic portion

Hydrophilic portion

Inner cytoplasmic surface

philic (water loving) parts of the molecules to the outside of the structure. This gives the membrane a "sandwich" appearance, with the hydrophilic portions of the phospholipids as the bread and the hydrophobic parts as the filling. The protein molecules, which may have hydrophilic and hydrophobic portions, may occur on one or both sides or protrude through the entire membrane thickness. These membrane-bound proteins serve many functions; for example, they are receptor sites which react with hormones and other chemicals and which help the transport of chemicals from extracellular space to intracellular space and vice versa.

A special characteristic of the plasma membrane, also called a *unit membrane* because of its peculiar structure, is that it allows some materials to pass into the cell and excludes others. Because of that characteristic the membrane is said to be *selectively permeable, semipermeable*, or *differentially permeable.* A membrane's permeability determines the ease with which it allows a certain substance to enter or exit the cell. Generally plasma membranes are freely permeable to water. The permeability of a substance is determined by its size, lipid solubility, and charge as well as the absence or presence of carrier molecules in the membrane. Some substances, such as complex molecules, have limited or no permeability. The size factor should be obvious: large molecules are not permitted to pass through the membrane. Smaller molecules such as water and amino acids pass through easily. Molecules that have a high *lipid solubility* pass through the lipid portion of the membrane more easily than those molecules with a low lipid solubility. *Charged* or *polar molecules* such as water pass through the protein portion of the membrane.

Plasma membranes contain different types of carrier molecules depending upon the type of cell in question. These carrier molecules act as a transport mechanism to allow the entrance and exit of specific molecules.

Contiguous membranes Another distinguishing characteristic of the plasma membrane is its contiguity with membranes on the interior of the cell and with projections on the exterior of the cell, made possible through a myriad of invaginations and evaginations. The connection with the inside of the cell is very important for communication between the interior of the cell and its surrounding environment. Various substances pass along and through those projections, thus forming a *communication* or *transport system* which conveys molecules into and out of the cell as well as within the cell itself, a storage place for various chemicals and a place for certain chemical reactions to take place. The projections within the cell form a complex of membrane-enclosed cavities called *cisternae*. This system of channels, called the *endoplasmic reticulum*, is continuous with the *nuclear membrane*, a portion of unit membrane which surrounds the nucleus. The endoplasmic reticulum also serves as a point of attachment for *ribosomes*, one of the cellular organelles. When ribosomes are attached, endoplasmic reticulum is referred to as *rough* or *granular reticulum* because of its appearance. *Smooth* or *agranular reticulum* is devoid of ribosomes.

Cellular Organelles

As previously mentioned, found within the plasma membrane is the cytoplasm, which contains various cellular organelles. These include the *ribosomes, Golgi complex, lysosomes, mitochondria, microtrabeculae* and *microtubules, nucleus, flagella* and *cilia*.

Ribosomes Ribosomes are the organelles responsible for the production of proteins. They are composed of two subunits: a larger subunit composed of thirty-four proteins and two molecules of RNA and a smaller subunit composed of twenty-one proteins and one molecule of RNA. These organelles may be attached to the endoplasmic reticulum or they may be found free in the cytoplasm. During protein synthesis, *messenger RNA* becomes associated with a ribosome and begins coding for a specific protein molecule. At this time more ribosomes may become attached to the messenger RNA as amino acids are added to the growing peptide chain. A number of ribosomes thus associated is called a *polyribosome*, or more simply a *polysome*. As proteins are synthesized, they are transported through the endoplasmic reticulum and stored in the cisternae and channels in the form of globules.

Golgi complex The Golgi complex, or *Golgi apparatus*, is closely associated with the endoplasmic reticulum; indeed, they are attached at a number of places. The Golgi complex is composed of a unit membrane but is devoid of ribosomes. Similar to the endoplasmic reticulum, the Golgi complex is composed of a number of cisternae stacked upon one another as well as expanded *vesicles* and *vacuoles*. In essence this organelle has somewhat the appearance of a stack of pancakes. The Golgi complex is important in the production and storage of complex molecules such as polysaccharides and lipids. They also seem to be important in the storage of proteins produced by the endoplasmic reticulum. The proteins are accumulated in the cisternae, which then expand to form the previously mentioned vesicles. Once the vesicles attain a certain size they pinch off and form discrete secretory granules or vacuoles. Thus, depending upon the chemicals involved, the vacuole may be either protein, lipid, or a glycoprotein in nature.

Lysosomes Lysosomes are organelles formed from the unit membranes that compose Golgi complexes. These organelles, saclike in structure, contain a myriad of hydrolytic enzymes capable of digesting many kinds of substances. Lysosomes are particularly predominant in white blood cells and are important in the destruction of phagocytozed bacteria. In other cells these organelles may be important in the resorption of bone or in the degradation of embryonic structures which are no longer needed.

Mitochondria Like the organelles previously mentioned, mitochondria are bounded by a unit membrane, but in this case the membrane is doubled. The inner membrane is greatly folded and gives rise to projections called *cristae*. Located on this inner membrane are the enzymes responsible for oxidative phosphorylation, and thus mitochondria are essential in the cell's ability to produce energy-rich compounds such as adenosine triphosphate (ATP). Because of its energy production function, this organelle is often called the "powerhouse" of the cell. In rapidly growing cells, where there is a high energy demand, large numbers of mitochondria can be found. In nerve cells the mitochondria tend to aggregate at the ends of the cells, where a large supply of energy is needed to synthesize, release, and degrade *neurotransmitters*, which relay information from one cell to the next. In muscle cells these organelles form ringlike structures. During cell division the mitochondria can be seen to align themselves and then to become fairly equally divided between the two new daughter cells. They have also been observed to fragment during cell division: the mitochondria contain DNA different from that found in the cell nucleus. The discovery of

DNA in these organelles indicates that they can be self-replicating.

Microtrabeculae and microtubules The *cytoskeleton*, or cell skeleton, consists of the *microtrabeculae system*. Microtrabeculae, minute filaments attached to the inner surface of the plasma membrane, form an intricate network, or *microtrabecular lattice*, giving structure to the cell (see Figure 2–4). These filaments help support and maintain the form of the cell and are especially abundant in certain types of cells, such as red blood cells. These structures also combine with ribosomes, which appear under the microscope as free-floating polysomes or as individual ribosomes. In addition to their function as support structures, the microtrabeculae also divide the cytoplasm into smaller areas where certain chemical reactions can take place and where specific pH conditions need to be maintained. The lattice is also important for intracellular movement. The proteins which make up these filaments (as well as other filaments in the cytoskeleton, such as the microfilaments and microtubules) are contractile in nature. These proteins include actin, myosin and tubulin.

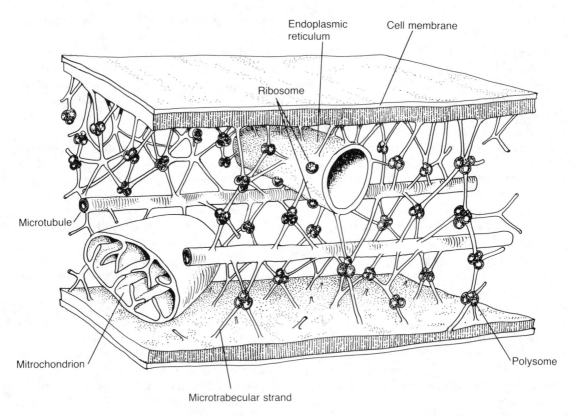

FIGURE 2–4
Microtrabecular lattice, which gives structure to the cell

Microtubules, found in all eucaryotic cells, are hollow cylinders, the periphery of which are composed of individual bundles of filaments. These structures often occur in an organized fashion along the axis of a cell, observable in nerve axons. Like microtrabeculae, microtubules are important in the intracellular movement of organelles. They are also responsible for the movement of certain structures (such as centrioles and chromosomes) during cell division and for the movement of cilia and flagella.

Nucleus The nucleus is the "reproductive" system and "brains" of the cell. This organelle contains the genes of heredity, which determine what kind of cell it is and how it will function. In the nucleus all of the major biochemical "decisions" are made. This is accomplished through the duplication of DNA and the ultimate division of the nucleus and remainder of the cell into two daughter cells. Also important in the functioning of cells is the production of RNA, which controls the various metabolic functions of the cell through its role in protein and therefore enzyme synthesis.

The nucleus is an ovoid, or spherical-shaped body, which is bounded by a double unit membrane called the nuclear membrane. The space between these two membranes is called the *perinuclear cisterna*. This membrane is somewhat modified from the plasma membrane in that it contains large pores up to 1.5 angstroms in diameter. These pores allow communication between the endoplasmic reticulum and the nucleus. The three basic constituents of the nucleus are the *karyolymph*, the *chromatin granules*, and the *nucleoli*. The karyolymph, also called the *nucleoplasm*, is the ground substance of the nucleus. This matrix contains enzymes, presumably used in the replication of RNA from the DNA and in the duplication of DNA during cell replication. It is the DNA that is the major constituent of the chromatin granules, which are thin threadlike masses when the cell is not undergoing the process of cell division. During cell division these threads become shortened and take on a wormlike appearance. Once in the shortened condition they are called *chromosomes*, and it is in that form that they can be observed going through the various stages of mitosis or meiosis, depending upon the cell type. It is also in the chromatin granules and the chromosomes that the bulk of the histones and other chromatid proteins are located. Nuclear DNA is tightly coiled around these proteins.

Generally, each nucleus contains one or more nucleoli, though they are either absent or inconspicuous in sperm and muscle fibers. These structures are highly visible in rapidly metabolizing cells, where there is a great deal of protein synthesis occurring. The nucleolus, predominately composed of RNA and protein, is thought to be the site of ribosome production and or assembly. The nucleolus may also be the site of histone production.

Flagella and cilia Some cells possess projections of the plasma membrane which may be important in the movement of the entire cell or which may move substances along the exterior of the cell. In the former case such structures are called flagella; in the latter they are called cilia. Flagella are longer and utilize a whiplike motion, whereas cilia are much shorter and employ a slower rowing motion. The overall composition of these two organelles is similar except that spermatozoan flagella contain a helical filament around the periphery of the flagellum. In general though, each flagellum (or cilium) is

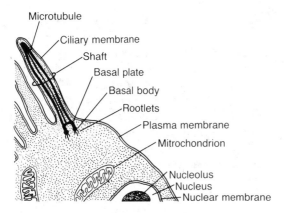

FIGURE 2–5
Generalized structure of a cilium

composed of nine bundles of microtubule *pairs*, or *doubles*, and are attached to the cell by a *basal body* (see Figure 2–5). Inside of this cylinder of filament pairs are two more groups of filament pairs. The flagellum is composed of two sets of pairs surrounded by nine pairs. The two central pairs are connected to the nine other pairs by a protein called *dynein*. It is through the contraction of dynein that a sliding motion is set up and movement of the flagellum is achieved.

Transport Across Membranes

The movement of water and other substances into and out of the cell is regulated through the plasma membrane which surrounds each cell. The integrity of this membrane is of prime importance to the well-being of the cell. As previously discussed, the permeability of a membrane to a substance is a function of the molecule's size, lipid solubility, and charge as well as the absence or presence of carrier molecules in the membrane. The actual mechanism whereby a substance moves across a membrane may be a *passive process*, in which the cell does not

expend energy or assist in the movement, or it may be an *active process*, in which the cell does expend energy in order to transfer the substance from one side of the membrane to the other. Passive processes include *diffusion, facilitated diffusion, osmosis,* and *filtration.* Active processes include *active transport, pinocytosis,* and *phagocytosis.*

Passive processes

Diffusion. A soluble substance, when placed in a solvent, will exhibit random movement as a result of its internal kinetic energy. Since there are more particles and kinetic energy at the concentrated center of the solute when placed in the solvent, the net random movement is from the area of highest concentration to the area of lowest concentration. When the substance finally becomes uniformly distributed in the solvent, movement becomes equal in all directions and a state of equilibrium is reached whereby a stable solute distribution is achieved throughout the solvent. Before such an equilibrium is reached, there exists a *concentration gradient*, or differential concentration. In other words, the distribution is not uniform and the solute exhibits a net movement from an area of higher to lower concentration (down its concentration gradient). Note that the concentration gradient is also called the *diffusion gradient.*

The rate of diffusion is affected by the kinetic energy and size of the molecule in solution. Hence, the rate increases when the temperature and thus kinetic energy increases. Size is a variable: the rate of diffusion is inversely proportional to the square root of the size of the ionic or atomic species. The rate of diffusion is, therefore, greatest when the temperature is highest and the particle size is smallest.

The difference in concentrations of a particular ion species divided by the distance (thickness of the membrane) between two concentrations constitutes a concentration gradient. The rate at which equilibrium is reached in diffusion across a cell membrane depends upon a number of factors imposed by the membrane and the particular ion species which surround it. These factors have already been discussed and will not be elaborated upon here.

A mechanism of passively maintaining equilibrium between different ion species on each side of a cell membrane is described by means of the *Gibbs-Donnan equilibrium.* The first premise of the Gibbs-Donnan equilibrium is that the products of the concentrations of the diffusible ions on each side of a differentially permeable membrane are equal. Suppose two solutions, A and B, are separated by a differentially permeable membrane and that the solutions contain identically diffusible anions and cations. In addition, solution A also contains a nondiffusible protein anion (see Figure 2–6). The conditions of the Gibbs-Donnan equilibrium are met when, after sufficient diffusion time, the products of the concentrations of the diffusible ions on each side of the membrane

are equal, as in the following equation (the subscripts refer to the solutions previously mentioned):

$$[K^+]_A [Cl^-]_A = [K^+]_B [Cl^-]_B \qquad (2.1)$$

In order to maintain electrical neutrality, the following assumption for solution B must be made:

$$[K^+]_B = [Cl^-]_B \qquad (2.2)$$

For solution A, which contains nondiffusible protein anions (Pr$^-$), the following assumption must be made:

$$[K^+]_A = [Cl^-]_A + [Pr^-]_A \qquad (2.3)$$

Therefore, in order to insure electrical neutrality, the sum of the negatively charged particles must be equal to the sum of the positively charged particles on each side of the membrane. However, it is obvious that the concentration of potassium ions in solution A is not equal to the concentration of chloride ions in that solution because some of the potassium must be associated with the protein anions for the maintenance of electrical neutrality. Thus, solution A must have some K^+Pr^- and some K^+Cl^-.

According to equation 2.1, the products of the concentrations of diffusible ions on each side of the membrane are equal. Yet their sums are not equal, since there is a disproportionate amount of potassium ions to chloride ions in solution A. This incongruity is easily understood when an analogy is drawn using a rectangle and a square. In Figure 2–7, the areas represented by the two polygons are equal: 16 in each case, the product of 2 × 8 and 4 × 4, respectively. But the sums of their sides differ. The sum of the rectangle's sides is 20; that of the square's, 16.

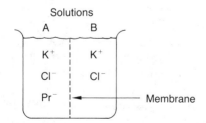

Solutions

FIGURE 2–6
Two solutions separated by a differentially permeable membrane: solution A contains diffusible potassium and chloride ions and nondiffusible protein anions; solution B contains only potassium and chloride ions

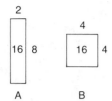

FIGURE 2–7
Rectangle and square: the products of the sides are equal, but perimeters are quite different

It is obvious that the potassium ion concentration is greater in solution A than in solution B. Therefore, a diffusion gradient for potassium ions exists between solution A and solution B. The diffusion of potassium ions along the diffusion gradient from A to B results in a negative charge in solution A. Eventually that charge becomes great enough to attract almost as many potassium ions back to solution A as will move to solution B, because of the diffusion gradient. Thus, there is a stable negative charge in solution A, and if solution A is negative then solution B must be positive. In that way a *membrane potential* is developed, in this case using a nonliving membrane and ion solutions. This model system shows how ion distribution can result in potentials or charge differences in the living cell. Such potentials are imperative in the proper functioning of certain cell types, such as nerve cells. The subject of membrane potentials will be covered in more detail in later chapters.

To review then, diffusion is the net movement of particles from an area of higher concentration to an area of lower concentration. Once the substance becomes uniformly distributed, a state of equilibrium exists for that substance. The development and maintenance of a diffusion gradient is required for a membrane potential to exist.

Facilitated diffusion. This is the movement of a particle with the aid of a carrier molecule from an area of higher concentration to an area of lower concentration. Molecules that are moved in this way are generally ones which are insoluble in lipid, such as sugars, and therefore do not easily pass through the lipid portion of the membrane. In such cases, the substance, which is said to have a low partition coefficient, combines with a *carrier molecule* and then becomes lipid soluble. The *carrier-substance complex* is then passively moved to the inside of the cell, where the molecule being transported is dumped into the cytoplasm and the carrier is freed once again to migrate to the exterior of the cell and pick up another molecule. There is no expenditure of energy by the cell in facilitated diffusion because the process is a function of the diffusion gradient for the particular molecule being moved.

Osmosis. Osmosis, a specific type of diffusion, is the movement of water molecules from an area of lower solute concentration to an area of higher solute concentration. This movement takes place across a differentially permeable membrane. The force with which the water moves is called *osmotic pressure.*

There are three different *tonicities*, or strengths of solutions, relevent to the solution in question (such as the cytoplasm of a red blood cell in blood plasma). These tonicities are: *isotonic, hypotonic,* and *hypertonic.* When a cell is placed in an isotonic solution, the concentration of the surrounding fluid is equal to the concentration of the cytoplasm. Thus, there is an equilibrium, and the net movement of water and solutes through the membrane is equal in both directions. When a cell is placed in a hypotonic solution, there is a net movement of water into the cell. Such is the case when a red blood cell is placed in distilled water. The distilled water is hypotonic with respect to the red blood cell, which has a higher solute concentration. The red blood cell would swell as the water passed through its plasma membrane, and *hemolysis*, or rupture, would result. In the opposite situation, when the red blood cell is placed in a solution containing a higher solute concentration than that of the cell, a hypertonic solution, there is a net movement of water out of the cell into the environment. The result would be *crenation*, or shrinkage, of the red blood cell.

Filtration. Filtration refers to the movement of substances, both solvents and solutes, across a semipermeable membrane due to pressure such as that exerted by water, or *hydrostatic* pressure. Again, the movement is from an area of higher pressure to an area of lower pressure, or down a pressure gradient just as osmosis and diffusion occur down a diffusion gradient. An excellent example of filtration may be observed in the kidney, where the pressure of the blood forces water and other molecules from the blood vessels into the tubules of the kidney.

Active processes The active processes by which cells move substances across the plasma membrane include active transport, pinocytosis, and phagocytosis. In all cases the cell must expend energy in order for the process to occur.

Active transport. The process of active transport is much like facilitated diffusion in that a substance in the cell's environment becomes attached to a carrier molecule on the plasma membrane. This carrier-substance complex is then transported to the inside of the cell, presumably through the lipid part of the membrane, where the substance is re-

leased from the carrier molecule by action of an enzyme. The energy for these processes is supplied by the cell, generally in the form of adenosine triphosphate (ATP).

Pinocytosis. The process of pinocytosis (cell drinking) involves the actual engulfing of liquid by the cell. In this case the plasma membrane forms an invagination and pinches off a portion of the surrounding liquid. That part of the cell membrane becomes detached from the rest of the membrane and forms a liquid vacuole inside the cell.

Phagocytosis. The process of phagocytosis (cell eating) is a process whereby *pseudopodia* extend from the body of the cell and eventually surround a particle (see Figure 2–8). Once the particle is surrounded, a portion of the plasma membrane detaches itself, as in pinocytosis, and forms a vesicle containing the particle. The material within this vesicle is later digested, usually by lysosomes which coalesce with the vesicular membrane. A prime example of phagocytosis occurs in white blood cells, one of the body's essential lines of defense against disease. These blood cells engulf substances such as viruses and bacteria and digest them, thus rendering them harmless.

The integrity of the plasma membrane is essential for the proper functioning of the cell. In certain systems of the body the cell membrane is important for the function of a specific cell type. In nerve cells and muscle cells the maintenance of a specific charge or electrical gradient is important in the transfer of information along their membranes (see chapter 3, The Neuron, and chapter 7, The Physiology of Muscles). As described earlier, the membrane is essential for energy production in the mitochondria and is also important for protein formation in conjunc-

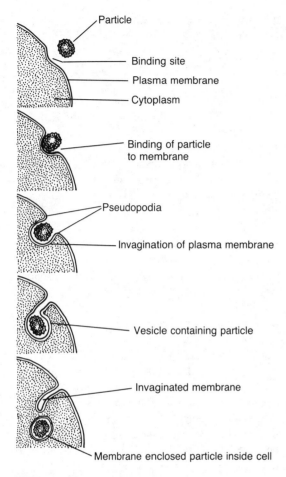

Particle

Binding site

Plasma membrane

Cytoplasm

Binding of particle to membrane

Pseudopodia

Invagination of plasma membrane

Vesicle containing particle

Invaginated membrane

Membrane enclosed particle inside cell

FIGURE 2–8
Phagocytosis occurs when a particle is surrounded by extensions of the plasma membrane called pseudopodia. Contents of the resulting vacuole may then be utilized by the cell.

tion with ribosomes and the endoplasmic reticulum.

SUMMARY

Living systems comprise both organic and inorganic compounds. Some of the inorganic substances include water (the universal solvent), acids, bases, and salts. Organic molecules include carbohydrates, proteins, lipids, and nucleic acids. Carbohydrates such as sugars and starch provide energy for the cell and are also important as building blocks for cellular components. Lipids are water insoluble and are essential in biological membranes. They also function as a storage form of metabolic fuel and as building blocks for some hormones and vitamins. Amino acids are linked together to form proteins, which are important in biological membranes, in the control of biological reactions (enzymes), as structural elements (connective tissue), as hormones (insulin), and as antibodies in the immune system. Nucleic acids are the major component of chromosomes and as such are essential in heredity.

The basic unit of living systems is the cell. A plasma or cell membrane surrounds each cell. It is this structure that is responsible for the passage of materials into and out of the cell. Within the confines of the plasma membrane are a number of organelles that tend to compartmentalize the cell interior. These include the nucleus (important in cell division and control of the cell), endoplasmic reticulum (cell communication system and site of ribosome attachment), ribosomes (site of protein synthesis), mitochondria (energy production), Golgi complex (production and storage of materials), lysosomes (contain high concentrations of hydrolytic enzymes), microtrabeculae and microtubules (cytoskeleton), flagella, and cilia.

Substances enter and exit cells through the plasma membrane. This is accomplished in several ways. Passive processes include diffusion, facilitated diffusion, osmosis, and filtration. Active processes include active transport, pinocytosis (cell drinking), and phagocytosis (cell eating).

3

THE NEURON: MORPHOLOGICAL AND PHYSIOLOGICAL PROPERTIES

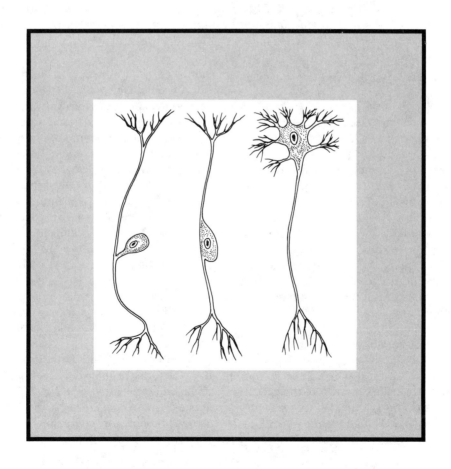

*T*he basic functional unit of the nervous system is the neuron, a cell which can respond to stimuli, deliver stimuli, or do both. The neuron has many forms and serves many functions, but underlying every function is the relay of information from one place to another within the organism. Neurons must be capable of responding to changes in the environment more rapidly than most cells and must be extremely sensitive, in most cases, to changes in the environment. That is, if a neuron receives a stimulus, it must act as a "triggering mechanism" that requires very little energy but is capable of inducing a widespread response which might involve the entire organism. Some neurons apparently have the ability to store information, whereas others are able to compare stored information with new sensory input. In that way a mammal's response to a stimulus is accomplished through comparison, integration, and action. In this chapter, the structure of a neuron, its parts and their individual functions, will be discussed. This generalized structure and function of the neuron will be applicable, with some modification, to nerve cells of all types.

THE STRUCTURE OF THE NEURON

All neurons in the mammal are composed of one or more *dendrites*, a *nerve cell body*, and one or more *axons* (see Figure 3–1). The dendrite receives information and carries it to other parts of the neuron. It is more diffuse in structure than the other neuron parts and has a large surface area, which gives it ample room for placement of the *terminal buttons* from other cells. In the case of sensory neurons, the dendrite allows for a large area for stimulus reception. The nerve cell body contains the nucleus and, therefore, the genetic information of the cell. Since the nucleus controls specific protein synthesis by the cell, it is responsible for synthesizing and replacing chemical elements necessary for nerve function. The axon is usually an elongated and specialized extension of the cell. It is this unique portion of the cell that has the ability to release a *neurotransmitter*, a sub-stance capable of inducing action in another neuron or muscle cell.

Nerve cells are generally separated into two structural types based upon the presence or absence of companion, or *glial*, cells. These companion cells are called either *oligodendrocytes* or *Schwann cells*, depending on their location. Oligodendrocytes are restricted to nerve cells found in the brain and spinal cord, whereas Schwann cells are found on cell extensions outside of those central areas. Both the Schwann cells and the oligodendrocytes contain a lipid called *myelin*. Myelinated neurons transmit information much more rapidly than the unmyelinated neurons by an adaptation, to be discussed later, called saltatory conduction.

A typical myelinated neuron, whose cell body and dendrite are unmyelinated, has on its axon Schwann cells separated by bare spaces known as *nodes of Ranvier* (see Figure 3–2). The Schwann cell primarily consists of

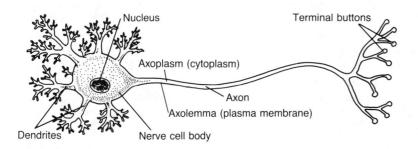

FIGURE 3–1
Generalized structure of a neuron

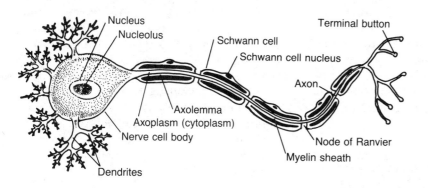

FIGURE 3–2
Myelinated neuron. This type of cell is characteristic of motor neurons whose nerve cell bodies are located in the ventral root of the spinal cord.

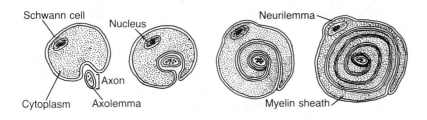

FIGURE 3–3
Cross sectional view of axon and Schwann cell showing growth of Schwann cell in spiral fashion around axon

many concentric layers of lipid membrane, which develop as a result of exogenic growth of the cell (see Figure 3–3). Ultimately, the spiraling growth of the Schwann cell is halted, leaving the layers of Schwann cell membrane around the axon core of the nerve cell. The *myelin sheath* formed by either the oligodendrocytes or the Schwann cells does not fully develop until a few days or months after birth, depending upon the species.

Such delayed development is typical in the altricial (immature) state of development seen in the newborn of many mammals.

CLASSIFICATION OF NEURONS

From a functional basis, neurons are classified as *sensory* or *motor*. Motor neurons *(efferent neurons)* carry impulses toward the periphery of the body, whereas sensory neurons *(afferent neurons)* carry impulses away from the periphery of the body. In the spinal cord, sensory information is sometimes carried directly to the motor neurons from the sensory neurons by means of an *interneuron,* or *internuncial cell,* located entirely within the grey matter of the spinal cord. Neurons can also be divided into a number of different types depending upon the structure and arrangement of their axons and dendrites. A single axon or a single dendrite is referred to as a *pole,* and cell classification can be determined on the basis of the arrangements of these specific units (see Figure 3–4). Figure 3–4A depicts a neuron type which appears to have a single cytoplasmic extension; ulti-

mately, that extension bifurcates into an axon and a dendrite. In such a case, the axon and dendrite do not originate in the typical fashion seen in other neuron types. Hence, it is not the obvious *monopolar neuron* one would expect when viewing the extensions of the nerve cell body. The neurons are thus known as *pseudomonopolar neurons.* True monopolar neurons are found only in lower organisms and are not known to exist in adult mammals. Figure 3–4B depicts a neuron that has a single axon and a single dendrite connected by a nerve cell body. Such a cell is, therefore, called a *bipolar neuron.* Bipolar neurons are found only in specialized sensory receptors such as the retina and the nasal mucosa. Figure 3–4C depicts the most frequent type of nerve cell found in mammals, the *multipolar neuron.* Such neurons are capable of interacting with a variety of nerve or muscle cells.

EARLY WORK ON NEURON MECHANISMS

In order to determine the function of a nerve and the mechanism by which it functions, a model had to be discovered which would allow relatively easy experimentation and manipulation. Early experiments by Galvani in the eighteenth century demonstrated that nerves could transmit a type of electrical impulse that would induce muscular contraction in the leg muscle of a frog. Numerous investigations concerning neuron function were subsequently carried out in the nineteenth and early twentieth centuries. A great deal of histological evidence was amassed, and it was generally accepted that the basis of neuron activity was the result of the electrical characteristics associated with it. That idea prevailed until the mid–twentieth cen-

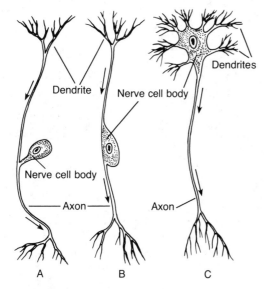

FIGURE 3–4
Different types of neurons based upon cell structure: (A) pseudomonopolar neuron associated with sensory transmission in the dorsal root of the spinal nerves; (B) typical bipolar neuron found in the organs of specialized senses; and (C) multipolar neuron typical of motor cells in the ventral root of the spinal nerves. Arrows indicate direction of transmission.

tury, when the giant squid axon was utilized as a physiological model and the basic mechanisms of nerve function were discovered. A. L. Hodgkin, A. F. Huxley, and Bernard Katz, who studied the giant squid axon in the early 1950s, were the first to describe the physiological mechanism of nerve transmission. The giant squid axon is large enough that electrodes can be strategically placed inside it in order to monitor transmembrane potentials. Also possible is the replacement of the axon's normal axoplasm (cytoplasm) with physiological solutions of known concentrations so that effects of individual ion species can be studied. The use of the squid axon has allowed scientists to manipulate the concentration gradients of specific ions across the membrane and to "clamp" the membrane voltage at specific potentials, thereby elucidating the ions involved in neural transmission. By placing two electrodes along the entire length of the axon, one on the inside and one on the outside of the neuron, an electrical polarity can be maintained (clamped) at any strength chosen by the investigators. After equilibration fluid samples can be taken from both sides of the membrane and analyzed for ion content. Other techniques using the squid axon have been refined and applied to mammalian systems with much success. Significant knowledge about mammalian systems was the result of diligent work by the early investigators in the fields of electro- and neurophysiology.

THE RESTING MEMBRANE POTENTIAL

In order that the student might better understand the electrical potentials developed around living membranes, a review of the principles of diffusion might help (see chapter 2, A Review of Basic Chemical and Cellular Concepts).

When electrodes are placed on either side of a nerve membrane, the potential developed by the diffusible ions can be measured by means of a sensitive voltmeter. In so testing nerves at rest, the outside of the membrane has been found to be positive relative to the inside of the membrane. (see Figure 3–5). The potential measured in the cell in its resting state is called the *resting membrane potential.* Analysis of the fluids on either side of the membrane quickly reveals a very regular distribution of specific particles. Sodium has been found to be in high concentration on the outside of the cell and in relatively low concentration on the inside. An opposite situation has been observed for potassium ion concentration. The concentrations of so-

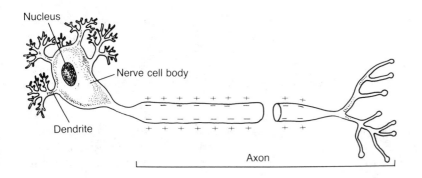

FIGURE 3–5
Potential across the resting membrane of the nerve cell is considered to be uniformly distributed during the resting phase, so that the external surface is positively charged while the internal surface carries a negative charge

$$E_k = \frac{RT}{FZ_k} \ln \frac{K_o^+}{K_i^+} = -61.5 \log \frac{K_o^+}{K_i^+} \quad \text{(at 37° C)}$$

where,

E_k = Equilibrium potential for K^+

Z_k = Valance of K^+ $(+1)$

K_o^+ = K^+ concentration outside the cell

K_i^+ = K^+ concentration inside the cell

R = Gas constant

T = Absolute temperature

F = The faraday (number of coulombs per mole of charge)

FIGURE 3–6
The equilibrium potential of potassium (E_k) as calculated from the Nernst equation.
The equation can be simplified by converting from the natural logarithm to log base 10
and substituting constants for R, F, Z_k, and T, at mammalian body temperature of
37° C. This becomes -61.5, as shown at far right.

dium and chloride ions are essentially equal, whereas the positive charge of the intracellular potassium ions are electrostatically attracted to nondiffusible, anionic proteins (Pr^-). Further analysis indicates that the nerve membrane is 100 times more permeable to potassium ions than it is to sodium ions. When the electromotive force (voltage) generated by the ion distribution is calculated by means of the Nernst equation (see Figure 3–6), it is found to be approximately -75 millivolts (mV). This is almost identical to the usual -70 mV measured by means of the oscilloscope. When the potassium ion concentration around the membrane is manipulated, it is found that an increase in external potassium ion concentration causes the resting membrane potential to decrease. Less obvious effects are observed when concentrations of sodium and chloride ions are manipulated.

How then is a resting membrane potential maintained? The potassium ion gradient from the inside to the outside of the mem-brane results in a negative charge supplied by the protein anion, which is too large to pass through the membrane. In essence, there is a diffusion gradient of potassium ions that is opposed by the electrochemical gradient it causes (see Figure 3–7). The two gradients, approximately equal and opposite in direction, tend to maintain a rather uniform membrane potential.

Over a period of time such a system would reach equilibrium due to the leakage of both potassium and sodium ions through the membrane. In order to prevent the leakage of these ions, a slow and constant active transport of potassium and sodium ions is achieved with a membrane-bound carrier called *sodium-potassium ATPase*, so called because the carrier is also an enzyme capable of splitting ATP. The function of the *sodium-potassium pump*, as the mechanism is called, is to pump sodium ions out of the cell and potassium ions into the cell. Active transport in the neuron requires the expenditure of energy by the cell in order to pump

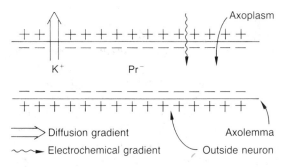

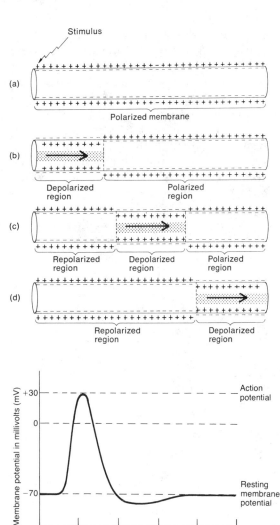

FIGURE 3–7
Diffusion gradient based upon ion concentration is from inside to outside of the nerve cell and is approximately equal (and opposite to) the electrochemical gradient, which is from outside to inside

these ions against their concentration gradients. Movement of these ions requires the participation of carrier molecules which must specifically bind sodium and potassium ions. The sodium-potassium pump is therefore responsible for the maintenance of the observed ion concentrations. For short periods of time, however, a nerve can continue to function under conditions in which activity of the sodium-potassium pump is blocked.

THE ACTION POTENTIAL

In order for information to be transmitted from one point to another, a change in potential must occur that is self-propagating. In other words, a potential must be developed that moves along the membrane and therefore transmits a message. An *action potential* is an ephemeral change in the membrane potential which progresses along the surface of the neuron. With microelectrodes placed on either side of the membrane, one can record the relatively rapid changes in membrane potential on the screen of an oscilloscope (see Figure 3–8). As the action potential

FIGURE 3–8
Changing ionic environment as an action potential moves down the membrane, which results in charge alterations as shown on the oscilloscope trace (lower graph). From G. J. Tortora and N. P. Anagnostakos, *Principles of Anatomy and Physiology*, 3rd ed. (New York, N.Y., 1981), 289, fig. 12–6. Reprinted by permission of Harper and Row Publishers.

approaches the electrode, it is preceded by a small change in potential, called the *prepotential*, which brings the membrane to threshold voltage. The action potential lasts only a scant four to five milliseconds and occupies a very small portion of the nerve membrane surface at any one time. At its peak, the polarity of the membrane potential is reversed: the inside of the membrane becomes positive and the outside becomes negative, or approximately +35 mV to the inside (see Figure 3–9A). The positive internal potential developed in this manner is some-

times called a *reversal potential.* The reversal potential is followed by a *negative after potential* (denoted by a change in slope of the oscilloscope trace), which terminates when resting voltage is reached. Subsequently, the potential falls below the voltage of the resting membrane for a few milliseconds and then returns to the resting level. The period in which the polarity exceeds the resting potential is called the *positive after potential.* During that time, the membrane is said to be *hyperpolarized* because the total charge across the membrane is greater than the charge

FIGURE 3–9
Typical monophasic action potential with (A) alterations in the action potential associated with (B) alterations in the potassium and sodium ion permeability. Duration of these phenomena are dependent upon the type of nerve fiber being tested.

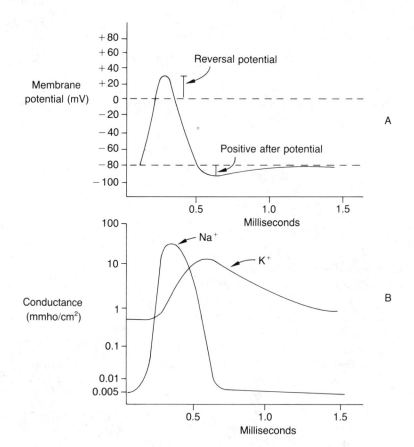

during the resting stage. The term "positive" in this case seems confusing at first, but it should be remembered that charges are relative and the positive or negative designations can be altered by reversing the position of the electrodes. The importance of this phenomenon and the ionic balances which cause it should not be overlooked in deference to convention.

The reversal potential is accomplished by a rapid change in the permeability of the nerve membrane to sodium ions (see Figure 3–9B). Apparently, the stimulus triggers a change in the membrane permeability, which suddenly allows sodium ions to move rapidly into the neuron. The rapid movement of sodium ions across the cell membrane is due in part to the large concentration gradient of sodium ions and to the extracellular positive charge and intracellular negative charge of the resting membrane. In other words, during the time of the reversal potential, sodium ion movement proceeds rapidly because the ion is moving with both its concentration gradient and its electrochemical gradient.

After sodium permeability has reached a maximum, the membrane becomes more permeable to potassium ions. Since the charge of the electrochemical gradient is opposite that of the resting membrane (i.e., negative outside) at this time, potassium ion movement to the outside of the membrane is increased. The movement of potassium causes the electrochemical gradient to return toward the normal resting state of -75 mV negative to the inside. The increased permeability of the membrane to potassium ions is prolonged for a few milliseconds after the decay of the reversal potential. This results in increased polarity, or hyperpolarization negative to the inside, and is responsible for the positive after potential.

Propagation of the Action Potential

The movement or propagation of the action potential involves the local flow of current between the edges of the action potential and its contiguous membrane, which is in the resting state. Currents flow locally from positive to negative (by convention), bringing the portion of the membrane near the site of the action potential toward *threshold* (see Figure 3–10). Threshold, as used here, is the electrical potential reached across a membrane that alters membrane conductance and allows a massive increase in sodium ion permeability. If the flow of current is insufficient to allow threshold voltage to be reached, no action potential occurs. The threshold varies with different types of neurons and under different experimental conditions. But once threshold is reached, the action potential achieves the maximum intensity in accordance with the "all or none law." The "all or none law" is exhibited by

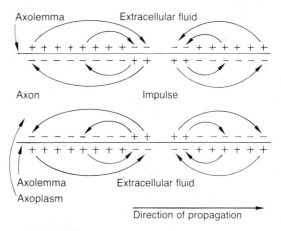

FIGURE 3–10
Local circuit flow around an action potential from positive to negative (by convention)

the neuron, since the action potential reaches its full capacity (governed by the distribution of ions around the membrane) or it does not occur at all: no partial action potential can be developed.

The action potential is followed by a *refractory period*, a period in which the membrane cannot be excited. This only lasts for a few milliseconds, but it insures that the action potential only moves in one direction. In other words, the membrane is excitable immediately in front of the action potential but is refractory immediately behind it. The refractory period can be divided into an *absolute refractory period*, during which no additional stimulation is possible, and a *relative refractory period*, during which additional stimulation is difficult. The absolute refractory period exists from the time that the firing level (threshold) is reached until repolarization is about one-third complete. The relative refractory period immediately follows the absolute refractory period and is complete at the beginning of the positive after potential.

Analogous to the propagation of the action potential is the lighted fuse of a firecracker. When one portion of the fuse is ignited, heat flow to an adjacent portion of the fuse brings the firecracker to the kindling point. When the kindling point is reached, the firecracker becomes ignited, and thus the combustion is propagated. In the neuron, local currents cause a change in the potential of the adjacent membrane. A point is reached at which membrane permeability to sodium ions is drastically altered. Again, this point is known as the threshold, and threshold is the point at which maximum sodium permeability allows for the influx of sodium ions and the reversal of the membrane potential. This movement of the charge down the surface of the membrane is referred to as the *local cir-cuit theory* of propagation. In this case, local circuit refers to the flow of current from positive to negative at the interface between action potential, or spike, and the resting potential. The local circuits are not ionic movements but represent flow of electrical current between areas of the membrane having different charges. This would be identical in nature to the flow of electrical current between the positive and negative poles of a battery if they were connected by a conductor. As the action potential moves down the membrane, portions over which it has traveled recover and return to the resting state.

Saltatory Conduction

The rate of transmission of an action potential is ten or more times as great in myelinated neurons than in the unmyelinated neurons. When an action potential is transmitted along a membrane in an unmyelinated neuron, the rate at which it is propagated is a function of the rate at which the respective ion fluxes occur about the membrane surface. Thus, electrochemical transmission is inherently slow when compared to the speed of transmission of electrical current in metal (which travels at the speed of light, approximately 186,000 miles per second). The relatively slow mode of propagation caused by ion fluxes which result in action potentials, is partially overcome in myelinated nerve cells. In these neurons there is direct electrical conduction from positive to negative positions of the nodes of Ranvier, both through the extracellular fluid surrounding the nerve cell and through the cytoplasm of the neuron (see Figure 3–11). It is only within the nodes that action potentials occur as they do in the unmyelinated neurons. Since the action potential jumps or skips from one node to the next, the process

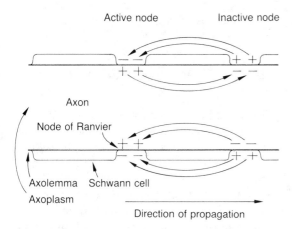

Active node   Inactive node

Axon

Node of Ranvier

Axolemma   Schwann cell

Axoplasm

Direction of propagation

FIGURE 3–11
Flow of current between nodes of Ranvier during saltatory conduction in myelinated nerve cell.

has been called *saltatory conduction*. The rate of transmission between the nodes is very rapid but then slows at the nodes because of the ion fluxes, which generate an action potential at those points. Electrochemical flow based upon diffusion rates occurs only at the nodes, where a typical action potential is generated. The areas between the nodes of Ranvier are shielded or "insulated" by the myelin, and the local circuits are extended, or jump, from one node to the next.

When an action potential causes a node to discharge, a reversal potential occurs. The charge on that node becomes opposite to the charge on the next node and flow can thus occur, as shown in Figure 3–11. When the second node in a series reaches threshold, it discharges, giving rise to a reversal potential, and the potential "hops" from one node to the next. In some of the larger myelinated neurons, transmission rate is known to reach 120 meters per second. This is hardly comparable to the transmission of electricity through metal, but it is admirably greater than the rate of transmission in unmyelinated neurons, which would not exceed two to three meters per second. Thus the validity of the rumor about the college athlete who was so fast that he could turn out the lights and jump into bed before the room became dark is answered.

THE SYNAPSE

A *synapse* is a junction between two nerve cells or between a nerve cell and a muscle cell. In Figure 3–12, the specific parts of the synapse are shown. At a typical synapse, a substance called a *neurotransmitter* is re-

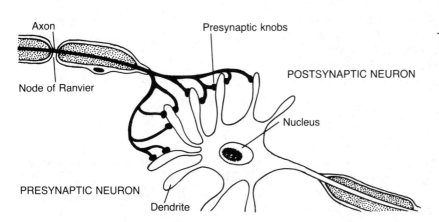

Axon

Presynaptic knobs

POSTSYNAPTIC NEURON

Node of Ranvier

Nucleus

PRESYNAPTIC NEURON

Dendrite

FIGURE 3–12
The synapse is a junction between two neurons or a neuron and a muscle cell, forming a definite structural relationship where communication by neurotransmitter is possible

THE NEURON: MORPHOLOGICAL AND PHYSIOLOGICAL PROPERTIES

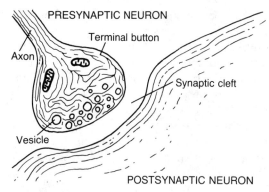

FIGURE 3–13
Typical synaptic relationship, in which the presynaptic neuron communicates with the postsynaptic neuron by means of small enlargements called terminal buttons, or presynaptic knobs. These structures release neurotransmitter from their vesicles.

leased which diffuses from the *presynaptic* cell to the *postsynaptic* cell and effects a change in the conductance of the membrane of the second, or postsynaptic cell. In most synapses the axon of the presynaptic neuron terminates on the postsynaptic neuron in a number of small lobular structures called *terminal buttons* or presynaptic knobs (see Figure 3–13). Each terminal button, when depolarized by an action potential, releases neurotransmitter from the vesicles into the *synaptic cleft*. *Quanta*, or units from the individual vesicles, are released from the presynaptic membrane as the result of the action of the nerve impulse. The impulse increases the calcium ion permeability at the presynaptic nerve ending, an increase essential to the quantal release of the transmitter. The neurotransmitter diffuses across the synaptic cleft and binds to specific receptor sites on the postsynaptic membrane, resulting in either an excitatory or inhibitory postsynaptic potential. The type of potential developed

(excitatory or inhibitory) depends upon the response generated by the neurotransmitter.

Excitatory Postsynaptic Potentials

An *excitatory postsynaptic potential (EPSP)* is a local potential which occurs when a small portion of the dendrite of the postsynaptic membrane becomes depolarized. The action of the neurotransmitter enhances the permeability of the postsynaptic membrane to sodium ions, causing a local reversal of the resting membrane potential. If sufficient depolarization occurs, an action potential will be set up on the membrane of the postsynaptic neuron (see Figure 3–14). The method by which an action potential is set up involves the flow of current between the polarized portion of the neuron and the area depolarized as a result of the action of the neurotransmitter. A typical neurotransmitter that causes EPSPs is acetylcholine. In order to terminate the action of the excitatory sub-

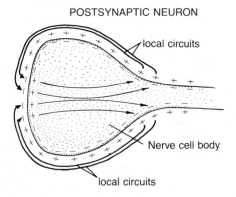

FIGURE 3–14
Postsynaptic membrane with graded local potential induced by neurotransmitter released from the presynaptic cell. Note that the local circuits run from the depolarized region of the postsynaptic membrane to the beginning of the axon rather than to adjacent areas of the postsynaptic membrane.

stance after it has been released, an enzyme (acetylcholinesterase in this case) present on the postsynaptic membrane catalyzes the breakdown of the neurotransmitter so that excitation takes place for a limited time only.

In many cases altered states of neural activity can be induced by exposing a neuron to a substance which competes with the normal neurotransmitter for the receptor sites. Such a competitor is usually a substance which imitates the structure of the natural neurotransmitter. When the receptor sites are blocked by a competitor, the acetylcholine or some other mediator produced by the presynaptic neuron cannot induce its normal effect, and a variety of reactions might result. First, since the competitor blocks attachment of the natural neurotransmitter, permeability to sodium might not be altered; in that case no reaction would take place in the postsynaptic cell. Second, the competitor may alter the sodium permeability to a greater degree than the natural mediator; in that case hyperexcitation occurs. In many cases the hydrolytic enzyme in the postsynaptic cell has no effect on the competing substance, and its action may be continued indefinitely.

Inhibitory Postsynaptic Potentials and Presynaptic Inhibition

Specific neurons within the central nervous system function only as *inhibitors*, or neurons that reduce the excitation of the postsynaptic membrane. Two morphologically distinct nerve cell types exert *inhibitory postsynaptic potentials (IPSP):* Renshaw cells and Golgi bottle neurons. Both cell types can bring about *presynaptic inhibition* and *postsynaptic inhibition* (see Figure 3–15). In vertebrates only, motor neurons and interneurons can be inhibited with postsynaptic inhibi-

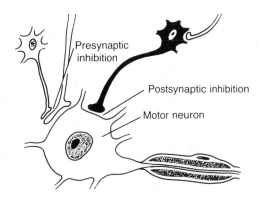

FIGURE 3–15
Examples of pre- and postsynaptic inhibition. Presynaptic inhibition is depicted here as affecting the nerve terminal; it frequently affects other parts of the nerve as well.

tion. The action of sensory neurons can be inhibited by means of presynaptic inhibition.

When the postsynaptic membrane is inhibited or an inhibitory postsynaptic potential is set up, potassium ion permeability is increased and the postsynaptic membrane becomes hyperpolarized. Hyperpolarization is the phenomenon seen in the positive after potential, when the membrane polarity becomes greater than normal (i.e., -80 mV as compared to -75 mV for the normal resting membrane potential). In such cases, the charge across the membrane is greater than the normal charge and is, therefore, further removed from the threshold voltage (see Figure 3–16). Where an inhibitor affects the postsynaptic neuron it is called postsynaptic inhibition.

Presynaptic inhibition can also occur where the inhibitory neuron affects the presynaptic neuron in a way that alters its normal function. As a result of presynaptic inhibition, the magnitude of the action potential reaching the nerve ending is reduced. That

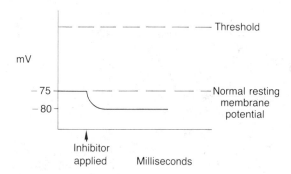

FIGURE 3–16
Changes in potentials at the membrane surface. Note hyperpolarization of the postsynaptic membrane which occurs at the time of inhibition.

reduction in turn results in a reduction of the amount of neurotransmitter released. Reducing the membrane potential causes the nerve to become more excitable, as might be expected, but it also reduces the size, or total magnitude, of the action potential reaching the nerve ending. Consequently, less neurotransmitter is released into the synaptic cleft, the postsynaptic membrane receives less neurotransmitter than normal, and less postsynaptic excitation occurs. The ionic basis for the action caused by the presynaptic inhibitor is unknown, but the action may result from either a slight increase in sodium ion conductance or a decrease in potassium ion conductance across the membrane of the presynaptic cell.

Many substances are suspected of functioning as inhibitory neurotransmitters. Such *mediators* are characteristic of specific portions of the nervous system. No specific substance has been isolated as an inhibitor, though *gamma aminobutyric acid (GABA)* is suspected in some cases to result in presynaptic inhibition. There are many additional substances which are possible inhibitors.

Arrangement of Synapses

Synapses can be arranged in ways that develop refinement of response to stimuli. In many cases, neurons diverge to affect more than one postsynaptic cell. Sometimes several neurons converge on a single postsynaptic nerve cell (see Figure 3–17). When a presynaptic neuron causes an action potential to be generated in a postsynaptic neuron, the postsynaptic cell is said to be in the *liminal area* of the stimulating nerve cell. If the postsynaptic membrane is partially depolarized but no action potential results, it is said to be in the *subliminal area* of the presynaptic neuron. Where two or more presynaptic neurons converge upon a postsynaptic nerve cell, the effects of the presynaptic neurons can be added, or *summated.* Since this

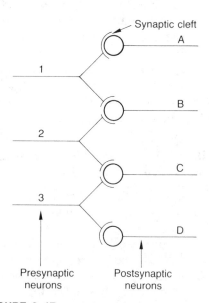

FIGURE 3–17
Convergence and divergence as they occur in neurons. Presynaptic neuron 1 diverges to synapse with postsynaptic neurons A and B. Both presynaptic neurons 1 and 2 converge on postsynaptic neuron B.

is the summation of effects from more than one neuron, it is referred to a *spatial summation*. The specific effect of each presynaptic nerve is called *facilitation*, since each moves the postsynaptic potential toward threshold voltage. In this case, presynaptic neurons are singly too weak to evoke a discharge. In Figure 3–17, if two action potentials occurred very rapidly in neuron 3, their effects could be summated and cause an action potential in neuron C. That would be an example of *temporal summation*, because the primary variable involved is time and the action can be accomplished with one presynaptic neuron.

Sometimes postsynaptic neurons do not behave as expected. If a neuron is stimulated and two postsynaptic neurons fire, and if another neuron is stimulated causing two more postsynaptic neurons to become excited, the expected result of the simultaneous stimulation of the two presynaptic nerves is the excitation of four postsynaptic cells. But if neurons 1 and 2 of Figure 3–17 were stimulated only three postsynaptic neurons would be excited. In that case, in which the number of postsynaptic potentials is less than expected after presynaptic stimulation, *occlusion* is said to have occurred.

NERVE FIBERS

An axon or dendrite that extends out from the nerve cell body is sometimes referred to as a *nerve fiber*. There is a wide variation in the sizes of nerve fibers, and myelination and nonmyelination contribute to differences in neuron morphology. Erlanger and Gasser have attempted to classify nerve fibers according to their type and function. The various types of fibers and their functions have been correlated with such structural and functional characteristics as fiber diameter and conduction velocity. Several types of fibers, based upon morphological and physiological characteristics can be distinguished in mammals (see Table 3–1). Myelinated fibers are classified as types A and B. Type-A

TABLE 3–1
Properties of different mammalian nerve fiber types

Type of Fiber	Diameter of Fiber (μ)	Velocity of Conduction (m/sec)	Function
A (myelinated)			
A (α)	13–22	70–120	Motor, muscle proprioceptors
A (β)	8–13	40–70	Touch, pressure
A (γ)	4–8	15–40	Touch, motor excitation of muscle spindles
A (δ)	1–4	5–15	Pain, heat, cold, pressure
B (myelinated)	1–3	3–14	Preganglionic autonomic
C (unmyelinated)	0.2–1.0	0.2–2	Pain, itch, heat(?), cold(?), pressure(?), postganglionic autonomic, smell

Source: From *Textbook of Medical Physiology*, 5th ed., by A. C. Guyton. Copyright © 1976 by W. B. Saunders Co. Reprinted by permission of W. B. Saunders, CBS College Publishing.

fibers are typically large in diameter and show a definite negative after potential. Type-B fibers are smaller in diameter than type-A fibers, and further differ from Type-A fibers in that Type-B fibers have no negative after potential. All unmyelinated fibers are grouped as type C. Since saltatory conduction does not occur in type-C fibers, they do not show the rapid conduction rates found in the myelinated fibers of types A and B. At least two-thirds of the total nerve fibers in the human are type C. Even though their conduction velocities are slow, type-C fibers provide an excellent example of space economy as the result of their small diameter.

Throughout the body, nerve fibers make up *nerve trunks*, where several fiber types may be grouped together to innervate a particular portion of the body. If these nerve trunks are examined by means of an oscilloscope, they can be separated by the voltage generated by the action potential of each and by the rate at which an action potential travels on each fiber type (see Figure 3–18). In general, larger fibers conduct action potentials more rapidly and with greater electromotive force than do the smaller fibers.

In many cases these fiber types differ in their sensitivity to hypoxia and anesthetics, as well as to other physical factors. For instance, in motor fibers pressure may retard conduction while pain sensations remain intact. Almost everyone has experienced the sensation of sitting in one position for an extended period of time and having a leg or foot "go to sleep." In this type of situation, pressure has inhibited conduction in type A fibers *(somatic motor fibers)*, which control movement, while type C fibers for pain and touch continue to function normally.

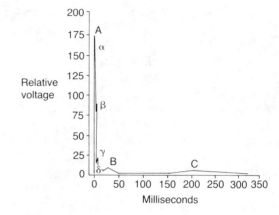

FIGURE 3–18
Record obtained from mixed nerve showing relative time-voltage relationships of individual neuron types. A (α, β, γ, δ), B, and C refer to fiber types of the mixed nerves. The complete record is known as a compound action potential.

SUMMARY

The basic unit of the nervous system is the neuron, which varies in structure as well as function. The most common characteristic of all types of neurons is their ability to transmit action potentials from one point to another within the body. Some neurons inhibit the activity of other nerve cells or muscle cells, whereas others excite or provoke activity. Nerve cells are connected to each other and to muscles by means of junctions called synapses. At the synapse, chemical substances called neurotransmitters are released which enable communication between cells to take place. Each neurotransmitter has a specific structure which binds to specific receptor sites on the postsynaptic membrane. Foreign chemicals with the same general structure can be introduced at the synapse as competitors. Competition of this type frequently leads to altered states of response.

Neurons differ structurally in the number of extensions projected from the nerve cell body. Adult mammals have pseudomonopolar, bipolar, and multipolar neurons, known by the number of cellular projections or poles which may be present. In addition, neurons can be classified on the basis of fiber size and myelination. Morphological characteristics based on such variables result in functional differences, which can be measured in intensity and rate of transmission.

4

THE CENTRAL
NERVOUS SYSTEM

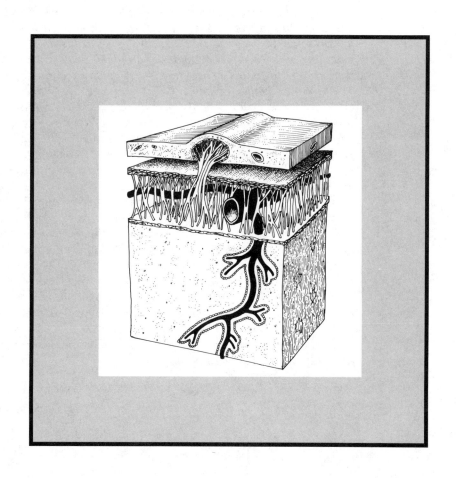

*T*he nervous system of mammals can be divided into a central nervous system (CNS), which consists of the brain and the spinal cord, and a peripheral nervous system (PNS), which comprises all of the nerves outside of the central nervous system that innervate the organs and tissues of the body. All nerve cell bodies, except some of those belonging to the autonomic nervous system and the organs of the specialized senses, lie within the central nervous system. The motor or efferent neurons carry information (impulses) to the organs and tissues, whereas the sensory or afferent neurons carry information to the central nervous system. The brain and the spinal cord provide most of the integrative functions of the mammalian nervous system. Exceptions to that rule occur in the autonomic ganglia and organs of the special senses.

The vertebrate brain has undergone a number of evolutionary changes since its beginning millions of years ago. Basically, it is derived from three distinct portions, readily seen in the primitive-appearing or embryonic brain (see Table 4–1 and Figure 4–1). The forebrain, or prosencephalon, has given rise to the most complex functions of the nervous system in mammals. Its derivatives allow the animal to recognize sensory stimuli and generate complex actions. The forebrain is divided into two distinct parts, the telencephalon and the diencephalon. The telencephalon gives rise to the allocortex, which is present in all vertebrates, and the neocortex or cerebral cortex, which is unique to mammals and is most highly developed in primates and cetaceans (whales, etc.). The diencephalon forms the epithalamus, the thalamus (or dorsal thalamus), ventral thalamus (or subthalamus), and the hypothalamus. In addition, the diencephalon gives rise to the posterior pituitary and the pineal gland. The midbrain, or mesencephalon, functions as an area of nerve passageways between the forebrain and the rest of the nervous system. The mesencephalon contains several extremely important nuclei that are needed for motor and integrative control (see Table 4–2). A nerve center, or nucleus, consists of a group of nerve cell bodies within the central nervous system that control a particular physiological function. Some parts of the center are excitatory whereas others are inhibitory, but all are associated with the function of a particular organ or organ system. The hindbrain, or rhombencephalon, gives rise to the medulla oblongata, pons, and cerebellum.

TABLE 4–1
The principal brain structures in the embryo and their derivatives in the adult brain

Embryonic or Primitive Parts of the Brain	Adult Structures of the Brain
Prosencephalon	
Telencephalon	Neocortex (cerebral cortex) and allocortex
Diencephalon	Epithalamus, dorsal thalamus (thalamus), ventral thalamus, hypothalamus, posterior pituitary, and pineal gland
Mesencephalon	Nerve passageways and certain nuclei
Rhombencephalon	Medulla oblongata, pons, and cerebellum

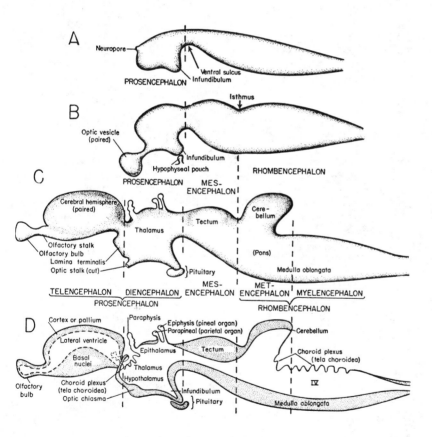

FIGURE 4–1
Developmental sequence of the brain from simple tube to the general structure found in higher vertebrates: (A) only the primitive forebrain (prosencephalon) is distinct from the remainder of the neural tube; (B) all three major divisions have been established; (C) more mature stage of the three principal parts; and (D) same as C, only in median section rather than lateral section. From *The Vertebrate Body,* by A. S. Romer. Copyright © 1956 by W. B. Saunders Co. Reprinted by permission of W. B. Saunders, CBS College Publishing.

TABLE 4–2
Main cell masses or nuclei of the mesencephalon

	Cell Masses	Connections		Possible Functional Associations
		Afferent	Efferent	
Tectum	Tectum opticum (called superior colliculus in mammals)	II, cord, bulb, sensory nucleus of V, isthmus, torus semicircularis or inferior colliculus, pretectum, thalamus, telencephalon	Cord, bulb, periaqueductal gray, reticular formation, nucleus isthmi, thalamus (especially birds and mammals), retina (teleosts, amphibians)	Correlation of visual, auditory, and somesthetic; feature extraction; localizing stimuli; formulation of higher reflex commands; eye and head movements, especially in orientation
Tegmentum	Torus semicirculairs (called inferior colliculus in mammals)	Lateral line nuclei (fish), cochlear nuclei (tetrapods), vestibular nuclei (less in higher groups), cord, V sensory nucleus	Tectum, thalamus, reticular formation	Correlation of information on equilibrium and near-field aquatic displacements (and electric fields); sound sources; localization
	Nuclei III, IV (including general somatic and general visceral efferent)	Vestibular nuclei, cerebellum, tectum (indirectly), reticular formation	Extraocular muscles, iris, and ciliary muscle (parasympathetic)	Movements of eyes; accommodation; pupillary constriction
	Periaqueductal gray matter, tegmental nuclei, interpeduncular nuclei	Complex, including tectum, hypothalamus, habenula, cord, telencephalon	Complex, including nuclei of III, IV, VI, pons, thalamus, hypothalamus	Limbic system; affect, visceral control

EVOLUTION OF THE BRAIN IN HIGHER VERTEBRATES

Among the vertebrates, the brain shows the greatest development and complexity in the mammals. That complexity is demonstrated by the highly developed social orders of human civilizations as well as by many of the complex behavior patterns found in other mammals. One way of assessing the increased role of the brain in mammals is to compare brain size with body size. Mammals with greater size have larger brains, but that may not, at first glance, seem meaningful because that says nothing about cell size or cell density within the brain. Closer observation reveals that neuron size does not vary tremendously among mammals. For instance, neuron size is only a few times larger in elephants than in mice. This situation, in general, holds true for other mammalian species as well. It is therefore safe to say that larger mammals have greater numbers of brain cells

TABLE 4–2
(continued)

	Cell Masses	Connections		Possible Functional Associations
		Afferent	Efferent	
Tegmentum	Isthmo-optic nucleus	Tectum	Retina (in birds only)	Horizontal cell response
	Nucleus isthmi (in nonmammalian forms)	Tectum, probably torus semicircularis	Tectum, torus semicircularis tegmentum, thalamus	Correlation of optic, equilibrium, acoustic influences
	Reticular formation, including tegmental reticular nuclei	Cortex, pallidum, reticular formation of other levels, cerebellum, vestibular nuclei, cochlear nuclei, tectum, cord	Reticular formation of other levels, thalamus, cord	Motor control; pupil; many functions; reticular activating system
	Red nucleus	Dentate, interposed nuclei, precentral cortex (somatotopically organized)	Cord, bulbar reticular formation, inferior olive, cerebellum, thalamus (especially from small-celled newer part of red nucleus)	Motor coordination, especially righting; flexor activity; well developed in carnivores, poor in primates
Intermediate zone	Substantia nigra (large in man, small in other mammals; only a forerunner in reptiles)	Caudate, putamen, subthalamus, pretectum,	Striate, pallidum, thalamus	Extrapyramidal motor; inhibition of forced movements; pathologic in Parkinsonism

Source: From *Introduction to Nervous Systems* by T. H. Bullock. Copyright © 1977 by W. H. Freeman and Company. All rights reserved.

than do smaller mammals. The largest neurons (in diameter) in the animal kingdom are found in relatively simple invertebrates such as mollusks.

One can, however, assume that a finite ratio can be determined between brain weight and body weight and that this ratio may be greater in animals which have greater learning and thought capacities. This increased ratio might also be reflected in some aspect of neural function associated with the intri-

cate communication system found in many communal animals. If one compares the brain weight to body weight ratio in existing vertebrates, the increased ratio is quite obvious in mammals, especially in primates (see Figure 4–2). This trend seems to have significant adaptive value. When the brain/body-weight ratio comparisons are made using the estimated values from primitive mammals and mammallike reptiles, it is clear that the mammalian brain/body-weight

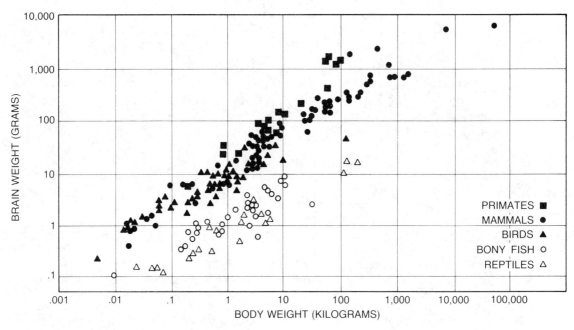

FIGURE 4–2
Differences in the ratios of brain weight to body weight in existing vertebrates. From
Paleoneurology and the Evolution of the Mind, H. J. Jerison. Copyright © Jan. 1976 by
Scientific American, Inc. All rights reserved.

ratio has been increasing in evolutionary sequence (see Figure 4–3). This increase in ratio, termed *encephalization*, signifies the increased importance of the brain as mammals
evolved. If one compares relative brain size of
various groups of animals through time, one
finds that all groups show an increase in
brain/body-weight ratio, an increase that invariably reaches a plateau at some point during each group's evolution (see Figure 4–4).
The sharpest increase through time has been
found in humans, though the degree of encephalization shown by porpoises is remarkably close to that found in humans (see Figure 4–5).

The significance of encephalization cannot be overemphasized. In humans it means
that very exacting movements of the hand

and facial muscles are possible, giving rise to
the abilities of tool utilization and self-
expression. Also, the role of the *facilitory neurons*, whose nerve cell bodies are located in
the brain, and their effect upon motor nerves
in the spinal cord are quite obvious. With
greater encephalization there is an increased
facilitory role played by the brain in *cordal
reflexes*, responses of the organism carried
out by the spinal cord. Primitive vertebrates
show relatively unaltered cordal reflexes
when the cerebrum is removed, or *decerebrated*, whereas advanced species show *decerebrate rigidity* or, in some cases, complete
absence of motor activity. *Spinal shock*, the
quiescent period of inactivity and unresponsiveness which occurs after *transection* of the
spinal cord, lasts for several days or weeks in

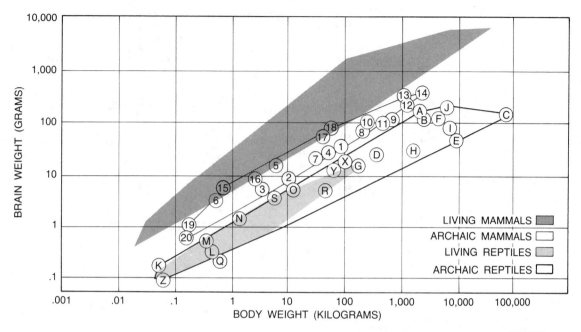

FIGURE 4–3
Evolutionary changes from primitive to advanced reptiles and mammals. Numbered points represent data from archaic ungulates and carnivores. Oldest is *Triconodon* (20). Fossil reptiles are dinosaurers (A–J), pterosaures (K–O), mammallike reptiles (Q–S), two amphibians (X, Y), and a fish (Z). From Paleoneurology and the Evolution of the Mind, H. J. Jerison.

humans and only a few hours in the cat. The lower the vertebrate, the less the effect of spinal shock; in many species it is difficult to demonstrate. Such differences, as well as many other phenomena, are a manifestation of the importance of the evolutionary process to the development of the mammalian central nervous system.

PARTS OF THE CENTRAL NERVOUS SYSTEM

The Telencephalon

The brain of man and higher primates epitomizes the evolution of the cerebral cortex (or neocortex) from the frontal lobe of the primitive brain, the allocortex. In mammals, the allocortex is often referred to as the *limbic system*. In other vertebrates, such as reptiles, birds, and amphibians, the neocortex is completely absent. Many neurological actions that would normally be associated with the neocortex in mammals are carried out by the allocortex in the lower vertebrates. The neocortex has evolved slowly, increasing in size with the evolution of higher mammals (see Figure 4–6). It would appear that in mammals the neocortex has taken over the more complex aspects of the neurological processes; the more primitive emotions and drives common to most mammals have remained with the allocortex. For instance,

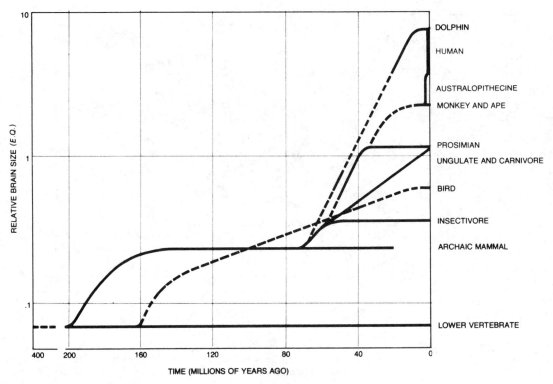

FIGURE 4–4
Evolutionary changes in brain/body-weight ratios. Note the definite plateau shown by each group, usually within the last eighty million years. From Paleoneurology and the Evolution of the Mind, H. J. Jerison. Copyright © Jan. 1976 by Scientific American, Inc. All rights reserved.

emotions such as anger as well as drives associated with hunger and libido are expressed as intensely in the lower mammals as they are in humans. But complex thought processes, as in humans, are foreign to those species lacking a neocortex or having a neocortex of noticeably less complexity than humans.

The cerebral cortex can be divided into six basic layers (see Figure 4–7). The first layer is devoid of neurons, whereas the second and third layers are formed by neurons important to the integration of different regions of the cortex. In related species, layer four appears to be fairly constant in thickness, whereas the outer three layers (layers one, two, and three) show a definite increase with increased body size (see Figure 4–8). Interestingly, layers five and six are also thicker in larger species of related mammals, but that relationship is not as consistently true for those two layers as for the first three layers. Function in the layers varies; information is usually received by the fourth layer, whereas the neurons of the fifth and sixth layers are involved in outflow of cortical information. It

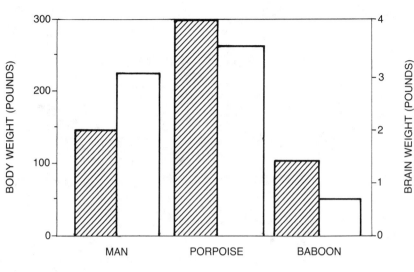

FIGURE 4–5
The greatest ratios of brain weight to body weight in mammals are found in primates and cetaceans. Here brain/body-weight ratios among man, baboon, and porpoise are compared. The brain of man occupies about 2 percent of total body weight. The brain weight of the baboon constitutes slightly less than 1 percent of its body weight, whereas the brain weight of the porpoise is slightly greater than 1 percent. Patterned bars denote body weight; open bars denote brain weight.

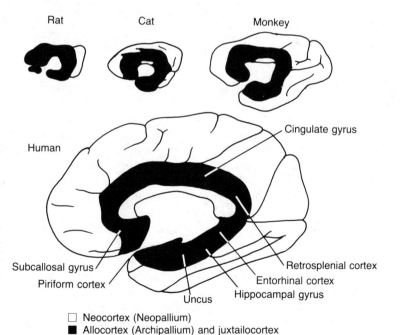

FIGURE 4–6
Relative increase of the neocortex with the increase in brain size in mammals. Dark areas indicate the allocortex, which has become the limbic system in higher mammals. From P. D. MacLean, The Limbic System and Its Hippocampal Formation, *J. Neurosurg.* 11(1954):29, figs. 1, 5, 8. Reprinted by permission of Dartmouth Medical School, Hanover, N.H.

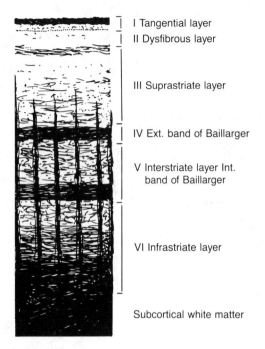

I Tangential layer

II Dysfibrous layer

III Suprastriate layer

IV Ext. band of Baillarger

V Interstriate layer Int.
   band of Baillarger

VI Infrastriate layer

Subcortical white matter

FIGURE 4–7
In the cerebral cortex there are six basic layers, which can be distinguished on the basis of cell type and function

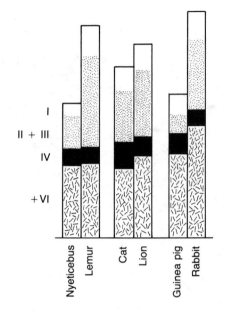

I

II + III

IV

+ VI

Nyeticebus   Lemur   Cat   Lion   Guinea pig   Rabbit

FIGURE 4–8
Relative thickness of different cortical layers in related species. From C. V. A. Kappers et al, *The Comparative Anatomy of the Nervous System of Vertebrates Including Man* (New York, N.Y., 1936). Reprinted by permission of Macmillan Publishing Co.

also should be noted that larger mammals have thicker cortexes, though the difference is not dramatic between species as are the differences in the weight of the entire brain (see Figure 4–9).

The mammalian cerebral cortex is divided into two basic halves, or *cerebral hemispheres*, which are connected by a dense group of transverse myelinated fibers known as the *corpus callosum*. Each hemisphere has specific activities usually not completely duplicated in the other. For instance, motor activity in humans is dominated by one of the cerebral hemispheres. The ability of one hemisphere to control movement, reducing that burden for the other hemisphere, is called *cerebral dominance*. The left hemisphere is usually dominant in motor abilities

in right-handed people, though the right hemisphere is dominant in only about 30 percent of all left-handed individuals. In cases where the dominant hemisphere is ablated, as in strokes or other types of trauma, the other hemisphere can in time achieve the ability to carry out the motor functions once controlled by the dominant hemisphere.

It appears that the hemisphere which is not dominant performs precise functions and is not merely a backup system to be used in case of loss of the other hemisphere. Evidence now points toward hemisphere specialization in humans: the one (dominant) half of the brain is specialized in motor and, consequently, language function, whereas the other (nondominant) half is specialized

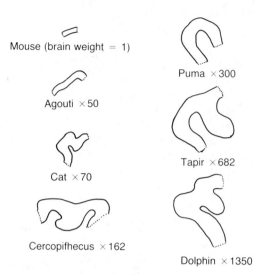

Mouse (brain weight = 1)

Agouti ×50

Cat ×70

Cercopifhecus ×162

Puma ×300

Tapir ×682

Dolphin ×1350

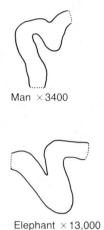

Man ×3400

Elephant ×13,000

FIGURE 4–9
The thickness of the cerebral cortex is greater in larger mammalian species, though it differs only by a factor of three between the mouse and the elephant. Brain weight differs by a factor of 13,000. From C. V. A. Kappers et al, *The Comparative Anatomy of the Nervous System of Vertebrates Including Man* (New York, N.Y., 1936). Reprinted by permission of Macmillan Publishing Co.

in recognition and visuospatial relations. That nondominant side also seems to be specialized to control spatiotemporal relations and is therefore important for a sense of time as well as for visual and auditory recognition. This has given rise to the term *categorical hemisphere* for the dominant hemisphere and *representational hemisphere* for the nondominant hemisphere.

Regions of the cortex are specialized, so distinct portions have specific actions. For instance, motor activity and sensory reception occur in separate areas of the cerebral cortex, known as the *motor cortex* and the *sensory cortex,* respectively. The recognition of sound and of light occur at separate sensory areas, known as the *auditory cortex* and the *visual cortex,* respectively (see Figure 4–10). In the sensory cortex there are sensory neurons which are innervated by specific receptors from the skin. The relative portion of the cortex devoted to a particular motor function or to a particular sensory modality is representative of the importance of that particular phenomenon or action in a partic-

ular species (see Figure 4–11). For instance, the area devoted to sound reception in the cetaceans, which have developed a very good echolocation technique, should be disproportionately large when compared to the size of the auditory cortex in humans, which rely less than cetaceans on sound reception as a means of communication.

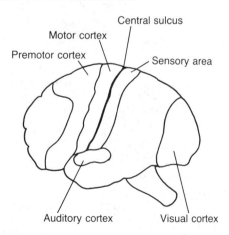

FIGURE 4–10
The primary motor and sensory regions of the human cortex

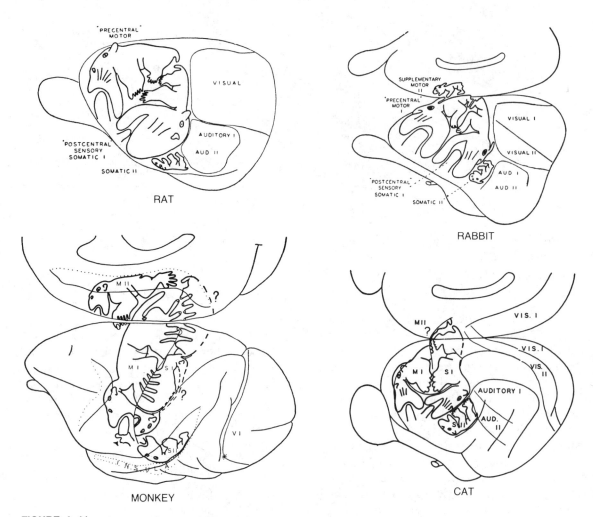

FIGURE 4–11
Somatic cortex of four mammalian species. MI, precentral motor; MII, supplementary motor; SI, postcentral sensory; and Somatic II, second somatic sensory areas. The areas of the cortex devoted to a particular part of the body vary among different species. From H. F. Harlow and C. F. Woolsey (eds.), *Biological and Biochemical Basis of Behavior* (Madison, Wis., 1958), 66–68, figs. 19, 20, 21 & 22. Reprinted by permission of The University of Wisconsin Press.

The Diencephalon

The several divisions of the diencephalon are believed to have visceral and pineal control, to control emotional expression, to relay function from both motor and sensory areas, and to provide association areas for visual and auditory stimuli. The various structural divisions of the diencephalon and the functional aspects primarily associated with each division are discussed in this section.

The epithalamus The functional significance of the epithalamus is for the most part unknown. It is clearly associated with the *pineal gland*, which is implicated in hormonal control of gonadal function, temperature acclimation, and perhaps dormancy with some species.

The thalamus (dorsal thalamus) The thalamus functions primarily as a relay center for impulses that originate elsewhere in the organism. Nuclei located in the thalamus act as relay centers for all sensory receptors in the body except for the nasal mucosa (the sensation of smell). The impulses transmitting the sensation of sound pass through the *median geniculate nuclei*, the sensation of light (vision) through the *lateral geniculate nuclei*, and the sensation of taste through the *ventral posterior nuclei*. Other nuclei of the thalamus are relay centers for neurons which innervate the skeletal muscles, and thus constitute the *somatic nervous system*. These are the *ventral lateral nuclei*, which control voluntary motor actions, and the *ventral anterior nuclei*, which act as relay centers to the neurons associated with voluntary motor actions and arousal. In essence, the thalamus acts as a relay center for all sensory information, except smell, and provides relay centers for the motor neurons which control the skeletal muscles.

Some sensory interpretation also occurs in the thalamus. Experiments with decorticate mammals, an animal whose cerebral cortex has been removed, indicate an awareness of certain stimuli in the absence of a cerebral cortex. These animals respond to painful stimuli and seem to recognize stimuli of temperature, touch, and pressure.

Several nuclei located below the cerebral cortex and associated with the thalamus are of obvious significance to movement in mammals. These nuclei are termed the *basal ganglia* and consist of the *caudate nucleus*, the *putamen*, the *globus pallidus*, the *subthalamic nucleus*, the *substantia nigra*, and the *red nucleus* (see Figure 4–12). The basal ganglia assume the role of the motor cortex in birds and reptiles and are responsible for movement in those animals, which lack a motor cortex. In mammals, humans in particular, these nuclei have a less significant role, and their exact functions are somewhat of an enigma. Research related to specific functions of the basal ganglia in mammals has been almost universally fruitless. Nevertheless, their functions are of extreme importance, since such conditions as Parkinson's disease and Huntington's chorea are definitely related to the malfunction or degener-

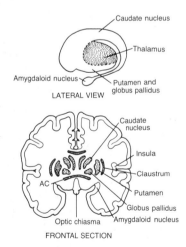

FIGURE 4–12
The basal ganglia of the human brain (AC, anterior commisure)

ation of the basal ganglia. It would appear that the basal ganglia have some role in the programming of movement, since activity in these areas precedes movement.

The hypothalamus The hypothalamus, a very complex region of the brain, is involved with numerous integrative responses of the animal. It is the principal area of control of homeostatic responses of the organism. Of major importance is its control of the autonomic nervous system and the pituitary gland. It functions as an endocrine gland in the sense that *releasing hormones* are produced in the hypothalamus which activate the production of trophic hormones by the anterior pituitary. Two hormones which affect water balance and smooth muscle contraction, *vasopressin* and *oxytocin,* are synthesized in the hypothalamus and released by the posterior pituitary.

Almost every action not associated with the somatic motor system in some way involves the hypothalamus. The hypothalamus controls food and water intake by responding to the stimuli of thirst and satiety. Even stressful stimuli seem to have subconscious effects which evoke responses through the hypothalamus. Individual functions of the hypothalamus, such as temperature regulation, control of the autonomic nervous system, and reproduction, will be covered in detail in other chapters.

The pineal gland The pineal gland is seated on the dorsal aspect of the brain in most mammals and is closest in position to the epithalamus (see Figure 4–13). Increased development of the cerebral cortex, as in humans, a few of the other higher primates, and the porpoise, has given it a more central and posterior position. In these mammals the pi-

FIGURE 4–13
The pineal gland of the rat

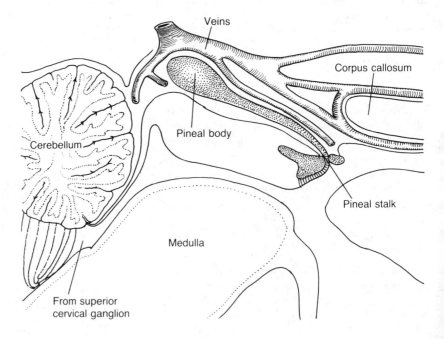

neal is covered by the cerebral hemispheres, which show phenomenal growth in comparison to other vertebrates.

The function of the pineal gland has been discussed for centuries, though little evidence was acquired about the nature of its function until the middle of the twentieth century. Galen, who described the pineal in the fourth century, considered it to be a secretory organ important for the process of thought. Its most famous proposed function was suggested by Descartes, who in 1662 extolled the pineal as the seat of the soul. In more recent times, it has been shown that the pineal is indeed secretory in birds and that its products are essential for birds' normal activity cycle. In both birds and mammals it contains *melatonin*, which is synthesized from the amino acid *tryptophan*. Ambient light inhibits *in vivo* melatonin formation in the pineal; its production is stimulated in some species by decreasing photoperiods associated with autumn. It has been shown by Reiter and others that melatonin produced by the pineal in some way blocks the action of gonadotropic pituitary hormones which control the reproductive cycles of rodents. It might also function in the process of temperature acclimation through enhancing the ability to sustain metabolic rate and, therefore, heat production. More information on the pineal gland is discussed in chapter 17, The Endocrine System.

The Rhombencephalon

The medulla oblongata The medulla oblongata, or simply *medulla*, forms the *brainstem* and provides relay centers for sensory information to the cerebellum and cerebral cortex. The medulla is the site of origin of several *cranial nerves*, which include the *ves-*

tibulocochlear or *auditory nerve* (VIII), the *glossopharyngeal nerve* (IX), the *vagus nerve* (X), the *accessory nerve* (XI) and the *hypoglossal nerve* (XII). A portion of the *vestibular branch* of the *auditory nerve* also synapses with neurons in the pons. Some motor axons from the motor cortex pass through the *pyramid* of the medulla and terminate on the motor neurons of the ventral horns of the spinal cord (see Figure 4–14). The motor neurons whose axons pass through the pyramidal system are varied in nature, with about 60 percent being myelinated and 40 percent

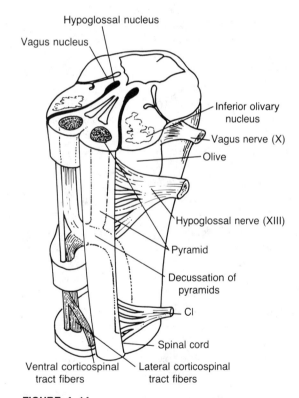

FIGURE 4–14
The medulla oblongata of the human brain showing transverse section and ventral aspect (CI, first cervical nerve)

being unmyelinated. The largest of these neurons are the *Betz cells*, which are 16 micrometers in diameter and make up about 2 percent of the total pyramidal neurons. Most of the motor neurons from the left side of the brain cross over to the right side in the pyramidal tract, and vice versa. The area of crossing over is called the *pyramidal decussation.*

Many nuclei which control visceral functions of the body are centered in the medulla. Its dorsal side contains the *nucleus grasilis* and the *nucleus cuneatus*, which receive sensory fibers from the spinal cord and relay sensory information to the cerebral cortex through the thalamus. Most sensory impulses cross over to the opposite side of the brain from the site of the stimulus. In addition to the centers involved in the integration of afferent neurons, the medulla contains centers which control heart rate *(cardiac center)*, rate and depth of breathing *(respiratory center)*, and blood vessel diameter *(vasoconstrictor center)*. It also houses centers which control swallowing, vomiting, coughing, sneezing, and hiccuping.

The *olives*, located on each side of the medulla, are oval-shaped projections containing the *inferior olivary complex*, which is responsible for relaying afferent somatic information to the cerebellum for comparative analysis with sensory and motor fibers from the cortex. The complex consists of the *principal olivary nucleus*, which is predominate in primates, the *dorsal accessory olivary nucleus*, which is predominate in some ungulates, and the *medial accessory olivary nucleus*, which is predominate in whales (see Figure 4–15).

The pons The pons (or *pons varolii*) is an oval structure located on the anterioventral aspect of the medulla (see Figure 4–16). The

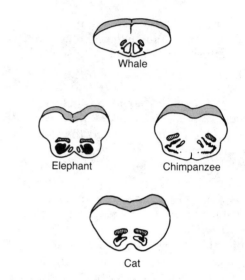

FIGURE 4–15
Relative areas of the inferior olivary complex in various mammals. Black areas denote principal olivary nucleus; dorsal hatched areas, the dorsal accessory olivary nucleus; and, open areas, the medial accessory olivary nucleus.

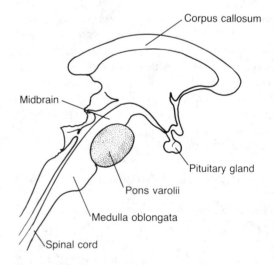

FIGURE 4–16
Sagittal section through the brain stem of the human showing the relationship of the pons varolii to the midbrain and medulla oblongata

term "pons" means bridge. True to its name, the pons provides a connection between the brain and other neurons in the body. It also forms bridges or areas of integration between different parts of the brain. The nuclei for several cranial nerves originate in the pons, including the *trigeminal nerve (V)*, the *abducens nerve (VI)*, the *facial nerve (VII)*, and the *vestibular branch* of the *auditory nerve (VIII)*. In addition to nuclei for cranial nerves and relay fibers, the pons contains the *pneumotaxic center*, which is essential for regulation of the breathing rate (see chapter 15, Respiration).

The cerebellum The cerebellum, formed from the roof of the rhombencephalon, provides a massive area of integration of both sensory and motor information. For many years it has represented an enigma to neuroscientists, being called a motor component of the extra–pyramidal system by some and the head ganglion of the *proprioceptive* (sensory) *system* by others. Most of the functional relationships were observed in mammals with *cerebellar lesions*. Lesions are usually made using high tension electrodes capable of destroying a small portion of neural tissue. *Lesioning* can be accomplished with a fair degree of accuracy by fixing the head of the experimental animal in a stereotaxic apparatus and carefully guiding the electrode into position in accordance with previously mapped regions of the brain. After the experiment has been completed, exact placement of the electrodes can be verified through histological examination.

Although the cerebellum occupies only about one-tenth of the brain weight in humans and one-fifth of the brain weight in whales, its surface area by comparison is quite significant, occupying an area comparable to 75 percent of the surface area found on the cerebral cortex. Its complex structure consists of external gray matter (composed primarily of unmyelinated fibers) and internal white (myelinated) fibers arranged in a number of lobules (see Figure 4–17). The cerebellum functions in the integration of muscular actions during complex movements. Skilled voluntary movements as well as many *phasic actions* (rapid reflex actions such as removal from painful stimuli) require interaction of antagonistic and synergistic muscles, and it is in such integration of motor processes in the central nervous system that the cerebellum seems to be most effective.

The cerebellum has both afferent and efferent connections with the motor cortex and the basal ganglia. It also receives information from the sensory receptors located in muscles and tendons. In general, it appears that some movements are preprogrammed through the cerebellum as muscular action occurs. It is in this sense that the cerebellum acts as an internal correcting mechanism that functions during an action of the body to allow for constant compensation. For example, in order to pick up an object with the hand, one must not only start the hand in motion but also constantly monitor and correct its position as the hand moves toward the object. Comparisons must be made between the action initiated and the action as it is being carried out. In order to do that, the cerebellum must be appraised of the motor stimuli causing the action, the sensory information about the hand's position, and the rate of speed that the hand is actually traveling. If the movement is not precisely equal to the stimuli, the motor input to the hand can be altered by the efferent connections of the cerebellum, which synapse with neurons in the motor cortex. In other words, the cerebellum appears to operate as a *servo sys-*

FIGURE 4–17
Superior and inferior views and sagittal section of the human cerebellum. The ten principal lobules of the cerebellum are marked with Roman numerals.

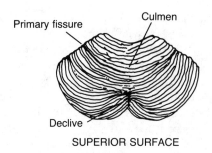

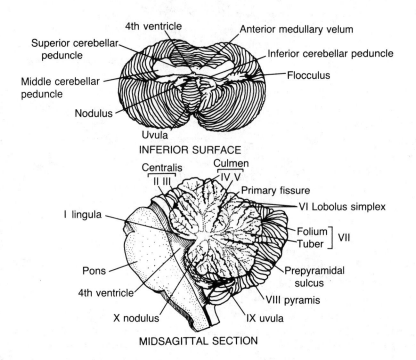

SUPERIOR SURFACE

INFERIOR SURFACE

MIDSAGITTAL SECTION

tem, a mechanism that perpetually monitors and corrects.

The cerebellum of mammals consists of three distinct units, when viewed from an evolutionary aspect. These are the *archicerebellum*, the *paleocerebellum*, and the *neocerebellum*. The archicerebellum, represented by the *flocculonodular lobe*, functions primarily in body equilibrium. The paleocerebellum can be divided into an *anterior lobe*, which includes the *lingula*, the *centralis*, and the *culmen*, and a *posterior lobe*, which comprises the *pyramis*, the *uvula*, and the *paraflocculus*. The paleocerebellum's primary function is in the maintenance of posture, including stance and orientation of the body with respect to its surroundings. The neocerebellum consists of the *ansiform*, the *paramedian tubes*, the *declive*, and the *simplex*. It is primarily associated with voluntary fine movements necessary in the control of the hands and face in primates and many of the refined movements characteristic of other mammalian groups as well.

The Reticular Activating System

Running throughout the brain and the anterior region of the spinal cord there is a system of neurons, diffuse in origin, that innervates almost every section of the brain (see Figure 4–18). This system of diffuse neurons is known as the *reticular activating system (RAS)*. It is not a distinct anatomical unit, as are other parts of the brain, but it instead composes a portion of almost every part of the brain.

The function of the RAS is principally facilitative, because when activated it maintains an organism's wakeful state through a general stimulation of many areas of the brain. When the organism is awake, the RAS also seems to be essential in maintaining concentration and alertness. Two centers of the RAS have been located: one in the brainstem and another in the thalamus. When the brainstem portion of the RAS is stimulated, the entire brain is activated. It appears that neurons in this region are essential for the maintenance of the sleep-wake cycle. When the thalamic portion is stimulated, a less diffuse reaction occurs in which specific regions of the cerebral cortex are stimulated. The thalamic portion of the RAS has the function of directing the animal's attention and of maintaining alertness.

The Cranial Nerves

As encephalization occurred through evolution, the spinal nerves located in the anterior aspect of the spinal cord became a part of the brain. With further encephalization, more spinal nerves became associated with the brain; twelve pairs were finally included in mammals. These cranial nerves became more specialized through evolution until some were purely sensory, some were purely motor, and still others were mixed sensory and motor. These nerves still retain similarity with spinal nerves in that the nerve cell bodies of the sensory neurons are located in ganglia outside of the brain, whereas the nerve cell bodies of the motor neurons are located in nuclei within the brain.

The twelve pairs of cranial nerves are denoted by Roman numerals to indicate their order from a *rostral* to *caudal* perspective (i.e., front to rear); their names generally denote innervation or function. They contain fibers which are a part of the somatic nervous system as well as parts of the autonomic nervous system. The largest of the cranial nerves is the *vagus nerve (X)*, which serves the viscera and contains both sensory and motor fibers. A detailed description of each nerve is not appropriate here; Table 4–3 provides information concerning innervation, function, and name of the cranial nerves as they appear in mammals.

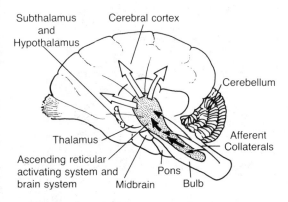

Subthalamus and Hypothalamus

Cerebral cortex

Cerebellum

Thalamus

Afferent Collaterals

Ascending reticular activating system and brain system

Pons

Midbrain

Bulb

FIGURE 4–18
The ascending reticular activating system projected on a sagittal section of the cat brain

TABLE 4-3

Brainstem nuclei of the cranial nerves: nuclei, main destination of motor components, and main function or source of sensory components (blanks indicate absence of components of that type) Roman numerals refer to specific cranial nerves: III, Oculomotor; IV, Troclear; V, Trigeminal; VI, Abducens; VII, Facial; VIII, Auditory; IX, Glossopharyngeal; X, Vagus; XI, Spinal Accessory; and, XII, Hypoglossal. Cranial nerves I (Olfactory) and II (Optic) are not included because they are not found in the brainstem.

	Medial					Lateral
Cranial nerve	Somatic efferent	Special visceral efferent	General visceral efferent	Visceral afferent	General somatic afferent	Special somatic afferent
III	III nucleus (extrinsic eye muscle)		Edinger-Westphal nucleus (iris and ciliary muscle)		Unknown (proprioceptive to eye muscle)	
IV	IV nucleus (extrinsic eye muscle)				Unknown (proprioceptive to eye muscle)	
VI	VI nucleus (extrinsic eye muscle)				Unknown (proprioceptive to eye muscle)	
V		Motor nucleus of V (masticatory muscle)			Main sensory and spinal nucleus (skin) Mesencephalic nucleus (proprioceptive to masticatory muscle)	Lateral line nucleus* (exteroceptive)
VII		Motor nucleus of VII (facial muscle)	Salivatory nucleus (salivary glands)	Solitary nucleus (taste and face)		Lateral line nucleus*

	Somatic motor	Branchial motor	Visceral motor	Visceral sensory	Somatic sensory	Special sensory
VIII						Vestibular nucleus (labyrinth) Cochlear nucleus (cochlea)
IX		Nucleus ambiguus (branchial muscle and stylopharyngeal muscle)	Salivatory nucleus (salivary glands)	Solitary nucleus (taste and pharynx)		Lateral line nucleus*
X		Nucleus ambiguus (branchial muscle of pharynx and larynx)	Dorsal motor nucleus of X (viscera)	Solitary nucleus ("vagal lobe") (taste, abdominal viscera)	Spinal nucleus of V (skin)	Lateral line nucleus*
XI		Nucleus ambiguus (branchial muscle of pharynx and larynx; Ventral horn, cervical 1–6 (trapezius and sterno-cleido-mastoid muscle)	Dorsal motor nucleus of X (viscera)			
XII	Hypoglossal nucleus (tongue muscle)				Unknown (proprioceptive to tongue)	

Source: From *Introduction to Nervous Systems*, by T. H. Bullock. Copyright © 1977 by W. H. Freeman and Company. All rights reserved.

*The lateral line nerves and their sensory ganglion cells are so distinct from the classical components of VII, IX, and X that we must either broaden the definition of those nerves or regard this major cranial inflow as supernumerary to the series of numbered cranial nerves.

The Meninges

The brain and spinal cord are surrounded by three membranes called *meninges*. The outer layer, known as the *dura mater* (hard mother), is a strong, thick layer which provides protection for the brain and associated circulation. The intermediate layer, called the *arachnoid* (spider layer), is well supplied with blood vessels and is an important element in the nutrition of the brain. The inner layer, named the *pia mater* (gentle mother), closely adheres to the surface of the underlying neural tissue and contains numerous blood vessels. Each of the meninges cover both the brain and the spinal cord (see Figure 4–19) and are continuous inside the skull and neural canal of the vertebrae.

Cerebrospinal Fluid

The brain is bathed in a liquid called the *cerebrospinal fluid (CSF)*, which contains glucose, salts, some proteins, and amino acids. It is quite different and distinct from other fluids in the body. This distinction is maintained by means of a filtration system known as the *blood-brain barrier*. It has been known for some time that vital dyes do not enter brain tissue when injected into the blood. The blood-brain barrier arises from the *atypical intercellular spaces* found in capillaries that supply blood to the central nervous system. These spaces between the cells of brain capillaries are much smaller than those found in capillaries of most other parts of the body, which probably allows filtration of molecules that would readily pass through the intercellular gaps found in other capillaries. In addition, some of the materials found in the cerebrospinal fluid are apparently obtained from a highly selective active transport system which allows specific substances to be accumulated at the expense of others.

Cerebrospinal fluid fills the lateral, the third, and the fourth ventricles of the brain and passes into the *subarachnoid space* through the *foramen of Magendie* and the lateral apertures, or the *foramina Luschka*. The fluid of the subarachnoid space, continuous over the spinal cord and brain, provides buoyancy and support for the central nervous system. Most of the fluid is produced by the capillaries of the *choroid plexus*, which is a dense network of capillaries found in the ventricles of the brain. The fluid circulates throughout the ventricles, central canal, and subarachnoid space and is ultimately filtered through capillaries of the arachnoid villi (see Figure 4–20). Blockage of the normal circulation or drainage can lead to excessive cranial pressure and sometimes a condition known as *hydrocephaly*, in which excessive pressure causes brain and cranial enlargement and ultimately, mental retardation.

The Spinal Cord

The spinal cord in mammals begins at the posterior edge of the medulla oblongata and passes through the *neural canal* of the vertebrae to about the second lumbar vertebra. A pair of spinal nerves is given off with each somite, or segment in the embryo, which amounts to a pair of nerves per vertebra in the adult. The principal functions of the spinal cord are to carry impulses both to and from the brain and to provide the *neural circuitry* for reflexes, circuitry that exit at specific levels in the cord.

The spinal cord consists of *gray* (unmyelinated) and *white* (myelinated) tissue (see Figure 4–21). The gray matter is made up of nerve cell bodies of motor neurons, unmye-

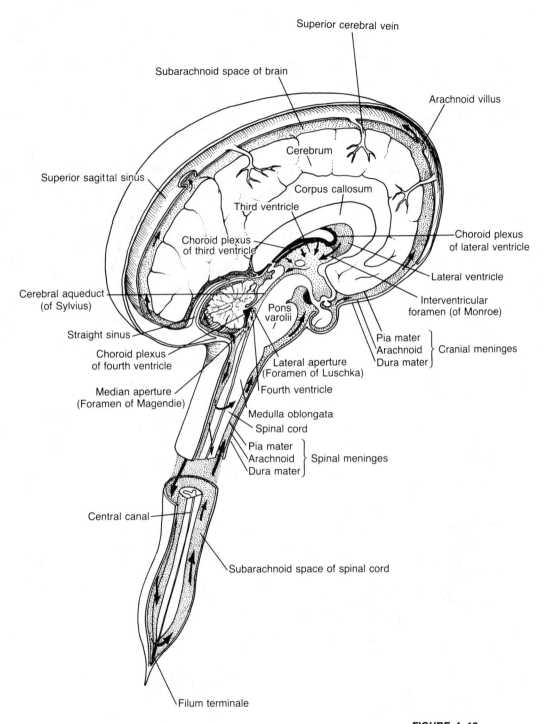

Superior cerebral vein

Subarachnoid space of brain

Arachnoid villus

Cerebrum

Superior sagittal sinus

Corpus callosum

Third ventricle

Choroid plexus
of lateral ventricle

Choroid plexus
of third ventricle

Lateral ventricle

Cerebral aqueduct
(of Sylvius)

Interventricular
foramen (of Monroe)

Pons
varolii

Straight sinus

Pia mater
Arachnoid   Cranial meninges
Dura mater

Choroid plexus
of fourth ventricle

Lateral aperture
(Foramen of Luschka)

Median aperture
(Foramen of Magendie)

Fourth ventricle

Medulla oblongata

Spinal cord

Pia mater
Arachnoid   Spinal meninges
Dura mater

Central canal

Subarachnoid space of spinal cord

Filum terminale

FIGURE 4–19
Human brain and meninges seen in sagittal section; the direction of flow of cerebrospinal fluid is indicated by arrows

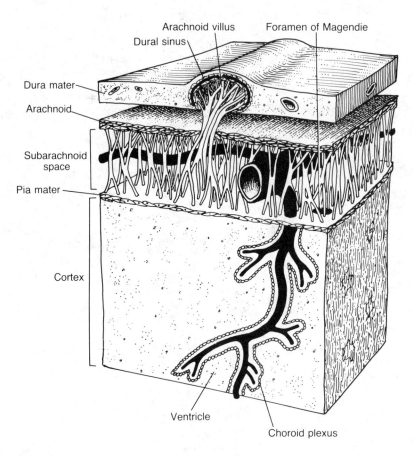

FIGURE 4–20
Section through cranium showing the subarachnoid space and the relation of the brain to the arachnoid villi

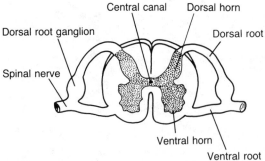

FIGURE 4–21
Cross section of the spinal cord showing gray matter (shaded areas) and white matter (light areas). Also shown are the various parts of the spinal cord, including the dorsal and ventral roots, the dorsal and ventral horns, and the central canal.

linated *internuncial cells* (or *interneurons*), and inhibitory neurons called *Renshaw cells*. It also includes a number of synapses and presynaptic terminals. The white matter is made up of myelinated axons of sensory and motor neurons, which form *tracts*, or specific bundles, that carry information to and from the brain.

In cross section the gray matter is shaped like a butterfly. At the center of Figure 4–21 is a small opening called the *central canal*, which is continuous with the ventricles of the brain and the subarachnoid space. The *horns* of the gray matter represent points of entry and exit for sensory and motor nerves.

Sensory nerves enter the gray matter through the *dorsal roots* of the spinal cord, and motor neurons exit through the *ventral roots*. Nerves of the dorsal and ventral roots communicate directly with the dorsal and ventral horns of the gray matter.

The white matter is located around the gray tissue and forms the *spinal nerves*, *spinal roots*, and *spinal tracts*. The relative amounts of white and gray matter in the

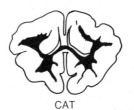

CAT

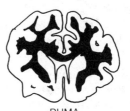

PUMA

FIGURE 4–23
Proportion of white matter (dark areas) to gray matter (light areas) in the brain of related species of different sizes. Note that the relative amount of white matter is greatest in the larger species. From C. V. A. Kappers et al, *The Comparative Anatomy of the Nervous System of Vertebrates Including Man* (New York, N.Y., 1936). Reprinted by permission of Macmillan Publishing Co.

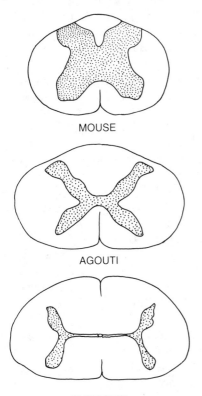

MOUSE

AGOUTI

ELEPHANT

FIGURE 4–22
When sections of the same spinal cord levels of different mammalian species are drawn nearly equal in size, the greater proportion of white matter in larger species is clear. From C. V. A. Kappers et al, *The Comparative Anatomy of the Nervous System of Vertebrates Including Man* (New York, N.Y., 1936). Reprinted by permission of Macmillan Publishing Co.

spinal cord differ vastly between mammalian species (see Figure 4–22). Larger mammals, even of related species, have a disproportionately greater amount of white as opposed to gray matter in the brain (see Figure 4–23). The functional necessity for this differential distribution of white and gray tissue is unknown.

The dorsal and ventral gray horns divide the white matter into three broad areas: (1) the *ventral white column*, (2) the *dorsal white column*, and (3) the *lateral white column*. Each column, or *funiculus*, is composed of distinct tracts. The ascending tracts contain axons of neurons which carry impulses to the brain. The descending tracts contain axons of neurons whose cell bodies are located in the brain; these axons carry information downward to various levels of the spinal cord. The fibers are isolated in the ascending and descending tracts, so the bundles are either motor or sensory.

The nerve cell bodies of sensory neurons are located in discrete regions of the dorsal roots known as *dorsal root ganglia.* The nerve cell bodies of motor neurons are located in the gray matter and provide axons that pass to the periphery through the ventral roots. Because of the direction of transmission of nerve impulses, the dorsal roots are said to be *afferent* or *sensory,* whereas the ventral roots are said to be *efferent* or *motor.* Normally, a number of presynaptic neurons synapse with a single motor neuron that is referred to as the *final common path.* Thus, a single physical action results from an integrated response in the central nervous system.

Sensory nerves form in relation to specific somites during embryonic development and are therefore associated with distinct regions of the skin known as *dermatomes* (see Figure 4–24). When receptors in a specific dermatome are stimulated, associated spinal nerves transmit the impulses to the central nervous system. The number of sensory receptors in each dermatome varies considerably, with the largest number being located in the skin of the face and hands and the fewest being found in the skin of the back.

FUNCTIONS OF THE CENTRAL NERVOUS SYSTEM

Movement

The role of the brain should be viewed as an essential element of movement in which coordinated effort is necessary. The cerebral cortex has two areas responsible for motor activity: the *premotor cortex* and the *motor cortex* (see Figure 4–10). Axons of the neurons located in the motor cortex pass through the pons and ultimately activate motor neurons of the spinal cord. These nerves, which form the *pyramidal system* in primates and the *corticospinal tracts* of other mammals, are responsible for transmitting motor activity from the cortex to the spinal cord (see Figure 4–25). Conventionally, nerve tracts are named with the origin of the nerve tract in the first half of the word and the termination of the tract as the second part of the word. For example, the corticospinal tract refers to a nerve tract that transmits impulses in the cerebral cortex to the spinal cord. Stimulation of individual neurons of the motor cortex activates individual motor neurons in the ventral root of the spinal cord. In other words, simple direct action can be brought about by the stimulation of a single nerve on the motor cortex. But even in the primates, these neurons are not able to transmit impulses to the motor neurons of the ventral horns in the comparatively rapid manner seen in other motor tracts, such as the *reticulospinal* and *vestibulospinal tracts* found in all mammals. Although small and feeble in many mammalian groups, the corticospinal tracts in carnivores approach that of the pyramidal tract in primates in effectively inducing action in the motor nerves of the ventral horn.

The premotor cortex is responsible for complex motor activity of the body. Its neurons are multipolar and can activate several neurons on the motor cortex. Such actions as driving a nail, running, or other complex movements involving motor coordination are possible through the association which exists between the premotor and the motor cortexes. The development of an integrated movement involving several muscles in the body requires the stimulation of many neurons of the motor cortex, but only a few neu-

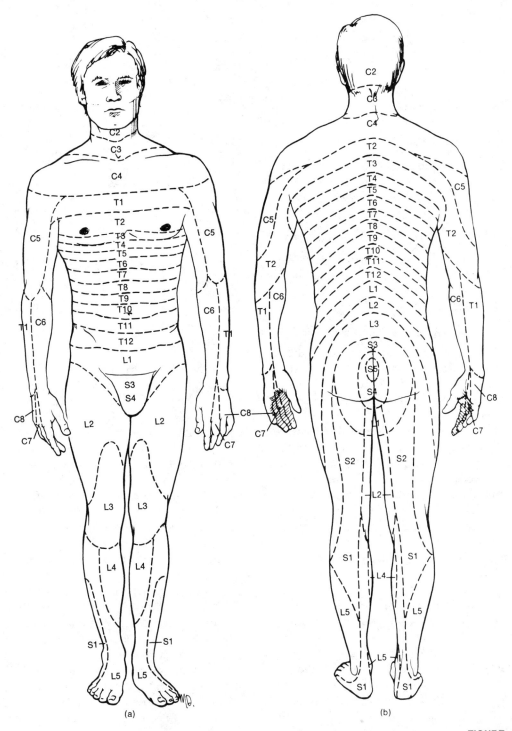

FIGURE 4–24

Distribution of spinal nerves to dermatomes in the human: (a) anterior view; (b) posterior view. Specific spinal nerves are listed for each dermatome. C refers to cervical, T to thoracic, L to lumbar, and S to sacral. Adapted from G. J. Tortora and N. P. Anagnostakos, *Principles of Anatomy and Physiology,* 3rd edition (New York, N.Y., 1981), 321, fig. 13–15. By permission of Harper and Row Publishers.

FIGURE 4–25
General distribution of tracts in the spinal cord of mammals: descending tracts (motor) are shown on the right and ascending tracts (sensory) on the left (dh, dorsal horn; ret, reticular substance; and vh, ventral horn)

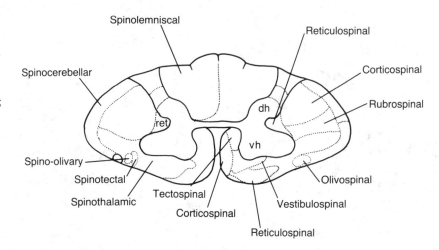

Reflex Action

rons of the premotor cortex must be active. The premotor cortex has no direct connection with the spinal motor nerves; it induces activity through stimulation of neurons of the motor cortex.

The most rapid and effective movement of the body is induced through the vestibulospinal and reticulospinal tracts. Fibers of the vestibulospinal tracts, which are parts of neurons that originate in the vestibular nucleus of the medulla, control balance and orientation of the body in space. They transmit information from the vestibular apparatuses of the ears through an integration process in the vestibular nucleus, and finally to the cerebellum. These fibers, largely excitatory, induce motor responses to regulate body orientation. The fibers of the reticulospinal tract transmit information related to a number of reflexes associated with posture and body movement. These actions are very crude and lack motor control from the motor cortex. For instance, if transection of the brain is performed leaving the lower reticular nuclei intact, the mammal might be able to walk but would completely lack purposeful locomotion.

Reflexes are the automatic responses that an organism makes to stimuli. They can occur at all levels of development of the nervous system that have the basic parts for reception of stimuli, transmission of the stimuli to the central nervous system, relay of information to the effector organ, and execution of a subsequent response. Where several neurons are involved or where several responses are evoked, sensory information is transmitted to the appropriate motor neurons by means of internuncial cells, which are located exclusively in the central nervous system.

Cordal reflexes *Cordal reflexes* are reflexes limited to the spinal cord. In such reflexes, circuits for reception and transmission of the stimulus and the action resulting from that stimulus occur without any of the information passing to the brain. The many different types of cordal reflexes are based upon the number of neurons involved, the types of receptors involved, and the part of the spinal cord affected.

The simplest type of cordal reflex is the *monosynaptic reflex*, which involves only two neurons, the *affector* and the *effector*. This kind of reflex is typified by the *stretch reflex* (see Figure 4–26). *Stretch receptors* in skeletal muscle are specialized muscle cells called *nuclear bag cells* and *nuclear chain cells*. These modified muscle cells, referred to as *intrafusal fibers*, have lost their ability to perform external work. The fibers which develop tension and perform work are termed *extrafusal fibers*. The nuclear bag cells have a clear, baglike central portion containing many nuclei and have typical *sarcomeres* at each end of the nuclear bag. Nuclear chain cells show no signs of striation or sarcomeric structure and usually do not extend over the entire length of the muscle (see Figure 4–27). Both types of intrafusal fibers contain a centrally located nerve ending called an *annulospiral ending*, which is capable of forming a generator potential when it is stretched from its normal helical configuration.

The *knee jerk reflex* often tested by clinicians is a good example of a *monosynaptic reflex*. This reflex commonly involves the sudden stretching of muscles attached to the *quadraceps tendon*, which is attached through the *patellar tendon* to the *tibia*. When the patellar tendon is tapped with a rubber mallet, intrafusal fibers in the group of muscles known as the *quadraceps* are stretched, which distends the annulospiral endings, increasing sodium ion permeability,

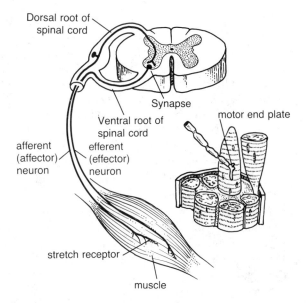

FIGURE 4–26
Stretch reflex in mammals. Note that there are only two neurons and one synapse.

which leads to generation of action potentials that are sent back to the spinal cord through afferent fibers of the *sciatic nerve*. In the spinal cord, afferent neurons synapse with motor neurons, which carry impulses back to the extrafusal fibers. Stimulation of the extrafusal fibers causes them to contract and results in the extension of the limb.

The contactile portions at either end of the nuclear bag cells provide an interesting

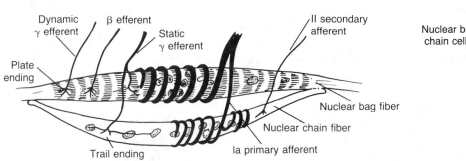

FIGURE 4–27
Nuclear bag cells and nuclear chain cells in somatic muscle

example of *threshold modification*. When these portions of the cell are stimulated by input from the *gamma efferent fibers* that innervate them, internal tension is developed in the nuclear bag, bringing the annulospiral ending toward threshold. In this way the *reflex time*, or the time elapsed between stimuli and muscle contraction, is reduced because the latent period of stimulation of the annulospiral ending is reduced. In addition, the minimum stimulus necessary to evoke the reflex is reduced.

Another type of receptor ending found in the nuclear chain cells is called a *flower spray ending* because of its peculiar shape. Flower spray endings are innervated by *Group II sensory fibers* instead of *Group Ia afferent fibers*, which innervate annulospiral endings. The annulospiral endings respond rapidly, and the time required for them to regain their resting potential is also rapid. This on-and-off display is called a *phasic response*. The flower spray endings, however, give rise to a *tonic response;* that is, they develop a generator potential slowly. The tonic response is then maintained for a relatively long period of time. For more information on fiber types see chapter 3, The Neuron.

Cordal reflexes may involve several neurons at once and involve more than one side of the spinal cord. A reflex that involves several nerves is termed a *polysynaptic reflex,* by nature a more complex response than the monosynaptic responses seen in the stretch reflexes. When action occurs on the same side of the spinal cord on which the stimulus arose, the reflex is said to occur on the *ipsilateral* side; when action occurs on the side of the spinal cord opposite to the side on which the stimulus arose, the reflex is said to occur on the *contralateral side*. Reflexes can also involve the action of several muscles, or effectors, which may have a *synergistic effect*

in some cases and an *antagonistic effect* in others. Reflexes involving movement are usually carried out after inhibition of motor neurons leading to *antagonistic muscles,* muscles that contract in opposition to the action expressed in a particular reflex. In the mammals, and in other vertebrates as well, muscles are not inhibited directly by inhibitory neurons. Inhibition always occurs in the central nervous system and results in a lack of activity in appropriate effector neurons. Therefore, the muscles that those neurons innervate do not contract.

The coordinated movement of walking is an example of a polysynaptic reflex which involves both sides of the spinal cord. Such involvement is typical of a *crossed extensor reflex,* in which one limb is extended while another is flexed (see Figure 4–28). In such a reflex, antagonistic action for both extension and flexion is inhibited, but corresponding muscles on each side of the body show opposing action. For instance, during flexion the appropriate muscles must be contracted while their antagonistic muscles are relaxed (inhibited) and stretched. In the extension of a limb, the opposite effect is seen: the flexors are stretched while the extensors are contracted.

Not all reflexes involve the contralateral side at the same level of the spinal cord. Four-legged animals, or *quadrupeds,* develop very complex limb rhythms involving different portions of the spinal cord that control action in both front and hind legs. Such a reflex in quadrupeds involves both the sacral and thoracic regions of the spinal cord rather than a single level of the cord, as seen in monosynaptic reflexes.

Nerve-hormone reflexes Some reflexes involve the integration of nerves and hormones in order to reach completion. The

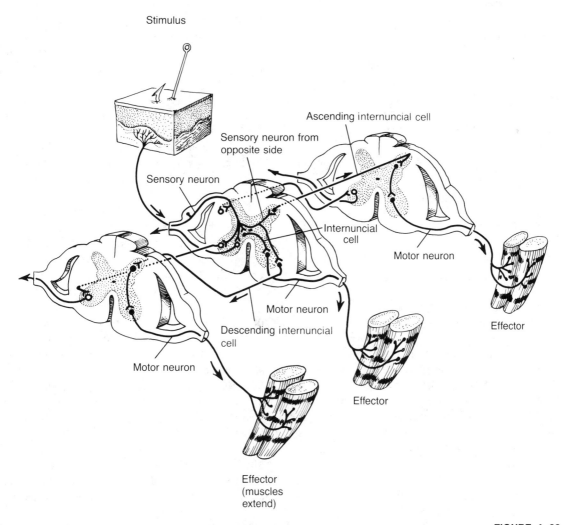

FIGURE 4–28

Crossed extensor reflex. Note that pain on one side of the body can cause action in extensor muscles on the contralateral side at more than one level of the spinal cord.

milk-ejection reflex of mammals is an example of this type of reflex. *Oxytocin*, a hormone released by the posterior *pituitary*, enhances contraction of smooth muscle and causes milk ejection in lactating females. During suckling, the young stimulates pressure receptors in the mother's nipples, inducing action potentials in sensory nerves in her teats. The action potentials thus generated are transmitted to her hypothalamus and cause oxytocin secretion by the posterior pituitary. After release, oxytocin circulates through the blood and affects smooth muscles in the mammary glands, causing them to eject milk.

This reflex is easily demonstrated, since the motor fibers to the mammary glands can be severed and milk ejection can still be induced with suckling. On the other hand, if all sensory neurons are severed, this reflex fails to occur. If the sensory nerves to only some of the teats are severed, milk ejection occurs from all of the teats because of the stimulation of one of the intact teats. In some species the sight or cry of the young provides adequate stimulation for oxytocin release and subsequent milk ejection. Thus, oxytocin release can be activated through sensory modulation other than pressure receptors in the teats.

Learning and Related Phenomena

The central nervous system has evolved as an area in which sensory input can be integrated and appropriate motor responses can be evoked by adding responses to new stimuli. Analogous to the central nervous system is a desk calculator that automatically adds numbers to give their sum to the operator. Additional circuitry could be developed in the calculator that would not only add the numbers but might also automatically divide by 100 to give percent. The calculator has circuitry which will give an automatic response for particular input. No matter how large the calculator, it will always do the same thing as a result of its fixed electrical circuitry. Similarly, in mammals fixed pathways are innate and are therefore not a part of the learning process. But mammals also have programmable pathways whose functions can be altered as a result of experience.

Mammals are in many cases born with the capacity to carry out certain innate behavior patterns. In other words, they react to the external world in a manner identical to the cal-culator example. They have specific acts which are carried out when the correct stimuli (key punches) are given. For example, in marsupials, which are born at a very undeveloped stage, the newborn starts climbing immediately towards its mother's pouch, guided by what is often referred to as an *instinct*, an innate behavioral pattern. The newborn marsupial only needs the stimulus of birth to go directly toward its mother's pouch and attach itself to one of her teats.

Many reflexes and instincts are difficult to modify through training because they occur infrequently, and change may be impossible because they are based upon a very rigid set of genetically programmed instructions. For example, the pouch-seeking reflex of newborn marsupials occurs only once in the life of the animal and is therefore practically unalterable. But when reflexes and innate behavior patterns are frequently repeated, the stimulus that initiates the reflex can be *conditioned* experimentally to a completely different stimulus. For instance, the Russian Pavlov, who worked with dogs, was able to substitute the sound of a bell for the sight or smell of food in order to evoke salivation. This is widely heralded as the first documented evidence of a *conditioned reflex*. The animals used in the experiment were fed at a particular time each day, and salivation was a regular response to the sight or smell of food. Pavlov rang the bell at each feeding, and the dogs began to associate the sound of the bell with food. Eventually the animals would salivate whenever the stimulus was given, regardless of the presence or absence of food. Pavlov continued to study reflexes associated with digestion and was able to show that the reflex controlling the secretion of hydrochloric acid by the mucosa of the stomach could also be conditioned. Indeed, naturally conditioned reflexes play a large role in our daily lives and are essential for survival in most mammals.

Pavlov taught his dogs to accept a stimulus not normally associated with the pertinent reward (i.e., the sound of the bell was substituted for the sight and smell of food). This is, indeed, a primitive type of *learning*. Perhaps learning can be defined as the ability to recognize and associate stimuli which are not innately programmed. In order for such recognition to occur again, it must somehow be retained. Therefore, *memory* must play a definite role in a complex learning system in which more than one set of circumstances or repetitions is involved. In other words, when an animal is conditioned, as in the experiments of Pavlov, the animal must retain its response. If an animal could develop the same response to the flash of light or the sound of a whistle as to the ring a bell, it would demonstrate a greater degree of complexity in its learning ability, since more stimuli are recognized. The fewer the number of trials necessary before a stimulus becomes conditioned, the faster will be the learning process.

Memory To continue the desk calculator analogy, electrical circuitry could also be developed for the storing of numbers for later display. This is an illustration of the memory of specific input. The calculator would be made even more complex by developing circuitry to store negative numbers separately from positive numbers. Note that the calculator has no ability to learn but merely has the ability to store numbers. In the same way, physiology students store the names and structures of the compounds which constitute the Krebs cycle.

A number of experiments have provided insight into the mechanism of the memory process. For instance, laboratory mammals develop thicker cerebral cortexes and a higher ratio of RNA to DNA when raised in a more complex, or *enriched*, environment. This would indicate that certain changes occur in the brains of mammals when information is received and stored. Furthermore, brain weight, as well as such cellular components as RNA and DNA, have been found to increase when mammals are trained or raised in an enriched environment. Far too little data have been collected, however, to make generalizations from rodents to humans.

Emotions and Behavior

Mammals show many innate activities which are quite complex and involve many neurons and several organ systems. These activities, though for the most part poorly understood, are too complex and too involved to be considered simple reflexes. We call these activities *emotions* in humans. Emotions often are displayed through precise actions, allowing one to refer to their expression as *behavior*. In order to establish objectivity when dealing with other animals, the outward signs of emotions and drives are referred to as behavior. In other words, behaviors are actions that an animal takes, and emotions and drives are internal feelings that an animal may have. Many human behavior patterns are grouped by terms defined, for the sake of simplicity, as emotions or drives. From an analytical standpoint, only the expression of such patterns can be measured quantitatively.

The allocortex of the primitive brain contains a number of nuclei or cell groups which constitute the limbic system. These are the *medial* and *lateral olfactory stria,* the *stria medullaris,* the *olfactory tubercle,* the *diagonal band of Broca,* the *septum anterior nucleus of the thalamus,* the *mammillary body,* the *interpeduncular nucleus,* the *habenula,* and the *medial forebrain bundle* (see Figure 4–29). Originating within these nuclei are the emotions of humans and many of the behavior patterns of other mammals. There are few connections between the neocortex and the limbic nuclei, making it difficult for emotions to be controlled by the conscious mind. Even if outward behavior patterns are restricted, the neurological activities which induce them may linger for long periods of time.

Within the limbic system originate all of the basic drives, such as reproduction, fear, hunger, and so on. The physiological basis of behavior has been established through the manipulation of nuclei within the limbic system in both humans and other animals. There follows a discussion of a few general behavior patterns; the discussion in no way is intended to be an exhaustive treatment of these behavior patterns.

Reproductive behavior In most mammals except higher primates, the basic behavioral patterns of reproduction are turned off and on through the natural change of some environmental variable, such as *photoperiod.* Such correlation allows for the development of a precise breeding period and an ideal time of birth, insuring a better chance for the survival of the young. The time of breeding readiness is usually referred to as the *rut period* in males and the *heat period* in females. The mechanisms whereby the rut and heat periods are initiated will be discussed in a

FIGURE 4–29
Nuclei of the allocortex that constitute the limbic system of mammals (M str, medial olfactory stria; L str, lateral olfactory stria; Str med, stria medullaris; Tub, olfactory tubercle; DB, diagonal band of Broca; Sep, septum; AT, anterior nucleus of the thalamus; M, mammillary body; H, habenula; IP, interpeduncular nucleus; MFB, medial forebrain bundle). Reprinted by permission of Elsevier Science Publishing Co., Inc., from Psychosomatic Disease and the Visceral Brain, by P. D. MacLean, *J. Psychosom. Med.,* 11:338. Copyright 1949 by the American Psychosomatic Society, Inc.

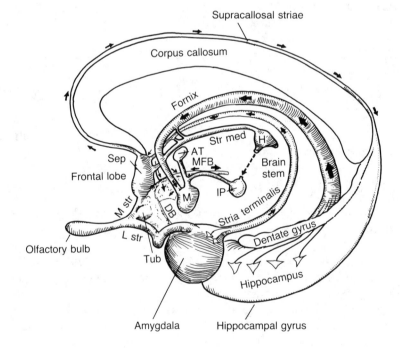

later chapter. The lack of a distinct heat or rut period in higher primates, a phenomenon most pronounced in humans, is of particular interest because of its significant evolutionary implications.

The manifestations of sexual behavior in both male and female mammals, except humans, is dependent upon the presence of the hormones *estrogen* or *testosterone*, respectively. Estrogen and testosterone, however, are said to increase libido in human males and females, and it has been observed that homosexual behavior in humans is intensified by the injection of either hormone into homosexuals.

In the male, bilateral *limbic lesions* in the *piriform cortex* overlying the *amygdala* (parts of the mammalian limbic system) intensify sexual activity. From that finding, it could be concluded that the neurological source of male sexual behavior is the amygdala and that inhibition of this behavior is evoked by the stimulation of the piriform cortex. When inhibitions have been blocked by appropriate lesions, males of one mammalian species have been known to copulate with females of other species and to attempt to copulate with inanimate objects. The quantity of testosterone available to the amygdala after bilateral piriform cortex ablation does not seem to be important, though a total absence of testosterone causes the behavior to cease.

The hypothalamus, also known to be active in the control of sexual behavior patterns in male mammals, is quite responsive to local testosterone implants. Anterior hypothalamic implants of testosterone restore normal sexual behavior in castrated rats, and ablation of the anterior hypothalamus abolishes sexual behavior entirely in some species.

In the female, the amygdala or surrounding structures do not seem to play an important part in sexual behavior but selective ablation of anterior hypothalamic areas destroys behavioral heat. The anterior hypothalamus is also sensitive to *sex steroids* (steroids that promote sexual activity), and implantation of testosterone or estrogen induces an increase in female sexual behavior.

Antagonistic behavior   Antagonistic behavior in mammals is usually associated with the defense of territory, food, or a mate. Such behavior is considered by some to be associated with the same physiological mechanism as is fear. The relationship of fear to rage stems from observation of the behavioral options available when an animal is attacked: an animal either becomes enraged or it attempts to flee. The two behavioral responses may indeed have similar physiological mechanisms, but the display of either under controlled circumstances does not necessarily mean that they have the same neurological origin.

Antagonistic behavior can be evoked by minor stimuli in *decorticate mammals*, or mammals whose cerebral cortex has been removed, a response which indicates that in the intact animal there is some control over such behavior by the cerebral cortex. However, lesions of the *ventromedial hypothalamic nuclei* also induce rage in intact animals, and *bilateral ablation* (destruction) of the amygdala erases all ability to express antagonistic behavior. Antagonistic response due to amygdaloid stimulation is usually abolished by lesions of the lateral hypothalamus or rostral midbrain.

In several species, antagonistic behavior is not apparently associated with any type of defense, such as protection of territory, food, or a mate. In these mammals antagonistic behavior requires little provocation other than the presence of another member of the same species, or in some cases only the presence of another mammal of any species. Typical examples of this phenomenon can be observed in the *American pit bull terrier* and the *fighting cattle* of Latin American countries and Spain. In such animals neither sex needs provocation to fight; fighting behavior is displayed in both males and females. In fighting cattle, electrical stimulation of the amygdala interrupts antagonistic behavior, and continued stimulation is said to cause the animals to become relatively tame. The wolverine, an undomesticated species, exhibits similar antagonistic behavior when kept in captivity.

Antagonistic behavior, as well as sexual behavior, can usually be modified by the sex steroids. In many species of rodents and ungulates, males castrated before sexual maturity do not show antagonistic behavior without a great deal of provocation. Males castrated after sexual maturity usually lose some aggressive tendencies, but they regain them with testosterone supplementation.

Pleasure (Motivation) When certain parts of the human brain are electrically stimulated, a sensation of "pleasure" or relaxation is felt. This is termed *motivation* in lower animals because it is unknown if they sense pleasure as humans know it. Experiments in the human were preceded by experiments in other mammals, in which the animal was allowed to electroschock certain parts of the brain at will. When the stimulating electrodes are placed in certain areas (*tegmentum, posterior hypothalamus, dorsal midbrain*, and *entorhinal cortex*), laboratory rats who are able to evoke the electroshock stimulus by pressing a movable bar inside the cage press that bar from 5,000 to 12,000 times per hour. Monkeys have been known to evoke the same stimulus 17,000 or more times per hour. The intensity of the stimulus seems to make little difference in the rate of repetition: even when the electrical potential is strong enough to stun the experimental animal, it will usually repeat the stimulus.

Visceral Functions Controlled by the Central Nervous System

Hunger The *hunger response* can be evoked in the absence of one or more dietary factors. Some evidence points to the reduction of *plasma glucose content* (the so-called *glucostatic hypothesis*) or to the reduction of *plasma lipid content* (the so-called *lipostatic hypothesis*) as effectors of the hunger response. It seems certain that some feedback mechanisms must function in regulating the appetite, since many mammals regulate food intake and thus control body weight at a fairly precise level. After being force-fed to induce excessive weight gains, animals will reduce food intake when returned to free-choice feeding regimens. Food intake usually plateaus after normal body weight is attained. Likewise, after starvation animals will increase food intake until normal body weight is regained. In both cases, poststarvation and post-force-feeding, plasma glucose and plasma lipid levels sometimes are maintained at the usual homeostatic levels. Such maintenance indicates that hypotheses other than the glucostatic or lipostatic hypotheses must be considered in explaining the hunger response.

The neurological factors affecting appetite can be located in at least two areas of the brain, the hypothalamus and the limbic system. Parts of the hypothalamus affect appetite in opposing fashions: the stimulation of the *feeding center* of the lateral hypothalamus causes increased appetite, and the stimulation of the *satiety center* of the *ventromedial nuclei* causes cessation of the feeding behavior (see Figure 4–30). Destruction of the satiety center while leaving the feeding center intact induces *hyperphagia*, or voracious appetite. Likewise, destruction of the feeding center while leaving other parts of the limbic system unaltered induces *anorexia*, or loss of appetite. In some experimental animals it has been shown that *lower blood sugar* reduces the activity of the satiety center and causes an increase in feeding. The satiety center is one of the few neurological regions dependent upon the hormone *insulin* for glucose utilization, which explains the increased appetite of diabetics despite their high level of blood sugar.

Hunger can also be associated with part of the limbic system. When the amygdala is lesioned, moderate hyperphagia can be produced. Also, animals with amygdaloid lesions become *omniphagic;* that is, they will eat almost anything. Hunger, when induced in this way, is not associated with a specific craving or an appetite for specific foods.

Thirst An increase in *plasma osmotic concentration*, whether from dehydration or from intake of osmotically active substances, is known to increase the desire for liquids. When tonicity of the blood plasma becomes elevated, *osmoreceptors* in the hypothalamus are stimulated and a desire for liquids occurs. The location of the center for this sensation appears to differ among species. In the rat osmoreceptors are found in the lateral hypothalamus, whereas in the dog and goat osmoreceptors are found in the dorsal hypothalamus and are located posteriorly to the paraventricular nucleus. The role of these areas in the sensation of thirst has been substantiated by ablation and direct-stimulation experiments.

Receptors on the surface of the lips and the lining of the mouth can also be involved with thirst. The thirst response can sometimes be

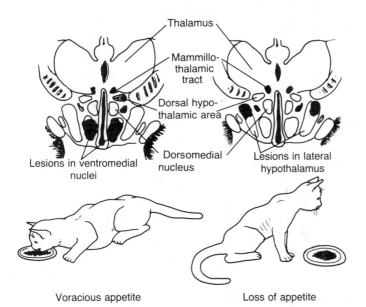

Thalamus

Mammillo-thalamic tract

Dorsal hypo-thalamic area

Dorsomedial nucleus

Lesions in ventromedial nuclei

Lesions in lateral hypothalamus

Voracious appetite

Loss of appetite

FIGURE 4–30

Effect of lesions in the ventromedial nuclei and the lateral hypothalamus on appetite. Reproduced, with permission, from Ganong, WF: *Review of Medical Physiology,* 9th ed. Copyright 1979 by Lange Medical Publications, Los Altos, California.

reduced in the human by wetting the inside of the mouth. Certain animals can determine in some way the amount of water necessary for restoring blood plasma tonicity without consuming an excessive amount. For instance, the camel, which can become so severely dehydrated that the volume of extracellular fluid is reduced, stops water consumption when the amount of water necessary to reestablish the usual tonicity of the blood plasma has been taken into the stomach. But in some animals, the consumption of water after dehydration can be very destructive; the horse is a notable example. After dehydration, horses have been known to consume water until the stomach ruptures. In less severe cases of overconsumption of water, the horse founders, or becomes lame. Frequently, the crippling of the horse is due to passive congestion of blood in the hoof caused by gastroenteritis or possibly excessive histamine release. Such congestion allows separation of the lamina of the hoof wall from the internal lamina, a condition called *laminitis*. When this occurs, the entire weight supported by the limb may be applied to the sole of the hoof rather than to the hoof wall. For more information on the horse hoof, see chapter 11, The Heart as a Pump.

SLEEP AND ACTIVITY CYCLES IN MAMMALS

The structural system required to maintain the sleep-wake cycle in mammals is the *reticular activating system (RAS)*. But the actual decrease in the neural activity associated with sleep may be due to the accumulation during the wakeful hours of a substance in the brain which reduces RAS activity and thus causes sleep to occur. In the early 1900s, a French scientist, Piéron, extracted

the cerebrospinal fluid from sleep-deprived goats. He found that the extracted fluid induced sleep when injected into the brains of animals that had previously received adequate sleep. Piéron's experiments were quite traumatic to the animal, since no anesthetics were used. Little notice was made of his data until 1939, when the experiments were repeated in dogs by Schendorf and Ivy. Results similar to Piéron's were obtained. But Schendorf and Ivy were not satisfied with their experiments since, in addition to sleep induction, the experimental animals showed other physiological changes not normally associated with sleep. The experiments were repeated in the 1960s by Pappenheimer and his associates at the Harvard Medical School with more reliable results, owing to the stable positioning of an indwelling catheter placed in the brain of goats (see Figure 4–31). In Pappenheimer's experiments it was possible to deprive the goats of sleep and extract cerebrospinal fluid with a minimum of trauma. Likewise, when the fluid was injected into other goats or even rats, a profound sleep was induced which was equivalent to the natural sleep seen in other individuals. Controls, which were injected with saline, did not show a similar response. Later attempts to purify the sleep-inducing factor were successful in showing that the substance was probably a protein whose molecular weight was between 350 and 500. This factor was able to induce sleep in experimental animals; its protein nature was confirmed when its potency was destroyed by means of *proteolytic enzymes*.

It would appear, then, that the apparatus for the sleep-wake state is provided by the RAS. The condition of sleep is brought about by means of a "tranquilizing" substance, which accumulates in the brain and cerebrospinal fluid during the awake periods and

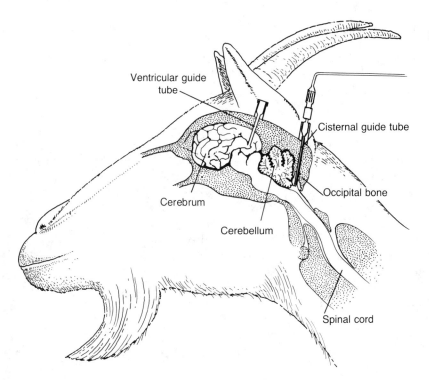

Ventricular guide
tube

Cisternal guide tube

Cerebrum

Occipital bone

Cerebellum

Spinal cord

represents another example of neural-hor-
monal integration in the central nervous system. When the animal is awake, the sleep-inducing substance continues to accumulate,
eventually reaching a critical level that induces sleep. In animals forced to stay awake
for abnormal periods of time, an excessive
amount of the sleep-inducing substance was
formed, producing a pronounced deep sleep.
The depth of sleep is confirmed by analysis
of brain waves in normal sleep and the sleep
of sleep-induced individuals.

SOME CLINICAL ABNORMALITIES OF THE CENTRAL NERVOUS SYSTEM

Many disorders associated with the central
nervous system have been known since antiquity. In many cases, a cure has not been
found; in some cases, even the causes remain
unknown. The following is a partial list of
some of the afflictions of the central nervous
system.

Cerebral Palsy

This condition has several causes, each of
which results in damage to specific portions
of the brain. Among the causes are *radiation*
during fetal life, *oxygen starvation* during
birth, and *hydrocephaly* during infancy. All of
these causes are associated with damage to
the cells of the cerebral cortex, the basal ganglia, or the cerebellum and are frequently
found to be related to malfunctions in the
three areas. Since cerebral palsy results from
loss of particular cells or parts of the brain,
damage is considered to be irreversible. Victims of this condition show a variety of

symptoms, so the disease is often difficult to diagnose in less severe cases. Usually, the individual will show loss of motor function, erratic motor function, mental retardation, blindness, or loss of hearing.

Parkinsonism

Parkinson's disease is marked by *hypokinesis*, *tremor*, and muscular rigidity. This condition, which results from the degeneration of the basal ganglia, was a common side effect of the influenza rampant during World War I. It normally strikes elderly people or those who receive treatment with the *phenthiozine group* of tranquilizer drugs. The symptoms of this disease can be alleviated by the use of *L-dopa*, which is able to pass the blood-brain barrier. In the brain L-dopa is converted to *dopamine*, which is deficient in individuals with Parkinsonism.

Multiple Sclerosis

This condition is associated with progressive degeneration of the myelin sheaths which surround the neurons of the central nervous system. *Plaques*, which remain after the destruction of the myelin sheaths, interfere with transmission of action potentials in the central nervous system. The cause or causes of this disease are unknown, though a *viral agent* is suspected. Multiple sclerosis normally strikes individuals between the ages of twenty and forty and most often occurs in countries with cool to moderate climates. The disease generally progresses in stages. It can show intermittent bouts of severe symptoms separated by periods of remission.

The symptoms of multiple sclerosis, which vary according to the portion of the central nervous system that is damaged, usually begin with a loss of sensory function followed by loss of muscular contractility. The

disease usually progresses over a period of seven to thirty years. Death most often ensues from a secondary destruction of the kidneys, which results from prolonged bladder infections.

Epilepsy

This disease of the central nervous system is characterized by *hyperexcitability* of the neurons. The symptoms may involve motor, sensory, and psychological malfunctions, depending upon which portion of the brain is involved. Massive discharge of neurons throughout the brain results in *grand mal seizures*, which are characterized by spasmodic contraction of skeletal muscles and loss of consciousness. Rather small areas of the brain are associated with *petit mal seizures*, which are associated with slow brain wave patterns and normally last for only a few seconds. Individuals with *petit mal epilepsy* generally do not show muscular seizures; they may appear to be daydreaming. Epilepsy, which has a number of causes, may exist for only a short period in the life of the individual. Causes include head injuries and such childhood diseases as mumps or whooping cough. There may be no obvious external induction of this disease.

SUMMARY

The mammalian brain has evolved from three basic parts of the brain of primitive vertebrates (i.e., the prosencephalon, the mesencephalon, and the rhombencephalon). The most recent elaboration has been the neocortex, which arose from the allocortex and shows its greatest development in the brain of primates. A significant evolutionary change seen in mammals has been the constant increase in brain size while body size decreased or remained the same. Many functions of the spinal cord have shifted to the brain in higher mammals and are exemplary of increased encephalization, or influence of the brain over other parts of the nervous system.

The mammalian brain is composed of several discrete structural units. The most obvious portion of the brain is the cerebrum (neocortex) which is highly developed in the higher primates and cetaceans. Portions of the cerebrum are devoted to movement (motor and premotor cortexes) and sensory reception (sensory, visual, and auditory cortexes). The basal ganglia, which control movement in the more primitive brains of birds and reptiles, are also present in mammals and are associated with movement and coordination. Their exact role in movement has not been clearly demonstrated.

The diencephalon consists of the epithalamus, thalamus (or dorsal thalamus), ventral thalamus (or subthalamus), and hypothalamus. Each has a separate but more primitive function than the derivatives of the telencephalon. Such functions as autonomic control and the production of releasing hormones and hormones of the posterior pituitary are associated with these portions of the brain.

The pineal gland has been poorly understood for many centuries. Its role in some vertebrate classes is definitely secretory but its function in the mammals is still not clear. In some mammals it regulates reproductive and activity cycles, and it may be important in temperature acclimation.

The midbrain, or mesencephalon, of mammals provides fiber tracts between the receptors of the retina and inner ear with other parts of the nervous system. Also, several nuclei of the cranial nerves are located here.

The cerebellum is derived from the hindbrain, or rhombencephalon. It functions in muscle coordination and makes integrated movement possible through analysis of both sensory and motor input. The cerebellum has both afferent and efferent neural connections with the motor cortex and is able to monitor muscular action as it occurs. Activity of the muscles is constantly compared to the motor stimuli from the cortex. The cerebellum tunes and controls the motor stimuli of the cortex based upon the comparative motor and sensory information available.

The brainstem, or medulla oblongata, is also derived from the rhombencephalon and contains a number of sensory relay centers. It also contains motor tracts from the cortex as well as the nuclei of origin of a number of motor cranial nerves. Relay centers for afferent nuclei occur on either side of the medulla in the olives. Each center relays information from the periphery to the cerebellum.

The pons is located on the ventral side of the medulla. It contains the nuclei of origin of some of the cranial nerves and contains nuclei which are associated with modification of the activities of several visceral organs.

The cranial nerves are analagous in derivation to the spinal nerves. But some specialization has occurred in the cranial nerves which has lead to purely sensory and purely motor nerves. Some cranial nerves, such as the vagus nerve, have mixed functions (both sensory and motor) and are associated with the function of a number of visceral organs.

The spinal cord lies within the neural canal of the vertebrae and is located between the first cervical vertebra and the second lumbar vertebra. It contains both gray and white matter and gives rise to a pair of spinal nerves for each vertebra. It contains all of the elements for reflexes and also contains sensory and motor tracts through which the brain and somatic muscular system communicate.

The central nervous system is enclosed and protected by three layers or meninges. The outer layer, or dura mater, provides protection and is anchored to the cranium and neural canal of the vertebrae. It covers the arachnoid, which is richly supplied with blood vessels and functions in removal of metabolic wastes and fluid from the cerebrospinal fluid (CSF). The innermost layer, or pia mater, covers the central nervous system tightly. It separates the cerebrospinal fluid from any direct contact with the neurons of the brain and spinal cord.

The cerebrospinal fluid supplies support for the central nervous system. It completely surrounds the brain and spinal cord and fills the spinal canal and ventricles of the brain. It is a distinct fluid and is isolated from the blood by means of the blood-brain barrier.

The part of the cerebral cortex devoted exclusively to movement is called the motor cortex. Other portions of the cerebral cortex receive sensory information; still others primarily remain as association areas. The motor and sensory areas of the cortex are integrated through the cerebellum, which cooperates to provide smooth, fluid movements constantly monitored for accuracy.

Neural responses are connected to sensory input through reflex actions. Reflexes can be specific and limited to only two neurons, as seen in the stretch or monosynaptic reflex, or they can be complex and involve a plethora of neurons all affecting one action by the organism, as seen in a polysynaptic reflex. Reflexes can be conditioned; that is, they can be initiated by an unrelated stimulus that is artificially associated with the usual or unconditioned stimulus. Such modification leads to a primitive form of learning.

In addition to simple cause and effect responses, mammals show complex activities of the central nervous system which are described as specific behavior patterns, or emotions. Emotion is a term that has explicit meaning in humans and can be related to other mammals through their behavior. Behavior is the expression of activity of the limbic system, which gives rise to emotions in humans. The limbic system is composed of specific nuclei within the allocortex. Some aspects of behavior modification have been brought about through chemical and physical manipulation of these brain centers.

Learning is a function of the cerebral cortex and can be defined as the ability to form associations among sensory inputs and to later apply these associations to different sets of circumstances. Such application implies an awareness and the ability to remember previous experiences. Memory, one of the principal functions of the central nervous system, has been correlated with increased RNA to DNA ratios in the cortex.

The sleep-wake cycle of mammals is controlled by the reticular activating system (RAS). This system of both afferent and efferent neurons is spread throughout the brain and upper portion of the spinal cord. It is essential for maintaining attention and concentration as well as the state of wakefulness. The sleep-wake cycle is affected by a protein which accumulates in the cerebrospinal fluid when the animal is awake. This substance, when injected into the cerebrospinal fluid of experimental animals, induces sleep.

Visceral functions such as hunger and thirst are also controlled by parts of the central nervous system. Many abnormalities of function of the nervous system have been discussed. Some of them, with possible treatments, are mentioned here.

5

THE AUTONOMIC
NERVOUS SYSTEM

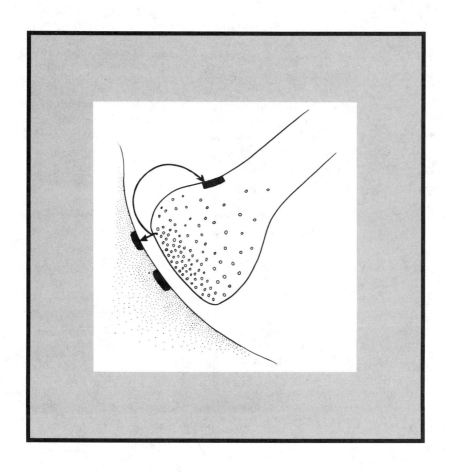

*T*he autonomic (*or* visceral*)* nervous system *probably evolved as a mechanism to coordinate the activities of specific visceral organs. As its name implies, the autonomic nervous system carries out numerous reflexes which are completely isolated from conscious control. It is present in very primitive chordates, such as amphioxi, and probably evolved as early or earlier than the central nervous system.*

The autonomic nervous system is an anatomical unit distinct from the somatic nervous system. *From a pharmacological perspective, the autonomic nervous system has more than one type of receptor, whereas the somatic nervous system has only acetylcholine at the motor end plates. In addition to possessing multiple receptors, the autonomic nervous system releases several chemically distinct activator substances, though only one type of substance is released from a single presynaptic neuron. The control of the system originates in the hypothalamus of the brain, and the system's effector neurons pass to the periphery of the body by way of the cranial nerves and the ventral horns of the spinal cord. The autonomic nervous system is unique because it has nerve cell bodies located outside of the central nervous system, either in* nerve plexi *or in the effector organs themselves.*

Two discrete divisions, or branches, of the autonomic nervous system, based upon structure, function, and pharmacology, are found in mammals: the sympathetic nervous system *and the* parasympathetic nervous system. *The two branches usually oppose each other in their functions. The sympathetic branch is normally responsible for preparing the animal for increased physical activity, also known as the* fight or flight response, *a term proposed by Walter Cannon in the early 1900s. The parasympathetic branch is more often associated with evoking vegetative or ruminative responses during an organism's quiescent period, when stressful or threatening situations are not imminent.*

STRUCTURE

The two branches of the autonomic nervous system exit the brain and spinal cord through distinct anatomical regions and differ remarkably in the lengths of their respective postsynaptic neurons. *Presynaptic sympathetic nerves* exit the spinal cord through *thoracic* and *lumbar motor nerves* and enter the *paravertebral sympathetic ganglia* through the *white ramus communicans* (see Figure 5–1). These paravertebral sympathetic ganglia lie on each side of the spinal cord in the thoracic and lumbar regions. Axons of the sympathetic ganglia may pass directly to the viscera, or they may reenter the spinal nerve through the *gray ramus communicans*.

STRUCTURE

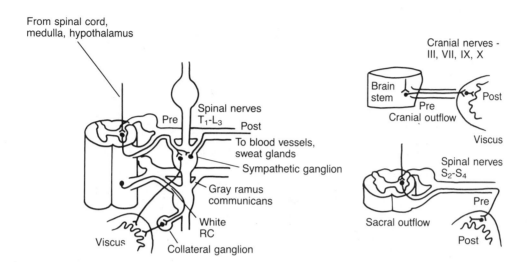

SYMPATHETIC DIVISION   PARASYMPATHETIC DIVISION

FIGURE 5–1
Relationship of the autonomic nervous system to the central nervous system (Pre, pre-ganglionic neuron; Post, postganglionic neuron; RC, ramus communicans; T, L, S re-fer to site of origin of spinal nerves, and thus T designates thoracic spinal nerve, L designates lumbar spinal nerve, and S designates sacral spinal nerve). Reproduced, with permission, from Ganong, WF: *Review of Medical Physiology*, 9th ed. Copyright 1979 by Lange Medical Publications, Los Altos, California.

Sympathetic neurons which reenter the spinal nerves synapse with effectors in the skin and blood vessels of the somatic mus-cles. Some presynaptic sympathetic fibers pass through the paravertebral ganglia and synapse with postsynaptic neurons in one of several *collateral ganglia*. Where the collateral ganglia are located near the viscera, the post-synaptic neurons are noticeably shorter than those which originate in the paravertebral sympathetic ganglia and directly innervate the visceral organs. A special system of short postsynaptic neurons of the sympathetic nervous system lies entirely within the *uter-ine myometrium.* In all other cases of the sympathetic branch, the synapse lies outside of the organ of innervation, either in a para-vertebral ganglion or in one of the collateral ganglia.

Effector neurons of the parasympathetic nervous system exit the central nervous sys-tem through the cranial nerves and the ven-tral roots of the sacral nerves (see Figure 5–2). Specifically, these nerves are cranial nerves III, VII, IX, and X and spinal nerves S_2, S_3, and S_4. The presynaptic nerves of the par-asympathetic branch are much longer than the postsynaptic neurons. Unlike the sympa-thetic branch, all postsynaptic neurons of the parasympathetic branch are located in the

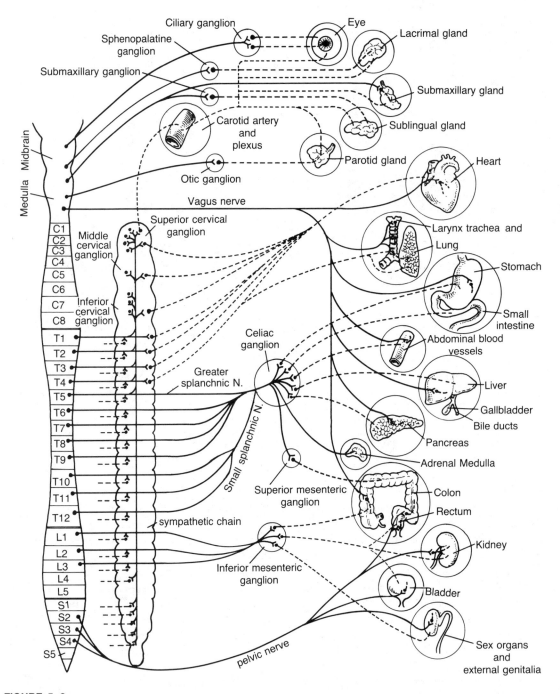

FIGURE 5–2
Diagram of the efferent autonomic pathways and organs innervated. Note comparative lengths of the pre- and postganglionic neurons of the sympathetic and parasympathetic nervous systems. Preganglionic neurons are shown as solid lines, postganglionic neurons as dashed lines. The heavy lines are the parasympathetic fibers, the light lines are sympathetic.

organs innervated. There are no ganglia outside of the effector organs; consequently, the postsynaptic parasympathetic nerves are quite short.

PHARMACOLOGICAL CHARACTERISTICS

Both branches of the autonomic nervous system utilize *acetylcholine* as a neurotransmitter in pre–effector synapses. The parasympathetic branch also releases acetylcholine at effector synapses. The sympathetic branch, however, releases the *catecholamines (norepinephrine* and *epinephrine)* at most effector sites. In the sympathetic branch, norepinephrine (or *noradrenalin*) and epinephrine (or *adrenalin*) are produced in a ratio of about 3:1, respectively. Consequently, it is convenient to use norepinephrine as an inclusive term even though both of the transmitters might be secreted by a particular neuron. Neurons which release norepinephrine and epinephrine are said to be *noradrenergic* (or, occasionally, *adrenergic*), whereas those which release acetylcholine are said to be *cholinergic.*

Acetylcholine is released from specific synaptic vesicles which are clear and spherical, quite unlike the structure of the vesicles which release the catecholamines. A small amount of acetylcholine is continually released from these presynaptic neurons during the resting phase of the nerve. This results in a nonpropagated local potential called a *miniature end-plate potential.* The amount of acetylcholine released during the resting phase of the nerve is directly related to the amount of *intracellular calcium* within the terminal button. When an action potential of the presynaptic neuron reaches the synapse, calcium ion permeability increases

dramatically and calcium ions in the extracellular fluid penetrate into the presynaptic terminal, which then induces the release of additional transmitter substance.

Acetylcholine is hydrolyzed at the postsynaptic membrane by *acetylcholinesterase.* There are a number of cholinesterases in mammals but only acetylcholinesterase is present in great enough quantity to be effective. The acetate and choline molecules produced from the hydrolysis of acetylcholine are, in turn, used in the resynthesis of acetylcholine in the presynaptic neuron in the presence of another enzyme, *choline acetyltransferase.*

The *adrenal medulla* functions as a group of postsynaptic neurons of the sympathetic nervous system. But it produces and releases significantly more epinephrine than norepinephrine, and its action is characteristic of an endocrine organ since its products are carried through the bloodstream to the target organs. Even though the adrenal medulla predominantly produces epinephrine, the circulating catecholamine in greatest abundance is norepinephrine.

Even though preganglionic fibers of both branches of the autonomic nervous system use acetylcholine as a transmitter substance, the two branches can be separated on the basis of their response to various drugs. In the sympathetic nervous system, postsynaptic neurons are excited by nicotine, which is able to mimic precisely the action of acetylcholine. But nicotine has no affect upon postsynaptic parasympathetic neurons. The parasympathetic effector organs, such as smooth muscle in the viscera, respond readily to *muscarine,* whereas those innervated by the sympathetic nervous system do not. Muscarine does not mimic in any way the action of the catecholamines. Therefore, the parasympathetic effector organs are said to have *muscarine receptors;* such receptors do not exist at the sympathetic effector sites. This further emphasizes the differences between the parasympathetic and sympathetic branches, since *atropine* acts as a competitor with acetylcholine at the receptor sites but does not compete with the catecholamines. The parasympathetic nervous system is said to exhibit *muscarine action;* the sympathetic nervous system is said to exhibit *nicotinic action.* The parasympathetic and sympathetic branches are pharmacologically identifiable based upon their responses to muscarine and nicotine.

Synthesis and Catabolism of Acetylcholine

Cholinergic neurons actively take up choline, which is able to react with the *acetyl-coenzyme A* present in most metabolically active cells. The reaction is catalyzed by choline acetyltransferase, which is abundant in cholinergic nerve cells (see Figure 5–3). This reaction is quite specific, and the presence of

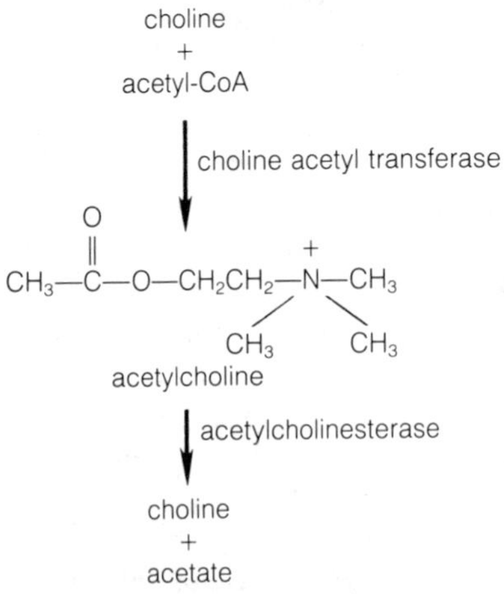

choline
+
acetyl-CoA

↓ choline acetyl transferase

$$CH_3-\overset{\overset{\displaystyle O}{\|}}{C}-O-CH_2CH_2-\overset{+}{N}-CH_3$$
$$\underset{CH_3 \quad\quad CH_3}{}$$

acetylcholine

↓ acetylcholinesterase

choline
+
acetate

FIGURE 5–3
Acetylcholine synthesis and catabolism

high concentrations of the enzyme is taken as evidence that the neurons in any given area are cholinergic.

Acetylcholine, whose release is activated by the increased permeability of the presynaptic nerves to calcium ion, is rapidly catabolized in the synaptic cleft by acetylcholinesterase. The acetylcholinesterase found at nerve terminals is known as *true,* or *specific, cholinesterase.* Cholinesterase found in the blood or other tissues of the body is called *pseudocholinesterase,* or *nonspecific cholinesterase.*

Synthesis and Catabolism of Catecholamines

The dietary precursors of the catecholamines are *phenylalanine* and/or *tyrosine* (see Figure 5–4). Phenylalanine is converted to *p-tyrosine* by the enzyme *phenylalanine hydroxylase.* Tyrosine is then converted to *dihydroxyphenylalanine (DOPA),* which is then converted to *dihydroxyphenylethylamine* (or *dopamine*) by the enzyme *dihydroxyphenylalanine carboxylase.* Dopamine forms norepinephrine in the presence of the enzyme *dopamine β-hydroxylase.* In parts of the sympathetic branch, such as the adrenal medulla, norepinephrine is converted to epinephrine by the addition of a *methyl group* in the presence of *phenylethanolamine-N-methyltransferase (PNMT).*

In some humans the enzyme necessary for the conversion of phenylalanine to tyrosine is absent because of a congenital metabolic defect. Deficiency of this enzyme causes phenylalanine and its derivative *phenylketonuric acid* (see Figure 5–5) to accumulate in the tissues. Unless detected shortly after birth, individuals born with this defect almost certainly develop signs of mental re-

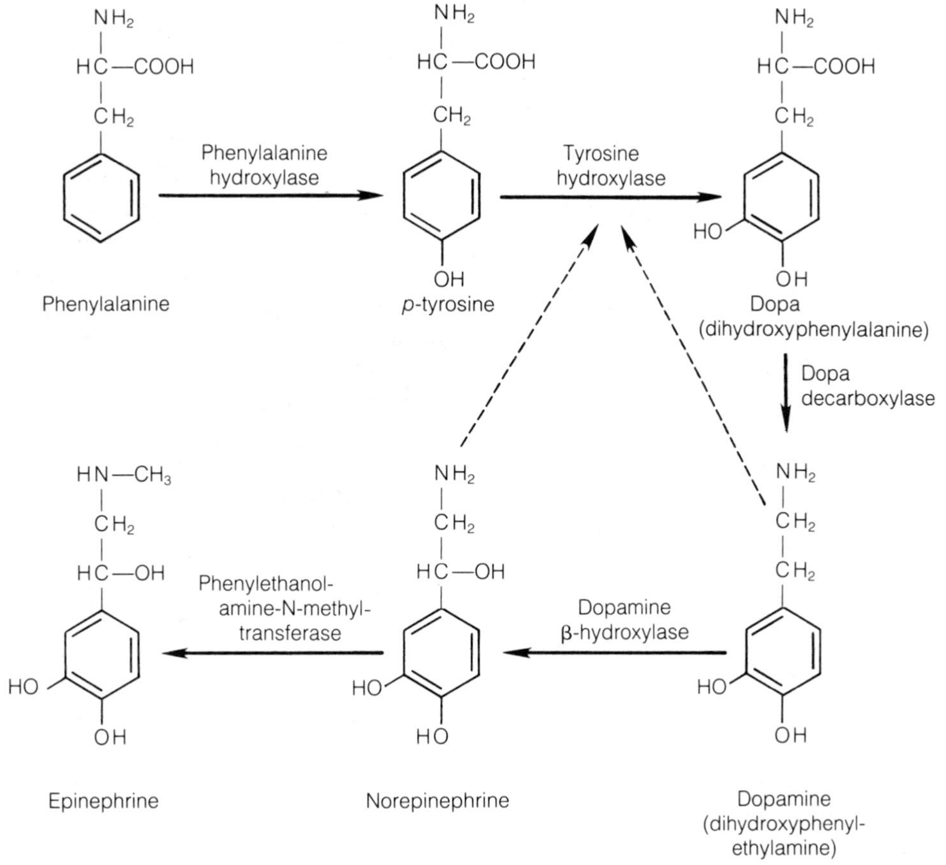

FIGURE 5-4
Biosynthesis of catecholamines

tardation. The disease, *phenylketonuria (PKU),* can be detected by a urine test. The urine of infants with PKU contains high levels of *ketone bodies,* which are formed by the cellular deamination of phenylalanine. When detection occurs in early infancy, mental retardation can be prevented by feeding the child a diet free of phenylalanine. When a phenylalanine-free diet is consumed, dihydroxyphenylalanine is derived solely from tyrosine, and the metabolic chain essential for

the formation of the catecholamines procedes in the normal fashion.

Both epinephrine and norepinephrine are stored in nerve terminals of the presynaptic neurons within granulated vesicles and are bound there to ATP by the protein *chromogranin.* When an action potential reaches the presynaptic nerve terminal, catecholamines are released from the cells by the process of *exocytosis* (or *emiocytosis*). Contrary to the situation in cholinergic neurons, norepi-

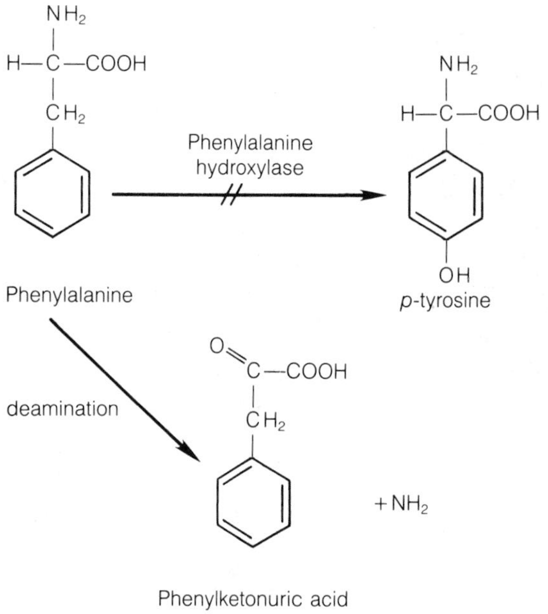

FIGURE 5–5
Biosynthesis of phenylketonuric acid

THE SYMPATHETIC NERVOUS SYSTEM

The sympathetic nervous system contains both adrenergic and cholinergic neurons, which innervate effector organs. Both cholinergic and adrenergic nerve endings of the sympathetic branch enhance energy utilization. Specific actions are induced by the sympathetic nervous system at specific sites in the body, contributing to the energy utilization of the organism as a whole (see Table 5–1). For instance, increased sympathetic activity induces dilation of the precapillary sphincter muscles in the arterioles that supply somatic muscles. Also, catecholamines cause smooth muscle relaxation in the intestines and contraction of the intestinal sphincter muscles. Acetylcholine is released by neurons of the sympathetic branch that innervate smooth muscle of the arterioles supplying blood to the somatic muscles and certain areas of the skin. These are the only known places where the sympathetic nervous system employs acetylcholine at effector terminals.

nephrine and epinephrine can be reabsorbed intact by the presynaptic nerves. These nerves can also synthesize additional catecholamines whenever necessary.

When not reabsorbed by the presynaptic neurons, there are two pathways of catecholamine catabolism. In one pathway, *monoamine oxidase (MAO)*, which is distributed throughout most of the body, oxidizes the catecholamines to form *3,4-dihydroxymandelic acid (DOMA)*, which is neurologically inactive. Most of the catecholamines, however, are converted to their *o-methylated derivatives*, such as *normetanephrine* and *metanephrine*, by *catechol-o-methyltransferase (COMT)*. Levels of normetanephrine and metanephrine in the urine are considered to be good indices of catecholamine secretion.

In skeletal muscle, energy is mostly expended through ATP hydrolysis. Therefore, in keeping with its role of enhancing energy utilization, the sympathetic nervous system acts to promote the production of energy in muscle tissue. This promotion is accomplished by dilation of the *precapillary sphincters*, which increases blood flow for oxygen and metabolite exchange, and by enhancing the formation of *cyclic AMP* in the muscle cells. Cyclic AMP is essential for glucose transport into the cell and is, therefore, necessary during times of stress (see Figure 5–6). Both epinephrine and norepinephrine are capable of entering the interstitial spaces of muscle tissue and can, therefore, enhance

Organ	Effect of Sympathetic Stimulation	Effect of Parasympathetic Stimulation
Heart muscle	Increases rate and force of contraction	Slows rate and decreases force of atrial contraction
Bronchi of the lungs	Dilation	Constriction
Blood vessels of the lungs	Somewhat constricted	No effect
Lumen of the gut	Decreases peristalsis and tone	Increases peristalsis and tone
Sphincters of the gut	Increases tone	Decreases tone
Pupil (eye)	Dilation	Constriction
Ciliary muscle (eye)	No effect	Excitation
Sweat glands	Copious sweating (cholinergic)	No effect
Basal metabolism	Greatly increases	No effect
Mental activity	Increases	No effect
Skeletal muscle	Increases strength and glycogenolysis	No effect
Abdominal blood vessels	Constriction	No effect
Skeletal blood vessels	Constriction (adrenergic) Dilation (cholinergic)	No effect

TABLE 5–1

Effects of the autonomic nervous system on various organs of the body

glucose availability through increased active transport.

In heart muscle, the sympathetic branch innervates both nodal tissue, such as the tissue of the A-V and S-A nodes, and *contractile fibers* (see chapter 11, The Heart as a Pump). Sympathetic neurons are interspersed within cardiac muscle cells, which allows for the uniform distribution of catecholamines within the heart tissue. As the sympathetic neurons pass through the *myocardium* (a part of the heart's wall), catecholamines are released at various positions or *varicosities* along the neurons rather than at specific *myoneural* (or *neuromuscular*) *junctions*. The catecholamines thus released increase both the rate of contraction and the force developed by the heart muscle. In the nodal tissue catecholamines enhance active transport of sodium and potassium ions, thus allowing the nodal cells to reach normal resting membrane potentials more rapidly after each discharge. Calcium transport from the sarcomeres of cardiac muscles is also heightened by the catecholamines, thus permitting a more rapid relaxation rate of cardiac fibers and, therefore, an increased rate of contraction. Both calcium transport from the sarcomere and metabolite transport into the cell are influenced by the action of catecholamines as a result of its role in the production of cyclic AMP.

As a generalization, gastric and intestinal activities of mammals are kept to a minimum

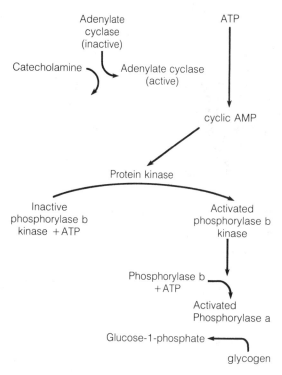

FIGURE 5–6
Cellular activation of glycogenolysis (or the breakdown of glycogen) by catecholamines

by the secretion of the catecholamines. Decreasing intestinal function maximizes the ability of the animal to concentrate all of its actions in preparation for the exertion of energy toward an emergency situation. Obviously, exertion of energy during flight or during an attack by an enemy requires maximum activity in skeletal and cardiac muscles and decreased activity of smooth muscles in the gastrointestinal tract.

Two seemingly opposite reactions occur during sympathetic stimulation of the eye. When stimulated by the catecholamines, the *radial muscle* of the iris contracts, causing the pupils to dilate (see chapter 6, Sensory

Reception). The radial muscle points toward the center of the pupil, like the spokes of a wheel. During contraction the "spokes" pull directly away from the center of the eye, causing pupil dilation, which allows more light to enter the eye. Unlike the radial muscle, the *ciliary muscle* of the eye relaxes when exposed to norepinephrine. This muscle functions like a sphincter muscle: when it contracts, tension of the suspensory ligament is reduced, which permits the lens to assume a more spherical shape. When it relaxes, as in norepinephrine stimulation, the internal pressure of the eye pushes outward, creating tension on the suspensory ligament, which in turn pulls the lens into the thinner shape necessary for distance vision.

The sympathetic stimulation of the eye is an excellent example of the respective roles of *alpha receptors* and *beta receptors.* The ciliary muscle of the eye contains beta-receptors, which cause relaxation when stimulated by the catecholamines. The radial muscle of the iris contains alpha receptors, which cause contraction when stimulated by the catecholamines. Two types of alpha receptors are found in animals: alpha-1 and alpha-2. Alpha-1 receptors are located on postsynaptic membranes, whereas alpha-2 receptors are located on the presynaptic neurons. The alpha-2 receptors provide a negative-feedback mechanism for the regulation of catecholamine release. In Figure 5–7, catecholamines secreted by the presynaptic neuron interact with the alpha-2 receptors to inhibit further release.

In adipose tissue, which contains beta receptors, catecholamines enhance *fatty acid mobilization* by activating *adenylate cyclase.* Fatty acid levels of the plasma are thus increased when catecholamines are released by sympathetic nerves in adipose tissue or

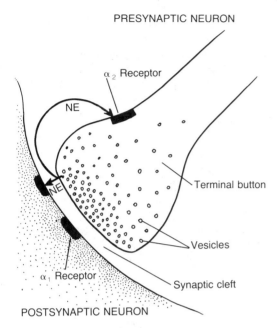

FIGURE 5-7
Role of alpha-1 and alpha-2 norepinephrine (NE) receptors at the synapse. Note that alpha-2 receptors function to inhibit the release of additional catecholamines.

THE PARASYMPATHETIC NERVOUS SYSTEM

Unlike neurons of the sympathetic nervous system, all parasympathetic neurons are cholinergic and actively promote functions of a sedentary or ruminating nature. In the heart the parasympathetic nerve endings are restricted to nodal tissue and do not have the diffuse distribution noted for the sympathetic branch of the autonomic nervous system. Acetylcholine acts primarily to reduce the rate of discharge of the nodes. It prolongs the permeability of nodal cells to potassium ions, thus increasing the duration of the prepotential and, consequently, decreasing the rate of nodal firing.

Secretion of acetylcholine by the parasympathetic nervous system causes the sphincter muscle of the iris to contract, thus reducing the aperature of the iris and restricting the entry of light into the eye. Acetylcholine also induces the ciliary muscle to contract, which then causes the relaxation of the suspensory ligament and allows the lens to assume a more spherical shape necessary for viewing objects close to the eye.

The smooth muscles of the intestine are innervated by two *nerve nets:* the *muscularis,* located between the two muscle layers, and the *submucosal,* located in the submucosa. These nerve nets affect activity in the smooth muscle layers, whose action is in turn modified by the autonomic nervous system. Whenever food is taken into the mouth, olfactory (smell) and gustatory (taste) sensations activate the parasympathetic nervous system through the vagus nerve, inducing the secretion of saliva and the increase of gastric motility. Pressure receptors located throughout the gastrointestinal tract initiate reflexes that facilitate autonomic responses.

when circulating catecholamines reach adipose tissue. These fatty acids are made available to skeletal and cardiac muscles through the circulation and allow for increased oxidative metabolism during situations of high energy demand.

During an asthma attack, the bronchial muscles of the lungs constrict and there is an increased mucous secretion, which severely restricts breathing. Catecholamines cause the bronchial muscles to relax and also inhibit the action of the bronchial glands, which secrete mucous into the lungs. The discovery that this effect could be induced through the direct application of epinephrine by means of a spray mist has been a boon to numerous asthma sufferers in the past few decades.

Parasympathetic activity causes the increase of gastric motility and hydrochloric acid secretion, as well as the production of other gastric juices, including *gastrin*. Gastrin secretion is enhanced by the acetylcholine released from parasympathetic neurons. The gastrin, in turn, enhances further gastric motility and secretion.

Acetylcholine stimulates both the emptying response of the gallbladder and the enzyme secretion by the intestinal mucosa. The acini of the pancreas also respond to parasympathetic stimulation by increasing the production and secretion of digestive enzymes (see chapter 17, The Endocrine System). In addition, acetylcholine activates production of the hormones insulin and glucagon by the islets of Langerhans. The mechanism of acetylcholine activity in the production of these hormones involves the stimulation of active transport of amino acids into the cells of the islets. The mechanism also enhances glycolysis, making more energy available to these cells.

Acetylcholine acts as an antagonist to the catecholamines in the lungs and induces the constriction of bronchial smooth muscles and the secretion of mucous by the bronchial glands. Activity in the lung appears to be a direct action of acetylcholine on the smooth muscle and bronchial glands; such activity is not associated with an intermediary nerve net, as seen in the gastrointestinal tract.

DRUGS AFFECTING THE AUTONOMIC NERVOUS SYSTEM

The autonomic nervous system is capable of many different and seemingly isolated actions. This is particularly true of the sympathetic branch. Hence, the pharmacological study of the adrenergic and cholinergic receptors, as well as the release mechanisms for acetylcholine and the catecholamines, have been extremely fruitful. Both acetylcholine and the catecholamines activate specific postsynaptic receptor sites. The response of postsynaptic neurons to acetylcholine and the catecholamines can be modified by drugs that affect their catabolism or their resorption by the presynaptic neurons and by drugs that compete for receptor sites on the postsynaptic membrane. *Anticholinesterase drugs* have been developed which inactivate acetylcholinesterase and therefore permit prolonged acetylcholine activity on the postsynaptic membrane. One of these drugs, *physostigmine* (or *eserine*) has been employed to reduce the effects of *myasthenia gravis* in humans. Characteristically, people with this disease have poor muscle tone and lack the normal sensitivity of the postsynaptic membrane to acetylcholine. "Tying up" or removing some of the acetylcholinesterase effectively promotes a greater response in the muscle cells, since less acetylcholinesterase makes available more of the active transmitter, acetylcholine. *Neostigmine* (or *prostigmine*), another substance related to physostigmine, also blocks the action of acetylcholinesterase, but neostigmine is not readily removed by metabolism. As a result, it is more potent than physostigmine and small amounts of the drug can be fatal. Exposure to neostigmine results in massive cholinergic action and causes clinical symptoms similar to grand mal seizures.

Many drugs promote the action of norepinephrine. Some enhance the release of norepinephrine, whereas others behave similarly to this catecholamine at the cellular level. *Amphetamines* are drugs that fall into both categories. Amphetamine itself is a compound very similar in structure to norepinephrine, a similarity that could have some bearing on amphetamine's physiological action (see Figure 5–8). Because of the widespread use of amphetamines both legally and illegally, its name is used to describe an entire class of compounds which have similar physiological effects in mammals. Compounds such as *ephedrine*, *benzadrine*, and *dexadrine* have amphetaminelike action and are, therefore, classified as amphetamines. Drugs of this type have varying degrees of potency and may not function at a cellular level in exactly the same way as norepinephrine, though their physiological manifestations in the intact organism are similar.

The *tricyclic antidepressants*, such as the commercially available *Tofranil* and *Elavil*, function at adrenergic synaptic terminals by inhibiting the uptake of excess norepinephrine. These drugs thus prolong the action of norepinephrine at the synapse. *Cocaine* employs the same mechanism. For reasons unknown, the various drugs which affect norepinephrine synapses affect totally different areas of the central nervous system. The tricyclic antidepressants appear to induce a mood elevation, but cocaine produces more behavioral stimulation and less mood modification; thus, each must affect a different area.

Another class of drugs widely used as antidepressants is the *monoamine oxidase inhibitors* (or *MAO inhibitors*), of which *tranycypromine* (or *Parnate*) is a prime example.

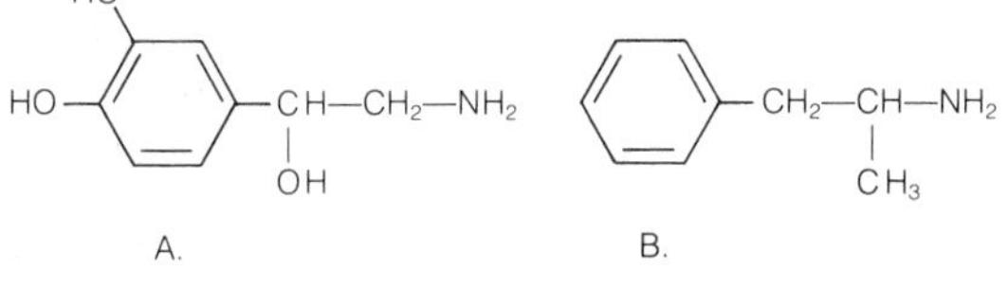

The MAO inhibitors function to inhibit the metabolic breakdown of the catecholamines at the nerve terminals. When the metabolic destruction of these transmitters is inhibited, their action is promoted for longer periods of time. Peculiarly, these drugs, as well as the tricyclic antidepressants, do not have a pronounced effect on the average individual. Both classes of drugs are mood modifiers in the sense that depressed individuals are relieved of their depression, but drastic behavioral modification, as produced by cocaine or amphetamine, does not occur. It is for this reason that MAO inhibitors and the tricyclic antidepressants have not become "street drugs."

SUMMARY

The autonomic nervous system consists of two distinct branches based upon structure, function, and pharmacology. The sympathetic branch exits the central nervous system through the spinal nerves of the thorax and lumbar regions. Sympathetic neurons may synapse with neurons of the paravertebral sympathetic ganglia or may synapse with nerves in other isolated collateral ganglia inside the body cavity. The parasympathetic nervous system has very long presynaptic neurons as well as short postsynaptic nerves limited to the organs innervated. Neurons of this branch exit the central nervous system through the cranial nerves and the nerves of the sacral region of the spinal cord.

The two branches also differ by producing different neurotransmitters, which are active in promoting distinct postsynaptic effects. The parasympathetic branch produces only acetylcholine; the sympathetic branch produces norepinephrine and epinephrine (the catecholamines) as well as acetylcholine. The

FIGURE 5–8
Structure of (A) norepinephrine and (B) amphetamine

sympathetic nerves innervating vascular smooth muscle of the skeletal musculature and certain areas of the skin are solely cholinergic.

Both acetylcholine and the catecholamines are produced from dietary precursors. Acetylcholine is formed as a result of the chemical bonding of choline and an acetyl group. The catecholamines are synthesized either from phenylalanine or from tyrosine, whichever is present in the diet. Where both are present, both can act as precursors.

The sympathetic nervous system is responsible for preparation of the organism for exertion of more energy. The parasympathetic nervous system is associated with ruminating functions of the animal and is active both during and after a meal, when the digestive processes are at their peaks.

Both the sympathetic and the parasympathetic branches of the autonomic nervous system provide a subconscious level of control within the body. Adjustments of the organism to changing physical and emotional situations are controlled through the autonomic nervous system. These mechanisms are essential to support systems for conscious actions carried out by the organism.

6

SENSORY RECEPTION

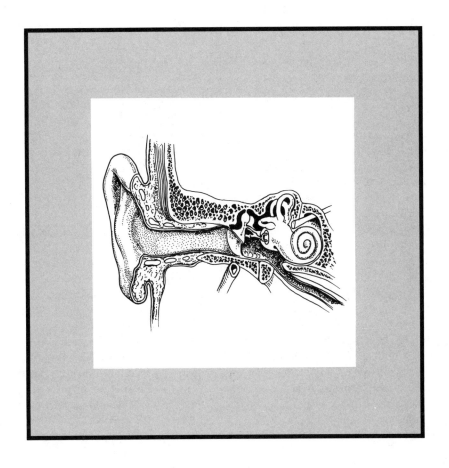

*T*he reception of external stimuli is one of the major functions of the nervous system, since it is a fundamental link with the animal's environment. An animal must not only be able to respond to specific stimuli, but also must be able to respond quantitatively to the intensity with which the stimulus is projected. Receptors have evolved in the skin of mammals which enable them to respond to tactile stimuli, pressure, pain, heat, and cold. In addition, specialized organs are present which enable the mammal to respond to light, sound, and chemicals carried through air or water. All of these receptors, whether individual cells (as in the case of receptors in the skin) or specialized organs (such as the eye and ear) respond to stimuli through local changes in membrane permeability and the resultant generator potentials. The differences in receptors lie in their ability to respond to certain stimuli, as opposed to the numerous other environmental changes that might be taking place. Most stimuli picked up by the sensory receptors are transmitted through sensory tracts in the spinal cord and base of the brain to specific locations on the sensory cortex of the cerebrum.

THE TYPES OF RECEPTORS AND THEIR FUNCTION

The *law of specific nerve energies* describes the relationship between receptors in the body and the *sensations* they generate. The law holds that for every stimulus there is a specific type of receptor best suited to receive it. It implies that for each modality there is a receptor that has evolved specifically for that modality. Consequently, receptors respond to very low levels of stimuli and are therefore very efficient. When *photoreceptors* are stimulated the animal perceives light. Likewise, when *Pacinean corpuscles* are stimuled pressure is perceived. But receptors can be stimulated by modalities for which they are not well suited or for which they do not readily respond. In any case, the organism still perceives the stimulus in a frame of reference or as a sensation for which the specific receptor has evolved. For instance, light at low intensities stimulates the rods of the eye, but pressure applied to the eye will also stimulate the light receptors. Although light receptors are not specifically adapted for pressure reception, they can nevertheless respond to pressure, albeit in an abnormal situation.

Specific identification of sensory modalities can be explained by examining the cerebral cortex. A portion of the cortex, called the *sensory cortex*, receives stimuli from sensory receptors located in the skin. Although the sensory cortex contains a variety of neurons which detect sensory stimuli from all portions of the body, each distinct sensation is represented by a specific group of *cortical cells*. Thus, specific neurons of the sensory cortex are stimulated when pressure receptors are stimulated. Stimulation of touch receptors activates a completely different set of neurons on the sensory cortex than those involved in photoreception. When photoreceptors are stimulated by pressure, the sensation of light is received by the organism. Therefore, stimulation of specific receptors results in specific sensations no matter what the modality of stimulus. As put by one eminent researcher, if the optic and auditory nerves could be switched one might hear lightning and see thunder.

Sensory receptors are divided into specific groups depending upon their location and function within the body. The receptors located in the skin for touch, pain, heat, and cold are called *exteroreceptors* since they give specific information about the external factors which immediately affect the skin. Many sensory receptors are located collectively in organs that maximize the effects of specific stimuli. Such receptors are collectively known as the *special senses*, even though they are exteroreceptors in that they receive information from outside the body. Other groups of receptors, which usually give the sensations of pain or pressure, are located within the organs of the body. These are called *interoreceptors* or *interoceptors* because of their position inside the body.

The various interoreceptors are not perceived by the conscious mind in the same way as are exteroreceptors. *Chemoreceptors* located in the aortic and carotid bodies respond to carbon dioxide and hydrogen ion concentrations in the blood. Receptors which describe body position are referred to as *proprioreceptors* or *proprioceptors*. *Stretch receptors*, proprioceptors found in muscles and in golgi tendon organs of the tendons, give quantitative as well as qualitative information about position and body movement.

Generator Potentials

The potential restricted to the receptor portion of the neuron and developed as the re-

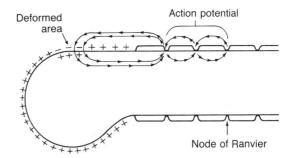

FIGURE 6–1
Excitation of sensory nerve fiber by a generator potential produced in a Pacinean corpuscle

sult of a stimulus is called a *generator potential.* For example, if the membrane of a Pacinean corpuscle is *deformed* by pressure, there is an increase in sodium ion permeability, producing a generator potential very much like the local potential on a postsynaptic membrane (see Figure 6–1). If the generator potential is large enough, local currents will induce an action potential on the axolemma of the sensory neuron and the stimulus will ultimately be received by the sensory cortex. Other receptors form generator potentials in the same way, though each type of receptor responds with maximum sensitivity to its associated modality.

Adaptation

Many, but not all, sensations originating from the sensory receptors decline in intensity over a period of time (see Figure 6–2). This process, called *adaptation* or *accommodation* of sensory receptors, involves recovery of the receptor's membrane to the original state even though the stimulus is still being applied. It is this phenomenon which allows an organism to respond initially to a stimulus and then grow accustomed to it, as if it were no longer present. An analogy might be the sensation of a hot shower: the water seems

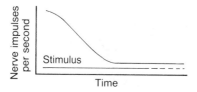

FIGURE 6–2
Adaptation of sensory neurons. The height of the curve indicates frequency of firing as a function of duration of stimulus.

to cool down after a period of time even though the water temperature remains the same. Receptors associated with critical sensations (such as pain) do not readily adapt. This seems to be an essential mechanism for the survival of the animal.

Intensity of Sensory Reception

Another factor which should be considered in sensory reception is the intensity with which a stimulus is perceived. The *Weber-Fechner law* states that the intensity of the sensation is proportional to the common logarithm (base 10) of the intensity of the stimulus. In other words, as the intensity of the stimulus increases, the sensation also increases, but only by the common logarithm of the stimulus. For example, if the *threshold pressure* of a Pacinean corpuscle is 10 grams, a pressure of 100 grams would not be perceived as ten times as great. According to the Weber-Fechner law, the magnitude of sensation from the 100-gram stimulus would only be twice as great as the sensation generated by the 10-gram stimulus, since the common logarithm of 100 is 2. The physiological basis of the law lies in how much the generator potential changes when the stimulus is increased: it is the generator potential which bears a logarithmic relationship to the intensity of the stimulus. On the other hand, the

number of impulses transmitted through a single sensory neuron is *directly proportional* to the size of the generator potential (see Figure 6–3). In other words, the intensity of the sensation received is a direct function of the rate of firing on the sensory neuron. But that rate (the number of action potentials per unit time) is controlled by the size of the generator potential, which bears a logarithmic relationship to the intensity of the stimulus.

An obvious benefit of this relationship can be seen in the latitude of the intensity with which stimuli can be received. If, for example, a neuron could transmit a maximum of 100 spikes (action potentials) per second, a

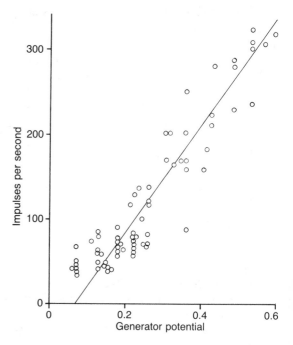

FIGURE 6–3
The number of impulses is directly proportional to the size of the generator potential. From B. Katz, Depolarization of Sensory Terminals and the Initiation of Impulses in the Muscle Spindle, *J. Physiol.* III(1950):261–282, fig. 10. Reprinted by permission of Cambridge University Press, London, U.K.

logarithmic relationship between stimulus intensity and sensation received affords a much wider range over which the receptor can respond than if the relationship were directly proportional. A tenfold increase in stimulus intensity only doubles the firing rate, and a one hundredfold increase only triples the firing rate.

Referred Pain

Pain perceived in the interior of the body by interoceptors is sometimes displaced from its site of origin. Frequently, pain felt in one part of the body is initiated in a completely different area. Such a sensation is called *referred pain*. This phenomenon is exemplified by the pain felt under the left arm by some victims of heart attacks or the pain felt near the navel in some cases of appendicitis (see

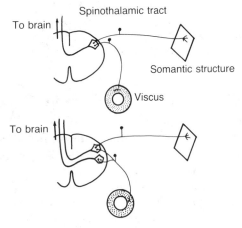

CONVERGENCE THEORY

FACILITATION THEORY

FIGURE 6–5
Diagram of convergence and facilitation theories of referred pain. Reproduced, with permission, from Ganong, WF: *Review of Medical Physiology,* 9th ed. Copyright 1979 by Lange Medical Publications, Los Altos, California.

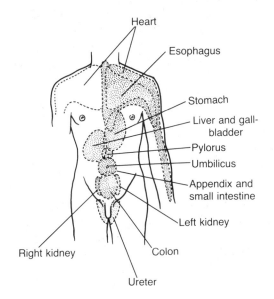

FIGURE 6–4
Surface areas of referred pain from different visceral organs. From A. C. Guyton, *Textbook of Medical Physiology,* 6th edition (Philadelphia, Pa., 1981), 670, fig. 50–7. Reprinted by permission of W. B. Saunders Publishing Co.

Figure 6–4). The physiological explanation of this phenomenon lies in the embryological origin of the receptors that innervate particular areas of the body. These areas are derived in the embryo from the same somite and therefore innervate the same afferent neuron in the spinal cord. In other words, neurons developed in very close proximity in the embryo are completely isolated in the adult, but their sensory terminals still retain their original positions in the central nervous system. According to the *facilitation theory,* sensory receptors originating in the same embryonic somite facilitate each other, and therefore little stimulus is needed to "refer" the pain from one part of the body to another (see Figure 6–5). According to the *convergence theory,* neurons developed from a particular somite converge on a single afferent neuron in the spinal cord, through which impulses are carried to the brain. Such convergence prevents opportunity for the differentiation between the two points of stimulus that might otherwise occur in widely separated regions of the body.

THE PHYSIOLOGY OF VISION

The electromagnetic spectrum comprises a wide range of oscillating energy units, or *waves* (see Figure 6–6). The distance between two consecutive oscillations is referred to as a *wavelength*. The energy range responded to by the mammalian eye is called the *visual spectrum* and in general includes all the wavelengths of the electromagnetic spectrum which lie between 400 and 800 nanometers. The visual spectrum differs among mamma-

lian groups. There is frequently more than one receptor type in the eye. Each type responds to a specific portion of the visual spectrum. Vision in mammals is an interpretive phenomenon developed in response to stimulation of these receptors, which are located on the retina.

In order to function as a light receptor, an organ or cell must in some way absorb energy from the electromagnetic spectrum. Absorption is made possible by *pigments* in the receptor cell, each capable of absorbing specific wavelengths. The pigments are arranged in overlapping *lamellae* within the receptor cells so as to maximize the amount of light which can be absorbed by a specific receptor (see Figure 6–7). Each receptor pigment absorbs light over a range of different wavelengths but characteristically has a maximum response in a very limited portion of the range. When these receptor cells are grouped, as they are in mammals, they constitute a *receptor organ*. Since these structures have evolved into receptors with a very specific function, they are referred to as *organs of the specialized senses.*

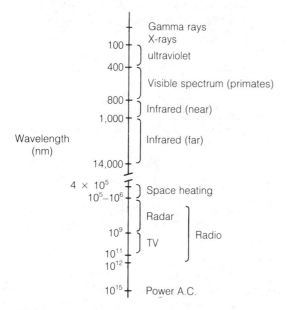

FIGURE 6–6
Wavelengths of radiation. Note that the visual spectrum for primates represents a very small portion of the electromagnetic spectrum.

Structure of the Mammalian Eye

The mammalian eye is situated in a depression within the skull called the *orbit.* In some mammals the orbit forms a complete circle around the eye to protect it laterally from physical trauma. In mammals with closed orbits the *zygomatic bone* unites with the *frontal bone* to complete the *arch.* Closed orbits are usually not found in the carnivores, though their eyes are protected to some degree by an incomplete zygomatic arch.

The eye can be exposed or covered by the *eyelids* (upper and lower), which are moved by very rapidly contracting muscles. Many

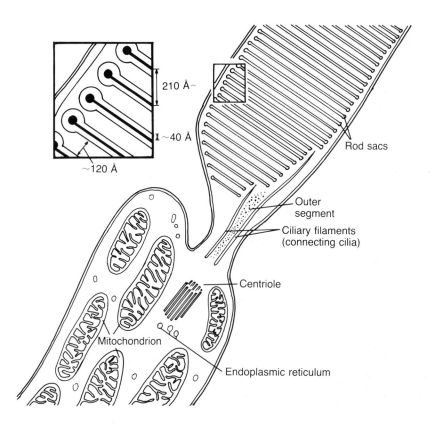

FIGURE 6–7
Electron micrograph of a longitudinal section through a photoreceptor cell (rod). Lamellae enhance the exposure area of pigment for light absorption.

210 Å~

~40 Å

~120 Å

Rod sacs

Outer segment

Ciliary filaments (connecting cilia)

Centriole

Mitochondrion

Endoplasmic reticulum

mammals, humans excluded, have a *third eyelid* which can be pulled across the cornea to give an added degree of protection. The third eyelid is extended by retracting the eye into the orbit. A layer of fat lying behind the eye is compressed when the eye is retracted. This layer of fat then pushes against the third eyelid, thus forcing it outward to cover the cornea. Third eyelids are present in all ruminants and in all carnivores except the skunk. It is particularly useful in the polar bear and seal, in which it can protect the eye underwater and still allow vision. In the caribou and horse the third eyelid probably is a protective device that prevents freezing of the cornea. These two species are capable of

running at speeds in excess of 20 miles per hour in ambient temperatures which may reach forty degrees below zero. The tremendous wind chill factor in such instances would cause the eye to freeze rapidly without some type of protection.

There are numerous variations in mammalian eye structure which are similar to the lens of a camera. The eye, like a camera, can direct light waves to a particular focus. It can also control the amount of light reaching the receptor cells in the same fashion as the shutter of a camera controls the amount of light reaching the photographic film. The ability to change the focal point of light rays entering the eye, called *accommodation*, is made possible by the refraction or bending of light rays by portions of the eye through which light passes.

The basic structure of the eye includes a *cornea* and *lens* for accommodation and a *pupil* which controls the amount of light received by the retina (see Figure 6–8). The *iris*, the pigmented portion of the eye, surrounds the pupil. In some species, particularly in such grazing animals as the ungulates, dark bodies called *corpora nigra* may appear to extend from the edge of the pupil (see Figure 6–9): These extensions apparently do not reduce the animal's vision and may provide additional shading from bright ambient light. The eye also contains two fluids called the *vitreous* and *aqueous humors*. These fluids, quite distinct from plasma, have refractive indices which differ from the cornea and lens.

The *choroid* and *sclera* are tough protective coats which resist trauma and assist in the maintenance of intraocular pressure. The *retina*, which lies on the inside of the cho-

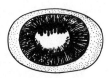
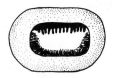

FIGURE 6–9
Corpora nigra, the "hanging" bodies which extend into the pupil of many ungulates (left, the horse; right, the camel)

roid, comprises several layers of neurons, which have a special arrangement (see Figure 6–10). The *primary layer* contains the receptor cells, which are pointed toward the sclera. The *secondary layer* contains neurons which allow information to be exchanged between the primary layer and the tertiary layer. The *tertiary layer* consists of afferent neurons, which form the *optic tract*. In some mammals the retina lies against a layer of pigmented cells called the *tapetum lucidum*, which reflects light after it passes through the retina and gives rise to the "eye shine" so frequently observed in nocturnal mammals. In most carnivores the pigment is contained

FIGURE 6–8
A cross section of the human eye

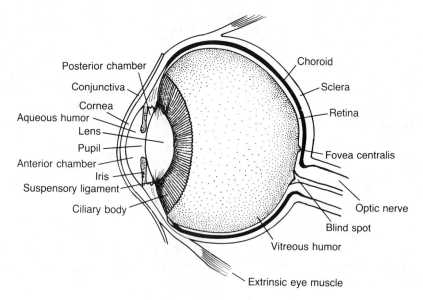

Posterior chamber
Conjunctiva
Cornea
Aqueous humor
Lens
Pupil
Anterior chamber
Iris
Suspensory ligament
Ciliary body

Choroid
Sclera
Retina
Fovea centralis
Optic nerve
Blind spot
Vitreous humor
Extrinsic eye muscle

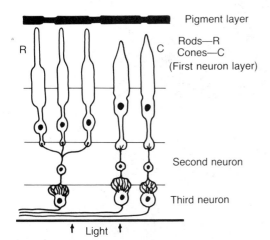

FIGURE 6–10
Three layers of neurons compose the retina. The primary layer contains the receptor cells (rods and cones). Note their association with the tertiary layer as a result of their synaptic relationship to the secondary neurons.

within iridescent cells called *iridocytes*, which collectively make up the tapetum cellulosum. The tapetum varies in shape among species and in some cases occupies only a small portion of the retinal surface. Certain breeds of dogs, such as the Pekingese and the pug, have *melanin granules* located in the lower portion of the tapetum, called the *tapetum nigrum*. The effective pigment in the tapetum lucidum of mammals is at present unknown, but it apparently is not related to *guanin*, which is found in the tapetum lucidum of lower vertebrates.

The pupil, which allows light to enter the eye, has a different shape depending upon the species and upon the amount of ambient light (see Figure 6–11). In nocturnal mammals the pupil is usually *elliptical*. This shape is better than the *concentric* shape found in many other species (including humans) because it enables the animal to change the pupil width from complete closure to a large opening for vision in dim light.

The pupils found in most species of foxes are in the form of a narrow *vertical slit*, which allows for a wide latitude of change depending upon ambient lighting conditions. In the fennec, a nocturnal fox of desert North Africa, and in the arctic fox, the pupils are *round* and resemble those of the domesticated dog. Interestingly, the pupil of the horse changes shape with age. The foal's *circular* pupil develops into a *horizontal slit* in the adult. It should be noted that the long axis of the pupil in the adult horse lies directly beneath the portion of the cornea which has the most perfect curvature.

The color of the iris in mammals is often quite distinctive, varying from almost black to

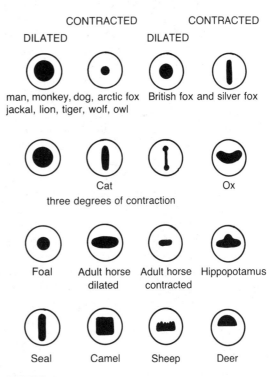

FIGURE 6–11
Pupil shapes in various mammals. From *Vision in the Animal World* by R. H. Smythe. © 1975: R. H. Smythe and reprinted by permission of St. Martin's Press, Inc.

light blue, and even pink in the case of albinos. Color shading is the result of the pigment *melanin* deposited in the cells of the iris. Melanin deposition is most prominent in the deeper cells of the iris. When melanin is absent from the upper layers, the color is lightened and becomes intermixed with the coloration of blood in the capillaries. Blue coloration is caused by the absence of melanin in the outer cell layers, whereas albino coloration is caused by a complete lack of melanin: the pink shade of the iris in albinos is due to the color of blood.

The central nervous system is primarily responsible for integration of the information generated by the receptors on the retina. Fibers in the optic tract carry information through the *lateral geniculate* of the thalamus to the *visual cortex* of the brain, which generates the sensation of vision. The optic fibers *decussate* (cross) to opposite sides of the cortex by way of the *optic chiasma* (see Figure 6–12). The degree of crossing, or the percentage of fibers that cross to different sides, varies according to species. In the dog, three-quarters of the optic fibers decussate. In the cat, only two-thirds of the fibers decussate, whereas in the rat and opossum decussation occurs in four-fifths of the fibers. Fibers also diverge from the optic tracts to nuclei associated with motor activity of the iris and other muscular activity controlling the corneal and vestibular reflexes. In addition, the *suprachiasmic nuclei* of the hypothalamus, which are essential in circadian and reproductive cycles, receive innervation from neurons which depart from the optic tract near the optic chiasma.

Accommodation

Light rays entering the eye are brought to a *focus* by the cornea and lens. The sclera is

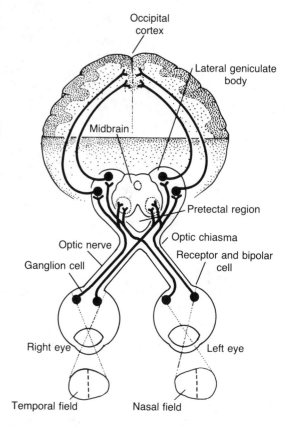

FIGURE 6–12
Visual pathways in the human. Note that fibers from the nasal half of each retina cross to the opposite side of the brain at the optic chiasma.

also essential to this process, since it provides a tough coat which maintains the fixed shape of the eye and thus produces a reliable plane for the projected image. Accommodation involves a reflex which results in alteration of shape of the lens, enabling light rays to be focused on the retina, the result of which is *image formation.*

The *refraction* (bending) of light rays is central to the process of accommodation. Refraction results from the change of the speed of light as it passes through different media. When light changes speeds as it passes through such transparent material as the cornea of the eye, it is bent from its original path. When light strikes a glass pane, part of the light waves slow down, and in doing so the entire beam is bent at an angle from the incident light (see Figure 6–13A). As the light reaches the glass-air interface on the other side of the glass pane, the opposite reaction occurs. The light beam is bent again, this time in the opposite direction, so that it resumes its original path. In a convex lens, both sides of the glass-air interface cause the light to take a path toward the center of the lens (see Figure 6–13B). Light rays which enter a convex lens are caused to converge at a point called the *principal focus*.

The cornea's curvature, which is fixed in the mammalian eye, causes light waves to bend inwardly (see Figure 6–14). The lens can cause additional curvature of the light rays, which ultimately reach a *focal point* in the normal eye. In the *emmetropic* or normal eye, light rays form an image, which is projected on the retina. In diving mammals, corneal accommodation is impossible because the *refractive index* of the cornea is identical to the refractive index of water.

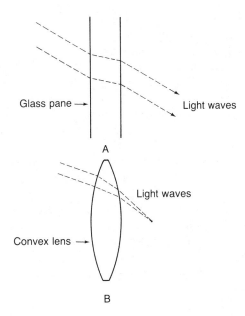

FIGURE 6–13
Refraction of light by (A) uniform glass pane and (B) convex lens

When the lens or cornea lacks perfect curvature, an *astigmatism* results. In some species the cornea naturally lacks perfect curvature and is therefore astigmatic. In the horse,

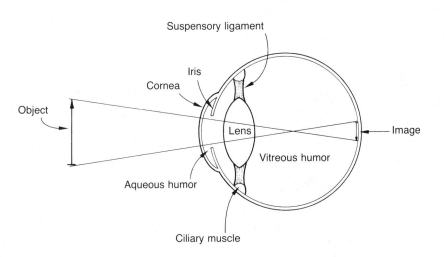

FIGURE 6–14
Convergence of light rays in the mammalian eye

for example, the *dorso-ventral axis* is always astigmatic, whereas the *horizontal axis* normally has near perfect curvature.

The *pupillary diameter* usually changes during accommodation. Because the lens and cornea have maximum perfection near their centers, visual acuteness is greatest when the pupil is restricted to a very small opening. The pupils of most mammals constrict when their vision is concentrated on a small object or on something that requires maximum visual acuity. Therefore, during accommodation the pupillary diameter usually changes, but the degree of change is also influenced by the amount of light present. Change of pupillary diameter caused by change of light intensity is usually referred to as the *pupillary reflex*.

Change in shape of the lens during accommodation is brought about through contraction and relaxation of the *ciliary muscle*. When the ciliary muscle is contracted, tension on the *suspensory ligament* is reduced, allowing the elastic lens to assume a more spherical shape. When the ciliary muscle relaxes, intraocular pressure pushes against the back of the lens, thus forcing it into a flatter shape. This action produces an elliptical rather than a round lens when viewed from the side. For *near vision*, the lens assumes a spherical shape, which causes greater convergence and allows the image to strike the retina. For *distance vision*, the lens assumes a flatter configuration so that image formation can be accomplished at the desirable site on the retina.

In some species the lens contributes little to the focusing apparatus. In these animals the lack of a smoothly curved retina allows for focusing by changing direction of light reception. The eye of the horse provides an excellent example of this process (see Figure 6–15). The horse is said to have a *ramp retina*, since different positions on the retina lie at different distances from the cornea. In order to accommodate, the animal simply raises or lowers its head to change the focal length and hence the site of image formation. This movement allows the focal plane to be brought closer to the focal point for near vision and moved further from the focal point for distance vision. By changing the distance from the focal point to the retina, the image can always be allowed to fall on the retinal surface. The ciliary muscles of the horse are apparently unable to alter the shape of the lens. This focusing method is found in sheep and perhaps other ungulates as well.

FIGURE 6–15
Section of the eye of a horse showing how different angles of entry of light into the eye alter distance from the cornea to the retina. From *Vision in the Animal World* by R. H. Smythe. © 1975: R. H. Smythe and reprinted by permission of St. Martin's Press, Inc.

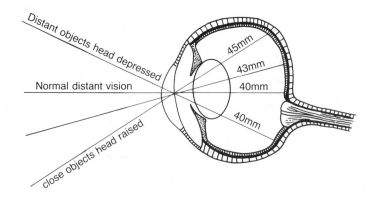

Visual Receptors

Two types of photoreceptor cells, *rods* and *cones*, are found in the mammalian retina. The rods, more sensitive to light than the cones, are grouped so that several rods synapse with one *secondary retinal neuron.* This arrangement makes convergence possible in the rods and aids in the ability of mammals to see in dim light. The pigment found in rods, called *rhodopsin*, is bleached in bright light, making rods unsuitable by themselves for adequate day vision. The cones contain pigments which require greater light intensity for bleaching to occur. As a result of the different absorption characteristics of the pigments found in rods and cones, the rods are much more sensitive to light (see Figure 6–16). Consequently, nocturnal mammals normally have a higher proportion of rods than cones in their retinas, enabling them to have maximum *scotopic* or *night vision.* Diurnal mammals usually have a higher proportion of cones than rods in their retinas, resulting in poor night vision.

In the primates, the cones are grouped in a portion of the retina called the *macula lutea*, or *yellow spot*, and have their greatest density in the *fovea centralis*, though some cones are scattered throughout the retina to provide peripheral vision in bright light. In nonprimates, areas of maximum sensitivity can be found on the retina, but there is no distinct region like the fovea in these species. Because the cones have a one-to-one relationship with the bipolar neurons of the secondary layer of retinal cells, they also have a one-to-one relationship with the neurons of the optic nerve (refer back to Figure 6–10). The arrangement of the cones with the secondary neurons provides for excellent *visual resolution*, the ability to distinguish between

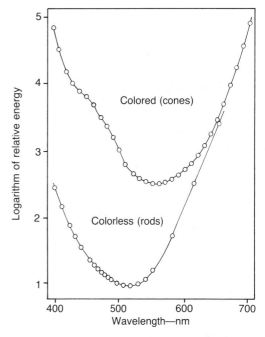

FIGURE 6–16
Relative sensitivity of rods and cones to different wavelengths of light. From S. Hecht and Y. Hsia, Dark Adaptation Following Light Adaptation to Red and White Lights, *J. Opt. Soc. Am.* 35(1945):262–267, fig. 2.

two points in space. The high density of the cones per unit area gives rise to the visual resolution necessary for the refined vision of the human species. This high density, as well as the one-to-one relationship of cones and bipolar neurons, enables humans to differentiate between two spots of light, as long as the spots fall on different cells of the retina.

The Visual Cycle

Chemical changes in the receptor cells of the retina result from stimulation by light and provide a mechanism of light reception, or vision. This cycle results in *bleaching* (breakdown) of the receptor pigment when light strikes the retina (see Figure 6–17). The result

FIGURE 6-17
The visual cycle as it occurs in the rods of the mammalian eye. From W. D. McElroy and B. Glass (eds.), *Light and Life* (Baltimore, Md., 1961). Reprinted by permission of Johns Hopkins University Press.

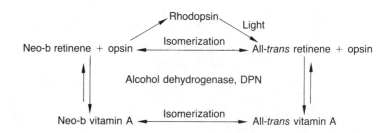

of the bleaching process is an increase in receptor membrane permeability and, ultimately, the formation of a generator potential. The sequence of chemical changes associated with this phenomenon was first described by Wald in 1954. The process is reversed in *dark adaptation*, when insufficient light is present to stimulate the rods and maximum quantities of rhodopsin are built up.

Examination of the rods has shown that rhodopsin absorbs light with the greatest efficiency at a wavelength of 510 nanometers, though it can respond to light at any wavelength between 400 and 620 nanometers. In mammals, there is great variation in the density of rods on the retina. Some mammals have pure rod eyes, whereas others have a mixture of rods and cones.

Color Vision

The ability to distinguish between different wavelengths of energy in the electromagnetic spectrum results in *color vision*. The primates are unique among mammals in this ability, though many nonprimate species are able to distinguish differently colored objects, apparently because of the different intensities of light reflected from them.

Long before pigments with different absorption characteristics were isolated, in the cones, a theory of color vision was devised based upon the supposed existence of different types of cones, or cones which respond to different wavelengths of light. This is known as the *tri-color theory*, or the *Young-Helmholtz theory of color vision*. The pigments of the cones are difficult to isolate, but analysis has been made by comparing the absorption of light by an intact cone with that of a cone in which the pigment has been removed by bleaching. As a result of these experiments, three different types of cones have been found in the primates, each having a different absorption spectra (see Figure 6-18). The three are characteristically called *red, green,* and *blue cones* because of the position of their absorption peaks. When an individual is exposed to monochromatic light at the absorption peaks of one of these cones, that individual sees red, green, or blue light. Other colors are generated as a combination of activities in more than one type of cone. True intermediate colors result from

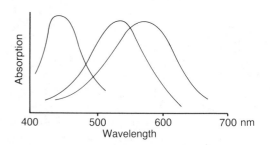

FIGURE 6-18
Absorption spectra of three cone pigments in the human retina. From C. R. Michael, Color Vision, *N. Engl. J. Med.* 288(1973):724, fig. 1. Reprinted by permission of the *New England Journal of Medicine*, 288:724, 1973.

integration in the central nervous system. White light results when all of the cones are stimulated simultaneously. Yellow monochromatic light (light of wavelength near 560 nanometers) is most obvious to the human eye simply because it stimulates some part of the absorption spectrum of each type of cone.

Binocular Vision and Depth Perception

The ability to see the three-dimensional form of an object requires a *triangulation process* which allows the subject to view an object from two different angles. When painting on a flat plane, depth perception can be simulated by allowing the viewer to see more than a single side of an object. Depth perception can be determined with one eye if the exact size of the object is known: comparison between the apparent size of a known object and its actual size gives clues about its distance from the observer. Such relationships provide another technique for artists to generate depth in a painting. Distant objects are simply reduced in size with reference to other figures in the painting. Another

method of determining depth perception with a single eye is to turn the head from side to side, so that two views of an object are presented to the brain (albeit at different times). This is neither as efficient nor as effective as the simultaneous viewing from different angles afforded by *binocular vision*, or vision with two eyes.

In the mammals, binocular vision has its greatest development in the primates. This adaptation is particularly necessary in arboreal mammals, since it is imperative that the distance between perches and branches be known. In humans, binocular vision allows for a multitude of finite and well-coordinated actions. Activities such as surgery, watchmaking, and various sports depend heavily on depth perception by the participants.

If a line is drawn through the center of each eye of an animal, in most species the two lines would meet behind the head to form an angle known as the *visual angle*. The visual angle is a useful tool as a means of comparison of binocular vision between species. Greater angles indicate more laterally positioned eyes and poorer binocular vision. The visual angles of several species are given in Figure 6–19. Note that in cats, most pri-

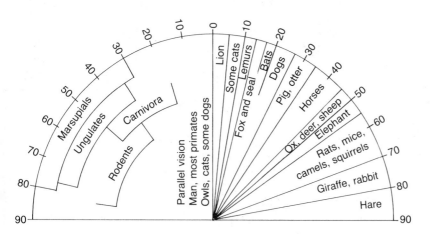

FIGURE 6–19
Visual angles calculated for several animal species. From *Vision in the Animal World* by R. H. Smythe. © 1975: R. H. Smythe and reprinted by permission of St. Martin's Press, Inc.

mates, and some dogs there is no angle. No angle indicates *parallel vision* and thus excellent positioning of the eyes for binocular vision. There is considerable variation in effective binocular vision among as well as within species, especially domesticated species. In dogs, for instance, such breeds as the Boston terrier and the Pekingese have reasonably good binocular vision because of the positioning of the eyes in the head. Many other breeds, such as the Great Dane and German shepherd, have eyes more laterally positioned, and the visual fields from the two eyes do not overlap except in a very narrow range some distance from the animal.

Clinical Disorders of the Eye

Myopia (nearsightedness) In some humans, the eyeball is longer than normal in its central axis, which causes the projected image to fall in front of the retina. In rarer cases, the lens is "too strong" (the curvature is greater than normal), which also results in the formation of an image in front of the retina. In myopia, if an object is near the eye, the image may fall on the retina; but as the object is moved farther away, the image moves in front of the retina, which results in an inability to see the object. For correction, a concave lens can be placed in front of the eye, causing the light rays to diverge and thus reducing the effective refractive power of the eye.

Hypermetropia (farsightedness) This condition can result from an eyeball which is too short or a lens system which is too weak when the ciliary muscle is completely relaxed. The result of either occurrence is the inability to form an image on the retina when the object is near the eye. Here, the image

falls behind the eye due to the curvature of the lens, the length of the eyeball, or both. Individuals with hypermetropia can frequently see distant objects quite well, because less refraction is needed in order to cause the image to fall on the retina. In order to view objects close to the eye, a biconcave lens can be used, aiding in normal light refraction and causing formation of the image in its proper place.

Cataracts and glaucoma A cataract is an opacity of the lens or its capsule. Because of the opacity of these structures, the light entering the eye which normally passes through the lens is reduced, so that only a degenerate image is formed. In severe cases no light can be transmitted to the retina. Glaucoma is another cause of blindness, especially in the elderly. In this disorder the fluid composing the aqueous humor accumulates more rapidly than it is returned to the blood through the *canal of Schlemm*. The resulting pressure restricts the flow of blood to the retina, which is progressively destroyed by anoxia.

THE PHYSIOLOGY OF SOUND RECEPTION

Sound is a neurological sensation resulting from stimulation of specialized receptors which respond to pressure changes in the surrounding medium. Sound received by mammals can be transmitted through air or water. These pressure changes, or the movement of *sound waves*, are analogous to the wave motion generated when a stone is tossed into a still body of water. If a stationary object is placed where the ripples are able to pass it, the number of ripples going by each second can be counted. This number constitutes a value of waves or ripples per second. Pressure pulses generated in air also follow the wave motion. The number of wave pulses per second, called the *frequency*, is measured as *cycles (hertz)* or *kilocycles (kilohertz)* per second, determined in much the same way as the counting of waves in water. Sound waves follow a pattern, with a trough or low point between each wave (see Figure 6–20). The distance between two pressure peaks constitutes the *wavelength* of sound. Sound always travels at the same speed under specific environmental conditions (i.e., same medium, same temperature). Thus, when the number of cycles per second is high the waves are short, and when the number of cycles per second is few the waves are long. As a result, one speaks of *high frequency* (high pitch) sound when the wavelength is short and low frequency (low pitch) sound when the wavelength is long.

Most sound is actually an accumulation of several frequencies. By very careful control one can generate pure pitch or a pure tone, but this is the exception rather than the rule. Sounds produced by animals and other sounds generated in the environment rarely if ever have pure pitch.

Anatomy of the Mammalian Ear

Although numerous modifications in ear structure exist among different species of mammals, the basic elements are approximately the same. The mammalian ear consists of three relatively distinct portions called the *external*, *middle*, and *inner ears* (see Figure 6–21). The external ear comprises the *pinna* and the *external auditory meatus*, which terminates at the *tympanum*, or ear drum. The middle ear is a cavity containing the tympanum and three distinct bones called *ossicles*. The outer or most lateral of the bones is the *malleus*, which connects the tympanum to the *incus*, the central of the three bones. The incus in turn articulates with the *stapes*, the most medial of the ossicles. The stapes, shaped like a stirrup, is positioned against the *oval window*, which is the opening into the inner ear. Two muscles are found in the middle ear. One is called the *tensor tympani* because it is inserted on the tympanum; and the other, which is attached to the stapes, is called the *stapedius*. When contracted, the two muscles tend to dampen sound-induced vibration of the ossicles.

The inner ear consists of the *cochlea* and the *vestibular apparatus*. The cochlea, spiral

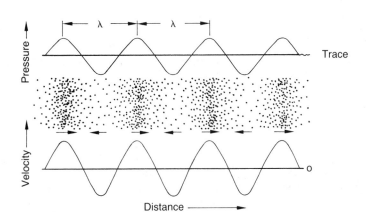

FIGURE 6–20
A diagrammatic depiction of sound waves. Lower figure shows crests and troughs represented by air molecules; pressure waves are graphed in the upper figure. From W. A. Van Bergeljk et al, *Waves and the Ear* (New York, N.Y., 1960). Reprinted by permission of Doubleday and Co.

FIGURE 6–21
Section through the human
ear showing external, middle
and inner portions. Middle ear
muscles have been omitted.

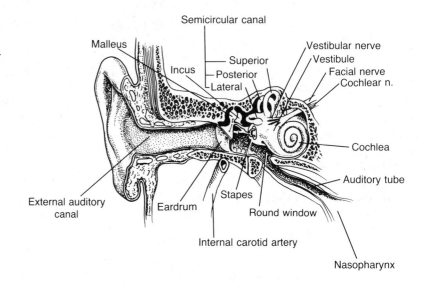

in shape, consists of essentially three tubes, which are separated by *Reissner's membrane* (or *vestibular membrane*) and the *basilar membrane*. The inner tube, called the *scala media*, houses the *organ of Corti* and is filled with a fluid called *endolymph* (see Figure 6–22). The outer tubes, called the *scala tympani* and the *scala vestibuli*, are filled with a fluid called *perilymph*. The scala vestibuli and the scala tympani are connected through a small opening called the *helicotrema* at the apex of the cochlea. The *organ of Corti*, which is poised on the surface of the basilar membrane, is innervated by the auditory branch of the eighth cranial nerve and consists of inner and outer rows of hair cells, which are embedded in the *tectorial membrane* lying above them (see Figure 6–23).

The vestibular apparatus contains three fluid-filled canals called the *semicircular canals*, which function in the detection of motion, and two round chambers called the *utricle* and the *saccule*, which function in the orientation of the body in space as well as in the detection of motion. Each semicircular

canal is oriented in a different direction: one horizontal (lateral) canal and two vertical canals at right angles to each other. One vertical canal lies in a posterior position, and the other lies in a superior position. Each semicircular canal has an enlarged portion at its base called the *ampulla*. A receptor organ called a *crista* is positioned inside each ampulla and is composed of hair cells which extend into its gelatinous portion called the *cupula* (see Figure 6–24). Because of inertia, the fluid of the semicircular canals does not move with the same speed as the rest of the body, causing the fluid to push against the cristae when the head is moved. Deformation of the hair cells in the cristae results in the formation of a generator potential. The movements of fluid in these canals enable the mammal to detect rate and direction of the body's movement with respect to the external environment.

The utricle and saccule contain tiny hair cells which extend toward the center of the chamber and support calcium carbonate concretions called *otoliths*. When a mam-

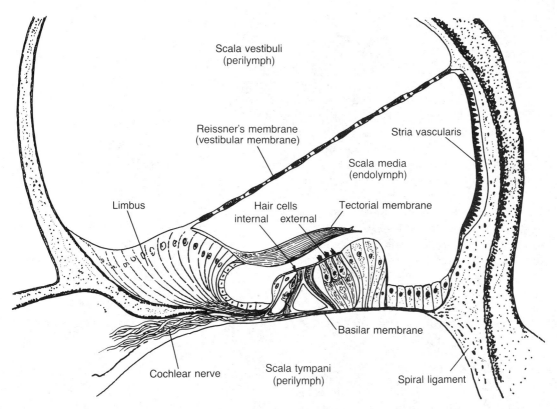

Scala vestibuli
(perilymph)

Reissner's membrane
(vestibular membrane)

Stria vascularis

Scala media
(endolymph)

Limbus

Hair cells
internal   external

Tectorial membrane

Basilar membrane

Cochlear nerve

Scala tympani
(perilymph)

Spiral ligament

FIGURE 6–22
Cross section through the cochlea of the guinea pig

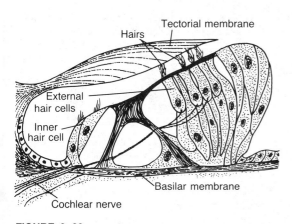

Tectorial membrane

Hairs

External
hair cells

Inner
hair cell

Basilar membrane

Cochlear nerve

FIGURE 6–23
The organ of Corti. Note relationship of the tectorial
membrane to the hairs projecting from the hair cells.

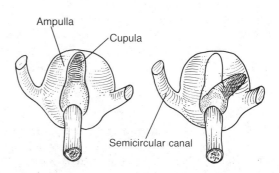

Ampulla

Cupula

Semicircular canal

FIGURE 6–24
Cross-sectional view of the crista showing position of the
cupula

mal's body is shifted in space, the position of the otoliths changes and different hair cells are stimulated. In this way, the mammal can monitor spatial orientation.

Information from the vestibular apparatus (which consists of the semicircular canals, utricle, and saccule) is transmitted by the VIII cranial (auditory) nerve through the vestibular ganglion to the vestibular nuclei, where information is carried to several important areas affecting motor control in the central nervous system (see Figure 6–25). The vestibular nuclei feed information directly to the muscles of posture and body orientation through the lateral and anterior vestibular spinal tracts. It also relays information to the cerebellum for integration with other input concerning body position from other areas of the body. The thalamus provides a second relay area for vestibular information transmitted to the cerebral cortex.

Mechanism of Sound Reception

The generation of sound waves in the environment can only be detected by animals which have specialized organs to receive them. In the mammal, sound waves are received by the outer ear, which directs sound into the external auditory meatus, where vibrations can be set up in the tympanum. These vibrations are transferred to the perilymph and then into the endolymph; they ultimately reach the organ of Corti. Sound initially causes the formation of generator potentials in the hair cells of the organ of Corti, which may result in action potentials in the auditory branch of the VIII cranial (auditory) nerve. Action potentials generated in the auditory nerves are transferred to opposite sides of the brain in much the same way as visual stimuli are transferred to opposite sides of the cortex through nerves crossing in the optic chiasma (see Figure 6–26).

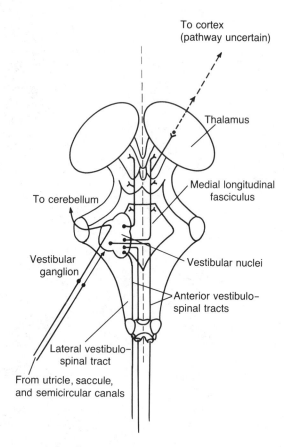

FIGURE 6–25
Information from the vestibular apparatus is transmitted to the vestibular nuclei, where the impulses travel to areas affecting motor control. Figure shows a dorsal view of the human brain with cerebellum and cerebral cortex removed. Reproduced, with permission, from Ganong, WF: *Review of Medical Physiology*, 9th ed. Copyright 1979 by Lange Medical Publications, Los Altos, California.

The middle ear in sound reception

Sound waves striking the tympanum cause it to oscillate at a frequency proportional to, but not identical to, the frequency of sound or pitch perceived by the animal. The *magnitude* of the tympanic vibrations is proportional to the magnitude (or loudness) of the sound. Vibrations are transferred from the

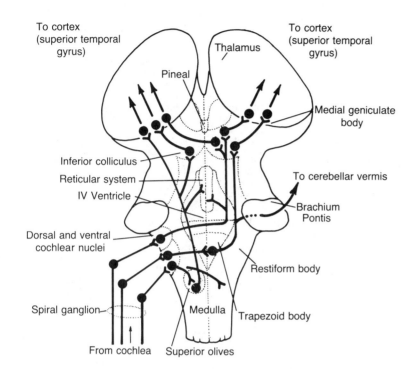

FIGURE 6–26
Auditory nerves cross to the opposite side of the brain, as shown in this simplified diagram of a dorsal view of the brain stem. Note that the cerebellum and cerebral cortex have been removed.

tympanum to the oval window of the cochlea through the vibrations of the ossicles. The function of the ossicles is twofold: they transduce sound waves into wave motion in the perilymph and then amplify the intensity of the sound waves which reach the tympanum.

Magnification of sound energy is proportional to the relative areas of the tympanum and the stapes where the latter encounters the oval window. In the human, the area of the tympanum is about 50 to 90 square millimeters, whereas the area of the stapes at the oval window is about 3.2 square millimeters. This relation provides a twenty- to thirty-fold amplification of sound from the tympanum to oval window. Any number of mechanical devices use the same principle: a force applied over a large area is transmitted to a smaller area and is thereby magnified. The knife and the splitting wedge are such devices, since each has a large area to which force is applied and a finer (sharper) surface of contact against the object to be cut or split. In some species the size of the *bulla*, the chamber surrounding the ossicles, appears to be of importance to hearing. Since the *eustachian tube*, the connection with the pharynx, is normally closed except when swallowing, the bulla acts as a closed system in most situations. It is thought by some that the greater the size of the chamber (as in such rodents as the geraboa and the kangaroo rat), the greater the sensitivity to sound, since greater oscillations of the tympanum and ossicles will occur if they are contained within a large chamber.

The inner ear in sound reception
Through a series of ingenious experiments, von Békésy was able to show that oscillation of the stapes at the oval window induced os-

SENSORY RECEPTION

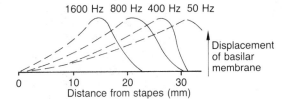

FIGURE 6–27
Displacement of the basilar membrane by the waves generated by the stapes. Vibration frequencies are shown at the top of each curve. From *Handbook of Experimental Psychology*, G. von Békésy and W. A. Rosenblith, S. S. Stevens, editor, copyright 1951, John Wiley and Sons, Inc. Reprinted by permission of John Wiley and Sons, Inc.

cillation of pressure waves in the perilymph and that subsequently the endolymph and basilar membrane were affected (see Figure 6–27). By altering the frequency of the stapedial oscillations, he discovered that various pressure waves reach a maximum at specific distances along the organ of Corti. High frequencies, those associated with high-pitched sounds, cause the wave to reach a maximum near the base of the cochlea, whereas low frequencies, those associated with low-pitched sounds, result in oscillations toward the apex of the cochlea. To substantiate the theory that a pure sound has a specific point on the basilar membrane at which maximum deflection occurs, von Békésy placed silver particles inside the cochlea and observed their movements when the stapes was mechanically oscillated. It was later shown that the reception of a particular pitch can be obliterated by selectively destroying the hair cells at appropriate points along the basilar membrane.

Generator potentials recorded from the neurons of the basilar membrane indicate that the greatest electrical activity occurs at the position of greatest deflection of the basilar membrane. As a result, it would appear that the oscillations caused by movement of the stapes result in deflection of the basilar membrane. When hair cells of the organ of Corti are deflected, the agitation between the hair cells and the tectorial membrane results in the formation of a generator potential. The animal perceives a particular pitch due to the point of maximum stimulation of the hair cells on the basilar membrane. Many hair cells are stimulated with each unit of sound; but with slightly different sounds, slightly different numbers of hair cells are stimulated. Thus, different frequencies induce selective stimulation of hair cells and thus can be distinguished on the basis of the specific hair cells activated.

The magnitude of sound discrimination

The human ear has received a great deal of attention because of the importance of the sense of hearing. The normal unhindered human ear can respond over a frequency range (pitch) of 20 to 40 kilohertz (KHz). But the different pitches are not all observed with the same facility. Therefore, many of the sounds must be very intense to be heard by the human ear, whereas others are heard only when a light intensity is used. An *audiogram* is a graph which expresses the perception of frequency as a function of intensity (see Figure 6–28). One *dyne*, the force necessary to accelerate a gram of mass one centimeter per second, is the typical measurement of sound intensity and is equal to zero decibels. The dyne is a pressure measurement, whereas the *decibel* is a logarithmic function based on a relative scale of intensity of sensation. Notice in Figure 6–28 that certain frequencies are much more audible and require less energy for stimulation than others.

The sound which is able to stimulate the mammalian ear varies considerably with species (see Figure 6–29). "Silent" dog whistles

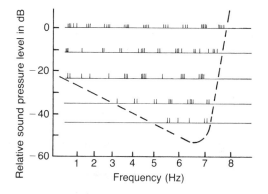

FIGURE 6–28
Responses of a single auditory nerve fiber of a guinea
pig to tones of different frequencies and intensities. A
similar curve is constructed when preparing a human
audiogram. From I. Tasaki, Nerve Impulses in Individual
Auditory Nerve Fibers of Guinea Pig., *J. Neurophysiol.*
17(1954):97–122. Reprinted by permission of the American Physiological Society, Bethesda, Md.

are sound generators that produce very intense sound but at frequencies to which human ears do not respond. Most dogs hear
over a range of 30 to 40 KHz, whereas bats,
which are exceptionally well known for their
hearing ability, can respond to sounds of up

to 200 KHz. Cats can hear frequencies of
sound as high as 50 KHz, and cetaceans,
which also utilize a type of sonar echolocation for navigation, can hear sounds whose
frequencies reach 150 KHz. As a general rule,
smaller mammals are more able to hear frequencies of higher pitch than are larger
mammals (excluding the forementioned adaptations). Animals with a very wide range of
pitch discrimination usually have longer basilar membranes, which provide better spatial
separation of wave motions generated by different sound frequencies in the endolymph.

Echolocation

Many mammals navigate in situations where
visibility is for all practical purposes impossible. Bats negotiate flight inside caverns in
total darkness and avoid hitting both the
walls of the cave and one another. They are
capable of detecting wire of only 0.3 millimeters in diameter strung in a meshwork
throughout a room. In addition, the insectivorous bats are able to collect small insect

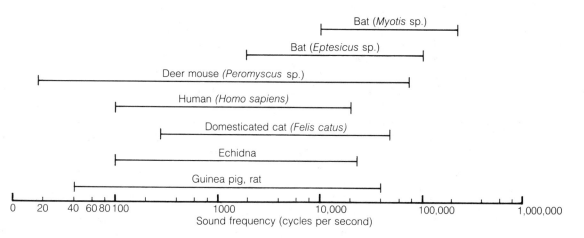

FIGURE 6–29
Sound frequency spectrum for several mammalian species

prey in complete darkness. The eyes of the "blind" river dolphin *(Platonista gangelica)* are small and lack lenses. Vision in these animals is very poor. In addition, its native habitat is limited to several muddy rivers of India and Parkistan where visibility is extremely restricted due to large concentrations of sediment. Even so, the river dolphin can swim rapidly in these waters, navigate, and survive without the predominant use of vision.

A great deal of work has been done concerning *echolocation,* or navigation by means of *self-generated sound* (a sonar mechanism), which is reflected from objects in the animal's environment. Lazaro Spallanzani performed experiments in 1793 which suggested that bats could navigate by means of such acoustical perception. It was not until much later that the work of Griffin and others during the 1940s bore this out. Such navigation is frequently quite complex and involves some very refined physiological mechanisms. Animals which navigate by echolocation produce intense sound impulses, usually undetected by the human ear because of their high pitch. The intensity of sound produced by bats, for example, can be as high as 200 dynes per square centimeter when recorded 5.0 centimeters from the bat's mouth. It is fortunate that human ears do not respond to the high frequencies produced by bats, because these frequencies would be very noticeable and perhaps hazardous. Not all bats emit such strong signals, however. Those bats that belong to the families Megadermatidae and Phyllostomatidae produce a sound of only one dyne per square centimeter when recorded 5.0 centimeters from the bat's mouth.

With such intense sounds being emitted, how then do bats withstand their own noises? The two muscles of the middle ear, the tensor tympani and the stapedius, dampen the oscillations of the bones of the middle ear by increasing muscle rigidity just before a sound pulse is emitted. Contraction of the tensor tympani increases the tension of the tympanic membrane; contraction of the stapedius muscle changes the angle at which the stapes contacts the oval window. A more acute angle of interface between the stapes and the oval window reduces the area of contact and thus lessens the force which can be exchanged between the stapes and the perilymph. The muscles apparently relax at the end of the sound pulse, and thus the reverberating sound can be easily detected.

Of interest in the echolocation of bats is their ability to increase the number of sound pulses, called *clicks* by some observers because that part of the pulse is audible to humans, as the prey is approached. The more rapid the rate of sound pulses, the greater the ability of the bat to follow an insect in flight. In some instances the sound pulses may be as short as one millisecond, and they may be emitted at a rate of 200 per second. Pulse production in the cetaceans follows a pattern somewhat similar to the sequence of clicks seen in bats. As the animal approaches an object of interest, the clicks become more frequent and can reach 70 to 80 per second in the Amazon dolphin *(Inia geoffrensis).*

Wavelength is very critical in echolocation. Smaller wavelengths (i.e., higher frequencies of sound) allow the animal to detect very small objects and impart better sonar resolution to the animal which uses it. As stated earlier, bats can detect wires only 0.3 millimeters in diameter. Experiments with bats indicate they can detect objects as small as one-tenth the length of a single sound wave. Other species, such as the dolphins, can discriminate between spheres which differ in diameter by ten percent and can avoid metal wires as thin as 0.2 millimeters in diameter. These mammals are able to resolve objects in their environment by the use of sound of a very high frequency.

Echolocation, a fairly widespread phenomenon, has been well documented in most bats, some insectivores, pinnipeds, and odontocete cetaceans; it is suspected in other mammals as well. Echolocation is best developed in bats and in such aquatic mammals as cetaceans and pinnipeds that are nocturnal or dive in water penetrated by little light or swim in murky water where vision is limited. Echolocation may be used by other mammals which navigate in murky or deep water. Perhaps freshwater species such as beavers and muskrats employ some navigation of this type.

Whales are interesting because of their ability to dive to great depths and endure tremendous hydrostatic pressure on their ears. The problem is overcome in several ways. First, the external auditory meatus is filled with wax in some whale species and reduced in size or covered with skin in others. Second, the tympanic bullae in cetaceans are not fused to the skull and are insulated by a system of unique sinuses. The sinuses are filled with an oil medium which apparently protects the sound detecting system from compression. It has been suggested by some investigators that cetaceans utilize the lower jaw as a collector of high frequency sounds, which can then be transferred to the inner ear and thus avoid the action of the ossicles altogether.

Although the sounds produced by cetaceans can be readily measured and described, their origin is an enigma. Porpoises, dolphins, and toothed whales lack vocal cords altogether but still are able to produce sounds in an extremely well-regulated fashion. Sound in these animals may be produced in some way by the muscular nasal plugs associated with the blowhole, though there are a variety of anatomical characteristics inherent to the blowhole that perhaps produce the required sound.

The blind river dolphin presents an interesting example of echolocation. It swims on its side with the lateral fin maintained only two to three centimeters from the bottom of the river. The pulses emitted from this mammal are concentrated in a projected angle which covers no more than ten degrees. This animal has a domed head (as do many dolphins) called the *melon*, which is supported by highly developed extensions from the maxillary bones. The sound produced through the blowhole is thought to be concentrated by the melon into a narrow beam. As the animal swims on its side, the head moves back and forth in a plane lateral to the river bottom and in this way sweeps the murky waters with a well-regulated locating device.

Several of the seals are also believed to echolocate, though a knowledge of the mechanisms and attributes of echolocation in these animals is rather limited. It is known that the Weddell seal (*Leptonycholis weddelli*) emits a sound of 30 KHz in frequency and can apparently find breather holes in the arctic ice by means of echolocation.

The shrews echolocate and emit sounds in the neighborhood of 50 KHz. There are also some cases on record of echolocation in humans, and humans have been able to use clicking devices to generate sound pulses that can be detected when reflected from objects in their environment. Additional research can still produce quite fruitful results in this area.

THE CHEMICAL SENSES: SMELL AND TASTE

The specialized senses in animals probably originated when primitive organisms began responding to the dissolved chemicals in the surrounding environment. Both protozoa and bacteria show strong *chemotactic responses* when exposed to certain chemicals. Even free-moving cells such as the white blood cells of mammals show a response to dissolved substances in their environment and migrate toward wounds or infections as a result of chemical attractants that may be liberated at the site of trauma.

The ability of the chemical senses, particularly smell, to evoke emotions and behavioral displays is a familiar phenomenon in a variety of mammalian species. Taste is closely related to the sense of smell chemically but is actually quite distinct neurologically, since entirely different portions of the brain are involved. But differentiation between taste and smell is extremely difficult in aquatic mammals because both senses are evoked by specific chemicals dissolved in the surrounding medium. In terrestrial mammals the two are more easily distinguished: smell involves transfer of chemicals through the atmosphere and taste results from stimulation by chemicals taken in as food.

Taste and smell probably evolved as different processes for entirely different reasons. The sense of smell evokes a *preparatory response* for things to come and probably conjures up physiological responses based upon previous experience. Thus, the smell of a particular food might evoke a variety of behavioral patterns in mammals and induce salivation and gastric action usually associated with the intake of food. Taste, on the other hand, is a sensation which describes an ongoing process, the process of food consumption, and is a sensation associated with fulfillment rather than anticipation. Thus, taste could be expected in some way to be associated with the sensation of satiety.

Smell

The olfactory powers of many domesticated mammals are well known. Hunting dogs rely on their olfactory ability to follow selected quarry. The use of bloodhounds for locating missing persons is probably the best example of profitable use of the mammalian ability to detect specific chemicals by smell. Olfactory senses of many species have been put to beneficial use. Both pigs and hounds have been used to locate truffles, a fungus which grows underground and leaves no visual clue as to its whereabouts. In one case in Britain, it was reported that a sow was taught to point and retrieve birds and was as effective as a dog in the field. This animal probably used olfactory cues to locate downed birds and retrieve them for her master. More recently, dogs have been trained to locate explosives and drugs by smell. In most cases these animals are responding to chemicals whose concentrations are so low as to be almost undetectable by modern analytical means.

Actions resulting from olfaction Many physiological changes occur as the result of olfactory cues given off by mammals. A variety of behavioral patterns in mammals are also evoked by smell, sometimes from great distances. In cattle, bulls become sexually aroused when exposed to vaginal odors emanating from females in estrus. In elk, the dominant male is thought to display physiological preparedness for breeding through odors emanating from his urine. In the rhesus monkey, the smell of vaginal secretions of the female during the time of ovulation promotes sexual excitement and copulatory behavior in the male. In ungulates, testosterone secretion in males is promoted by the odor of a female in heat.

Domesticated cows recognize their newborn calves purely by odor. Sometimes when the odor of an orphaned calf is masked by a strong aerosol perfume it will be more readily accepted by a foster mother. In herding species, odors can alert the entire group of animals to impending danger. Some species, such as the peccary *(Tayassu tajacu)*, when frightened give off a strong odor from a scent gland located in the skin of the back. This odor acts to alert the rest of the herd and prepares them for escape. Horses, also herd animals, are naturally frightened by the smell of blood. These animals will usually not readily approach a recently killed animal. This seems to be a reaction to the smell of blood and can be easily eliminated by applying menthol to the olfactory sensory areas.

Physiological mechanisms of olfaction

Olfaction results from the generation of action potentials in the *olfactory nerve* when compounds come in contact with the *terminal cilia* of the *olfactory fibers* (see Figure 6–30). The receptor cells extend through the *cribiform plate*, where they are exposed to the nasal cavity and synapse with cells of the olfactory tract, which carry information to the central nervous system.

Substances belonging to a family of compounds frequently give rise to entirely different odors. Yet substances with quite different molecular structures may produce identical odors. The most promising theory explaining the functional mechanism of the sense of smell is founded upon the premise that each compound has a characteristic *steric config-*

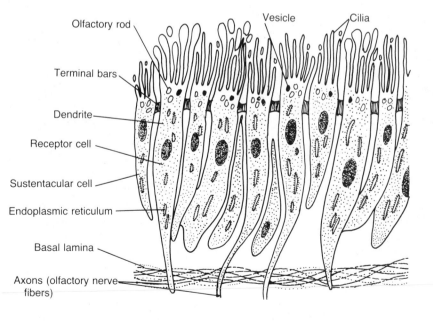

Olfactory rod
Vesicle
Cilia
Terminal bars
Dendrite
Receptor cell
Sustentacular cell
Endoplasmic reticulum
Basal lamina
Axons (olfactory nerve fibers)

FIGURE 6–30
Structure of the olfactory receptors. Note terminal cilia.

uration recognized by receptor sites on the *olfactory epithelium*. This theory implies that the receptor cells of the *olfactory mucosa* have specific sites where molecules can become trapped. But no entrapment occurs unless there is a perfect fit between the molecular structure of the potentially odorous substance and the "trap" on the surface of the receptor cell. In this way olfactory stimulation is brought about in the same fashion as the lock and key relationship seen in enyzme-substrate reactions (see Figure 6–31). Both the shape of the molecule and the charge distribution on its surface probably affect the molecule's compatability with the relevant sites on the olfactory receptors. Other properties of the molecule, such as volatility and solubility in the mucous membranes of the olfactory epithelium, could also be involved.

Of interest here is the connection between the central nervous system and the olfactory

FIGURE 6–31
Lock and key relationship of odorous substances with olfactory epithelium. Figures on left and center represent odorous substances. Olfactory epithelium is represented on the right. From J. E. Amoore, Elucidation of the Stereo Chemical Properties of the Olfactory Receptor Sites, *CTFA Proc. Sci. Sect., Spec. Suppl.* 37(1962):1–20. Reprinted with the permission of CTFA, the Cosmetic, Toiletry and Fragrance Association, Washington, D.C.

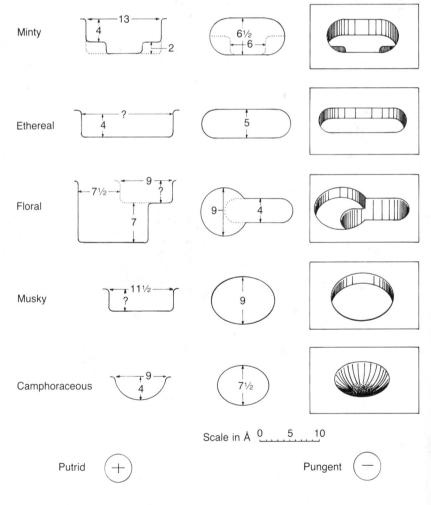

nerves. The limbic system of the brain of modern mammals has evolved from the *rhinencephalon*, or small brain, of primitive vertebrates. This provides a probable relationship between olfaction and the emotions, which are seated in the limbic system. The role of olfaction in emotions is well known. In many cases odors are known to incite mammals to sexual arousal, fear, or hunger. One of the obvious functions in this relationship is seen in the *pheromones*, airborne substances produced by one member of a species to evoke a hormonelike effect in another. Olfaction may well be the source of the numerous subliminal stimuli that affect humans as well as other species on a regular basis.

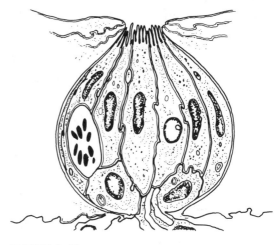

FIGURE 6–32
Vertical section through taste bud of a rabbit

Taste

In terrestrial vertebrates taste becomes a very distinct sensation quite different from the olfactory senses. The receptors for taste in mammals are short-lived cells which usually survive for ten days or less. They are generally of the *phasic-tonic type* (i.e., they induce a burst of spikes followed by spikes of slower frequency that are sustained for the duration of the stimulus). These receptors have a short burst of intense activity followed by a phase of relatively subdued activity. They are grouped into units called *taste buds* and are usually uniform in that they contain cells responding to a specific taste modality (see Figure 6–32).

In the human, four basic taste modalities are recognized: sour, sweet, bitter, and salt. The *sweet sensation* appears to be associated primarily with carbohydrates and alcohols. The *salt sensation* is induced primarily by sodium chloride but can also be induced by other compounds, such as potassium chloride, ammonium chloride, sodium bromate,

sodium fluoride, and calcium chloride. Some variation from the "pure" salt taste is also noticed with any of the other compounds. The *sour sensation* is caused by hydrogen ions and is usually evoked by weak acids. The *bitter sensation* is not as clearly defined as the other tastes; the standard for its modality is quinine. A number of other substances are known to produce bitter sensations with results somewhat comparable to that of quinine. In humans the taste buds for bitter sensations are located near the back of the tongue, with the tip of the tongue containing sweet receptors and the sides containing sour receptors. The taste buds for salt seem to be uniformly distributed among the other taste buds. But no particular area is exclusive for a particular taste because there is some degree of mixing of the basic tastes in all of the areas.

The number of sensations which can be demonstrated in species other than humans is difficult to describe. Some species, cats for instance, appear not to have sweet receptors.

Dogs can taste sugars but do not respond to saccharine. Many mammals, excluding humans, have receptors sensitive to distilled water. Little is known about the sensations of taste or about the substances which induce them. Specific tastes probably differ among individuals of a species, though little data has been accumulated on this point. Also within the realm of probability is that certain tastes could be modified by previous experience and training. Again, little evidence has been acquired to give logical conclusions to this question.

Physiological mechanisms of taste The cells of the taste buds act as receptors for chemicals dissolved in the solution which bathes them. The exact mechanism by which these receptors are stimulated is still unknown, but it is known that these cells have the typical charge distribution about their membranes, are negatively charged inside, and have an external positive charge. It is believed that when the taste cells are stimulated, the chemical tasted becomes loosely bound to a protein on the surface of the cell. This binding alters the relative distribution of charges on the membrane surface, which in turn allows sodium penetration. Consequently, a generator potential is produced. The binding between the chemical substance tasted and the protein of the cell membrane is weak, and the taste can be removed by washing with distilled water.

The nerve fibers which innervate the taste buds are enveloped by the membrane of the taste cells. In some as yet undetermined way the generator potentials of the receptor cells are transferred to the nerve fibers which innervate them. As long as the taste substance is in place, the generator potential is maintained. But the innervating neurons show an initial burst of activity followed by adaptation to a less frequent but constant level of firing.

SUMMARY

The sensory receptors give input to the central nervous system about the external and internal environment. It is in the central nervous system that the stimuli are both identified and quantified. Many types of receptors are located throughout the body, whereas others are collected into distinct sensory organs. All sensory receptors are adapted to specific modalities of stimuli (the law of specific nerve energies), and the intensity of the sensations perceived are a function of the common logarithm of the intensity of the stimulus (Weber-Fechner law).

In mammals the eye is a specialized organ which allows light to be focused on the retinal cells, the result of which is image formation. The retina comprises three layers of neurons. The primary layer may contain two different types of cells, called rods and cones. Some species have only rods, which endows them with excellent night vision. But most mammals, like the primates, have a mixture of rods and cones in the retina. The secondary and tertiary layers of neurons transmit impulses from the rods and cones to the brain, where they are interpreted.

The receptor cells of the retina contain pigments which absorb light. The process of light absorption produces generator potentials, which cause impulses to be carried to the brain by the optic nerve. The rods, the principal cells in nocturnal mammals, contain a pigment called rhodopsin. The cones, characteristically used in day vision, contain one of three different pigments, giving rise to three different types of cones based upon the specific pigment present. These cone types are red, green, and blue. The maximum absorption peak of the pigment contained in the cone denotes its color designation.

Light rays converge to form an image on the retina. Convergence of light is the result of refraction by the cornea and lens. The cornea provides a fixed curvature, whereas the lens in most species can change shapes in order to accommodate. Some species lack the ability to alter lens curvature and accomplish accommodation by changing the position of the head and thus the angle through which light strikes the retina. Present in these species is a ramp retina, one that lacks spherical curvature. By moving the eye, the distance from the lens to the retina in the focal axis can be changed.

Binocular vision is, to some extent, characteristic of most mammals. Its development is dependent upon the position of the eyes in the head. Humans and most other primates have excellent depth perception because both eyes are directed straight ahead in parallel fashion.

Sound is the sensation generated as the result of reception of pressure waves carried through water or air. Sound is both a common mode of communication and a means of navigation in mammals. Sound waves oscillate in characteristic frequencies, which are detected by mammals as pitch. Sound rarely occurs as pure frequency but is usually a mixture containing many different wavelengths.

Sound is received by the mammalian ear, which consists of three distinct portions called the external, middle, and inner ears. The external ear functions to funnel sound into the middle ear. The middle ear contains three bones, or ossicles, which amplify the pressure waves and cause vibration of the tympanum. The inner ear consists of the cochlea, the semicircular canals, the utricle, and the saccule. The semicircular canals function as organs for reception of body motion, whereas the utricle and saccule function primarily in the detection of body position. The cochlea contains the organ of Corti, which consists of hair cells and the tectorial membrane. When vibrations of the stapes set up pressure waves in the cochlea, specific hair cells on the organ of Corti are stimulated as a result of their shearing force on the tectorial membrane. Sounds of different pitch activate different hair cells, with high-pitched sounds having their greatest activity near the oval window and low-pitched sounds affecting hair cells near the apex of the cochlea.

Most mammals are able to hear a wide variety of sound frequencies, though a great deal of variation exists among species in their ability to detect specific frequencies. Animals which utilize sound as a detection or sonar device can hear and emit sounds as high as 150 KHz or higher.

Echolocation is a widely observed navigational technique employed by seals, whales, bats, and other mammals. It is very well developed in bats, with almost all species using this technique for navigation and feeding. Bats not only emit high frequency sounds but also produce sounds of phenomenal intensity, which gives them excellent ability to echolocate very small objects at a distance.

Both taste and smell provide mammals with a means of detection of chemicals in their environment. In terrestrial animals the sensation of smell is induced by airborne chemicals, whereas taste is caused by dissolved substances which bathe the sensory cells. Many substances are known to induce the sensation of smell, and it is believed that distinct odors are differentiated as a result of their geometric as well as electrical configurations. Odors are responsible for many behavioral as well as physiological responses in mammals.

Taste sensations are limited to fewer specific modalities than those producing the sensation of smell. The basic taste observed in humans arises from stimulation of cells located in units known as taste buds. All taste buds are not capable of responding to all of the specific taste modalities, and certain portions of the tongue contain groups of taste buds which respond primarily to one type of substance. The specific taste modalities of humans are salt, sweet, sour, and bitter, though considerable variation can be found in other species.

The physiological mechanism for taste reception is unknown. It is thought that specific proteins in the membranes of the taste cells become loosely bound to dissolved chemicals. Binding alters the charge distribution at the surface of the cells and hence induces a generator potential and, subsequently, an action potential, which relays the information to the central nervous system.

7

THE PHYSIOLOGY
OF MUSCLES

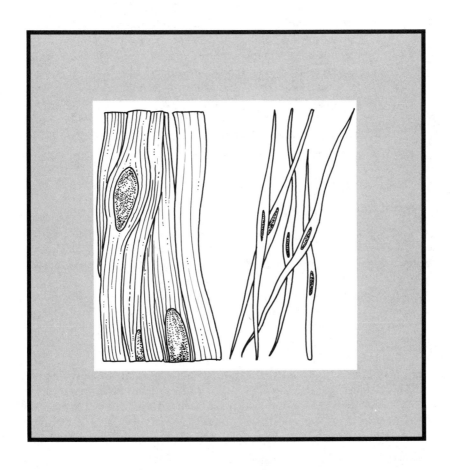

In mammals, muscles make up the largest portion of the body mass and provide most of the heat for maintenance of body temperature. Muscle contractions are responsible for body movement, for the propulsion of such fluids as blood and chyme within the body, and for the control of the direction and flow of peripheral blood, lymph, and other body fluids.

There are three basic types of muscles in mammals, named primarily for their appearance and location: skeletal muscle, cardiac muscle, and smooth muscle. *Skeletal muscle, the best known and most widely understood muscle type, is striated in appearance and is generally attached to the skeleton. The principal functions of skeletal muscle are in voluntary movement and heat production. Cardiac (heart) muscle is also striated in appearance, but it can easily be distinguished from skeletal muscle by the presence of membranes interdigitated between adjacent cells, called* intercalated discs. *Smooth muscle surrounds cavities in the body, such as the gastrointestinal tract, major arteries and veins, and the uterus. It is usually found in two layers: an outer, longitudinally oriented layer which causes shortening of the cavity; and an inner, concentrically oriented layer which causes constriction. Smooth muscle also forms most of the valves within blood vessels and intestines. Regardless of the type of muscle, individual muscle cells are known as* fibers.

In this chapter we will discuss skeletal muscle in detail, from both a structural and functional view. Cardiac and smooth muscle will be described at the cellular level.

SKELETAL MUSCLE

Skeletal muscles are composed of individual, multinucleated fibers. The fibers are arranged in parallel, and thus the force of contraction of each cell is additive. The fibers of a muscle are grouped together, and several fibers may be innervated by a single motor neuron. A motor neuron and all of the fibers it innervates is called a *motor unit.* Based on the duration of muscle contraction and the rate of conduction of the motor neuron, a motor unit can be classified as *fast* (phasic) or *slow* (tonic). Most skeletal muscles contain a mixture of fast and slow units. Muscles that contain a predominance of fast units are referred to as *fast muscles.* Because of their pale color, fast muscles are sometimes called *white muscles.* Fast muscles have a relative lack of the pigment *myoglobin,* which results in the lighter color.

Muscles that contain a predominance of slow units are called *slow muscles.* Slow muscles, usually darker in color, are also called *red muscles.* This darker color is due to their rich supply of myoglobin. Red muscles are adapted to activities that require endurance. They have more mitochondria and mitochondrial enzymes than do white muscles, which are capable of bursts of contraction but fatigue easily. Muscles of the back, which are primarily used for posture, are usually red muscles; whereas the *extraocular muscles* around the eyeball and the muscles of the hand are of the white variety. Most muscles of the body are a mixture of both white and red units.

The degree to which fast and slow units are distributed within a muscle varies with the species. Mammals with great endurance usually have muscles with greater quantities of slow units than do mammals that move with a burst of speed but tire rapidly. Many of the canids, such as the wolf, are able to search for prey for prolonged periods of time at a slow lope. Such animals have an abundance of red muscle. Members of the cat family (Felidae) are capable of short but intense bursts of speed. Their muscles are predominantly of the white type.

The difference between fast and slow muscle units can be altered through *cross innervation*. In other words, if the nerve from a fast muscle is transferred to a slow muscle and allowed to regenerate, the slow muscle becomes fast. The reverse is also possible. The effect of the nerve in changing the muscle is apparently caused by the pattern of its discharge.

In many cases, conditioning muscles for endurance are associated with the intracellular storage of energy-rich compounds and myoglobin. Further, it has been shown that exercise not only increases the amount of stored metabolites and contractile protein but also induces changes in the number of muscle fibers. When cats are taught to exercise for food, for instance, there is an increase in the number of muscle fibers in the *flexor carpi radialis*. Such evidence indicates that an increase in muscle fiber number with exercise might be possible in other mammals and has great significance for situations in which muscle fiber numbers are reduced by disease or inactivity. The type of fiber produced in this way is not clear, and development may possibly be governed by the type of exercise performed.

Connective Tissue

Muscles, as well as other organs of the body, are covered by fibrous connective tissue termed *fascia*, which provides protection as well as support for blood vessels, lymphatics, and nerves. The fascia are quite variable in thickness and can be divided into three types depending on their nature and position in the body. The *superficial fascia*, or *subcutaneous layer*, lies immediately below the skin and covers the entire body. It is variable in thickness and usually contains adipose cells and numerous blood vessels. The *deep fascia* is distinct in both structure and function. It is composed of dense connective tissue and does not contain fat. It serves an important function in holding muscles together and separates them into functional groups. The *subserous fascia*, of much less importance to the musculature of mammals, serves primarily as a lining of the thoracic and abdominal cavities and the external surfaces of the viscera.

Muscles are covered and strengthened by heavy layers of deep fascia sometimes called the *epimysium*, which are arranged so that they bind together specific muscle bundles and connect muscle cells to other structures such as blood vessels and nerves (see Figure 7–1). Muscles are divided internally by extensions of the epimysium called the *perimysium*. The perimysium provides a flexible framework whereby nerve and blood vessel connections are secured in position within the muscle. Each muscle fiber is isolated from the adjoining muscle fibers by extensions of the perimysium called the *endomy-*

FIGURE 7–1
Section of skeletal muscle showing the relation of connective tissue to contractile fibers

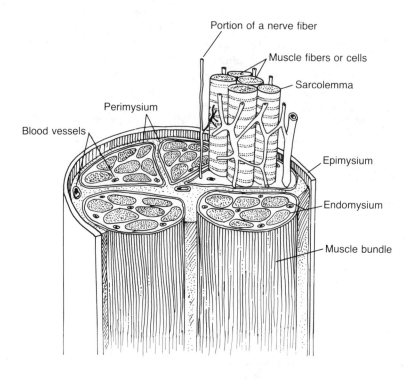

sium. Through these somewhat tough layers of connective tissue each muscle is secured in its internal arrangements and maintained as an integrated unit. In skeletal muscle these layers of connective tissue are extended beyond the muscle cell and are collated into units for attachment to the *periosteum* of the bones. Hence these extensions compose the connecting elements known as *tendons* and serve as the mechanical device for transferring the force of contraction to the skeleton (see Figure 7–2).

Muscle Fiber Structure

Each skeletal muscle cell consists of longitudinally oriented strands called *myofibrils*, which are composed of *sarcomeres* connected end to end. Each muscle cell within a muscle is innervated by a motor neuron and has connections with the circulatory system. These connections are stabilized in position by the perimysium.

The muscle fiber is surrounded by a membrane called the *sarcolemma*, which is intimately associated with each sarcomere by small tubules that penetrate the fiber at an angle transverse to its length. These *transverse tubules*, or *T-tubules*, terminate near the *sarcoplasmic reticulum* (see Figure 7–3). The sarcoplasmic reticulum forms cavernous structures adjacent to the tubules called the *terminal cisternae*. The terminal cisternae along with the T-tubules are referred to as the *triad*.

The basic contractile unit of the muscle is the sarcomere, which is composed of proteins arranged to form two types of filaments,

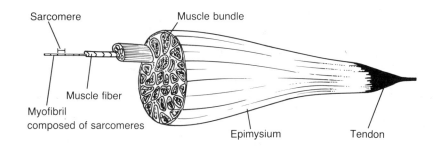

Sarcomere

Muscle bundle

Muscle fiber

Myofibril
composed of sarcomeres

Epimysium

Tendon

FIGURE 7–2
Relationship of the sarcomere
to the myofibril, muscle fiber,
and bundles of fibers. Note
the formation of the tendon at
the end of the muscle.

FIGURE 7–3
A muscle cell. The sarco-
meres are shown in relation
to the transverse tubules and
the sarcoplasmic reticulum.

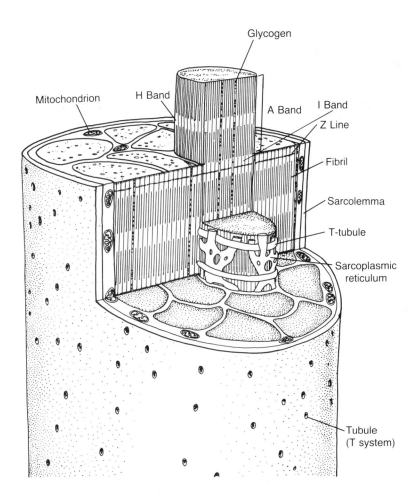

Glycogen

Mitochondrion

H Band

A Band

I Band

Z Line

Fibril

Sarcolemma

T-tubule

Sarcoplasmic
reticulum

Tubule
(T system)

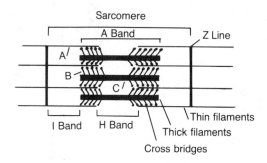

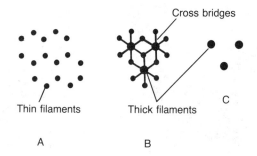

FIGURE 7–4
The sarcomere showing the interrelationship of the filaments. Lower diagrams represent cross sectional areas of the sarcomere (A, cross section through the I band; B, cross section through the A band; and, C, cross section through the H band).

called the *thick* and *thin filaments* (see Figure 7–4). They are named for their characteristic structure as revealed by electron micrographs. Each sarcomere terminates at the *Z lines,* to which are attached several thin filaments extending inward toward the center of the sarcomere. The thin filaments, more numerous than the thick filaments, form a hexagonal arrangement around the thick filaments when viewed in cross section.

The sarcomere is arbitrarily divided into several regions based upon the positions of the thick and thin filaments. The area where there are no thick filaments, at each end of the sarcomere, is called the *I band*. This term is derived from the band's *isotropic,* or clear, characteristic. In the middle of the sarcomere, thick and thin filaments overlap to form a dense area that does not allow light to pass through easily. This region is called the *A band* because of its *anisotropic* nature. In the center of the A band is another distinct area, devoid of thin filaments, termed the *H band.*

The Myoneural Junction

The normal mode of excitation of skeletal muscle involves the formation of an action potential on the sarcolemma. This is induced at the junction of the muscle membrane and the motor nerve. The terminal branches of the motor axon, free of myelin, are intimately aligned with the sarcolemma at specific sites known as *motor end-plates.* This arrangement, the *myoneural junction,* allows for a large area of contact between the two membranes (see Figure 7–5). At the myoneural junction the sarcolemma forms a number of convoluted ridges, which essentially increase the surface area for connection with the motor fiber membrane. Although closely interdigitated, the muscle and nerve fibers retain the integrity of their respective membranes, which are separated by a distinct space or synaptic cleft of twenty to sixty nanometers.

The terminal button of the axon membrane contains numerous *synaptic vesicles,* of some fifty nanometers in diameter, which are positioned near the synaptic junction. In mammals these vesicles contain acetylcholine which, when released, diffuses across the synaptic cleft and binds to the specific acetylcholine receptor sites on the surface of the sarcolemma. Acetylcholinesterase, the enzyme which catabolizes acetylcholine, is in abundance on the postsynaptic membrane near the motor end-plate.

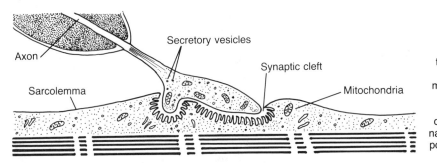

FIGURE 7–5
The myoneural junction. An increased surface area for contact is made possible through an irregular relationship of adjacent nerve and muscle membranes. The motor end-plate is part of the motor nerve, which consists of the branching nerve terminals which make up the nerve portion of the myoneural junction.

Myoneural Activity

Excitation of the presynaptic motor neuron causes the release of acetylcholine, which is able to traverse the synaptic cleft and induce ion-specific changes in permeability of the sarcolemma. When acetylcholine is added to the sarcolemma at sites other than the motor end-plate, no reaction occurs. This indicates that the region of the sarcolemma at the motor end-plate has specific receptor sites for acetylcholine not present on the remainder of the sarcolemma. At the motor end-plate a series of diffusion reactions occur in a way quite similar to the diffusion previously discussed at the nerve-nerve synapse. Sodium ions diffuse through the cell membrane along their concentration gradient and in a direct relationship with the electrical gradient, maintained primarily by the flux of potassium ions.

The potential which develops at the myoneural junction is local and of low magnitude in comparison to either the resting membrane potential or the action potential which may ensue. The intensity of the end-plate potential varies according to the quantity of acetylcholine released. Charge flows between the adjacent part of the sarcolemma, which is in the resting phase, and the recently depolarized area of the sarcolemma. Where sufficient current flow occurs to reach threshold in the adjacent membrane, an action potential is developed which is propagated both throughout the sarcolemma and within the sarcomere, and thus the contractile process is activated. The action potential on the sarcolemma is similar in mechanism to the action potential of the neuron, though the former is usually slower. Also, in some muscles the action potential on the sarcolemma is more persistent than the similarly activated portions on the typical axolemma (see chapter 3, The Neuron).

The Sliding Filament Theory

The *sliding filament theory* of contraction was first published in the 1950s. Early electron micrographs showed that the filaments of the sarcomere seemed to "slide" past each other during different stages of contraction. Further magnification showed that the filaments were connected by *cross bridges*, whose movements seemed to generate a mechanical force that resulted in the sliding mechanism. Analysis of the thick filaments has subsequently showed that they are composed of *myosin*, a protein consisting of many molecules laid parallel to one another to form a single thick filament. Each subunit of the thick filament is divided into two parts. One portion, called *light meromyosin*, forms the main body of the thick filament. The cross bridges, known as *heavy meromyosin*,

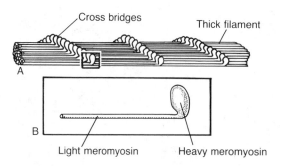

FIGURE 7–6
Thick filaments with cross bridges indicated on the surfaces (A). Note that the cross bridges are arranged in a spiral around the long axis of the filament. Myosin molecules make up the thick filaments which are thus composed of light and heavy meromyosin subunits (B).

are actually the second portion of the molecule and are directed away from the thick filament towards the thin filaments (see Figure 7–6).

Detailed analysis shows the thin filaments to be composed of *actin* molecules arranged in a double helical strand. The specific sites for cross bridge attachment are covered by another protein called *tropomyosin* and are held in place by smaller *troponin* molecules (see Figure 7–7).

Mechanism of Contraction

When an action potential of the motor nerve reaches the myoneural junction, a local membrane potential, called the *end-plate potential*, is generated at the synaptic junction of the muscle fiber. If an action potential,

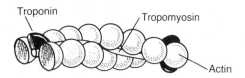

FIGURE 7–7
Thin filament showing the arrangement of actin, troponin, and tropomyosin

which follows the all-or-none law, is formed in the muscle, it moves along the sarcolemma to the interior of the cell by way of the T-tubules. The action potential alters the permeability of the terminal cisternae of the sarcoplasmic reticulum, and calcium ions are released into the sarcoplasm, where they come in contact with the filaments and interact with troponin. The troponin molecule has three subunits which react independently with other molecules in their environment. In the resting phase, the *I subunit* is attached to the actin molecule and the *T subunit* is attached to the tropomyosin (see Figure 7–8). The *C subunit* is not attached in the resting phase, but when calcium ions are introduced they are quickly bound to this subunit. The binding of calcium to the C subunit results in a redistribution of the charges on the troponin molecule, which shifts its position to free the activity sites on the actin filament. The activity sites thus exposed are able to react with the cross bridges from the thick filaments. *Actomyosin*, formed from the joining of the actin and myosin filaments, acts as a catalyst for the hydrolysis of ATP to ADP and inorganic phosphate, providing energy for contraction of the muscle. Contraction is the result of movement, or *flexion*, of the cross bridges. That flexion in turn pulls the actin filaments toward the center of the sarcomere and thus reduces the distance between adjacent Z lines. The total force of contraction of any myofibril is a function of the sum of the contraction of all of the sarcomeres activated. The total force of contraction of any muscle is generated from the number of fibers thus activated.

Muscle Contraction

The complete cycle of muscle contraction and relaxation is termed the *muscle twitch*

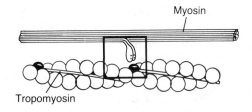

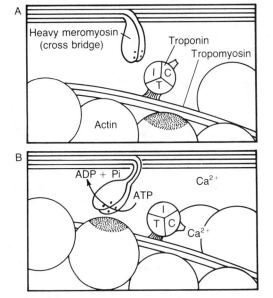

FIGURE 7–8
(A) The relationship between the thick and thin filaments during relaxation, and (B) the rearrangement of troponin and tropomyosin after calcium binding

(see Figure 7–9). Each phase of the twitch represents a complex series of chemical and physical phenomena. When a muscle is stimulated, a short pause called the *latent period* occurs. There follows a period of contraction and then a period of relaxation. The latent period is associated with acetylcholine diffusion across the synpatic cleft and the alteration of the sodium permeability of the sarcolemma, thus generating a local potential. The end-plate potential is responsible for the ensuing action potential, which in turn is trans-

mitted to the interior of the fiber, where calcium ion release from the terminal cisternae occurs. The calcium ions then diffuse into the sarcoplasm and react with troponin, where the activity sites on the actin molecules are released for the formation of actomyosin. Each of the aforementioned steps is associated with a part of the delay observed as the latent period.

It should be noted that the absolute *refractory period*, the time in which a second stimulus cannot be generated, only occupies that portion of time between the stimulus of the muscle (and formation of the end-plate potential) and the return of the membrane to threshold voltage. This period is relatively short in comparison to the time spent in active contraction, which occurs in the sarcomere. For this reason it is possible to summate skeletal muscle contraction.

The moment of contraction begins with the hydrolysis of ATP by the actomyosin catalyst, which is thus an *ATPase*. Simple contraction ends when flexion of the cross bridges is complete. Full contraction requires repeated opening and closing of the acto-

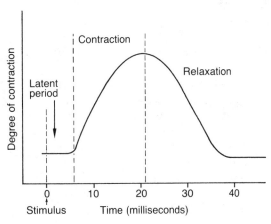

FIGURE 7–9
Muscle twitch showing different phases after stimulation

myosin bridges. Relaxation requires a series of reactions: (1) calcium ion removal by active transport, (2) breakage of the actomyosin linkage, and (3) resumption of the so-called extended position of the cross bridges. Note that all phases of contraction and relaxation require energy, which is ultimately given off as heat. That energy can be conveniently grouped as the *heat of contraction* and the *heat of relaxation*. Additional preparation of the muscle for further contraction occurs through the generation of additional ATP from glycolysis (the breakdown of glucose). The heat thereby given off is the *heat of regeneration*.

Energy Relations

Healthy muscle tissue ultimately receives its energy from two dietary substances, carbohydrates and lipids. These principal sources of energy may be stored in the muscle as *glycogen* and *triglycerides*, respectively, or they may be absorbed directly from the blood. Glycogen is broken down, or catabolized, into smaller components which yield chemical energy in the form of ATP. Glycogen catabolism proceeds either through the *anaerobic pathway* (i.e., the *Embden-Meyerhoff pathway*) or through the *aerobic pathway* (i.e., the *Krebs cycle* and the *cytochrome system*). In the anaerobic pathway, most of the net energy is used in the formation of ATP by *substrate phosphorylation*. In the aerobic pathway, ATP is produced by oxidative reactions. Lipids that contribute to the energy of contraction are stored as triglycerides in adipose tissue and in muscle cells. Lipids, utilized as energy sources only in the aerobic metabolic pathway, have a principal role in *tonic muscles*, where slower, sustained activity requires synthesis of ATP during contrac-

tion. Tonic muscles have the oxidative (aerobic) capacity because of a greater density of mitochondria and myoglobin. Phasic muscles, on the other hand, have reduced amounts of these substances but store quantities of high-energy phosphates for quick release of energy.

In addition to ATP, whose production is derived from carbohydrates and lipids, high-energy phosphates are also stored as *creatine phosphate (CrP)*. Creatine phosphate readily exchanges chemical energy with ADP to form ATP. The reaction is apparently controlled by a mass-action relationship of substrates involved. When ADP and CrP are in abundance, ATP and creatine are formed. When ATP and creatine are in abundance, after sufficient catabolism of the lipid and carbohydrates substrates is complete, creatine phosphate is stored and the ADP formed is able to pick up additional energy to form more ATP from oxidative and substrate phosphorylation.

Characteristics of Muscle Contraction

Treppe   When a well-rested muscle is stimulated sequentially (with ample time for relaxation), the degree of *muscle shortening* increases in a stepwise fashion, termed *treppe* after the German word for staircase (see Figure 7–10). The *staircase phenomenon* may be attributed to the viscosity characteristics of the sarcoplasm. It is believed that increased stimulation results in increased availability of internal calcium ions for binding with troponin. In addition, successive stimulation results in the production of heat, which is in turn absorbed by the sarcoplasm. As is characteristic of many fluids, the viscosity of the sarcoplasm is reduced when heated. It is

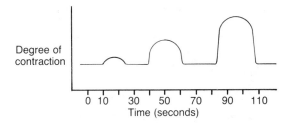

FIGURE 7–10
Treppe (staircase phenomenon) during stimulation of a well-rested muscle. Each contraction is greater than the preceding one, though the force returns to zero at the end of each contraction.

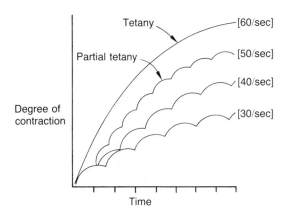

FIGURE 7–11
Wave summation in skeletal muscle as recorded on a polygraph. Each line is produced by a different stimulus frequency. The greater the frequency of stimulation, the greater the degree of shortening.

therefore more pliable and can respond readily to force within the cell. The force generated by the muscle can then be wholly expended on the process of shortening instead of being used in part to reshape the sarcoplasm. In other words, the sarcoplasm is more easily redistributed when the muscle is warmed by previous contractions and can therefore conform more readily to the new shape of the muscle in the contracted condition. Thus, the internal resistance to contraction is reduced and additional energy can therefore be expended on the shortening process. The beneficial effects of this phenomenon are frequently taken advantage of by humans prior to an atheletic event or a situation which requires maximum muscular performance. "Warm-up exercises" should always be designed to affect the muscles most used in the task at hand, since an increase in efficiency is the purpose of those exercises.

Wave summation When a muscle is stimulated successively without sufficient time for relaxation, each new twitch is added to the contraction of the previous twitch (see Figure 7–11). Consequently, the muscle becomes shorter as the rate of stimulation in-

creases even though a constant number of sarcomeres is involved. As the sarcomere becomes shorter, the H band becomes smaller and more area is available for the formation of cross bridges between actin and myosin. Thus, during such *wave summation* there is an additive effect: as each new stimulus arrives, the contraction resulting from cross-bridge formation and ATP hydrolysis is added to the previous contraction. It is this additive effect which makes wave summation entirely different from treppe, since in treppe a complete relaxation must occur between successive stimuli.

When a muscle is stimulated at a maximum frequency so that no relaxation is possible, a constant shortened muscle length is achieved. Under such conditions the muscle is said to show *tetany*. If stimulation is continued, the expenditure of energy becomes greater than its synthesis and metabolic wastes accumulate. The result is the decrease in contractile force known as *fatigue*. Where circulation to the muscle is maintained, lactate (the principal metabolic product of anaerobic glycolysis) is removed or oxidized and ATP is resynthesized. Within a few minutes the fatigued muscle's stored high-energy phosphates are resynthesized, and contraction can proceed again with vigor.

Multiple-fiber summation When a muscle-nerve preparation is made using a large *nerve trunk* such as the *sciatic nerve*, many motor units can be involved. Each motor nerve and the muscle fibers it innervates constitute a single motor unit. If the intensity (voltage) of stimulation is increased, the force of contraction increases proportionally. The explanation for this phenomenon lies in the anatomical relationship of nerve to individual muscle fibers in the muscle bundle (see Figure 7–12). In such a situation, each motor neuron has a decidedly different threshold of stimulus. As the voltage of successive stimuli is increased, additional motor units are activated and the force of contraction increases. This phenomenon of *multiple-fiber summation* differs from wave summation which can be performed by a single fiber or sarcomere. Multiple fiber summation, by definition, always involves the recruitment of two or more individual motor units.

Length, Velocity and Tension in Muscle Contraction

In the laboratory, muscle fibers and their components can be manipulated to function in precisely predictable ways. When the muscle is treated as an intact unit, characteristics of contraction which were unnoticed in the fiber or its fraction can be observed, giving particular insight into the function of the muscle tissue in the intact organism. Physical factors which modify specific activities in the intact organism are muscle *length*, *tension*, and *velocity of contraction*.

Tension When a muscle contracts, its force is dissipated by two elements: (1) its internal *elastic elements* and (2) the weight of the object being moved. The elastic element of a muscle consists of membranes and noncontractile fibers (i.e., nuclear bag and nuclear chain cells, and tendons) which must be stretched before the force of contraction can be delivered to the point of insertion. During contraction, tension in the elastic element is increased until it becomes equal to the tension developed in the contractile element. Additional force, in excess of that taken up by the elastic element, is imparted to the work of moving the load.

Length The length to which a muscle is stretched has a decided effect upon the amount of tension developed (see Figure 7–13). Stretching of the muscle reduces the amount of energy that must be expended in the shortening process, because it lessens the amount of energy wasted in the development of tension in the elastic element. The amount of stretch placed on a resting muscle

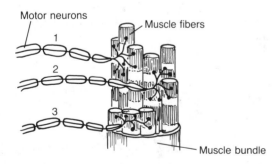

FIGURE 7–12
Cross section of skeletal muscle showing motor units. Each motor neuron and the muscle fibers it innervates constitute a single motor unit.

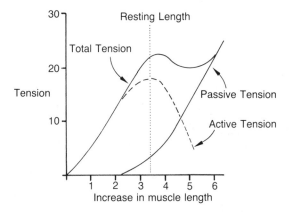

FIGURE 7–13
Length-tension curve for skeletal muscle. Passive tension denotes stretch. Active tension signifies the force generated by muscle contraction. Total tension is the sum of active and passive tension. Data reproduced, with permission, from Ganong, WF: *Review of Medical Physiology*, 9th ed. Copyright 1979 by Lange Medical Publications, Los Altos, California, and from Fundamental Studies of Human Locomotion and Other Information Relating to Design of Artificial Limbs, Report to NRC, Committee on Artificial Limbs 2(1947), reproduced by permission of University of California (Berkeley) Press, Berkeley, Calif.

is referred to as *passive tension*. The tension resulting from the contractile process of a stimulated muscle is called *active tension*. These two forces together form the *total tension* developed. The magnitude of active tension is thus dependent upon the number of cross bridges which can collectively be formed in the sarcomere. The maximum number of cross bridges is thought to occur when the muscle is at its normal resting length. As the muscle is stretched, total tension increases until the development of active tension becomes impossible, because the thick and thin filaments do not overlap to a sufficient degree for cross bridge formation.

Velocity of contraction The velocity with which a muscle contracts is also a function of the number of cross bridges in the sar-

comere that can be formed at any particular time. As a load is applied to a muscle, the rate of tension development after stimulation is a function of the rate at which the muscle overcomes the inertia of the load to be moved. As the load applied to the muscle increases, its inertia increases proportionately, and contraction velocity is reduced.

The Function of Muscles

Muscles frequently develop greater force in the intact animal than is expected from the amount of contractile tissue, or bulk of the muscle. This magnification of the force of contraction in the intact organism is the product of levers formed by the position of muscles and tendons around specific joints in the skeleton. Such levers in mammals provide a mechanical advantage which improves performance beyond that ordinarily associated with a muscle.

Three factors are involved in all levers: (1) the weight to be moved, (2) the position of the *fulcrum*, and (3) the force of application. The fulcrum is a pivot around which forces and weight are applied. There are three basic classes of levers found in mammals (see Figure 7–14). Classification depends upon the placement of the three factors of weight, fulcrum, and force. A first-class lever exists where the fulcrum lies between the weight or resting force (R) and the contractile force (energy) applied (E). An example of this type of lever is provided by the *semispinatus capitis* muscle, which attaches to the occipital protuberances and inserts on the vertebral spines of the cervical vertebrae. Here, the *occipital condyles* provide the fulcrum while the weight of the head is the resistance weight to be moved. The force supplied by the *semispinatus capitis* elevates the head and completes the action characteristic of a

THE PHYSIOLOGY OF MUSCLES

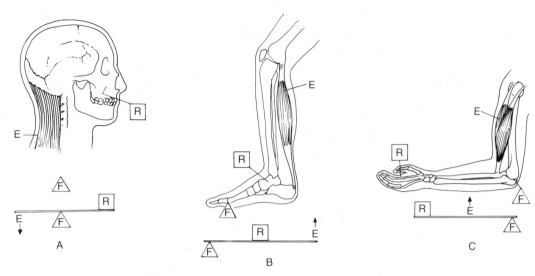

FIGURE 7–14
Types of levers found in mammals: (A) first-class lever, (B) second-class lever, and
(C) third-class lever (E, contractile force; R, weight; and F, fulcrum). From G. J. Tor-
tora and N. P. Anagnostakos, *Principles of Anatomy and Physiology*, 3rd edition (New
York, N.Y., 1981), 727, fig. 28–17. Reprinted by permission of Harper and Row
Publishers.

first-class lever. In grazing animals this system provides the action necessary for elevat-
ing the lower incisors so that grass may be
cropped during eating. In carnivores this system provides a tremendous mechanical advantage which enables them to rip flesh from
their prey.

The second-class and third-class levers
are most easily demonstrated in movement
of the limbs. When a human stands on tip-
toes, a second-class lever is activated; the
gastrocnemius and *soleus* muscles provide
the force of application, the ball of the foot
acts as a fulcrum, and the weight of the body
applied to the ankle is the force which must
be moved. Third-class levers are found in the
forearm and the foreleg; in flexion, the elbow
or knee provides the fulcrum and the limb
becomes the weight to be moved.

The positioning of the muscles to provide
greater speed or strength can be seen when
comparing, for example, movement of the
limbs of the wolverine and the cheetah (see
Figure 7–15). In the wolverine the *teres major*
is placed at a distance from the fulcrum, allowing the strength of the limb to be used in
digging. In the cheetah the same muscle is
closer to the fulcrum, allowing for greater
speed when running.

Many organisms that employ great speed
in running also utilize the mechanical effects
of joints to reduce the elastic element of a
muscle before contraction begins. In the
horse, when the weight of the animal is applied to the hoof in running, the *fetlock joint*
stretches the ligaments attached to the hoof
before contraction in the flexor muscles begins. Once the elastic elements are so

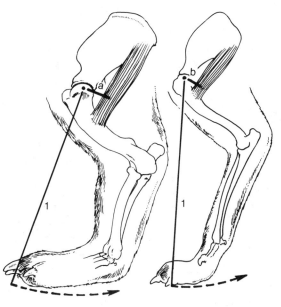

FIGURE 7–15
Power and speed are alternatively achieved in the wolverine (left) and the cheetah (right) by placement of the *teres major* muscle. In the cheetah, the small distance (b) between the muscle insertion and the joint it moves yields a higher rate of oscillation than in the wolverine, in which the distance (a) is greater.

stretched, the force generated can be applied directly to the bones involved. In turn, the reverse snap of the ligament causes the hoof to snap back into its normal position when the weight is removed (see Figure 7–16).

Specific Actions of Skeletal Muscles

Muscles seldom act individually during movement of the body. More often two or more muscles work together to perform a particular action. The unified contraction of two or more muscles is referred to as *synergism*. Frequently, a limb must be "locked" in place when performing certain activities. Such action requires the contraction of muscles which work against each other. Such muscles are called *antagonistic muscles*. Antagonistic muscles apply forces to opposite sides of the joint that they manipulate, and thus a limb or part of the body can be made rigid, as in the leg muscles when standing or the muscles of the arm when holding a weighted object at length.

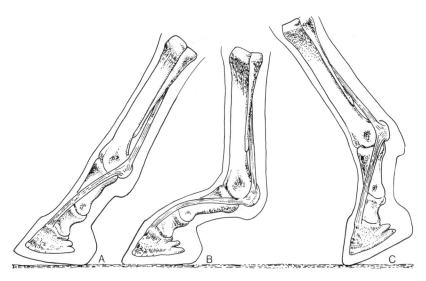

FIGURE 7–16
Springing ligaments in the legs of horses (shown here) and in other hoofed runners reduce the need of heavy leg muscles. The impact of the foot against the ground (A) bends the fetlock joint (B) and stretches the elastic elements, which then snap back when the foot leaves the ground (C). The springing action straightens the foot and gives the leg an upward thrust. From How Animals Run, M. Hildebrand. Copyright © 1960 by Scientific American, Inc. All rights reserved.

Muscles make possible such complicated movements as spreading the toes or moving a limb toward or away from the midline of the body. When a limb is moved away from the midline it is said to be *abducted*. When it is moved toward the midline it is said to be *adducted*.

In many animals a great degree of coordination is present, enabling a limb to be rotated around a central axis. Such movement can be observed in the human leg when rotation is caused by the contraction of the *sartorius* muscle, which originates on the lateral aspect of the pelvic girdle and is inserted medially at the knee (see Figure 7–17). Contraction therefore gives rise to lateral rotation of the knee.

The facial muscles of mammals show complex movement, which permits the expression of emotions, the consumption of food, and the avoidance of injury to certain parts of the face. For example, aggressive displays require a complex action involving contraction and relaxation of several facial muscles. Both the *obiscularis oris* and the *obiscularis oculi*, which are *constrictor muscles*, reduce the diameter of the mouth and orbit, respectively, when contracted. Other muscles, such as the *nasalis*, allow the tip of the nose to be lowered. The *buccinator* retracts the lips in a snarl and is an essential muscle involved in exposing the teeth during hostilities in some animals.

Movements such as *extension*, the enlargement of the angle of a joint, and *flexion*, the reduction of the angle of the joint, require that some muscles contract while their antagonistic muscles are inhibited. That is, the motor neurons which excite the antagonistic muscles are inhibited so that less resistance from antagonistic contraction develops.

Coordination of all muscle movements is only possible through the activity of the central nervous system. Wave summation in the intact organism is induced through increased activity of a fixed number of motor neurons. Conscious effort, on the other hand, may allow an animal to increase the number of motor units during contraction and thus perform multiple-fiber summation. In essence, contractions of both the number of muscle fibers and the specific muscles are central nervous system phenomena. Mechanical force is developed by the combined interplay of the muscles themselves and the lever systems they utilize.

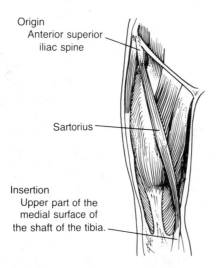

Origin
Anterior superior
iliac spine

Sartorius

Insertion
Upper part of the
medial surface of
the shaft of the tibia.

FIGURE 7–17
Musculature of the human leg showing the origin and insertion of the *sartorius* to give the rotating movement of the leg

CARDIAC MUSCLE

Cardiac muscle is briefly discussed here to acquaint the student with the nature of cardiac tissue and some of its characteristics. It is intended that the material presented will be of a particular use in understanding the mechanical factors of blood flow (see chapter 11, The Heart as a Pump).

Structure

Cardiac muscle is similar to skeletal muscle in that it contains striations due to the presence of thick and thin filaments (see Figure 7–18). The contractile unit, the sarcomere, is also of similar structure as that discussed for skeletal muscle. Cardiac muscle cells, however, are distinctly branched and have only one nucleus per cell. Cell membranes are juxtaposed at tightly fitting junctions known as *intercalated discs.* The advent of the electron microscope has revealed that the discs are formed by an extensive series of interdigitated folds of adjacent cell membranes. Close adhesion at these cell junctions allows the force of contraction of adjacent cells to be transmitted from one to another. In this way an entire portion of the heart muscle, such as the ventricles, can be excited and contract as a single unit. The close junction and large surface area at the intercalated discs allows the action potential of one cell to be transmitted to the adjacent membrane without the use of an excitatory substance such as that found at synaptic junctions (e.g., acetylcholine). The close interaction of the intercalated discs allows direct depolarization of adjacent muscles. This characteristic, along with the lack of evidence of distinct cell membranes at the intercalated discs prior to the advent of the electron microscope, prompted the theory that the heart was a *syncytium,* a multinucleate structure formed by the merging of cells.

In cardiac muscle cells the T-tubules are always positioned at the the Z lines instead of at the junction of the A band and the I band, as seen in the skeletal muscle. Cardiac muscle cells are richly endowed with myoglobin and contain many mitochondria. These characteristics are consistent for tissue almost completely dependent upon oxidative metabolism.

Physiological Characteristics

Cardiac muscle must contract repeatedly and with a somewhat constant rhythm throughout the life of the animal. Such traits have resulted in metabolic, mechanical, and electrical properties quite different from those of skeletal muscle, even though both types have a number of morphologically similar features.

Metabolism Cardiac muscle is well vascularized and has a high concentration of *myoglobin,* which is used in oxygen storage. Under normal conditions sixty percent of the energy used in the human heart is derived from lipid metabolism. Carbohydrates provide thirty-five percent, and the remaining five percent is the result of ketone and amino acid metabolism. The use of lipid stores may be quite phenomenal in some species, as in the ruminants, which have characteristically low levels of plasma carbohydrates and high plasma concentrations of short-chain fatty acids. Arctic mammalian species also generally have high levels of plasma lipids and low levels of carbohydrates in their diets. These animals may therefore utilize plasma lipids to a surprisingly high degree in cardiac metabolism. Little data are available on the ability of different species to store oxygen in cardiac muscle or to alter the source of energy by diet or need. In the human, less than one percent of the total energy liberated by car-

FIGURE 7–18
Electron micrograph of cardiac muscle (A); diagram of cardiac muscle as seen under the light microscope (B); diagram of cardiac muscle as revealed by the electron microscope (C). Photograph by Carolina Biological Supply Company.

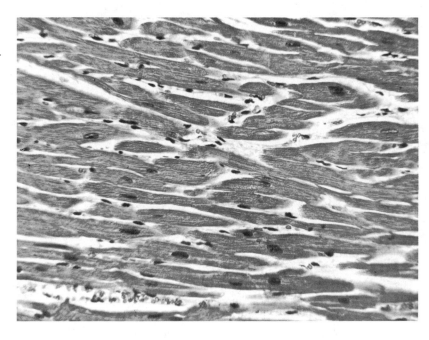

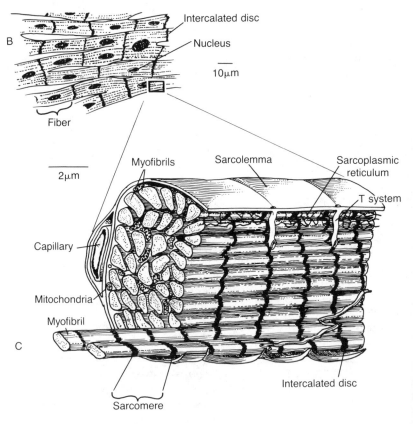

B

Intercalated disc

Nucleus

10μm

Fiber

2μm

Myofibrils

Sarcolemma

Sarcoplasmic reticulum

T system

Capillary

Mitochondria

Myofibril

C

Intercalated disc

Sarcomere

diac muscle metabolism is normally derived from anaerobic metabolism. But during hypoxia as much as ten percent of the energy requirement can be derived by anaerobic means.

Electrical properties The resting membrane potential of cardiac muscle lies well within the limits outlined for the resting membrane potential of nerve and skeletal muscle cells. It is maintained primarily by means of potassium ion flux (as described for neurons) and is of about − 80 mV, negative relative to the inside of the membrane.

Stimulation of cardiac muscle is possible by means of a weak electrical current, but the ensuing action potential differs remarkably from the action potential portrayed in nerve cells (see Figure 7–19). In intensity, the maximum potential generated is far in excess of the reversal potential in nerves, and a distinct plateau is generated, which allows the

potential to be maintained above the resting level for approximately 200 more milliseconds than that of a typical nerve action potential. The absolute refractory period is thus extended over most of the time occupied by the action potential. The long refractory period of the cardiac action potential is critical in preventing the development of tetany, as seen in skeletal muscle. When there is no tetany, there is also no summation, and thus there is ample time for the chambers of the heart to fill at the end of each contractile wave. The plateau in electrical potential is the result of a prolonged increase in calcium ion permeability. In other words, calcium ions enter the cell at the beginning of the spike and conductance is maintained for an extended period of time. The potential returns to the resting level at the end of the plateau as a result of a delayed increase in potassium ion permeability.

The mammalian heart contains *pacemaker tissue*, or *nodal tissue*, which is unable to contract. Nodal tissue exhibits electrical properties distinct from the action potentials of typical cardiac muscle cells (see Figure 7–20). The modified muscle cells of the nodal

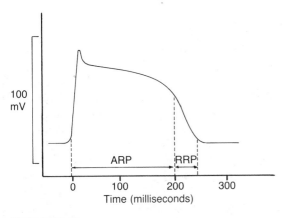

FIGURE 7–19
The action potential in cardiac muscle sarcolemma. Sharp discharge (upward peak) is caused by an increase in sodium permeability. The absolute refractory period (ARP) is the period maintained by calcium ion flux. The relative refractory period (RRP) is the result of partial repolarization due to an increase in potassium ion permeability.

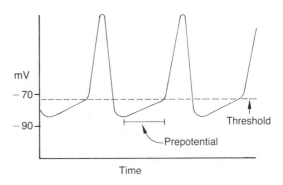

FIGURE 7–20
Rhythmic discharge seen in the heart nodal tissue. The rhythm is controlled by the rate at which the prepotential approaches threshold level.

tissue have recurring action potentials and are therefore able to exhibit *tonic*, or repetitive, qualities. In these cells there is a distinct prepotential which is caused by a progressive decrease in the potassium ion permeability, thus reducing the membrane potential toward threshold. When threshold is reached, the membrane discharges and an action potential ensues which lacks the plateau phase seen in the other cardiac muscle cells. The pulse generated by the nodal tissue is thus repetitively induced by the changing potassium permeability. It is otherwise similar to the action potentials of neurons, albeit somewhat slower. In mammals the rate at which the pacemaker, or *S-A node*, discharges controls the rate of heart contraction. The rate varies from about 30 to 600 pulses per minute under normal circumstances, depending upon the species. The slower rates are found in larger animals, whereas the rapid rates are encountered in the smaller mammals.

SMOOTH MUSCLE

Smooth muscle can be distinguished from cardiac and skeletal muscle by its lack of striations, even though both actin and myosin are present (see Figure 7–21). Smooth muscle contains only one nucleus per cell and lacks myoglobin. Lacking myoglobin, it has a poor capacity to store oxygen. At least two classes of smooth muscles, based upon structure and function, are found in mammals: *visceral smooth muscle* and *multiunit smooth muscle*. The function of smooth muscle varies considerably since it is used both in gross (bulk) movement in digestion and in fine control of pupillary changes in the eye during the light reflex.

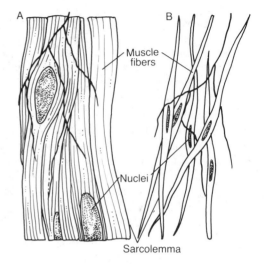

FIGURE 7–21
The histology of smooth muscle tissue: (A) visceral smooth muscle tissue and (B) multiunit smooth muscle

Visceral Smooth Muscle

Visceral smooth muscle is found in the viscera, uterus, and ureter. It is made up of sheets of cells which have the ability to function as a syncytium because of the presence of closely adhering, low-resistance intercellular bridges where the membranes of adjacent cells are united. These bridges, referred to as *gap junctions*, permit cell-to-cell conduction of action potentials through the smooth muscle. Visceral smooth muscle tissue is responsible for slow, graded contraction maintained for long periods of time without relaxation.

Most of the smooth muscle in an organism is of the visceral type, which is innervated by both the sympathetic and parasympathetic divisions of the autonomic nervous system. Nerve activity in smooth muscle has the role of modifying contraction rather than inducing it. Visceral smooth muscle contracts spontaneously in a manner very much like that of cardiac muscle. In this case the contractions are initiated from several different foci of electrical discharge, in contrast to a simple pacemaker such as the S-A node of the heart.

In visceral smooth muscle the modifying actions of norepinephrine and acetylcholine are in opposition. Acetylcholine enhances the frequency of contractions by depolarizing the membrane and thus shortening the time between spontaneous action potentials. Stimulation of the sympathetic nerves innervating smooth muscle results in the release of norepinephrine, which has the opposite effect of acetylcholine in that it causes membrane hyperpolarization and thus decreases the basal contraction rhythm.

Multiunit Smooth Muscle

Multiunit smooth muscle does not act as a syncytium. The cells within any group, such as those found in the iris of the eye, act as groups of motor units and share many characteristics of contraction with skeletal muscle. Contraction of this type of smooth muscle is usually not spontaneous, and no foci for intrinsic pacemaker-type stimulation are present. Contraction may be induced by either the release of epinephrine from the adrenal medulla or by direct stimulation via innervation of noradrenergic neurons from a branch of the autonomic nervous system. In this way multiunit smooth muscle functions in a fashion similar to skeletal muscle, except that the membrane potentials and contraction waves are comparatively much longer. A multiple fiberlike action similar to the fiber recruitment seen in motor units of skeletal muscle can be observed in multiunit smooth muscle, which enables it to exhibit very exact and refined movements such as those in the

iris. The pupillary reflex, which controls iris activity and thus the diameter of the pupil, is a very finely graded response. The ciliary muscle of the eye is controlled by the autonomic nervous system, so that a precise amount of light is allowed to strike the retina even though the eye may be exposed to a wide range of light intensities.

SUMMARY

The significance of muscle contraction cannot be underrated, for it is an integral part of every expression or action of an organism. Although thoughts may originate and develop in the human mind, there is no documented method of expression except through the accurate and proper coordinated action of muscle tissue. Muscles provide the force for movement of the body and act through lever mechanisms which often create a mechanical advantage far greater than could be expected from the tension developed directly. The action of muscles is not only integrated with the skeletal system to provide movement but also innervated by the nervous system to provide a means of enhancing efficiency. Such efficiency is enhanced by controlling both the number of fibers contracting at any particular time (multiple-fiber summation) and the rapidity of successive contractions (wave summation).

With the advent of the electron microscope, the intimate structure of the contractile machinery has been determined, and scientists have been able to develop a theory of contraction based upon the detailed structure of the sarcomere. Chemical analyses of protein elements within the sarcomere have been responsible for understanding the interrelationship of muscle proteins in the contractile process. Additional chemical and microscopic information has laid the groundwork for the roles of calcium ions and the sarcoplasmic reticulum in muscle activation.

Additional information concerning the role of skeletal muscle in the production of heat for the control of body temperature in mammals will be discussed in a later chapter. Muscle comprises the greatest portion of body mass capable of producing heat in most mammals. It is the most significant user of respiratory oxygen on a percentage basis, though some contraction is possible through anaerobic mechanisms of glycolysis.

8

THE SKELETAL SYSTEM

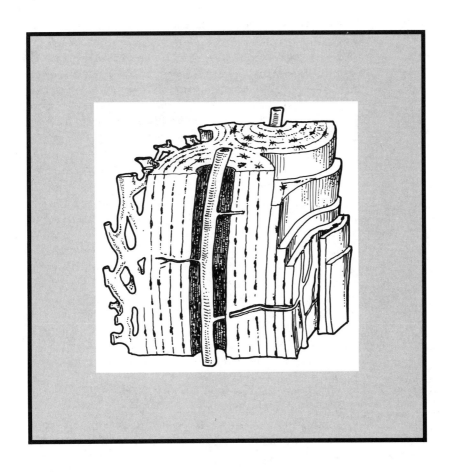

*I*n mammals the skeleton *provides both a calcium reservoir and a structural framework for body form, support, protection, and movement. A mammal's characteristic shape is largely a function of the framework provided by the skeletal system and reflects many things about its environment, such as climate, food sources, and terrain. For example, mammalian species from arctic climates usually have shorter limbs and more compact bodies than species from warmer climates. Development of specific body types in different climates is primarily a function of the skeleton. If the animal is a browser it may feed on twigs or leaves high above the ground. Such feeding behavior implies that the animal evolved with good climbing skills or with the height needed to feed on tree branches. An animal's form is also a reflection of the terrain. Plains or grassland grazing animals usually avoid danger by rapid escape mechanisms and are therefore endowed with skeletal proportions which allow them to run swiftly. Length of stride, so important in movement, is related to the length of the long bones in the limbs. In an animal whose mode of self-preservation is to outrun its predators, the ratio of limb length to body length is high. Mammals whose method of self-defense does not involve speed usually have shorter limbs, which are developed for activities other than running. Climbing mammals are usually well equipped with prehensile forelimbs, which are developed for grasping. Mammals that occupy subterranean habitats have powerful forelimbs, which provide the strength necessary for digging.*

In general, the support provided by the skeleton is reflected in the diameter of the bones, particularly the limbs. The upper limit of size in terrestrial animals is restricted by the cross-sectional area that can be attained by the bones of the legs. Weight increases as a function of the cube of the animal's approximate linear dimensions, whereas the cross-sectional area of the limb bones, which is proportional to the weight that the bone can support, increases as a function of the square of their radius. If the limb bones and body weight grew in a one-to-one fashion, there would be a disproportionate increase in weight compared to bone strength, a disparity that would lead to collapse of the limbs. Thus, long bone growth generally exceeds the whole body growth. Aquatic mammals, whose weight is partially supported by the buoyancy of water, avoid this problem and therefore can achieve much greater size than their terrestrial counterparts.

Movement is an inherent function of the skeletal system, which forms a rigid framework for muscles to pull against and provides the structural elements for levers, which can be important in speed as well as strength. The primary contribution of the skeletal system is to form a lever mechanism. *In doing so, it must provide both a site for muscle attachment and a fulcrum about which the lever can move.* Joints *are the principal fulcrums in the lever systems of mammals. Their design reduces friction, and thus maximum mechanical advantage is attained.*

The skeleton is used for protection in several different ways. The internal organs are protected by the bones of the thorax and sacral girdle. The protection for the central nervous system provided by the skull and vertebrae is of the utmost importance because of the fragile nature of the brain and spinal cord.

The skeletal system is also important in the synthesis of both red and white blood cells. Red blood cells, or erythrocytes, *are produced in the red bone marrow, or* myeloid tissue, *through a series of cell divisions, which allows the mature erythrocytes to be released into the blood. Red blood cells only survive for about three to four months in most mammals. Therefore, red blood cell production is a constant process carried on throughout life. Several types of white blood cells, or* leucocytes, *are also produced by the red bone marrow of the adult animal. The myeloid tissue shares the production of white blood cells with* lymphoid tissue, *such as that found in the spleen, tonsils, and lymph nodes. All of the blood cells, both red and white, produced by the red bone marrow originate from undifferentiated* mesenchymal cells *(see chapter 9, Blood as a Tissue).*

The bones are essential in maintaining homeostatic levels of plasma calcium ions. The crystalline structure of the skeleton is a dynamic reservoir of calcium storage. Calcium ions are removed from the bone when plasma levels fall below the optimum. In order to maintain homeostatic levels of calcium, any ions removed from the bone must ultimately be replaced from dietary sources. This storage function of the bone is constantly utilized in order to stabilize plasma calcium levels. In the bone, inorganic calcium carbonate *and* calcium phosphate *form* hydroxyapatite crystals, *which provide about 25 percent of the weight of bone and give it its characteristic hardness. The crystals of hydroxyapatite are laid down in an orderly fashion along a protein framework synthesized by the bone cells.*

COMPOSITION OF SKELETAL TISSUE

Cartilage

Cartilage is found throughout the vertebrates and forms a portion of the skeletal elements in mammals. The articulating surfaces of bone at the *synovial joints*, joints having a fluid-filled sack for connection of adjacent bones, are covered by a hard cartilage layer called *hyaline cartilage*, which is very smooth and has a glasslike appearance. Hyaline cartilage reduces the friction between surfaces of joints and therefore aids in increasing the efficiency of movement. It forms the *embryonic skeleton* and is the most abundant cartilage type in the adult. Hyaline cartilage also forms part of the sternum, ribs, nose, larynx, trachea, bronchi, and bronchial tubes in the adult.

Cartilage, in some cases, contains bundles of *collagenous fibers*, which provide strength and resilience. This type of cartilage, called *fibrocartilage*, is usually restricted to joints where only a small amount of movement is possible. Fibrocartilage is found in the pubic symphysis and in the discs between the vertebrae.

A third type of cartilage, called *elastic cartilage*, consists of a threadlike network of elastic fibers. These fibers are freely branching and can stretch and return to their original shape. Elastic cartilage is found in the larynx, the external ear, and the eustachian tube.

Bone

Bones fall into one of two categories based upon their internal structure. These two types of bone tissue include the *compact (periosteal* or *dense) bone*, which provides most of the support elements of the body, and the *spongy (endochondral* or *cancellous) bone*, which is supplied with numerous marrow-containing *cavities*. Most bones are composed of both spongy and compact tissue (see Figure 8–1). Spongy bone is arranged in plates called *trabeculae* which form cavities filled with *red bone marrow*. The red bone marrow of spongy bone is essential for the production of both red and white blood cells. Compact bone surrounds the *medullary* or *central cavity* of the bone, which contains a fatty, acellular substance called *yellow bone marrow*. As animals age, the relative amount of yellow (inactive) marrow increases.

Regardless of which category of bone tissue is involved, the entire bone is surrounded by a delicate, well-vascularized layer of tissue called the *periosteum*. The periosteum is noticeably thicker at each end of the long bones, where it forms the *articular cartilages* (see Figure 8–2). Blood vessels and nerves pass from the periosteum into the *Haversian canals* by means of the *Volkmann's canals*. The Haversian canals run parallel to the marrow cavity and are surrounded by concentric layers of bone called *Haversian lamellae*. Blood vessels and nerves which supply the bone cells and the cells of the marrow pass through the Haversian canals.

The cells which are found in bone are quite specific in their functions. *Osteoblasts*, located immediately beneath the periosteum, are important in the formation of new bone material. As the hydroxyapatite crystals become deposited, the osteoblast becomes restricted to a tiny cavern called a *lacuna*, which is connected to other lacunae by small passageways called *canaliculi*, or "little canals." When a cell is completely enclosed in a lacuna it is called an *osteocyte*. The innermost cells lining the marrow cavity are called *osteoclasts*. The osteoclasts are involved with

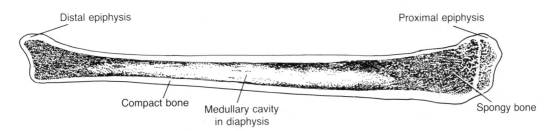

Distal epiphysis

Proximal epiphysis

Compact bone

Medullary cavity
in diaphysis

Spongy bone

FIGURE 8–1
A longitudinal section through the tibia to illustrate the differences between spongy
(cancellous) and compact (dense) bone

the demineralization of bone, a process that allows the marrow cavity to grow as the girth of the bone increases and allows calcium ions to be released from storage in the bone when plasma calcium levels fall below normal. As the mammal develops, modification in the bone structure frequently occurs to accommodate the phenomenon of growth. Osteocytes can then be converted to osteoclasts, which are able to reabsorb the bony matrix while it is being formed anew in another place within the membrane.

Classification of Bone

Bones are placed in categories according to their shapes and arrangements in the organism. The most obvious parts of the skeleton are the *long bones* of the limbs. These bones consist of a pillar of compact bone attached on either end to pieces of spongy bone. Long bones are round in cross section and have well-developed articulating surfaces.

The *flat bones* consist of two plates of compact bone separated by a layer of spongy bone. Flat bones provide wide areas of protection from physical injury. In the skull they protect large sections of the brain, which contains delicate nerve cells. Bones such as the *sternum* in the thoracic region and the *ilium* in the sacral region not only protect the soft tissues of the internal organs but also provide valuable areas for muscle attachment.

Short bones, such as the *carpals* and *tarsals* in the wrists and ankles, respectively, are small and have several articulating cartilages. In the hooved mammals such as the orders Artiodactyla and Perissodactyla, bones forming the fetlock joints (ankles) are actually derived through evolution from the phalanges in ancestral species. Because they are comprised of *multifaceted bones,* joints of the wrist and ankle of many mammalian species, and in particular the primates, are capable of complex movements.

The *irregular bones* found in the skull form most of the face and make up such bones as the *sphenoid* and the *turbanates.* Irregular bones consist of both compact and spongy elements. They give rise to the shape of the face and provide a rigid framework around the organs of such special senses as the eyes, ears, and nose. Irregular bones also provide numerous *processes* (projections) for muscle attachment. The muscles of the face are essential for the complex movements associated with facial expressions and communication.

The *sesamoid bones,* so named because of their seedlike appearance, function to guide tendons and reduce friction between ten-

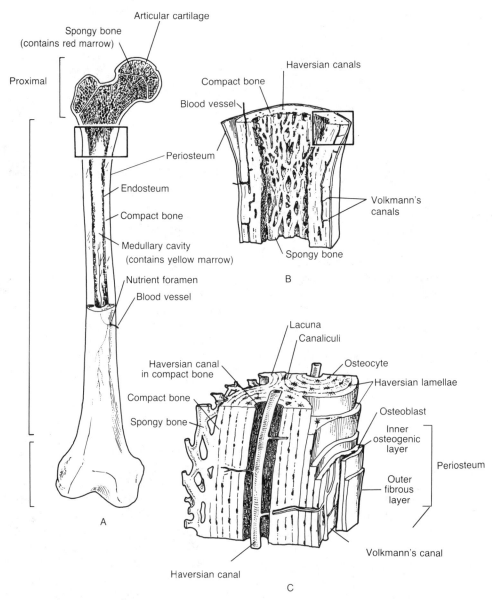

FIGURE 8–2
Bone tissue: (A) macroscopic appearance of a long bone that has been partially sectioned lengthwise; (B) histological structure of bone; and (C) enlarged aspect of Haversian canal systems in dense bone

dons and bones. They are located within tendons and have no direct articulation with the rest of the skeleton.

Wormian or *suture bones* are variable in both shape and number among different species as well as among members of the same species. They are found between the joints of several bones of the skull. Suture bones form at unpredictable rates and in unpredictable order because *ossification* (bone-formation) rates and growth rates are quite different among members of a species. Their formation follows a path somewhat similar to the clotting process in a large quantity of blood, in which different epicenters of clotting occur at different points in the mixture. In other words, ossification occurs sporadically and in unpredictable sites during the formation of these bones.

PARTS OF THE SKELETON

The skeleton can be divided into several units, each of which is composed of bones associated with specific functions. The central portion of the skeleton is known as the *axial skeleton* and comprises the skull, vertebral column, ribs, and sternum. Its primary functions are the protection of the central nervous system and the provision of places of attachment for muscles. Many variations have evolved among axial skeletons of mammalian species. These variations reflect the different habitats and ecological niches filled by these animals. The extended vertebrae in the neck of the giraffe give it the ability to browse on treetops. In most quadrupeds the *neural arches* of the thoracic vertebrae are extended to give space for attachment of the muscles which control the forelimbs. The number of bones in the axial skeleton is also quite variable. Among the primates, for instance, many have prehensile tails, whereas others lack tails or only have a few *coccygeal vertebrae.*

The limb bones of mammals, along with the bones of the *pectoral* and *sacral girdles*, which allow the long bones to articulate with the axial skeleton, are collectively called the *appendicular skeleton*. Most terrestrial mammals are quadrupeds, and the bones of the limbs are specifically designed for support and movement. But in many cases the *anterior limbs*, or forelimbs, have a reduced function in movement and support and have been variously adapted as appendages for grasping and manipulating. In the primates the anterior limbs have lost much of their locomotive role and are employed in feeding and communication. The forelimbs of *saltatory animals*, animals whose primary mode of locomotion is jumping or hopping, such as the hares and kangaroos, have reduced function in locomotion. In addition, in one order of mammals, the Chiroptera (the bats), the anterior limbs are adapted for support and movement by flying rather than the traditional mode of terrestrial locomotion. In true aquatic mammals the limbs have lost much of their support function and are specifically designed for swimming. Aquatic mammals such as the seals, sea lions, and walruses (suborder Pinnipedia) have flippers, which have limited use on land. The limbs of whales and other cetaceans are strictly designed for swimming, and these mammals have adapted to a completely aquatic existence.

The *heterotopic skeletal elements* comprise the sesamoid bones and other bones dissociated from the rest of the skeleton, such as the bony plates in the diaphragm of the camel, the heart of ruminants, the snout of hogs, and the *baculum* or *os penis* found in many mammals. The os penis is found in members of the orders Rodentia, Carnivora, Chiroptera, Cetacea, and some of the infra-human primates. In some species of cetaceans the baculum may reach a length of six feet. A similar structure composed of cartilage is found in various herbivores.

Articulations

The site where two bones meet or *articulate* is referred to as a *joint*. There are several types of joints found in mammals, named according to the relative amount of movement they are capable of performing (i.e., classified by function). Immobile joints are termed *synarthroses*. Joints of this type form the sutures of the skull and hold the individual bones of the sacral girdle together. Slightly mobile joints are referred to as *amphiarthroses*. Joints of this type unite the *splint bones* (or *metatarsals*) to form the *cannon bone* in the foreleg of perissodactyls. Freely movable joints are called *diarthroses*. The diarthrotic joint is exemplified in most mammals by such major articulations as the knee and elbow (see Figure 8–3).

Joints are also classified according to the material from which they are formed. *Ossified joints*, joints that are rigidly held together by bone, are referred to as *synostoses*. This type of joint is typified by the joints in the sacrum and skull. Synostoses are entirely made up of bone and do not contain a cavity. Joints that hold bones together by dense fibrous tissue are called *syndesmoses*. Joints of this category are slightly movable and do not form lever systems in the body. Amphiarthrotic joints are usually syndesmoses. Constant action of syndesmoses causes them to become irritated. This phenomenon is sometimes seen in race horses, where excessive force on the legs for extended periods of time results in irritation of the joints connecting the splint bones in the foreleg. This condition, when severe, must be treated by a process called "firing," which involves heating the cannon bone near the fibrous connections of the metatarsals. Heat induces the formation of more fibrous tissue and gives the bones a stronger bond.

Amphiarthrotic joints made of cartilage are called *synchondroses*. This type of joint is found in a *symphysis*, in which the connecting material forms broad flat discs of fibrocartilage. For example, the bones of the *pubic symphysis* are connected by means of a synchondrosis.

The most commonly recognized articulation is the *synovial joint* (see Figure 8–3). This type of joint is freely movable because the bones are united by means of a fluid-filled cartilagenous sack. It is this type of joint

FIGURE 8–3
The diarthrotic joint of mammals is freely movable due to the presence of a cavity filled with synovial fluid, which lubricates the adjacent bones

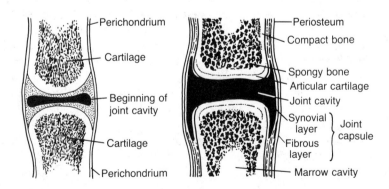

which allows the free mobility necessary for the limb action, which is characteristic of vertebrate movement. The synovial joint is classified by function as a diarthrosis.

DEVELOPMENT AND GROWTH OF BONE

Bones form in two basic ways in mammals. The simplest and most direct method occurs when osteoblasts begin to form in membranous tissue in the embryo. This type of ossification, known as *intramembranous ossification*, is responsible for formation of the flat bones of the skull, the mandible, and part of the clavicles. The second mode of bone formation, called *endochondral ossification*, occurs within cartilagenous tissue (see Figure 8–4). In this case *chondrocytes* (mature cartilage cells) are formed which produce a cartilagenous structure in the shape of the bone, which forms later.

Intramembranous Ossification

In this process, mesenchymal cells are converted to osteoblasts, which cluster together to form a center of ossification. A matrix of collagenous material, secreted by the osteoblasts, forms the framework for sequestering calcium salts. Calcium carbonate and calcium phosphate precipitate to form hydroxyapatite crystals on the collagenous fibers. A

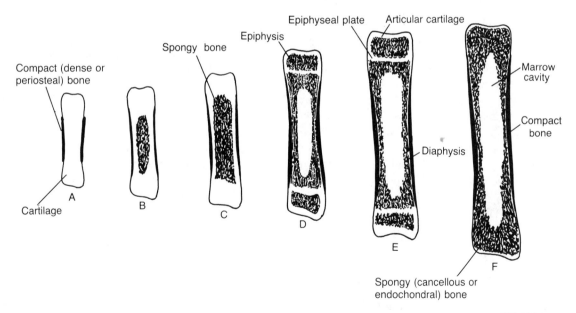

FIGURE 8–4
Ossification of long bones follows a progressive order: (A) collar of compact periosteal bone forms in the center; (B) primary ossification center begins with formation of endochondral bone; (C) marrow cavity begins to form; (D) appearance of secondary ossification centers in the epiphyseal cartilages; (E) bone growth occurs at epiphyses where cartilage moves away from the center of the diaphysis as a result of ossification; (F) closure of epiphyses with the union of primary and secondary ossification centers and disappearance of epiphyseal plates

single ossification center forms a trabecula, which becomes interconnected with other trabeculae to form the rigid structure of spongy bone. The outer layers of the membranous tissue become the periosteum, and a layer of compact bone forms beneath it. Osteoblasts are converted to osteocytes when they become enclosed within ossified tissue. Again, the small cavity which surrounds the osteocyte is called a lacuna. The osteocytes are not able to sequester the hydroxyapatite crystals and their function in growth ceases.

Endochondral Ossification

This process of bone formation is typical of the long bones of the body. In embryonic development *chondroblasts* (immature cartilage cells) lay down cartilage in the approximate shape of the bone. The cartilage is then covered by a membrane called the *perichondrium.* Later a blood vessel enters the structure about midway between each end. This entry appears to stimulate the cells of the internal layer of the perichondrium to become osteoblasts. The process involves the enlargement of the cells of the perichondrium and their conversion to a new cell type capable of laying down the organic matrix of bone. The osteoblasts are also able to sequester hydroxyapatite crystals from the surrounding medium that form the inorganic portion of bone. This initial ossification results in the formation of a *bony collar* around a cartilagenous interior.

The formation of long bones provides an excellent model for endochondral ossification, since such formation follows a predictable pattern over a very regular structure (see Figure 8–4). In the long bones there are two centers of ossification. Ossification begins in the central portion of the bone, the *diaphysis,* where the bony collar is formed and where

cartilage cells of the interior enlarge and eventually burst. Rupture of the cartilage cells probably provides a more alkaline pH, which induces the intercellular substance to become calcified.

Ossification prevents the penetration of nutritive material into the region and any remaining cells die. Blood vessels follow the cavities left by the dead cartilage cells. The cavities expand in size and coalesce to form the original *marrow cavity* (central or medullary cavity) of the bone. The perichondrium is now called the *periosteum.* Osteoblasts continue to be formed, resulting in the formation of an osseous core called the *primary ossification center.* This initial site of ossification quickly develops and covers the entire diaphysis, leaving two large cartilages, one at either end of the diaphysis, known as the *epiphyseal cartilages.*

The point of attachment of cartilage and the long bones is called the *epiphyseal plate. Secondary ossification centers* start in each of the epiphyseal cartilages. As the bone continues to grow, chondroblasts at either end of the diaphysis divide rapidly to form new cartilage cells. The layer of cartilage cells adjacent to the bone becomes isolated by intercellular ossification, and dies. The matrix is infiltrated and absorbed by osteoclasts. Osteoblasts move into the area and lay down new bone which is well vascularized.

The primary and secondary ossification centers are separated by the epiphyseal plates. Chondrocytes multiply and the epiphyseal plates move farther from the center of the bone, while the size of the secondary ossification centers also increases. The plates become thinner with age until the primary and secondary ossification centers are firmly united. The union of these ossification centers terminates the lengthening process of bone formation and fixes the stature or height of the organism at that point. The union of these two centers, called *epiphyseal closure*, is regulated by several endocrine processes. Both growth-stimulating hormone from the pituitary gland and steroids produced in the gonads affect growth (see chapter 17, The Endocrine System). For most mammals, epiphyseal closure signifies the termination of growth and is triggered by the release of large quantities of sex steroids such as estrogen and testosterone. Growth hormone from the pituitary causes lengthening of the bones without inducing epiphyseal closure. Insufficient growth hormone results in the small stature seen in *chondroplastic dwarfism;* an excess results in *giantism.* An excess of growth hormone after epiphyseal closure causes *acromegaly,* which is characterized by abnormal growth of the bones of the face and hands, which are not completely ossified at adolescence. In humans, growth of the long bones is usually complete by age twenty-five. In the dog and horse, growth is completed by age five in most breeds.

As mentioned earlier, as an organism grows the bones must also become larger in cross section. Increase in diameter of the bone occurs as osteoblasts are formed in the inner layer of the periosteum. As the diameter of the bone increases, the marrow cavity must also increase in size. Diameter of the marrow cavity is increased through the formation of osteoclasts at the margins of the cavity: osteoclasts erode the bone tissue and thus increase the diameter of the cavity.

CALCIUM METABOLISM

Homeostatic Function of Bone

The bones act as a reservoir of calcium, which can be released when plasma calcium levels drop below normal. Bone is therefore a dynamic tissue which can contribute calcium to the blood and consequently to other tissues. Calcium from bone can be replaced when dietary sources are sufficient. It is important to note that there is a constant turnover of calcium, and in healthy individuals bone calcium is constantly being removed and replaced. Throughout the life of an animal, plasma calcium levels are maintained at a rather constant level. Although there is some individual variation, in humans the normal plasma calcium level is approximately 10 milligrams per 100 milliliters plasma, or approximately 5 milliequivalents per liter. For mammals in general, calcium concentration in the plasma varies quite widely among species.

Plasma calcium ion concentration is controlled through several independent mechanisms in different organs of the body (see Figure 8–5). In maintaining a normal homeostatic level, calcium exchange among bone tissue, the gut, and the kidneys must be modified depending upon the demand for calcium by the tissues and calcium's availability in the diet. Subadult animals need calcium for growth and development in excess of the quantity necessary for the normal maintenance of the adult body.

Vitamin D is necessary for calcium absorption from the gut. It is produced in most mammals by the skin in the presence of sunlight. In areas of the world, such as the Arctic, where the quantity of sunlight is inadequate, vitamin D must be obtained from the diet. Fish is a good source of this vitamin, and mammals living in the Arctic, including humans, are very dependent upon the sea as a source of vitamin D. Insufficient absorption of calcium during development leads to the depletion of the crystalline portion of bone and a loss of rigidity. This condition can lead

FIGURE 8–5
Schematic diagram of plasma calcium regulation: the solid arrow designates action when plasma calcium ion concentrations are above homeostatic levels; the outlined arrow designates action when plasma calcium ion concentrations are below homeostatic levels

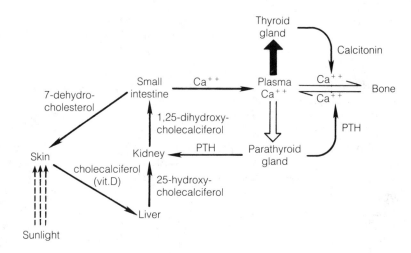

to gross changes in bone shape, which are easily recognized (see Figure 8–6). This condition, known as *rickets* in juveniles, has been found in almost epidemic proportions in some areas of the world where dietary supplies of vitamin D are inadequate and where atmospheric pollution resulting from increased industrialization reduces the availability of sunlight. In the adult the disease is known as *osteomalacia*, or "adult rickets." Untreated, rickets can lead to bone deformation and death.

The mechanism by which calcium balance is maintained in the body is controlled by means of two hormones which affect the metabolic pathways of calcium mobilization (i.e., release to the plasma) and storage: *parathormone*, or *parathyroid hormone (PTH)*, which is produced by the parathyroid glands; and *calcitonin*, which is produced by the thyroid gland.

Parathyroid Hormone

The *parathyroid glands* are small structures located close to the thyroid and vary in number among species of mammals. For example,

in the human there are two pairs of these accessory glands, whereas in the rat and the mouse there is but one pair. In herbivorous animals such as cattle, rabbits, sheep, and goats, there are numerous parathyroid glands, usually located in the neck region. These glands contain two types of cells: the *chief cells* and the *oxyphil cells*. Parathyroid hormone is produced by the chief cells and is a comparatively small protein molecule consisting of approximately eighty-four amino acids. The molecular weight of PTH varies among species but the activity site on the molecule remains the same. Therefore, in cases of PTH deficiency, replacement could be made with a hormone isolated from the parathyroid glands of another species.

The overall effect of parathyroid hormone in mammals is to maintain the homeostatic levels of calcium ions in the blood by enhancing the reabsorption of calcium in the kidney, the absorption of calcium from the gut, and the mobilization of calcium from the bone. Although its role in reabsorption from the renal filtrate is poorly understood, it is fairly certain that parathyroid hormone promotes the formation of *adenyl cyclase*, which

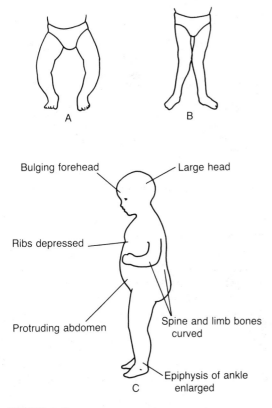

FIGURE 8–6
Some characteristic effects of rickets in the human: (A and B) leg deformities; (C) other deformities, not all to be seen in one individual. From L. J. Harris, *Vitamins* (London, U.K., 1952). Reprinted by permission of Churchill-Livingstone, Inc.

and the mobilization rate of calcium from the bone is reduced. Therefore, parathyroid hormone must cause the production of some substance by the osteoclasts that is able to augment calcium removal from bone and make it available to the plasma.

Although it is not completely known how the osteoclasts produce their effect of leaching the mineral portion of bone, it is thought that they produce locally high levels of citrate (a product of the Krebs cycle). The citrate chelates, or combines with, calcium ions and, therefore, removes them from the effective concentration in the area immediately surrounding the osteoclast. Since the concentration of calcium salts in solution is due to a mass-action effect, the chelation of calcium ions induces the ionization of additional calcium ions to take their place. Citrated calcium ions are then removed from the deossification sites by the circulatory system, and the process is continued until homeostatic calcium levels are reached in the plasma. Another hypothesis is that parathyroid hormone increases the production of cyclic AMP in osteoclasts, an increase that in turn increases calcium absorption from bone and, therefore, increases the rate at which it is transported into the plasma.

Calcitonin

It has been demonstrated that when the thyroid region is perfused with solutions which contain levels of calcium higher than normal plasma levels, peripheral levels of calcium in the plasma decrease. This has been interpreted to mean that a substance must be secreted from some structure in the region of the thyroid that actively accentuates the rate of clearing of calcium from the blood. This substance, *calcitonin*, is produced by the *parafollicular cells*, or *C cells*, of the thyroid.

acts as a catalyst in the production of *cyclic AMP*. Cyclic AMP in both the kidney and the gut is essential for the active transport of calcium ions.

In bone it appears that parathyroid hormone is necessary for the conversion of osteocytes to osteoclasts, which then induce calcium mobilization. PTH is also necessary for the continued activity and maintenance of the osteoclasts. When the concentration of plasma calcium ion reaches the homeostatic level, both parathyroid hormone formation

These cells are so named because of their clear appearance. Calcitonin comprises approximately thirty-two amino acid residues and varies in specific amino acid composition among species.

The action of calcitonin increases calcification of bone, probably by increasing the formation of osteoblasts from the chondrocytes. Those osteoblasts can then promote the precipitation of calcium and its salts on the protein matrix in bone. The precipitation of calcium in bone depends upon the relative concentrations of both calcium and phosphate ions. It is believed that hydroxyapatite crystals are precipitated as a result of the local increase in phosphate ions near the osteoblasts. When the solubility product of calcium phosphate is exceeded, precipitation occurs. Although the exact mechanism for creating a favorable environment for precipitation is poorly understood, it is thought that the osteoblasts produce *alkaline phosphatase*, which hydrolyzes phosphate esters and creates a locally high concentration of phosphate. When enough phosphate is in solution around the osteoblasts to exceed the solubility product of calcium phosphate, the solution is saturated and bone mineralization occurs. It is probable that both the organic matrix and the alkaline phosphatase are involved in the production of bone. Hydroxyapatite crystals exactly like those found in bone are not precipitated unless the organic matrix is present.

Vitamin D

Vitamin D, or *cholecalciferol*, is produced in the skin of mammals from *7-dehydrocholesterol* in the presence of ultraviolet light (see Figure 8–7). It can also be obtained from the diet, an essential dietary ingredient in those

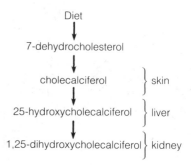

FIGURE 8–7
Biosynthesis of 1,25-dihydroxycholecalciferol, the active form of vitamin D

species which receive insufficient sunlight. Cholecalciferol is converted in the liver to *25-hydroxycholecalciferol*, which is transported through the blood to the kidneys. In the kidneys, the biologically active compound *1,25-dihydroxycholecalciferol* is synthesized from the 25-hydroxycholecalciferol. It is 1,25-dihydroxycholecalciferol which is necessary for the absorption of calcium from the gut. If this compound is unavailable a negative calcium balance results.

The formation of 1,25-dihydroxycholecalciferol by the kidneys is enhanced by parathyroid hormone, whose level is in turn controlled by calcium levels in the blood. The formation of 1,25-dihydroxycholecalciferol is dependent upon the active state of the renal enzyme *1,α-hydroxylase*. Interestingly, both the hormone prolactin and the hormone estrogen increase the activity of this enzyme which is necessary for maintaining an adequate supply of plasma calcium during lactation. The concentration of plasma phosphate also enhances the formation of active 1,α-hydroxylase, apparently through a negative feedback mechanism which exists in the kidney. The mobilization of calcium ion from bone is promoted by 1,25-dihydroxycholecalciferol, though its exact role is unknown. Calcium abosprtion from the gut is initiated by this compound. Such absorption stimulates the formation of messenger RNA, which is necessary for the formation of the enzyme that binds calcium in the mucosa of the gut.

A deficiency of vitamin D in mammals results in softer, more pliable bones due to the decreased calcification. This situation also occurs in lactating females. During lactation a dietary deficiency of calcium can lead to decalcification of bone. The sex steroids, estrogen and the androgens, are known to be important in calcification as well as organic matrix formation in bone. Postmenopausal reduction of estrogen formation is thought to be responsible for the weakening of bones, known as *osteoporosis*, which is seen in older women. It is not a disease which results in bone decalcification, as is the case in some forms of rickets, but instead results in a reduction of the total quantity of bone. It is usually associated with increased age or other factors which interfere with normal protein metabolism.

DISORDERS OF THE SKELETAL SYSTEM

Arthritis refers to a group of related diseases which involve inflammation of the joints. *Rheumatoid arthritis* is the most common form of arthritis. This particular disease is characterized by inflammation and swelling of the synovial membrane and subsequent loss of function of the joint. These symptoms are accompanied by a great deal of pain in many individuals. Rheumatoid arthritis should not be confused with *rheumatism*, a very general term which refers to any painful condition of the bones, joints, ligaments, ten-

dons, or muscles. *Osteoarthritis* is characterized by the degeneration of the articular cartilage, particularly of the weight-bearing joints. New osseous tissue is formed on the ends of the exposed bone and results in *spurs*, which then decrease the mobility of the joints.

Other diseases of the joints and their supportive tissues include *bursitis* and *tendinitis*. Bursitis is the inflammation of a *bursa*, a fluid-filled sac or saclike cavity which reduces friction during movement of the joint. Excessive friction in the area results in local inflammation and swelling due to the accumulation of fluid. Tendinitis, on the other hand, involves inflammation of tendons, especially in the wrist, knee, ankles, shoulders, elbows, and fingers.

SUMMARY

The skeleton provides support, form, protection of internal structures, and a storehouse for calcium and gives the rigidity necessary for movement through muscular contraction. Structurally, the skeletal system can be divided into an axial or central portion, which consists of the skull, the vertebral column, the ribs, and sternum, and the appendicular portion, which consists of the limbs, the pectoral girdle, and the sacral girdle. The heterotopic skeleton comprises those bones and cartilages not attached to other parts of the skeleton.

Bones connect with each other by means of articulations or joints. The joints are classified on a functional basis as synarthrotic (immovable), amphiarthrotic (slightly movable), and diarthrotic (freely movable). Each joint is a union of two or more bones connected by means of dense fibrous tissue (syndesmosis), by bone (synostosis), by cartilage (synchondrosis), or by a fluid-filled chamber (synovial).

Bones are formed within membranes by a process called intramembranous ossification and within cartilage by endochondral ossification. The bone-forming cells, or osteoblasts, lay down a protein matrix which is hardened through the precipitation of calcium salts in the form of hydroxyapatite crystals. When the osteoblasts become completely enclosed in small cavities called lacunae, their ability to form bone ceases and they are referred to as osteocytes. A third type of bone cell, the osteoclast, is formed from osteocytes adjacent to the bone marrow cavity. These cells have the function of mobilizing calcium salts from bone when calcium ions are needed by other parts of the body or when an increase in marrow cavity diameter is necessary.

The external dimensions of an organism are usually increased through an increase in the length and the diameter of the long bones. Growth of the long bones occurs as a result of the formation of osteoblasts, which are capable of forming bone tissue where cartilage previously existed. Growth of the long bones ceases with the union of the primary and secondary ossification centers, a process known as epiphyseal closure. High plasma concentrations of hormones such as testosterone and estrogen are known to be causative agents in epiphyseal closure.

Plasma calcium levels are regulated by means of parathyroid hormone and calcitonin. When plasma levels drop below normal homeostatic levels, parathyroid hormone is released, which induces the mobilization of calcium ions from bone. When the plasma calcium levels rise above the normal homeostatic levels, calcitonin is released from the thyroid gland. Parathyroid hormone is also necessary for adequate function of vitamin D in its role of enhancing intestinal absorption of calcium. The kidney, site of production of the active form of vitamin D (1,25-dihydroxycholecalciferol), is also important in the regulation of the plasma calcium levels. Parathyroid hormone enhances reabsorption of calcium ion and loss of phosphate from the kidneys.

Lactating animals have an increased rate of calcium loss through the milk, and insufficient dietary intake of calcium during lactation leads to the decalcification of bone. Two well-known diseases seen in mammals result from calcium ion deficiency. Rickets, frequently seen in younger animals, results in the formation of pliable bones due to the loss of rigidity provided by calcium salts. A second disease, osteoporosis, results from loss of bone material in older animals or in animals which have a protein deficiency. Its progress is usually tied to the decreased production of sex steroids with age or menopause.

9

BLOOD AS A TISSUE

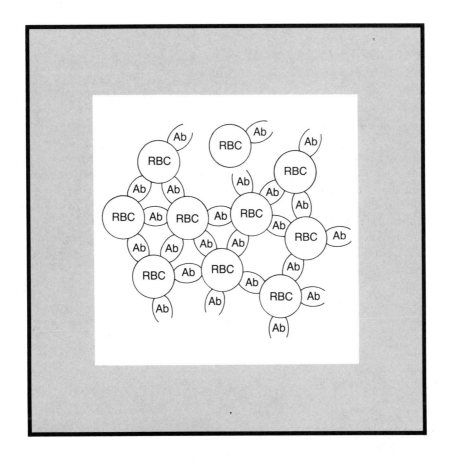

*T*ransportation of nutrients and waste materials in mammals is accomplished through the movement of dissolved and suspended substances in the bloodstream. Blood occupies approximately 7 percent of the animal's body weight and consists of liquid and solid components. The liquid portion of blood, called plasma, contains dissolved ions and organic substances in solution. When the proteins associated with the clotting process are removed from the plasma the remaining fluid is called serum. Blood cells, which constitute the formed elements of blood, are suspended in the plasma and are of two types: the erythrocytes, or red blood cells (RBC), and the leukocytes, or white blood cells (WBC). The erythrocytes are far more numerous than the leukocytes (5×10^6 and 7×10^3 per cubic millimeter of blood, respectively). The percent of blood volume occupied by the red blood cells is called the hematocrit. The hematocrit, which varies with the species and the physiological condition of the animal, is an extremely important factor in the adaptability of mammals.

FORMED ELEMENTS OF BLOOD

Erythrocytes

In essence, the mammalian red blood cell is a bag of *hemoglobin* molecules and other chemical elements necessary for oxygen transport. The red blood cells are not nucleated in mammals, but they are produced from nucleated cells in the red bone marrow that lose their nuclei immediately before being released into the bloodstream (see Figure 9–1). Mammalian erythrocytes are generally *biconcave*, rounded structures which are slightly larger than the diameter of the capillaries. In the family Camelidae, which includes the camel of Africa and the alpaca and guanaco of South America, the erythrocytes are *elliptical* rather than round in shape. The function of this peculiarity has not been determined. The size of the erythrocytes, which varies somewhat among species, for the most part ranges between 5.0 and 7.0 micrometers in diameter (see Table 9–1).

There is very little information about the role of size in erythrocyte function. It has

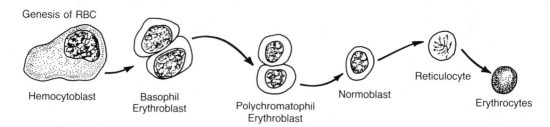

Genesis of RBC

Hemocytoblast   Basophil Erythroblast   Polychromatophil Erythroblast   Normoblast   Reticulocyte   Erythrocytes

FIGURE 9–1
Genesis of erythrocytes and principal precursor forms in mammals

TABLE 9–1
Erythrocyte diameters vary among species, but most range between 5.0 and 7.0 micrometers in diameter

Species	RBC Diameter (Micrometers)
Homo sapiens	7.5
Bos taurus (cattle)	5.9
Canis familiaris (dog)	7.0
Cavia porcellus (guinea pig)	7.4
Equus caballas (horse)	5.5
Felis catus (domesticated cat)	6.0

Source: From P. L. Altman and D. S. Dittmer, *Biology Data Book* (Bethesda, Maryland: Federation of American Societies for Experimental Biology, 1964)

been hypothesized that smaller red blood cells can be packed more densely than can larger ones, and therefore an animal with smaller erythrocytes has greater oxygen-carrying capacity. Also, small red blood cells might pass through capillaries more easily, therefore reducing peripheral resistance in some species. But small red blood cells are not necessarily associated with animals that have a high metabolic requirement. For example, in sheep the erythrocyte diameter is 4.8 micrometers, whereas the sheep's hematocrit is 31.7 percent and the hemoglobin concentration is 10.9 grams per 100 milliliters. The house mouse, on the other hand, has a much greater metabolic rate than the sheep but has red blood cells 6.0 micrometers in diameter. The mouse has a hematocrit of 41.5 percent and a hemoglobin concentration of 14.8 grams per 100 milliliters. The significance is that the animal with the highest metabolic rate has a greater oxygen-carrying capacity of blood. Carrying capacity is a function of the hematocrit and the plasma hemoglobin concentration, but carrying capacity is reflected neither in the diameter of the erythrocytes nor in the volume of individual

cells. It can be shown that the rate of oxygenation is affected by erythrocyte size and that smaller erythrocytes can be oxygenated more rapidly than larger ones (see Figure 9–2). But this still does not seem to have a functional basis, because metabolic rate does not appear to be correlated with either rate of oxygenation or erythrocyte size.

Significant hematocrit changes in most mammalian species require several days or weeks. In these species, the change results from increased production by *hemopoietic tissue*. In some species, however, the hematocrit can be altered rapidly depending upon biological need. Such animals store red blood cells in the spleen, from which they are readily released during strenuous exercise or other situations which require higher than normal oxygen transport. It should also be noted that such animals as the dog, cat, and horse, which can alter hematocrit in a short period of time, have comparatively low hematocrits at rest. Such rapid alteration of hematocrit cannot be carried out in human

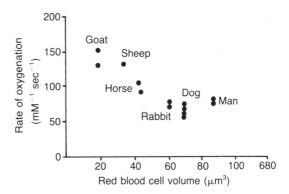

FIGURE 9–2
Relationship between rate of oxygenation and size of red blood cells. Notice that body mass does not follow a pattern here. From R. A. Holland and R. E. Horster, The Effect of the Size of Red Blood Cells on the Kinetics of their Oxygen Uptake. Reproduced from the *Journal of General Physiology*, 1966, 49:727–742, by copyright permission of the Rockefeller University Press.

athletes. But the process may be performed artificially during athletic training. Following periodic withdrawal of blood over several weeks during the conditioning period, the human athlete can be infused intravenously with his own erythrocytes immediately before an athletic event. This process is equivalent to storing red blood cells in the spleen and releasing them as the level of exercise increases.

Hemoglobin The red pigment that binds oxygen in mammals is called hemoglobin. It consists of an iron-containing *porphyrin*, or *heme portion*, and a protein, or *globin portion* (see Figure 9–3). Its molecular weight, approximately 64,450 daltons, varies slightly with different types of hemoglobin due to alterations in specific amino acids in the protein fraction. Hemoglobin comprises four

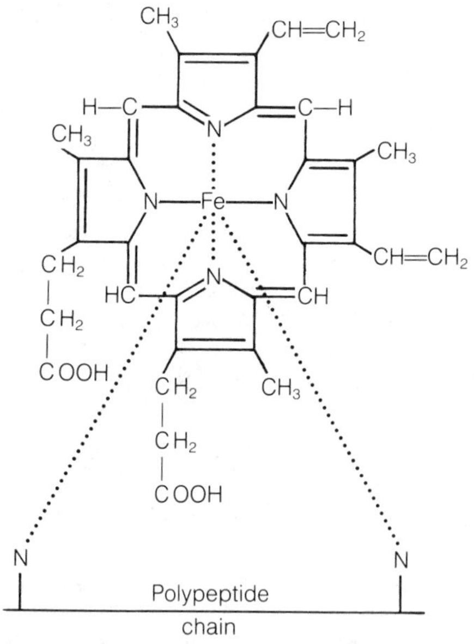

FIGURE 9–3
Diagram of deoxygenated hemoglobin

heme molecules and four protein subunits called the *alpha* and *beta chains*. Interspecific variations in oxygen affinities of hemoglobin are the result of minor alterations in these peptide chains. The most common hemoglobin type in humans is called *hemoglobin A* or *adult hemoglobin*, which normally consists of two alpha chains, each with 141 amino acid residues, and two beta chains, each of which is composed of 146 amino acids. Some individuals contain a second type of hemoglobin called *hemoglobin A_2*. In this second type, the beta chains are replaced by alpha chains which contain 146 amino acids, but at least 10 specific amino acids differ from the amino acids found in normal hemoglobin A beta chains. In other types of human hemoglobin, similar amino acid substitutions are found. For instance, some people of African descent have a hemoglobin which causes red blood cells to crenate and assume a sickle shape, hence the name *sickle cell anemia*. Since the sickle cell hemoglobin is a poor oxygen carrier, people with this condition suffer from insufficient oxygen, or anemia, at altitudes not stressful to people with hemoglobin A. Sickle cell hemoglobin (*hemoglobin S*) differs from hemoglobin A by having one amino acid residue in the beta chain, *glutamic acid*, replaced by *valine*. Individuals who are heterozygous for the gene that causes sickle cell anemia have greater survival rates in malaria infested areas than persons with normal adult hemoglobin. The homozygous condition, however, is usually fatal.

Sickle cell hemoglobin is not the only abnormal hemoglobin found in the human species. In fact, at least eighty different types of hemoglobin have been found. Given the number of total intraspecific variations in humans, other types different from hemoglobin

A will probably be discovered. In some of these hemoglobin types, deleterious effects such as poor ability to bind oxygen are balanced by an equivalent or more important survival factor (e.g., individuals with hemoglobin S have higher survival rates in malaria infested regions).

Hemoglobin F, or *fetal hemoglobin,* has a greater *oxygen affinity* than does adult hemoglobin. This is necessary for the fetus to obtain oxygen from the placenta during gestation. This characteristic is true of all mammalian species studied thus far. In *viviparous mammals,* in which the fetus develops in the mother's womb, oxygen must be extracted from the maternal circulation to supply the fetus. In order for oxygen to be retained by the fetus and used in its metabolism, a hemoglobin with greater oxygen affinity than that of the maternal blood is necessary. Even nonmammalian vertebrates such as amphibians have hemoglobin in the larval or embryonic stages that differs from the adult form. In the human species, the beta chains of the adult hemoglobin are replaced by the gamma chain in the fetus. The gamma chain consists of 146 amino acid residues, but 37 of them are different from the residues found in the beta chains of the adult. In some individuals fetal hemoglobin persists throughout adult life without obvious deleterious consequences.

Such examples point to the critical nature of the *quaternary structure* of hemoglobin. Hemoglobin has a very regular structure, with intermolecular binding between amino acids of the four peptide chains (see Figure 9–4). If a portion of the hemoglobin molecule is changed through the substitution of some amino acids, the normal binding properties of the protein chains are altered. The result is a modification of the quaternary structure

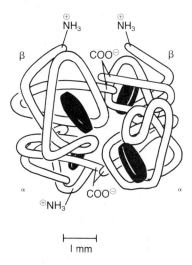

FIGURE 9–4
Quaternary structure of hemoglobin showing the relationship of alpha and beta chains. Heme moieties are represented by dark discs. From H. A. Harper et al, *Physiologische Chemie,* überarb. Aufl., Z völlig, (Heidelberg, Germany, 1979). Reprinted with permission from Springer-Verlag.

as it exists in the normal animal. Since oxygen is loosely bound by the hemoglobin, the quaternary structure of the hemoglobin molecule is very important. An alteration of this structure causes a redistribution of the molecular charges essential to oxygen binding and consequently results in a change in oxygen affinity.

Specific differences in hemoglobins among species are easily compared by determining the oxygen affinity of the blood. Oxygen affinity is assessed by measuring the partial pressure of oxygen at which 50 percent saturation of hemoglobin occurs. This is commonly known as the P_{50} *value.* The higher the P_{50} value, the lower the affinity of hemoglobin to oxygen. Normally, smaller mammals have higher metabolic rates than larger mammals, and the P_{50} values of their hemoglobins are correspondingly greater. Decreased oxygen affinity makes it easier for oxygen to unload at the tissue level, and therefore mammals with hemoglobin having a lower affinity for oxygen can deliver oxygen more easily to the tissues (see chapter 11, The Heart as a Pump).

As expected, mammals adapted to higher altitudes have hemoglobin with high oxygen affinity. Most of these species belong to the family Camelidae. The common dromedary of the Sahara and the Nile Valley, a member of this family, has hemoglobin with elevated oxygen affinity. No explanation is apparent in this case. One would expect mammals from areas such as the Nile Valley to have hemoglobin traits distinct from high altitude species found in the Andes Mountains of South America. In this case it is apparent that genetic background overrides environmental adaptation.

Leukocytes

The white blood cells are variable in size, function, and structure. All of the leukocytes are nucleated, and they are produced in the red bone marrow from *hemocytoblasts* or from other white blood cells in circulation (see Figure 9–5). The leukocytes fall into two major groups based upon structure. The *granulocytes* have granulated cytoplasm and possess lobed nuclei. Three types of granulocytes, based upon staining characteristics of the granules, are found in mammals: *neutrophils*, which have a lack of affinity for both acidic and basic strains; *basophils*, which have an affinity for basic dyes; and *eosinophils*, which have an affinity for acidic dyes. The second major group of leukocytes, the *agranulocytes*, lacks cytoplasmic granules and usually possesses a spheroid nucleus. Two types of agranulocytes are found in mammals: *lymphocytes*, which have large nu-

clei and very little cytoplasm; and *monocytes*, which have an abundant cytoplasm with small, kidney-shaped nuclei.

The life of circulating white blood cells is fairly short. Under normal conditions their lifespan does not exceed several weeks, but in the case of infection they might not live for more than five or six hours. New leukocytes are produced very rapidly during an infection, so in some cases there may be a doubling or tripling of the circulating number of white blood cells. Usually the type of infection is indicated by the relative number of particular leukocytic types. Bacterial infections are accompanied by increases in neutrophils and monocytes. Allergic reactions usually cause an increase in the number of eosinophils. A selective count of the different types of white blood cells is referred to as a *differential count*.

Functions of white blood cells   The white blood cells function in the production of *immunity*. They are considered to be the body's second line of defense, after the integrity of body surfaces, against infection: leukocytes inactivate foreign materials such as bacteria and viruses. They carry out their function by producing *antibodies*, which deactivate the foreign substances, called *antigens*. An antigen is a molecule or particle which stimulates the production of specific antibodies, cell mediated immunity, or both. The antibodies are serum or cell-bound proteins produced in response to an antigen and able to react specifically to that antigen. Some leukocytes also have the ability to engulf foreign particles by phagocytosis. White blood cells also produce and release substances which attack bacterial cell walls. Certain plasma fragments also modify the infecting particles, after which they may be more easily phago-

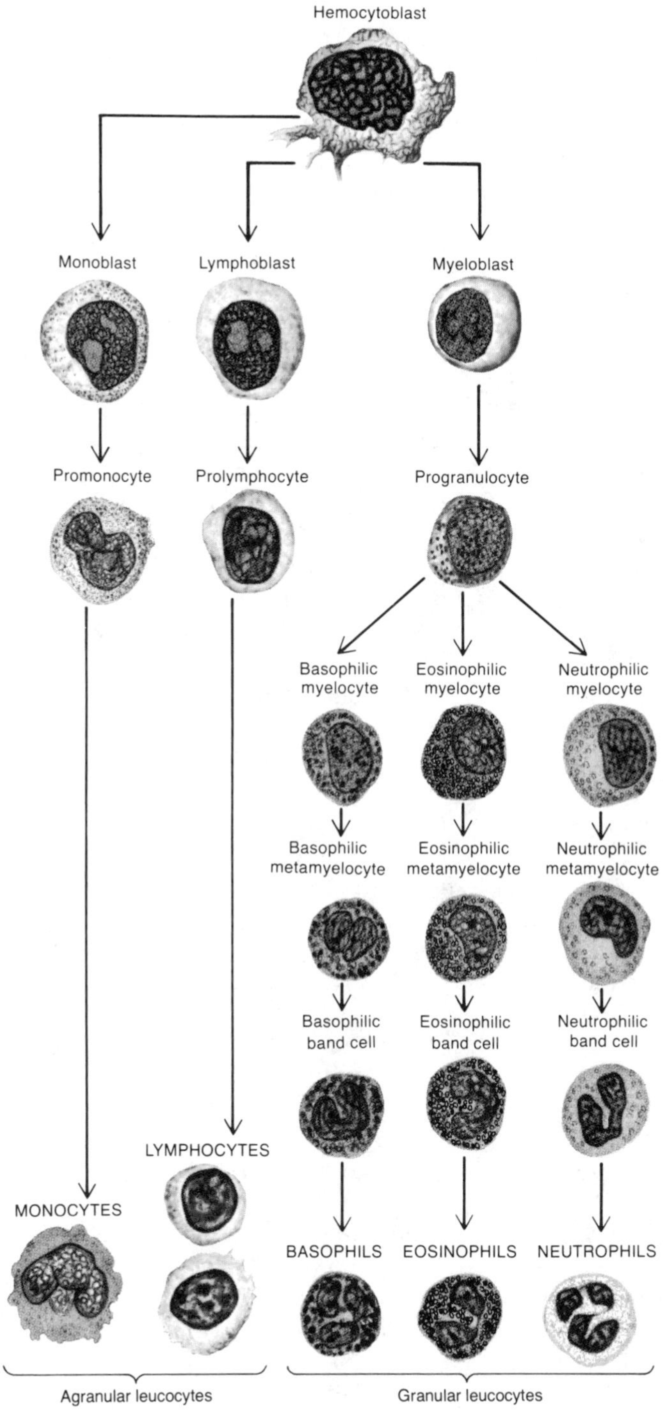

Hemocytoblast

Monoblast   Lymphoblast   Myeloblast

Promonocyte   Prolymphocyte   Progranulocyte

Basophilic   Eosinophilic   Neutrophilic
myelocyte   myelocyte   myelocyte

Basophilic   Eosinophilic   Neutrophilic
metamyelocyte   metamyelocyte   metamyelocyte

Basophilic   Eosinophilic   Neutrophilic
band cell   band cell   band cell

LYMPHOCYTES

MONOCYTES

BASOPHILS   EOSINOPHILS   NEUTROPHILS

Agranular leucocytes   Granular leucocytes

FIGURE 9–5
Schematic of leukocyte synthesis. Adapted from G. J. Tortora and N. P. Anagnastakos, Principles of Anatomy and Physiology, 3rd edition (New York, N.Y., 1981) 443, fig 19–1. Reprinted by permission of Harper and Row Publishers.

175

cytized by the leukocytes. This enhancing of phagocytosis is called *opsonization*. The plasma particles which act as *opsonins* are usually part of the plasma protein fraction.

White blood cells have the ability to exit the circulatory system and accumulate at the site of infection. They pass through the endothelial wall of the capillaries by a process known as *diapedesis*, which is similar to ameboid movement. Location of the site of infection is accomplished through a process called *chemotaxis*, whereby the leukocytes are attracted to the area of infection. In this way the white blood cells, usually neutrophilic granulocytes, can home in on the site of infection.

Phagocytosis is usually carried out by neutrophils. When phagocytosis of the foreign particle occurs, the phagocytic vesicle formed unites with granules in the cytoplasm. This process ultimately decreases the number of granules in the cytoplasm (degranulation) and effects an increase in oxygen uptake by the leukocyte. This *oxygen burst*, the rapid uptake of oxygen, leads to the production of *hydrogen peroxide* and the *peroxide radical*. Both hydrogen peroxide and peroxide radicals combine with the substances in the granules to lyse (disintegrate) the bacteria or other particle type after phagocytosis.

Monocytes Monocytes are phagocytic and contain peroxidases and lytic enzymes. Their function is very similar to that of the neutrophils, except that their reaction time is usually slower. During an infection, they enter the tissue and become *tissue macrophages*. The tissue macrophages collectively form the *reticulo-endothelial system*. This system includes cells bound to the endothelium of certain parts of the circulatory system.

Lymphocytes Lymphocytes are formed in bone marrow and lymph glands. Some migrate to the bloodstream, where they populate the thymus gland and are converted to *T lymphocytes*, which are then transferred to various parts of the body. The T lymphocytes, which become incorporated into most body tissues, are responsible for cellular immunity. They participate in tissue rejection and allergic reactions.

Some of the lymphocytes are probably affected by the gut-associated lymphoid tissue and become *B lymphocytes*. These cells produce plasma-borne antibodies and are therefore involved in *humoral immunity*. When the B lymphocytes contact a particular antigen, they are in some way modified to produce specific antibodies against that specific antigen. The antibodies have a characteristic molecular structure which "recognizes" (reacts with) their specific antigen. The recognition process between antigens and antibodies is very much like the reaction between enzymes and their substrates. In other words, the antibody has a steric configuration which recognizes proteins or other antigenic substances that have very specific characteristics. Once a lymphocyte begins to produce a particular antibody, it becomes a *committed lymphocyte* and will produce only one type of antibody. These committed lymphocytes are also capable of dividing and thereby producing many identical cells which also produce the specific antibody. This process, called *cloning*, enables cells activated by antigens to produce additional antibody-producing cells without the latter's having come in contact with the antigen themselves.

If an antigen is not reintroduced into the animal for a period of time, specific cells of that clone, which produce the antibody against that particular antigen, will continue to decrease in number. But some of the cells may continue to be produced. Such cells are called *memory cells* as the result of their ability to recognize their specific antigen. A similar process exists for the multiplication of T lymphocytes. It is in this way that organisms are able to maintain an immunity for long periods of time. The second introduction of the antigen usually results in a massive increase in the number of circulating antibodies and antibody producing cells, known as a *secondary* or *anamnestic response* (see Figure 9–6).

When an animal has developed sufficient antibodies to prevent a successful invasion of a particular strain of bacteria or virus, it is said to be *immune* to that particular disease-causing organism. In many cases immunity to a disease arises as a result of the animal's having contracted the disease or contracted a nonvirulent form of the disease. Such resistance is called *acquired immunity*. If an animal has resistance to a disease at birth or shortly thereafter as a result of heredity, it is said to have a *natural immunity* to that disease. A number of mammalian species have natural immunity to the invasion of specific disease-causing organisms. All mammals have certain types of cell-mediated and humoral immunity at birth or shortly thereafter, except in cases of genetic immunodeficiencies.

There is a great deal of variation in the degree of natural immunity among species. A list of such is outside of the scope of this text, but the following example should give some indication of the growing importance of research in this area. Tetanus toxin is a substance produced by the bacterium *Clostridium tetani*. This toxin has its main action on the motor horn cells in the spinal cord and on certain neurons in the brain stem. Individuals who have contracted an active culture of *C. tetani* usually show spasmodic activity because of the hypersensitivity developed in the spinal motor nerves. Such hypersensitivity is believed to result from the blockage of the release of inhibitory transmitter, though the exact inhibitory substance has not been identified. Most vertebrates are not susceptible to tetanus toxin, but most mammals do react to it to some degree. Little statistical data on the relative susceptibility of most species have accrued. Among the domesticated mammals, *C. tetani* infestations are most prevalent in the horse, which is said to be 800 times more susceptible to the disease than are humans. With only rare exceptions, humans who have contracted the bacterium have not survived.

For the most part, comparative data illustrating the susceptibility of mammalian species to different diseases or to the actions of specific toxins produced by the disease-forming organism are difficult to acquire. The

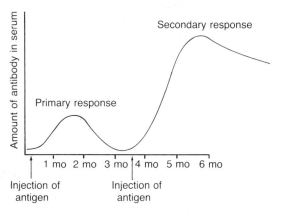

FIGURE 9–6
The anamnestic (secondary) response of mammals to an antigen after becoming sensitized earlier to the same antigen (primary response)

physiological mechanisms by which bacterial toxins are manifested are extremely interesting, and their mode of action should be of the utmost importance in developing adequate treatment and prophylaxis.

BLOOD COAGULATION

In order for a fluid system such as blood to be useful over long periods of time it is essential that it contain a *sealing mechanism* to prevent loss during trauma. A useful sealing mechanism, such as *blood clotting* or *coagulation*, must be triggered by a reliable indicator of trauma. In the normal sense, blood clotting is triggered by a substance released from damaged cells which compose part of the blood vessel wall or from adjacent tissue. The trigger is known as an *external clotting factor*, and the sequence of chemical reactions which proceed from it are known collectively as the *external clotting mechanism* (see Figure 9–7). The chemical events shown in Figure 9–7 ultimately terminate in the formation of the insoluble protein *fibrin*, which aligns itself into strands (see Figure 9–8). The fibrin strands adhere to the walls of the injured vessel, where they form a meshwork capable of collecting blood cells and *platelets* to form a solid plug, called a *clot*. The clot becomes denser due to contraction of the fibrin strands when stimulated or activated by *serotonin* (5-hydroxytryptamine). The serotonin necessary to induce this process, called *clot retraction*, is released from the platelets trapped in the meshwork of the clot.

After retraction of the clot, the vessel is normally *rechanneled*, or *recanalized*, to install adequate circulation to the area of the body previously isolated by the clot. Recanalization requires from several hours to several

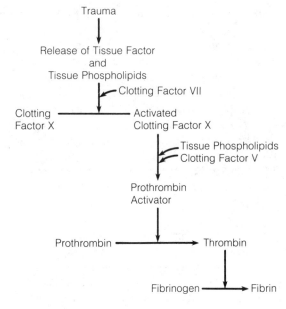

FIGURE 9–7
Steps responsible for thrombus formation by the external (extrinsic) clotting mechanism

days, depending upon the size of the vessel and the adequacy of collateral circulation to supply life support for the tissue in question. Some tissues, such as the heart and brain, have a constant demand for oxygen. Since the function of these tissues is essential to the function of the organism as a whole, any malfunction resulting from loss of circulation to these areas is usually noticeable.

A second type of clotting trigger sometimes activated in mammals can have a devastating effect. In this mechanism an *internal* or *intrinsic clotting factor* is formed in the absence of trauma (see Figure 9–9). If the clot forms in or travels to the vessels of the brain or heart, a reduction of blood flow may occur which results in *ischemia*, or a localized tissue anoxia, to the area that normally receives blood from the obstructed vessel. If the ischemic or oxygen-depleted area is large

Blood vessel wall

A. Blood escaping through severed blood vessel.

FIGURE 9–8
Steps in clot formation and
retraction in an injured blood
vessel

B. Formation of fibrin strands across vessel opening.

C. Entrapment and attachment of the formed
elements in blood by the fibrin strands.

D. Decrease in vessel diameter during
clot retraction.

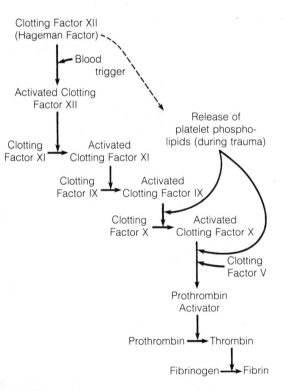

FIGURE 9–9
Thrombus (or clot) formation by the internal (intrinsic)
clotting mechanism

enough, partial or complete loss of function can occur. If the ischemia occurs in the brain or heart, the result is either a stroke or heart attack, respectively. Clots which result in tissue damage may be formed in other parts of the body and carried to an *arteriole*, or small artery, where they block circulation and blood supply. If the resulting clot or thrombus adheres to the walls of vessels in relatively nonvital tissue like adipose tissue or skeletal muscle, a critical decrease in function may not be noted. A floating clot, known as an *embolus*, can be formed from both external or internal clotting pathways. Ischemia can be caused by situations other than the intrinsic clotting mechanism. For instance, in some cases ischemia can result from arteriole spasms and schlerotic disease.

The *internal* or *intrinsic clotting mechanism* is of significant medical importance since an understanding of the exact causes of clots in the untraumatized individual could lead to significant reduction in the number of heart attacks and strokes, which are the major killers of humans in North American and European societies. Blood-borne substances such as cholesterol, triglycerides, and fatty acids have all been linked in one way or another to the problem, but little definitive data as to cause and effect have accumulated. It is obvious that a multitude of factors may be involved. Some of these, such as cigarette smoking and alcohol consumption, are societal and can be controlled; whereas others, such as climate and seasonal changes, must be tolerated until a method of controlling the response of the individual to these factors can be found.

Quite a bit of variation in clotting factors has been found in humans. Many of these are quite noticeable because the absence of certain factors has been associated with several of the bleeder diseases. Other factors such as *Hageman's factor* (Factor XII) are absent in some humans with no apparent ill effects. As a matter of fact, Hageman's factor is thought by some to be the principal culprit in the internal clotting mechanism and therefore is primarily responsible for the thrombotic diseases previously mentioned. A number of mammalian species lack Hageman's factor altogether and seem to have no problem with thromboembolic diseases.

BLOOD GROUPS

In the mammals, proteins on the surface of the red blood cells vary widely and may be capable of inducing antibody formation among individuals of the same species. In most cases, blood *agglutinins* (antibodies) are produced at a very early age and do not require exposure to the red blood cells of another animal. But in several cases, as in the *Rh blood group* in humans, prior exposure of an Rh-negative individual to Rh-positive blood is necessary for antibody formation.

The ABO blood-grouping system is perhaps the most widely known. These blood types are of the utmost importance in cases of blood transfusion because of the natural presence of agglutinating antibodies in the serum. Blood types characterizing this group are based upon antigens, or *agglutinogens*, carried on the red blood cells of each individual. Basically this blood-grouping system comprises the blood types *A*, *B*, *O*, and *AB*. Agglutinogen (antigen) A occurs in two principal forms: A_1 and A_2. Type B blood produces antibody A against the A antigen, and type A blood produces antibody B against the B antigen. Cross reaction among these blood types results in *agglutination* or tying together of the red blood cells to form the antigen-antibody complexes (see Figure 9–10). Antibodies in these blood groups have two reaction sites and are thus said to be *divalent*. They can bind together two antigens present on two different red blood cells. In this way, when two erythrocytes are bound by one end of the divalent antibody and enough antibodies are present, the red blood cells clump together to form a latticework structure which results in agglutination.

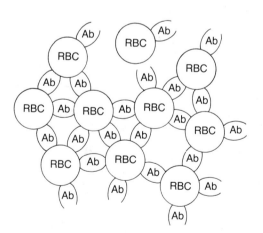

FIGURE 9–10
Agglutination of erythrocytes in the presence of divalent antibodies

Since type AB contains both A antigens and B antigens and the serum contains neither A nor B antibodies, individuals with AB blood can receive blood transfusions from any of the other ABO blood groups without ill effects. For this reason individuals with AB blood are known as *universal recipients.* Type O blood can be used to transfuse individuals with other blood types because of the lack of antigens which could react with antibodies present in the blood of the recipient. Therefore, individuals with O blood are known as *universal donors.*

In humans, blood types vary considerably among people of different racial and ethnic origins (see Table 9–2). In the ABO blood-grouping system there are eleven genotypes possible, based upon four alleles. Certain diseases are more prevalent in people of certain blood types than in others. This by no means implies that disease resistance is inherent to certain blood groups.

Another well-known blood-grouping system in humans is the Rh group. The etymology of *Rh factor* derives from its original discovery in the rhesus monkey. There are two basic phenotypes found in humans: *Rh-positive* individuals, who possess the *D antigen*

on their red blood cells; and *Rh-negative* individuals, who do not possess the D antigen. Antibodies to the Rh-positive blood types are acquired after exposure to the antigen, instead of being formed naturally as are the ABO antibodies. These antibodies are produced in Rh-negative individuals after they come in contact, by transfusion or other means, with the D antigen of the red blood cell. If an individual having Rh-negative blood is exposed to the D antigen, antibodies to the D antigen are synthesized so slowly that the recipient is not placed in any immediate danger. But because D antibodies eventually build up and may be retained for many years, further cross matching between the Rh-positive donor and the Rh-negative recipient is dangerous.

Transfusion between Rh-positive and Rh-negative individuals is normally avoided in clinical situations. But cross matching can naturally occur in situations where an Rh-negative mother carries an Rh-positive fetus. Small amounts of blood may be exchanged between the mother and fetus due to rupture of local vessels in the placenta during parturition. When blood transfer occurs, antibodies are formed in the maternal circulation in

TABLE 9–2
Distribution of blood groups in various human populations

Population	Location	Number of Subjects	Frequency (%)			
			O	A	B	AB
American Indian (Blackfoot)	Montana	115	23.5	76.5	0	0
Australian aborigine	Australia	805	53.1	44.7	2.1	0
Bedouin (Iraq)	Baghdad	338	40.8	26.6	25.8	6.8
Chinese	Peking	1,000	30.7	25.1	34.2	10.0
English	S. England	106,477	45.2	43.2	8.5	3.1
Eskimo	SW Greenland	1,063	46.0	46.1	4.9	3.0

Source: From P. L. Altman and D. S. Dittmer, *Biology Data Book* (Bethesda, Maryland: Federation of American Societies for Experimental Biology, 1964)

response to the foreign fetal antigens. The mother has thus been sensitized to (produced antibodies against) the D antigen. In this case, an active immunity will be produced over a period of time. During the first pregnancy involving an Rh-negative mother and Rh-positive fetus, there is usually little difficulty from Rh factors unless the mother was previously sensitized to the D antigen. If there is a second or third pregnancy with an Rh-positive fetus in a sensitized mother, she may begin to produce large quantitites of antibodies. The Rh-positive antibodies, *immunoglobulin G (IgG)*, are capable of crossing the placental barrier, where they cause fetal blood to agglutinate. Agglutinated red blood cells are *hemolyzed* (ruptured), and the hemoglobin which is released is converted to a bile pigment called *bilirubin*. Since the fetal liver is not capable of removing large quantities of bile pigments, bilirubin is released into the plasma and taken up by various tissues within the body. The absorption of bile by the skin results in a jaundiced appearance. The babies from this type of pregnancy are usually born with D antibodies from the mother and generally continue to lose red blood cells for six to eight weeks after birth. The hemopoietic tissue is stimulated to produce erythrocytes to replace the ones hemolyzed and as a result produces nucleated pre-erythrocytic forms such as hemocytoblasts. The increased number of *blastic* (nucleated) forms present in the blood gives the characteristic name of *erythroblastosis fetalis* to this disease.

When it is known that the mother is Rh-negative and has just had a miscarriage, abortion, or birth of an Rh-positive fetus, erythroblastosis fetalis can be prevented in future pregnancies. Since the mixing of fetal and maternal blood usually only occurs during parturition (if at all), antibodies usually only begin to form after parturition, rather than during a first pregnancy. If the mother is injected with a massive dose of D antibodies (a *Rho gam shot*), usually within 24 hours postpartum, the Rh antigens which may be present will be bound by these antibodies and cleared from the mother's circulation. Because of the clearing action, the mother will not become sensitized and therefore will not form her own antibodies against the D antigen. If these shots are given following subsequent pregnancies as well, the possibility of erythroblastosis fetalis is virtually eliminated.

The hemolysis of erythrocytes due to A and B antibodies crossing the placental barrier occurs only in very rare instances. In some cases, however, these factors pass the placental barrier and induce fetal blood agglutination. Also rare is the situation in which Rh-positive mothers produce D antibodies. Since the Rh factor depends upon multiple alleles, it has been hypothesized that these mothers have only one of the Rh-positive genes and are essentially Rh negative for all other alleles of the D antigen. This implies that they are genetically Rh-negative but have enough of the genetically dominant Rh-positive alleles to show an Rh-positive phenotype.

CALCULATION OF PLASMA AND BLOOD VOLUMES

The blood volume of domesticated mammals is fairly well known (see Table 9–3). In these species the range is usually between 6.0 and 8.0 percent of total body weight. But in such species as the thoroughbred horse, blood volume occupies a higher percentage, presumably essential to the excessive respiratory demands when racing. "Cold-blooded"

TABLE 9–3
Cellular constituents in blood of several species of domesticated mammals

Species	WBC* (× 10^3)	RBC† (Cell/mm^3 × 10^3)	Hb‡ (g/100 ml)	RBC Diameter (μm)	Total Plasma Protein (g/100 ml)
Cattle	4–12 8	5.0–10.0 7.0	8–15 11	4.5–8.0 5.8	6–8
Horse Cold-blooded Thoroughbred	6–12 8.5 5.5–12.5 9.0	5.5–9.5 7.5 6.5–12.5 9.5	8–14 11.5 11–19 15	4.0–8.0 5.9–5.8	6–8
Sheep	4.0–12.0 8.0	8–16.0 12.0	8–16 12	3.2–6.0 4.5	6–7.5
Goat	4.1–13.0 9.0	8.0–18.0 13.0	8–14 11	2.5–3.9 3.2	6–7.5
Swine	11.0–22.0 16.0	5.0–8.0 6.5	10–16 13		
Dog	6.0–7.0 11.5	5.5–8.5 6.8	12–18 15	6.7–7.2 7.0	6–7.5
Cat	5.5–19.5 12.5	5.0–10.0 7.5	8–15 12		6–7.5

Source: From *Veterinary Physiology* by J. W. Phillis. Copyright © 1976 by W. B. Saunders Co. Reprinted by permission of the author. After J. Bentinck-Smith (1969), *Hematology: A Textbook of Veterinary Clinical Pathology*, vol. 2. Baltimore: Williams & Wilkins.
*White Blood Cells
†Red Blood Cells
‡Hemoglobin

horses (draft horses) perform at a slower pace and hence place a lower demand upon the respiratory function of blood.

Plasma volume is normally measured by injecting a known amount of an easily detectable substance into the blood. The material ideally should be retained in the bloodstream and not leak into the surrounding tissues. The substance should also dissolve in the plasma and not enter the erythrocytes. After equilibration, a blood sample can be taken and centrifuged, and the plasma can be analyzed to determine the concentration of the injected material. Plasma volume can then be calculated by use of the following formula:

$$PV = \frac{S}{C} \qquad (9.1)$$

where,

PV = plasma volume (liters)
S = amount of the injected substance (milligrams)
C = concentration of the substance in the plasma after equilibration (milligrams/liter).

In most cases a vital dye such as Evans blue dye is used which remains in the plasma and causes no apparent harm to the animal.

In order to determine total blood volume using Evans blue dye, the volume taken by the red blood cells must be considered. Blood volume can be calculated by use of the following formula:

$$BV = \frac{\dfrac{S}{C}}{1 - \text{the hematocrit fraction}} \quad (9.2)$$

where,

BV = blood volume (liters)
S = amount of the injected substance (milligrams)
C = concentration of the substance in the blood after equilibration (milligrams/liter).
1 − the hematocrit = fraction of plasma.

As an example, let us determine the blood volume of a mammal using this method. First, five milligrams of Evans blue dye is dissolved in a milliliter of plasma or isotonic salt solution. This mixture is then injected into the test animal's bloodstream, and a time lapse of a few minutes is allowed for the dye to become equally distributed throughout the animal's circulatory system. Then a blood sample is drawn into a heparinized syringe and centrifuged to separate the cells from the plasma. A plasma sample is analyzed for dye concentration, and the plasma volume is computed using equation 9.1. Total blood volume is then calculated using equation 9.2. If the concentration of dye in the plasma is found to be 1.85 mg/l, the plasma volume is 2.7 liters. This is derived from equation 9.1, where S = 5 mg and C = 1.85 mg/l; then PV

$= \dfrac{5 \text{ mg}}{(1.85 \text{ mg/l})}$ = 2.7 liters. The total blood vol-

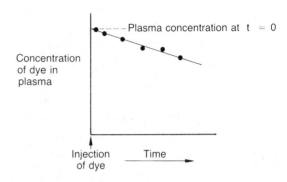

FIGURE 9–11
Determination of dye concentration by extrapolation to time zero

ume can be determined by dividing the plasma volume by 1 minus the hematocrit, as shown in equation 9.2. In this example, if the hematocrit is 0.45, 2.7 liters divided by 0.55 (i.e., 1 − 0.45) equals a blood volume of 4.9 liters.

A problem with this technique is that most dyes slowly leak out of the bloodstream and into the tissues. Such leakage is progressive and becomes greater with time. Thus, to measure blood volume accurately, one must know the concentration of dye in the bloodstream at the instant it is fully equilibrated, or at *time zero*. To determine plasma volume at time zero a progression of concentrations is determined as a function of time (see Figure 9–11). By extrapolating dye concentration to time zero, plasma and blood volumes can be more accurately determined.

Equation 9.1 will suffice in blood volume determinations if erythrocytes *labeled* with a radioactive substance are injected instead of a dye. The injected cells will become dispersed among the nonlabeled red blood cells. After dispersal of the labeled erythrocytes, whole blood can be analyzed for radioactivity. The equation for blood volume determination becomes:

$$BV = \frac{C_{IR}}{C_E} \qquad (9.3)$$

where,

BV = blood volume (liters)

C_{IR} = injected erythrocytes (counts/min)

C_E = blood sample after equilibration (counts/min/liter)

Plasma volume can also be assessed more accurately without the need of extrapolation by using labeled red blood cells instead of a dye. Red blood cells do not diffuse out of the circulatory system as a dye does.

SUMMARY

The primary functions of blood are the transport of substances and the defense against disease. Blood is a mixture as well as a solution, and its viscosity is not uniform in each part of the system through which it passes. When whole blood is allowed to stand in a test tube or is centrifuged, the cells settle out, leaving a clear liquid called plasma. The percentage of whole blood which is occupied by red blood cells is known as the hematocrit. Blood represents about 7.0 percent of the animal's body weight, and the erythrocytes occupy about 45.0 percent of the total blood volume.

The red blood cells are not nucleated and contain hemoglobin. The erythrocytes are produced from hemocytoblasts in the bone marrow of the adult mammal. The red blood cells are slightly larger in diameter than the smallest vessels through which they pass. Size of the cells does not seem to be correlated with metabolic rate. Some mammals can alter the concentration of erythrocytes in their bloodstream by storing them in the spleen and releasing them into the bloodstream during exercise or other situations which produce a high oxygen demand.

Hemoglobin is a blood pigment capable of binding oxygen and comprises porphyrin (heme) and protein (globin) portions. Hemoglobin structure differs both among and within species and has different affinities for oxygen depending upon the structure of the molecule. Several different hemoglobin structures are found in the human species. These differ primarily in the arrangement of only a few amino acids in the protein fraction. In general, mammals with high metabolic rates have hemoglobin with low oxygen affinity. This facilitates oxygen release at the tissue level.

The white blood cells are less numerous than the red blood cells. They are produced not only from the hemocytoblasts of the bone marrow but also from other white blood cells. These cells are always nucleated. They provide the body's second line of defense against disease. Leukocytes can remove bacteria by the process of phagocytosis and can produce antibodies capable of binding foreign substances in the blood and other tissues of the body. White blood cells also have the ability to leave the capillaries and proceed to an area of infection. They are therefore able to combat bacteria and other insults from foreign materials in most locations of the body. When leukocytes become sensitized to a particular foreign substance, many more cells capable of producing the same type of antibody are produced by cloning. Leukocytes called memory cells are retained for long periods of time and can produce new cells capable of producing the same specific antibody.

Many mammals produce antibodies beginning at birth which cause the red blood cells of individuals to agglutinate. This provides the basis for some very distinct blood-grouping systems. Still other blood groups are present which lack native antibodies but which are produced after sensitization to the antigen. All mammals have specific blood groups, but data concerning them in mammals other than humans are meager.

Blood contains a clotting mechanism known as coagulation and requires a complete series of chemical reactions before completion. Many variations occur in the clotting process of different species and among animals of the same species. For the most part, clotting is induced by a trigger substance from outside the blood which is released from traumatized cells. Blood occasionally coagulates as the result of an internally triggered mechanism.

Plasma and blood volumes can be determined after injecting a dye into the circulatory system. After equilibration, plasma samples can be taken and analyzed for concentrations of the injected dye. The plasma volume can be determined by dividing the amount of dye injected by the concentration of the dye in the sample taken. Total blood volume is equal to the plasma volume divided by the fraction of plasma in whole blood. Blood volume can also be determined after injection of red blood cells labeled with a radioactive substance. Once equilibrium is reached, blood volume can be determined by dividing the total counts injected by the total counts of radioactive material per cubic milliliter of whole blood.

10

THE CIRCULATORY SYSTEM AND BLOOD PRESSURE

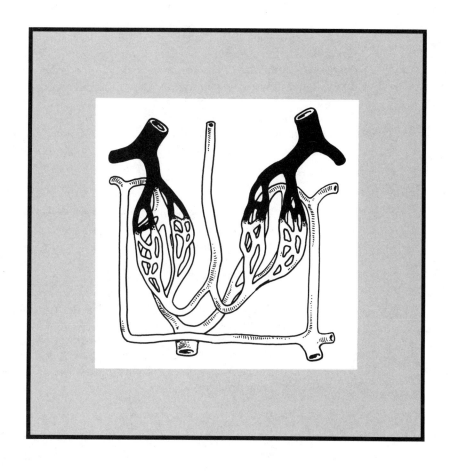

*T*he circulatory system of mammals represents the primary transport mechanism for metabolic substances and respiratory gases. In addition, it provides defense against invading microorganisms and harmful chemicals and maintains a uniform balance of fluids throughout the body. It is essential in communication through its transport of hormones within the body and provides a vital link for heat transfer between the organism and its environment.

The circulatory system of the vertebrates is a closed circuit of interconnected channels, or vessels, which carry blood to all parts of the body. Vessels carrying blood to the tissues from the heart are called arteries; those carrying blood back to the heart are called veins. A four-chambered heart is present in mammals which allows complete separation of venous and arterial blood. This system can be divided into two distinct cycles with respect to the heart and therefore into two separate units, called the systemic (greater) and pulmonary (lesser) circulations. In pulmonary circulation, deoxygenated blood is pumped from the right ventricle of the heart to the lungs and is carried back to the left atrium of the heart through the pulmonary veins. In systemic circulation, the left side of the heart pushes blood through the aorta to all parts of the body except the lungs. Blood flows from the tissues back to the heart through the venae cavae to complete the systemic circulation.

Two distinct features of the circulatory system have allowed the mammals to maintain a relatively high metabolic rate compared to other vertebrates: (1) the complete separation of oxygenated and deoxygenated blood and (2) the development of a vascular system capable of delivering blood to the tissues under comparatively high pressure. Complete separation of oxygenated and deoxygenated blood imparts greater efficiency to the mammalian circulation over that of most lower vertebrates. Since there is no mixing of oxygenated and deoxygenated blood in the heart, as occurs in some reptiles and amphibians, maximum oxygen tension is present in the blood pumped into the systemic circulation. In other vertebrate classes such as fish and amphibians, blood must initially pass through the respiratory capillaries of the gills before its delivery to the tissues. The large drop in pressure across the gills results in a very low pressure in blood circulating to the tissues. As a result of the relatively high pressure developed by the mammalian heart, blood can be delivered to the tissues in a shorter amount of time than could be achieved with a low-pressure system.

FUNCTIONS OF THE CIRCULATORY SYSTEM

The circulatory system is used primarily for the transport of oxygen, carbon dioxide, various nutrients, and other dissolved substances essential to the maintenance of metabolism and of blood cells. It is responsible for the transfer of metabolic wastes and excess salts to the kidneys for removal through the urine. Any excess water, ions, or other materials obtained from the gut are also transported to the kidneys for elimination.

Heat transfer by the circulatory system is one of the principal mechanisms involved in *thermoregulation*. During exercise, excess heat from muscles is transferred to the circulatory system and dissipated to the external environment by increasing the flow of blood to the periphery. Conversely, in a cold environment the rate of heat loss from the body can be reduced by retarding the transport of warm blood from the core to the peripheral tissues (see chapter 16, Thermoregulation).

Elements of the circulatory system prevent the development of infectious substances and enhance their removal from the body. When the body is exposed to toxic agents, antibodies may be present in the blood which are capable of deactivating the foreign substances by binding with them to form a nontoxic complex. Certain white blood cells phagocytize foreign substances in order to remove them from the organism. These phagocytic cells, transported by the circulatory system to sites of infection, thereby provide the body's second line of defense, after integument, against disease.

COMPONENTS OF THE CIRCULATORY SYSTEM

The Heart

The force that is necessary to pump blood to all parts of the body is provided by the heart. In terrestrial mammals, the heart varies in size from about 0.2 grams in the shrew to over 20 kilograms in the elephant. In general, heart mass bears a very close relationship to the body mass (see Figure 10–1). The equation for that relationship is:

$$M_h = 0.0059 \, M_b^{0.98} \qquad (10.1)$$

where,

$$M_h = \text{mass of the heart (kilograms)}$$
$$M_b = \text{mass of the body (kilograms)}$$

This tells us that heart mass is about 0.59 percent of the animal's body weight regardless of the animal's size. In other words, smaller mammals have essentially the same relative heart mass to propel blood through the circulatory system as larger mammals. This is certainly not what one would expect given the tremendous variation in mobility, endurance, metabolic capacity, and body fat content among different species of mammals. But, oxygen-transport capacity of blood pigments and their concentration in whole blood is variable among species and among individuals within a species. Such variation gives some organisms tremendous advantages in aerobic capacity over others even though heart-to-body-mass ratios are identical. In other words, differences in circulatory potential are accounted for, in part, by changes in blood constituents rather than by changes in heart size. It should be noted that

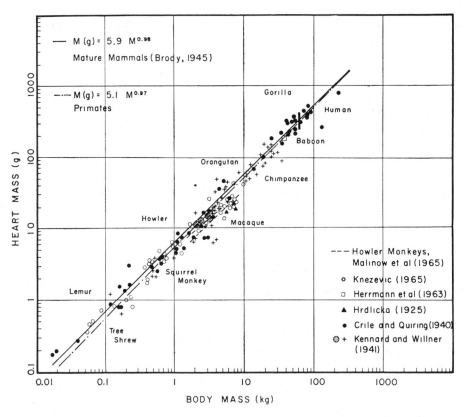

FIGURE 10–1
Heart size of mammals in relation to body weight: rather uniformly, heart size is about 0.6% of body mass. From W. R. Stahl, Organ Weights in Primates and Other Mammals, *Science* 150 (1965):1039–1042. Reprinted with permission. Copyright 1965 by the American Association for the Advancement of Science.

small mammals have higher resting heart rates than do their larger counterparts, compensating for the increased oxygen demand which results from the elevated metabolism of smaller mammals. Such factors only represent generalities, since heart hypertrophy occurs in a number of species during physical training and other conditions resulting in a chronic increased demand for oxygen. Thus, increase in heart size relative to body mass is apparent under certain environmental conditions.

The Blood Vessels

The blood vessels are tubes which carry blood throughout the body of mammals. Most of the vessels are composed of rather complex tissue layers which are resilient and allow the vessel to expand or contract depending upon the amount of blood passing through. Specific types of vessels recognized in mammals include: the *aorta;* the *arteries,* which bifurcate into smaller *arterioles;* the *metarterioles,* smaller arterioles which contain *precapillary sphincters;* the *capillaries,* the smallest vessels in the circulatory system; the *venules,* which coalesce to form veins; and the *venae cavae.* More than half of the blood of an organism at any particular time is held within the veins. The capillaries, though the smallest vessels, are possibly the most important of these vessel types because they are responsible for the actual exchange of nutrients and wastes between tissues and the circulatory system. Because of the muscular nature of their walls and the presence of precapillary sphincters, the arterioles and metarterioles are the principal controllers of blood pressure within the circulatory system.

The walls of the arteries, veins, arterioles, and venules are composed of three major layers (see Figure 10–2). The outer layer, the *tunica externa,* which is formed by connective tissue, isolates the blood vessels from the tissues through which they pass. The central layer, the *tunica media,* is composed of elastic fibers and smooth muscles. When stretched by the pressure of blood, the elastic tissue and smooth muscles rebound against the internal force. This rebounding action or contraction resonates against the internal pressure essential for the maintenance of uniform blood pressure. The inner layer of the blood vessels, the *tunica interna,* consists of a *basement membrane* and a single layer of *endothelial cells,* which provide a smooth surface over which blood flows. It is

important that the *endothelium,* which comes in contact with the blood, remains smooth and intact to reduce friction between blood and vessel walls.

The capillaries are very numerous and usually fairly short; their length rarely exceeds a few millimeters. They are also very narrow, so that erythrocytes (red blood cells) must pass through them in single file. In most mammalian species the red blood cells are compressed or folded as they pass through the capillaries. A group of capillaries in a particular tissue, known as a *capillary bed,* is usually fed by a single metarteriole (see Figure 10–3). A thick band of circular smooth muscle located in the wall of the metarteriole forms a *sphincter.* This precapillary sphincter can either contract or relax to control the flow of blood into the capillary bed.

Dilation and contraction of precapillary sphincters is, to a large extent, controlled by the microenvironment of the local blood flow through the tissue. When the sphincter is contracted, blood is usually diverted directly into a venule via another vessel, which functions as an *arteriole-venous shunt (A-V shunt).* In tissues which have a high metabolic rate, as in specific skeletal muscles of the body during exercise, metabolic by-products such as carbon dioxide and hydrogen ions are produced in greater than normal amounts. The local elevation in concentration of these

Artery

Arteriole

Capillary

Venule

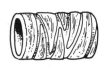
Vein

FIGURE 10–2
Except for thickness, tissue layers surrounding the arteries and veins are identical. Capillary walls, constructed of only endothelial cells, are one cell thick.

THE CIRCULATORY SYSTEM AND BLOOD PRESSURE

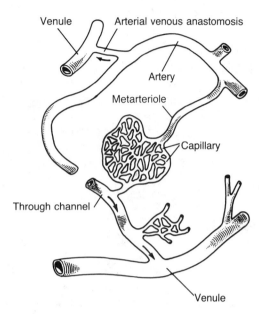

FIGURE 10–3
A mammalian capillary bed is fed through metarterioles and drained by means of venules

substances provides a signal which dilates the precapillary sphincter, thus producing capillary blood flow. Capillaries supplying active tissues during times of rapid metabolism are flushed with blood while those capillaries in less active tissues receive a sufficient blood flow for basal maintenance. In addition to the by-products of metabolism, other local substances are capable of affecting the contractile state of the arterioles and metarterioles. For instance, *mast cells* are present in practically all tissues, and their products are effective in controlling smooth muscles at the local level. Mast cells release *histamine,* which is a *vasodilator,* and *serotonin,* which is a *vasoconstrictor.* In addition to local substances, catecholamines and angiotensin released into the general circulation are potent *vasoactive compounds,* which cause arterioles to dilate or constrict depending upon

the tissue and the substance to which they are exposed. The precapillary sphincters and the arterioles are also innervated by vasoconstrictor fibers from the autonomic nervous system. Innervation of precapillary sphincters by the autonomic nervous system allows for alteration in the circulation before the initiation of physical activity. For example, even before muscular exertion athletes are capable of significantly increasing blood flow to the skeletal muscles.

Blood from the capillaries flows into the venules, whose walls are composed of three layers similar to those found in the arteries and arterioles. In the venules and veins, however, the muscle layers are much thinner, causing these vessels to be both more flexible and more fragile than the arterioles and arteries. Blood from the venules flows into the veins and ultimately into the venae cavae, which carry blood directly to the heart. The vena cavae, the largest veins in the body, have thin flexible walls compliant to the pressure of the blood carried and to the pressures within the abdominal and thoracic cavities.

Valves provide a distinguishing characteristic of veins (see Figure 10–4). Their presence

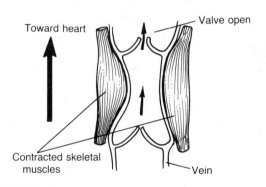

FIGURE 10–4
Venous valves allow a unidirectional flow of blood; distal pressure allows them to open, medial pressure forces them closed

allows blood to flow toward the heart and prevents backflow. Together with skeletal *muscle pumps*, valves greatly facilitate the return of blood to the heart. Excessive venous pressure sometimes causes the veins to become so distended that the valves can no longer prevent backflow. Permanent distention of the veins in humans can cause conditions such as *varicose veins* and *hemorrhoids.*

Lymphatic Tissue

In addition to the portions of the typical circulatory system described here, the *lymphatic system* drains tissues throughout the organism. That system is also responsible for producing certain white blood cells and for trapping bacterial debris and antigen-antibody complexes. The lymphatic system comprises: vessels; small masses of gut associated tissue known as *Peyer's patches;* lymph nodes; and three organs, the *tonsils,* the *thymus gland,* and the *spleen.* The lymphatic vessels originate in blind-ended sacs located in the tissues. In the intestines these sacs, called *lacteals,* are involved in the absorption of long-chain fatty acids. Elsewhere, these sacs are called *lymph capillaries* and are slightly larger than the blood capillaries. The lymph capillaries are more permeable to proteins than are the blood capillaries; they drain *interstitial spaces* of substances which cannot penetrate the blood capillary endothelium.

Two basic lymphatic circuits are functional in the mammals. Most of the lymphatic vessels anastomose (join together) to form the *left thoracic duct,* which enters the bloodstream through the left subclavian vein. A second circuit drains a small portion of the right side of the body. Vessels from this portion of the lymphatic system coalesce

to form the *right lymphatic duct,* which enters the circulation through the right subclavian vein.

The *lymph nodes,* or *lymph glands,* are strategically located so that all lymph fluid passes through them. Each node is covered by a capsule of connective tissue which extends into the node with fingerlike projections called *trabeculae.* Within this framework, the lymph node is organized into an outer *cortex* and an inner *medulla* (see Figure 10–5). The cortex contains masses of densely packed lymphocytes called *lymph nodules.* Inside the medulla, lymph cells are less densely packed and are arranged in strands called *medullary cords.*

Lymph fluid flows into the nodes through the *afferent vessels* which contain valves similar to those found in veins. These valves insure one-way flow of fluid toward the node. After entering the node, lymph flows into the *medullary sinuses,* which lie between the medullary cords. The fluid then exits the node through the *efferent vessels,* which also contain valves. The valves in the efferent vessels insure lymph flow away from the nodal area and result in lymph drainage into the venous circulation. Muscular contraction increases the pressure in the lymph vessels which, with the one-way flow insured by the valves, forces the lymphatic fluid toward the thoracic duct.

CAPILLARY EXCHANGE

The capillaries provide an area where dissolved substances and fluids of the blood can be exchanged with the surrounding tissues. The capillary membrane consists of a single layer of endothelial cells which allow water and solutes (except fairly large molecular species) to pass through the layer's intercel-

FIGURE 10–5
A lymph node

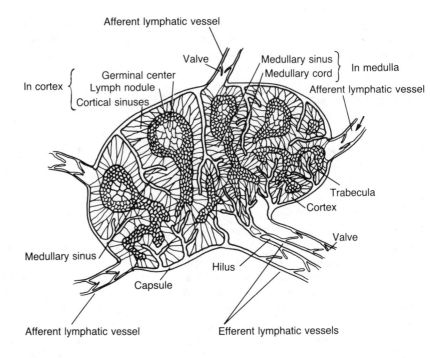

Afferent lymphatic vessel

Valve

Medullary sinus
Medullary cord
In medulla

Afferent lymphatic vessel

In cortex
Germinal center
Lymph nodule
Cortical sinuses

Trabecula

Cortex

Valve

Medullary sinus

Hilus

Capsule

Afferent lymphatic vessel

Efferent lymphatic vessels

lular spaces. In most capillaries, and in those found in the circulation to the skeletal muscles in particular, intercellular spaces allow passage of molecules up to 10 nanometers in diameter. Larger intercellular gaps occur in the capillary endothelium of endocrine glands and presumably aid in the extrusion of various secretory products. Larger gaps of this type, which may reach 100 nanometers, are also found in the capillary endothelium of the kidney and small intestine. But the size of the particles which penetrate these membranes is usually quite small when compared to the diameter of the intercellular gap. For instance, the basement membrane and the *podocytes* of the kidney restrict the size of molecules which will actually pass to particles about 8 nanometers in diameter or smaller. In the liver, large gaps in the *sinusoid membranes* may occur, since the endothelium is actually discontinuous.

Plasma proteins and other colloids do not normally pass through the endothelial membrane of most capillaries. But some proteins pass the capillary wall and enter the lymph. The mechanism by which they enter the interstitial fluid is only partially understood. From studies utilizing labeled proteins, it would appear that they pass directly through rather than between the endothelial cells by a method known as *vesicular transport* or *transcytosis (cytopempsis)*. This process involves the formation of a vesicle containing the protein on the inside of the capillary *(endocytosis)* and then the passage of the protein out through the opposing cell membrane *(exocytosis)*.

Filtration Pressure

The relationship of fluid exchange between plasma and tissue was poorly understood until 1896, when E. H. Starling proposed a system of forces governing this exchange. This became known as *Starling's hypothesis of capillary exchange*, or simply *Starling's hypothesis*. Exchange at the tissue level requires a balance of several different forces which results in a net pressure, the algebraic sum of all of the pressure components about the capillary. The net pressure, known as the *filtration pressure*, can be either negative or positive depending upon the quantitative values of individual force components. Positive filtration pressure results in fluid movement into the tissues; negative filtration pressure results in fluid movement into the capillaries.

The complementary forces which give rise to the filtration pressure are (1) *hydrostatic pressure*, (2) *colloidal-osmotic pressure*, and (3) *tissue pressure* (see Figure 10–6). Hydrostatic pressure is the pressure generated by a combination of the contraction of the heart and the recoil of the smooth muscles and elastic fibers in the arteries. The pressure is usually about 35 to 40 millimeters of mercury (mm Hg) at the site of entry of blood into the capillary. Colloidal-osmotic pressure (or *oncotic pressure*), the pressure generated by the colloids retained in the plasma after filtration, is considered to be negative at the arterial end of the capillary bed because its action opposes the hydrostatic pressure of the blood. Tissue pressure, the hydrostatic pressure generated from the weight of the tissue, is also considered to be negative because like colloidal-osmotic pressure it opposes the action of the hydrostatic pressure in the capillaries.

Filtration pressure can be calculated with this formula:

$$FP = HP - (COP + TP) \qquad (10.2)$$

where,

$$FP = \text{filtration pressure (mm Hg)}$$
$$HP = \text{hydrostatic pressure (mm Hg)}$$
$$COP = \text{colloidal-osmotic pressure (mm Hg)}$$
$$TP = \text{tissue pressure (mm Hg).}$$

Note that filtration pressure is positive when hydrostatic pressure exceeds the sum of colloidal-osmotic pressure and tissue pressure, and that it is negative when the reverse is true. When filtration pressure is positive, fluid can be filtered into the tissues from the capillaries. Negative filtration pressure results in the drainage of fluid from the interstitial spaces back into the capillaries. In the hypothetical example of Figure 10–6, the situation is idealized to show an approximately equal flow into and out of the capillary. Such is usually not the case; the total flow across the capillary bed is usually slightly positive.

Later work in essence demonstrated that Starling's analysis was not completely correct because he failed to recognize that certain

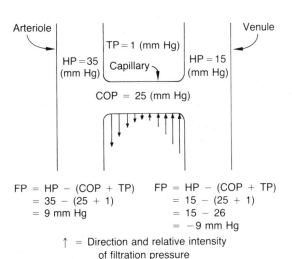

$$FP = HP - (COP + TP)$$
$$= 35 - (25 + 1)$$
$$= 9 \text{ mm Hg}$$

$$FP = HP - (COP + TP)$$
$$= 15 - (25 + 1)$$
$$= 15 - 26$$
$$= -9 \text{ mm Hg}$$

↑ = Direction and relative intensity of filtration pressure

FIGURE 10–6
Filtration pressure is a net pressure resulting from hydrostatic, colloidal-osmotic, and tissue pressures

proteins cannot reenter the capillary from the interstitial spaces. Some of the drainage which occurs must then be accomplished by the lymphatics. But the drainage component contributed by the lymphatics merely functions in addition to capillary exchange and does not alter the physical principles governing the exchange of fluids within a capillary bed.

For cases in which excessive hydrostatic pressure is generated, the tissues can become distended with excess fluids. This condition, known as *edema,* can be produced in the lower limbs when healthy animals are restrained in the upright position for long periods of time. Lack of movement due to restraint reduces the lymphatic and venous flow and prevents lymphatic drainage by creating high venous pressure in the *subclavian veins,* where the lymphatic fluids enter the venous system. When adequate exercise is possible, muscular contraction in conjunction with the venous valves enhances *venous return* to the heart and consequently results in better tissue drainage. Reduction in venous return causes the entire system to back up and therefore prevents lymphatic drainage; tissue edema results. Where the lymphatics are blocked by parasites (as in the disease *elephantiasis*), poor fluid drainage results in gross body deformation.

It would be interesting to observe the effects of restraint upon venous return in the giraffe. It has been reported that the giraffe has a very tight skin on the legs, a tightness that may aid in venous return. But since there are no muscles below the knee (or *hock*) it is difficult to see how tight skin might benefit, other than to reduce the volume of the vessels into which the venous blood can drain. Tight skin on the lower leg is simulated by humans who wear tight hose or stockings, which should effectively prevent

pooling of blood in the leg. If use of tight-fitting stockings is persistent, it should effectively prevent occurrence of varicose veins.

Diffusion of Gases

Whereas the movement of fluids from the blood into the tissues is dependent upon three independent pressure variables, the exchange of dissolved gases is a function of the gases' relative concentrations. Diffusion rate in a liquid medium is a function of a *diffusion gradient,* where other factors remain constant. The ability to deliver oxygen to the tissues is a critical factor in the maintenance of the metabolic rates found in mammals. Thus, diffusion rates must be greater in mammals with high metabolic rates than they are in mammals with more sluggish metabolism. In small mammals, metabolic rate normalized to body weight may be 20 to 40 times the metabolic rate of a larger mammal. The principal method available to mammals for modifying diffusion rate is to alter the diffusion gradient. A diffusion gradient is defined as the change in solute concentration over a distance through a permeable medium. Diffusion rate is increased if the concentration gradient increases. The diffusion gradient for delivery of oxygen to the tissues can be achieved either by increasing the oxygen content of the capillaries or by reducing the distance over which diffusion must occur (see Figure 10–7).

It has been found that both of the mechanisms mentioned for increasing the diffusion gradient are employed in mammals. But the latter method, changing the diffusion distances, shows the greatest variation among species that show widely differing metabolic rates. In the muscles of the mouse, for example, *capillary density* is about 2,000 capillaries per square millimeter of tissue,

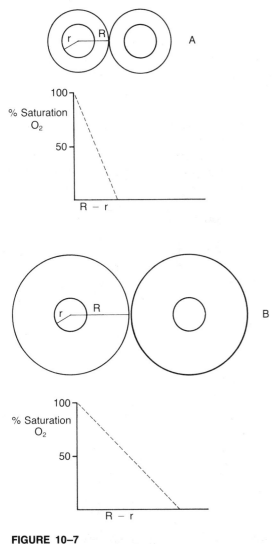

FIGURE 10–7
By shortening the distance over which metabolites and oxygen diffuse, mammals have essentially elevated the diffusion gradient (i.e., slope of the dashed line). In many cases, as with the horse compared with the mouse, the diffusion gradient is doubled by doubling the muscle capillary density, which reduces the diffusion distance by half. The top figure (A) represents the condition found in the mouse, where R − r is taken as one. The bottom figure (B) represents the horse, where R − r is two since the capillary density is halved in this species. Radius of the capillary (r) is approximately equal in both mouse and horse.

whereas in the horse it has been found to be less than 1,000 capillaries per square millimeter of tissue. It would be interesting to know if organisms which have high work capacity also show elevated capillary densities when compared to slower, more lethargic animals. In fact, muscles which have greater endurance, such as the flight muscles of the bat, would be expected to have a higher capillary density than those muscles which are used more sparingly in the same animal. It would be important from the standpoint of exercise physiology to determine if capillary densities change with increased physical fitness.

COMPARATIVE RATES OF FLOW

Since the mammalian circulatory system is closed, each portion of it contains a uniform volume of blood at all times. Thus, the same volume of blood must flow through each portion of the circulatory system simultaneously. In other words, if 5.0 liters of blood pass through the heart each minute, then 5.0 liters must pass through the capillaries each minute. This is not to say that the same amount of blood is present in each unit of the circulatory system (i.e., arteries, veins, capillaries, etc.) at all times. If one determines the volume of blood in each segment of the circulatory system, the largest volume is found in the veins (70 to 80 percent). The second largest volume is found in the arteries (10 to 25 percent). The approximate volume of blood which occupies the capillaries is 7 percent. These figures are affected by exogenous and endogenous factors such as physical activity, environmental temperature, disease state, and anesthesia. Especially large variations may occur among different species.

The velocity at which blood flows in a linear fashion (cm/sec) is inversely proportional to the total *cross-sectional area* (cm²) of any major division (e.g., arterioles, capillaries) of the circulatory system. This means that blood must flow at different velocities through the arteries, veins, and capillaries in order for blood flow (e.g., liters/min) to be constant (see Figure 10–8). This change in cross-sectional area among different segments of the circulatory system can be likened to a series of lakes connected by streams. The water in the streams has a high velocity because of the streams' limited capacity for volume, whereas the velocity of water in the lakes is very slow because of their huge capacity for volume flow, albeit total flow through the lakes and streams is constant.

In humans, the cross-sectional area of the aorta is approximately 4.5 cm², and the cross-sectional area of the capillaries (collectively) is 4,500 cm². The velocity of flow is less than 0.1 cm/sec in the capillaries, which have a much larger cross-sectional area. In the aorta it is approximately 40 cm/sec. This difference in velocity between arteries and capillaries is accentuated in small mammals. In these animals the capillary density is greater than it is in larger mammals, and therefore the ratio of the total cross-sectional area of the capillaries is relatively greater when compared to other parts of the circulatory system. If the total cross-sectional area of the capillaries is greater relative to cross-sectional area of the other parts of the circulatory system, then velocity of flow in the capillaries must be reduced in these species.

FIGURE 10–8
Differences in cross-sectional areas among various parts of the circulatory system, as related to velocity of flow. From R. F. Rushmer, *Cardiovascular Dynamics*, p. 10, fig. 1-4. Copyright © 1976 by W.B. Saunders Co. Reprinted by permission of W.B. Saunders, CBS College Publishing. Developed from data from O. Glasser, *Medical Physics* (Chicago: Year Book Publishers), 1944.

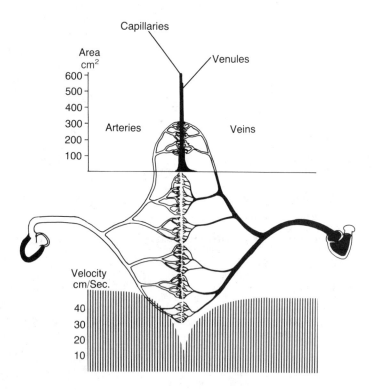

Very little comparative data concerning blood velocities among species are available but such information may be extrapolated based upon measurements of cardiac output and capillary density. The advantage of reduced blood velocity in the capillaries is great. Exchange of materials between blood and interstitial spaces is a process dependent upon filtration and diffusion. With slower rates of flow more time is available for diffusion and filtration, and capillary exchange is therefore more efficient.

CIRCULATION THROUGH SPECIALIZED AREAS

Coronary Circulation

Coronary circulation begins with the *coronary arteries*, which are the first branch off the aorta (see Figure 10–9). These arteries develop from the sixth pair of aortic arches of the embryo. Blood flows through the coro-

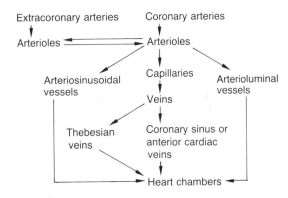

FIGURE 10–10
Coronary circulation. Reproduced with permission, from Ganong, WF: *Review of Medical Physiology*, 9th ed. Copyright 1979 by Lange Medical Publications, Los Altos, California.

nary arteries into various channels which lead to coronary capillaries, where exchange occurs between the blood and the *myocardium*, or heart muscle. Blood leaving the myocardium ultimately drains into the heart chambers instead of passing into the venae cavae and entering the right atrium, as is the case for other parts of the systemic circulation (see Figure 10–10).

Perfusion of the myocardium is extremely important because of the dependency of the heart muscle upon oxidative metabolism for production of high-energy phosphates. More than 50 percent of the chemical energy used in contraction of the heart is derived from lipids, placing a significant demand on the heart muscle for oxygen. In fact, less than 1.0 percent of the total energy used in myocardial contraction is derived from anaerobic glycolysis. In order for blood to flow to the myocardium a positive *perfusion pressure* must exist. That is, blood must enter the coronary circulation at a relatively high pressure and exit under lower pressure. Thus, pressure must be greater in the aorta than it is in the chambers of the heart. This favorable per-

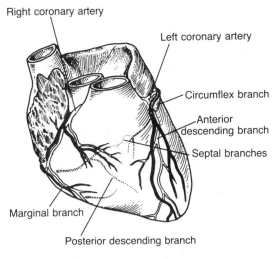

FIGURE 10–9
Coronary vessels seen on the surface of the human myocardium

fusion pressure exists only during ventricular *diastole* (relaxation). Perfusion actually begins shortly after closure of the semilunar valves, which occurs very early in ventricular relaxation. It continues until shortly after the beginning of the next ventricular *systole* (contraction), when pressure in the ventricles is again equal to the pressure in the aorta. As the ventricles contract, pressure is uniformly distributed to the myocardium. At maximum contraction, the pressure in the ventricular chamber, aorta, and myocardium is the same. After closure of the aortic semilunar valves, the ventricular pressure falls to 0.0 mm Hg, whereas pressure in the aorta falls to a fairly uniform diastolic pressure, near 80 mm Hg in most species. Systolic and diastolic pressure may differ in absolute value among species, but the principles given here for development of effective coronary perfusion are the same in all mammals.

Since blood flows to the heart during relaxation, the time spent in diastole becomes an extremely critical factor. When heart rate increases above the resting value, it usually does so at the expense of diastolic time. That is, systolic time (contraction time) remains fairly constant while the diastolic time (relaxation time) becomes shorter as the heart rate increases. At maximum heart rate the amount of time spent in systole has decreased very little in comparison to the normal. On the other hand, diastolic time has been reduced drastically in order to obtain the maximum contractile rate. The ultimate result of elevated heart rate is to reduce the amount of time available for blood to flow to the heart. This reduces the relative amount of blood which can flow to the heart and enhances the likelihood of coronary ischemia.

The *lumen* (cavity) of the coronary blood vessels is sometimes reduced in size as the result of lipid accumulation. Such reduction inhibits coronary flow, extremely important during exercise. The accumulation of lipids in the arteries, known as *atherosclerosis*, can be found in a number of species, particularly humans and domesticated animals. During times of relaxation, the restriction to flow caused by atheroschlerosis is usually not critical. But during exercise, when greater oxygen demands are placed on the heart, any reduction in normal flow is significant. It is for this reason that the causative factors of coronary ischemia usually prevail during exercise, when time available for coronary perfusion is reduced.

Hepatic Circulation

About 20 percent of the total circulating blood volume which reaches the heart is derived from the liver. Blood flows into the liver from the *hepatic portal vein* and the *hepatic artery*. The hepatic portal vein supplies about 80 percent of the total blood flowing into the liver; the additional 20 percent is supplied by the hepatic artery. Blood from the hepatic portal vein mixes with arterial blood from the hepatic artery in rather large cavities known as the *hepatic sinuses* (sinusoids) (see Figure 10–11). The sinuses have the same function as capillaries located in other parts of the body, in that fluid movement is slow and there is exchange between the hepatic cells and the blood filling the sinuses. The sinus walls differ drastically from the capillary endothelium. The cells forming the walls are, for the most part, *phagocytic Kupfer cells*, which are part of the *reticulo-endothelial system* of the body. The sinuses drain into central veins which anastomose to form *lobular veins*. Blood in the lobular veins ultimately enters the hepatic vein, which returns blood to the vena cava.

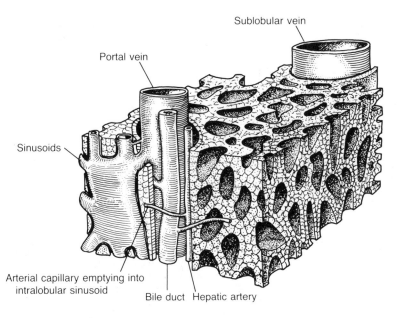

FIGURE 10–11
Internal structure of the normal human liver

Fetal Circulation

Since the *placenta* must function as a fetal lung, the fetal circulation must be organized to use a completely different source of oxygen from that seen in the adult. Oxygenated blood from the placenta is carried by the *umbilical vein* to the *inferior vena cava* of the fetus (see Figure 10–12). Blood enters the right atrium, where most of it is transmitted to the left atrium through the *patent* (open) *foramen ovale* (a flap of septal tissue). The blood which enters the right ventricle is transported through the pulmonary artery toward the lungs. Since the lungs are collapsed in the fetus, resistance to the flow of blood is high. Because of the residual high pressure in the lungs, blood entering the pulmonary artery can be diverted through a fetal vessel, the *ductus arteriosus*, into the aorta. The net result of a patent foramen ovale and ductus arteriosus is that oxygenated blood from the placenta is transported directly to the tissues. The fetus in essence lacks what is re-

ferred to as *pulmonary circulation* in the adult; the fetal heart functions as a two-chambered pump. It is in this case similar to the heart of a fish except that the placenta which acts as a gill is placed in parallel with the rest of the circulatory system rather than in series with it, as are the gills of most teleosts (see Figure 10–13).

Changes in fetal circulation At birth the circulatory system changes to allow for the acquisition of functional lungs and complete separation of oxygenated and deoxygenated blood. One of the first postpartum events is contraction of the placental blood vessels, which forces blood into the fetus. Placental circulation falls rapidly, and the newborn experiences asphyxia. Apparently the hypoxia at this time stimulates the respiratory center, which causes the neonate to take its first few gasps for breath. At these first gasps, *intrapleural pressure* (or pressure within the lungs) falls, providing a favorable perfusion

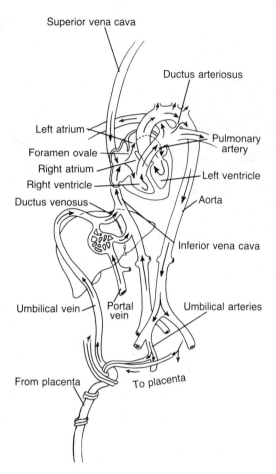

FIGURE 10–12
Fetal circulation. Reproduced with permission, from
Ganong, WF: *Review of Medical Physiology*, 9th ed.
Copyright 1979 by Lange Medical Publications, Los Al-
tos, California.

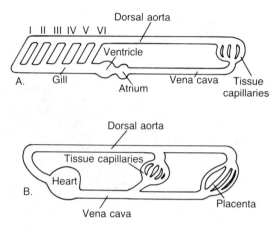

FIGURE 10–13
Comparison between (A) circulatory system in a gilled
vertebrate and (B) the fetal circulation of a mammal.
Note that the gill capillaries are in series with the tissue
capillaries, whereas the placental capillaries are in parallel with the tissue capillaries.

pressure between the heart and lungs. Decreased intrapleural pressure therefore results in blood flowing into the vascular system of the lung. As blood returns from the
lungs in significant quantities, it fills the left
atrium and causes an elevation in atrial pressure. Increased atrial pressure forces the
valve of the foramen ovale to close. The blood
now flows to the lungs through the pulmo-

nary artery and to the systemic circulation
through the aorta. As a result, the blood does
not flow through the ductus arteriosus but is
instead shunted back and forth without
passing through ·the ductus as pressure
changes in the aorta and pulmonary artery.
Shortly after birth the ductus closes in most
mammals. The mechanism by which closure
occurs is not completely understood, but
closure can be induced by injecting *prostaglandin synthesis inhibitors*. It is probable
that *prostaglandin,* a fatty acid, maintains the
ductus in the patent state during fetal development. A reaction, as yet unclear, appears
to occur at the time of parturition, which in-
terferes with prostaglandin synthesis or utilization and therefore initiates ductus closure.

Placental Circulation

The placenta in mammals presents an excellent example of an area where comparatively

massive volumes of gases and nutrients must be transferred from one circulatory system to another by means of diffusion. This is accomplished in one of two different ways depending upon the species. In primates, sheep, and goats, the maternal circulation forms huge blood sinuses which encapsulate the fetal capillaries (see Figure 10–14). In this system, blood passes from a maternal arteriole into the sinuses, which are drained through the veins back into the maternal circulation. The volume of the sinuses is very large, and blood therefore moves very slowly. The slow movement of blood in both circulatory systems gives ample time for exchange of materials by diffusion. In some species the maternal endothelium erodes away and leaves the fetal capillaries directly exposed to maternal blood. In the rabbit, cat, squirrel, cow, and dog, diffusion occurs between two systems of parallel capillaries called *countercurrent exchangers* (see Figure 10–15). Through this mech-

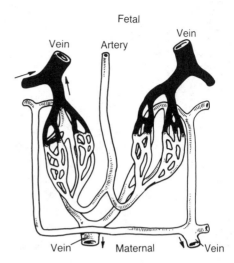

FIGURE 10–15
Countercurrent exchanger found in the placenta of many mammalian species

nism diffusion efficiency is intensified as a result of the two parallel vessels, which have opposite directions of flow. The opposing vessels maintain a stable diffusion gradient (i.e., uniform over their entire length), over which the slow velocity of blood gives ample time for diffusion to occur (see chapter 14, The Excretory System and Water Balance).

Cerebral Circulation

In mammals, blood is delivered to the brain through arteries that branch from a circular vessel called the *circle of Willis*, which surrounds the *hypophysis*, or pituitary gland (see Figure 10–16). In primates and rodents, blood is supplied to the circle of Willis through the *internal carotid arteries* and the *basilar artery*, which is formed from the right and left *vertebral arteries*. In artiodactyls (e.g., cattle, deer) and carnivores (e.g., dogs, cats), the carotid artery divides into a number of smaller vessels called *rete* prior to reaching the circle

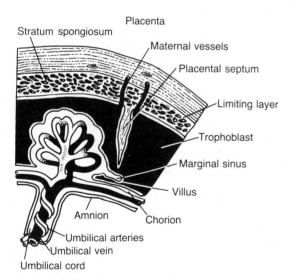

FIGURE 10–14
Relationship of the maternal sinuses with the fetal capillaries in the human placenta

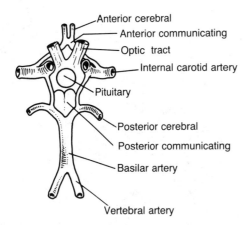

FIGURE 10–16
Circle of Willis and the related arteries in the human

of Willis (see Figure 10–17). In these species venous blood, cooled in the nasal passages, is carried into a venous sinus, the *cavernous sinus*, which surrounds the carotid rete. This provides an important cooling mechanism for the brain during exercise or ambient heat stress, when body temperature might rise to a height dangerous to neural tissue. Excessive warmth from blood in the carotid artery is dissipated to the relatively cool venous blood in the venous sinuses, resulting in a brain temperature several degrees cooler than the core temperature. In those mammals which have a carotid rete, blood is received predominately from the external carotid arteries since the internal carotid arteries are sparsely developed. These species have vertebral arteries, but they are reduced in size and transport only a minor fraction of blood to the brain. Species lacking carotid rete (e.g., rodents, humans) receive most of the brain blood flow through the internal carotid arteries. Among the carnivores, members of the cat family (Felidae) have an extensive rete; in dogs, wolves (Canidae), and pinnipeds, it is reduced in size and contains

only a few branches. The rete is absent in monotremes and marsupials and is surprisingly not found in the lagomorphs (e.g., rabbits) or perissodactyls (e.g., horses).

Blood entering the brain is transmitted to a unique capillary system which has reduced intercellular spaces and is surrounded by a continuous *basement membrane*. This arrangement of the capillary space and basement membrane restricts the diffusion of many substances that normally penetrate the membranes of capillaries in other parts of the body. This factor along with reduced interstitial spaces between the endothelial cells forming the capillaries provides the basis for the *blood-brain barrier*. Large groups of capillaries fashion a network, the *choroid plexus*, in the third and fourth ventricles of the brain, the location for the formation of most of the cerebrospinal fluid. Metabolites are ultimately drained from the cerebrospinal fluid through capillaries located in the arachnoid villi.

Testicular Circulation

The *testes* of most mammals must be maintained at a temperature below normal body temperature in order to insure viability of the sperm. In all mammals except elephants and cetaceans this task is achieved in part by keeping the testes outside of the body in a pouch called the *scrotum*. In such mammals as the horse and pig the testes, though maintained in the scrotum, are held near the body in a manner that makes cooling difficult. In these species, as well as in many others, cooling is enhanced by means of a countercurrent exchanger known as the *pampiniform plexus* (see Figure 10–18). Here, warm arterial blood loses heat and perhaps other substances to the venous blood returning to the body. This system is able to maintain the temperature of the testes as much as five to

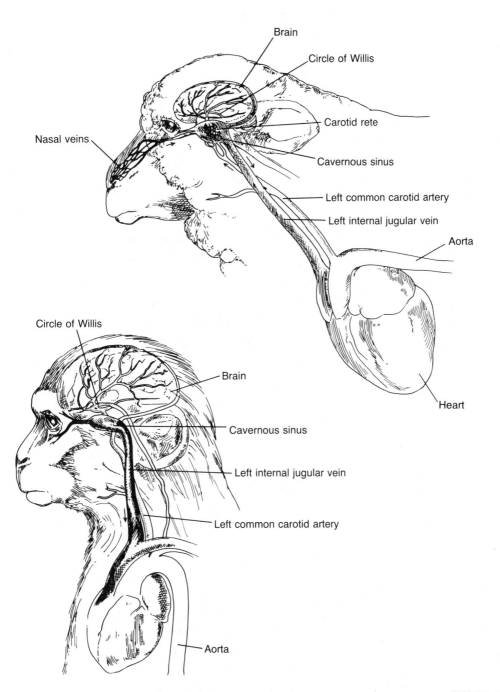

FIGURE 10–17

Blood supply to the brain of the sheep (which has a rete) and to the brain of the monkey (which lacks a rete). In the monkey, blood supplied to the brain is at heart temperature in the cavernous sinus. In the sheep, some blood reaches the circle of Willis through the basilar artery, though most of it is derived from the cooled blood of the internal carotids. From A Brain-Cooling System in Mammals, M. A. Baker. Copyright © May 1979 by Scientific American, Inc. All rights reserved.

205

FIGURE 10–18
The pampiniform plexus is an effective countercurrent exchanger which aids in cooling the scrotum of most mammalian species. This example is taken from a sheep.

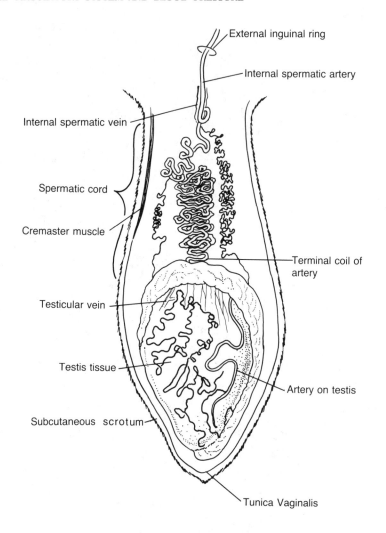

External inguinal ring

Internal spermatic artery

Internal spermatic vein

Spermatic cord

Cremaster muscle

Terminal coil of artery

Testicular vein

Testis tissue

Artery on testis

Subcutaneous scrotum

Tunica Vaginalis

six degrees below the temperature of the body core.

CLINICAL DISORDERS OF THE CARDIOVASCULAR SYSTEM

Some of the most serious and debilitating disorders concerning the cardiovascular system include *arterioschlerosis, aneurysms,* and *hypertension.* Arterioschlerosis is a group of diseases distinguished by a loss of elasticity and a thickening of the arterial walls. Such effects may be brought about by extensive deposition of calcium (as in *Mönckeberg's arterioschlerosis*) or fatty deposits or by other causes. Regardless of the cause of the thickening, there is a reduction in the amount of blood flow and also an increase in blood pressure. In atheroschlerosis, an added problem is that the *atheroma* (the mass of fatty material) may break loose from the vessel wall and become an *embolus*, which may subsequently become lodged in a smaller artery or capillary. The area served by this blocked vessel is then deprived of oxygen and becomes ischemic.

An aneurysm is a local distention or dilation of an artery or vein. The resulting structure is saclike in appearance. Any major blood vessel may be affected in this way, though aortic aneurysms account for the largest incidence of the disease. An aneurysm occurring in a cerebral artery, called a *berry aneurysm*, may result in a hemorrhage below the dura mater.

Hypertension, or high blood pressure, has received much attention as the "silent killer." It has been cited as the most common cardiovascular disease. There are two basic types of hypertension, commonly referred to as *primary* and *secondary hypertension.* In primary hypertension the elevated blood pressure cannot be attributed to any specific agent. On the other hand, secondary hypertension is associated with other maladies such as kidney disease, arterioschlerosis, and hypersecretion of such adrenal hormones as *aldosterone* from the adrenal cortex and epinephrine and norepinephrine from the adrenal medulla. Hypertension, regardless of the cause, may bring about kidney damage due to the thickening of the arteriole walls, which decreases the amount of blood flow to this organ. Hypertension may also cause the rupture of cerebral arteries, which results in a stroke. In many cases of hypertension, the heart becomes enlarged because of the added strain required for pumping blood at a higher pressure.

BLOOD PRESSURE

The blood pressure of mammals was first measured in the 18th century by the Reverend Stephen Hales, who placed a glass catheter directly into the carotid artery of his personal steed. Blood rose in the tube to a surprising height of 9 feet 6 inches above the heart. This value is somewhat on the high side when compared to more recent data on blood pressure in the horse. But considering that it was the first recording of blood pressure in any mammal and that the animal was not anesthetized, the Reverend Hales's finding was remarkable.

Pressure in liquids can be determined by the amount of water which can be displaced in a tube, hence the term *hydrostatic pressure.* In modern analysis, data are usually recorded in *millimeters of mercury (mm Hg),* or the pressure necessary to raise a column of mercury in a vertical tube. The increased weight of mercury allows the *manometer* (a device used to measure blood pressure) to be used in small areas since only a small volume of liquid is required. The mercury manometer has thus become a standard tool of both clinicians and researchers because of its portability and its use of the standard pressure unit called millimeter of mercury.

Blood pressure varies widely among different components of the circulatory system. In the human, blood pressure is fairly constant throughout the arteries but drops in the arterioles to about 35 mm Hg as it enters the capillary beds (see Figure 10–19). As blood passes out of the capillaries, its pressure is about 15 mm Hg. The pressure decreases progressively in the veins, with the lowest pressure occurring in the venae cavae.

The peak arterial pressure generated by the heart, called *systolic pressure,* occurs during ventricular contraction, or systole. The minimum pressure in the arteries, called *diastolic pressure,* occurs during ventricular relaxation, or diastole. In most mammals, blood pressure in the arteries increases with

THE CIRCULATORY SYSTEM AND BLOOD PRESSURE

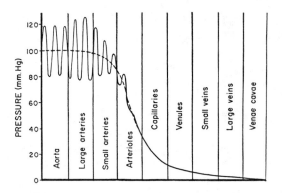

FIGURE 10–19
Pressure of blood in the various portions of the circulatory system. Although pressure begins to change in the arteries, the most dramatic change occurs in the arterioles. Pulse pressure is indicated by the broken line; mean pressure is shown by the solid line. From A. C. Guyton, *Textbook of Medical Physiology*, 6th edition (Philadelphia, Pa., 1981), 239, fig. 19–2. Reprinted by permission of W. B. Saunders Publishing Co.

age. In the human, the ideal blood pressure characteristic of a healthy twenty-five-year-old male is approximately 120/80 mm Hg, or 120 mm Hg systolic pressure and 80 mm Hg diastolic pressure.

Mean blood pressure designates the average of the pressure exerted in a particular vessel; *median blood pressure* designates the midpoint between maximum and minimum pressure. *Mean arterial pressure* is computed by adding the product of the average systolic pressure times the duration of time spent in systole to the product of the diastolic pressure times the duration of time spent in diastole, and then dividing that sum by the total time required to complete one cardiac cycle (i.e., total time of systole and diastole). This volume is given by the following equation:

$$MAP = \frac{(SP \times t_1) + (DP \times t_2)}{t_1 + t_2} \quad (10.3)$$

where,

$$
\begin{aligned}
MAP &= \text{mean arterial pressure (mm Hg)} \\
SP &= \text{systolic pressure (mm Hg)} \\
DP &= \text{diastolic pressure (mm Hg)} \\
t_1 &= \text{duration of systole (sec)} \\
t_2 &= \text{duration of diastole (sec)}
\end{aligned}
$$

Mean arterial pressure is usually lower than the median pressure because more time is spent in diastole than in systole when the animal is at rest.

Arterial pressures are amazingly close among different species of mammals (see Table 10–1). A notable exception on the low side is the duckbilled platypus, which has a systolic pressure of 14 mm Hg as opposed to the usual distribution in mammals of about 90 to 120 mm Hg. In contrast, the giraffe has a systolic pressure of 200 to 300 mm Hg and a diastolic pressure of 100 to 170 mm Hg at heart level. The average value for the giraffe taken at heart level is 260/160 mm Hg. If one realizes that the giraffe is supporting a vertical column of blood at least 7 feet above its heart and that the density of blood is near that of water, the problem becomes clear. In order to get blood to the cerebral capillaries, force must be created by the heart which is sufficient to lift the column of blood in the carotid arteries and still maintain a mean hydrostatic pressure in the head which is sufficient in magnitude to provide a positive filtration pressure in the capillaries of the brain. If one foot of water or blood is approximately 22 mm Hg, a giraffe whose head is 7 feet above its heart requires a pressure of 154 mm Hg to support the blood column from the heart to the brain. This value substracted from 260 mm Hg recorded for systolic pressure at the heart level appears surprisingly close to the systolic pressure of 120 mm Hg

	Blood Pressure		**TABLE 10–1**
Species	Systolic	Diastolic	Blood pressure in several mammalian species
Cattle *(Bos taurus)*	134	88	
Dog *(Canis familiaris)*	112	56	
Goat *(Capra hircus)*	120	84	
Guinea pig *(Cavia porcellus)*	77	47	
Horse *(Equus caballas)*	98	64	
Cat *(Felis catus)*	120	75	
Rhesus monkey *(Macaca mulatta)*	159	127	
House mouse *(Mus musculus)*	113	81	
Platypus *(Ornithorhyncus* sp.*)*	14	—	
Norway rat *(Rattus norvegicus)*	129	91	
Swine *(Sus scrofa)*	169	108	
Rabbit *(Oryctolagus cuniculus)*	110	80	

Source: From P. L. Altman and D. S. Dittmer, *Biology Data Book* (Bethesda, Maryland: Federation of American Societies for Experimental Biology, 1964)

recorded at the head of the giraffe. In fact, it has been found that blood entering the brain of the giraffe has a pressure of 120/75 mm Hg.

FACTORS AFFECTING BLOOD PRESSURE

The Blood and the Circulatory System in Relation to Pressure

A useful equation showing the relationship between pressure, flow, and resistance of liquids is named after 19th-century French physiologist Jean Poiseuille for his work concerning the basic principles of hydraulics and the flow of liquids in tubes. *Poiseuille's equation* is the following:

$$P = F \times R \qquad (10.4)$$

where,

$$P = \text{pressure (mm Hg)}$$
$$F = \text{rate of flow (vol/unit time)}$$
$$R = \text{total peripheral resistance}$$

This equation can be applied either to a particular part of the circulatory system or to the entire system. If one chooses the entire system, for the sake of simplicity P becomes arterial pressure and F becomes *cardiac output*, or the milliliters of blood pumped per minute. Resistance refers to the *total peripheral resistance*, or the entire impedance to flow in the circulatory system. Resistance in the system is a function of blood viscosity (V), length of the blood vessels (L), and the radius of the blood vessels (r). Resistance is usually expressed as:

$$R = \frac{8VL}{r^4} \qquad (10.5)$$

where,

R = resistance
V = viscosity of blood
L = length of the blood vessels (mm)
r = radius of the blood vessels (mm)

Let us direct our attention to the components of resistance and how they might be modified in the organism.

Viscosity of blood   *Viscosity* of a fluid is defined as its resistance to flow. Blood is a liquid which contains some dissolved substances, some suspended cells, and some emulsified particles. As a result of blood's unique characteristics, blood viscosity is different from that of water and from that of a solution of hemoglobin (see Figure 10–20). The presence of red blood cells drastically increases the viscosity of blood above the level derived from a solution which does not contain erythrocytes. Viscosity increases with increasing concentrations of red blood cells.

The percentage of blood volume occupied by erythrocytes is estimated by determining the hematocrit or, more simply put, by determining the percentage of red blood cells in a sample of whole blood. The hematocrit of mammals varies considerably both within and among species. In most mammals it is found to lie between 45 and 50 percent, though several external factors are known to alter it. In some species, hematocrit can vary in an individual within a very short period of time. Some mammals store erythrocytes in the spleen and extrude them into the bloodstream when they are needed. In the horse, for instance, hematocrit at rest can be as low as 33 percent but increases to 47 percent within a few minutes during strenuous exercise. The hematocrit can also increase as a

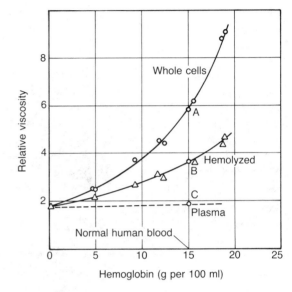

FIGURE 10–20
Comparison of viscosities of water, a hemoglobin solution, and whole blood. Even where hemoglobin concentrations are identical, the presence of blood cells in whole blood increases the viscosity over that of a hemoglobin solution. From K. Schmidt-Nielsen and C. R. Taylor, Red Blood Cells: Why or Why Not?, *Science*162 (1968):274–275. Reprinted with permission. Copyright 1968 by the American Association for the Advancement of Science.

result of cold acclimation, increased physical fitness, and acclimation to low atmospheric pressure. Such change in hematocrit occurs over several weeks or months, as opposed to a few minutes in mammals capable of extruding erythrocytes from the spleen.

Hematocrit will also increase in most species following dehydration. Humans usually die when as little as 20 percent of their body water has been lost. The dehydrated individual suffers from *hemoconcentration,* which causes an increase in blood viscosity, an increase in blood pressure, and ultimately death from cardiac failure. The camel is an exceptional animal for resisting severe dehydration: during water deprivation, moisture lost is derived from the interstitial fluid rather than from the blood and as a result there is little hemoconcentration.

Again, an increase in hematocrit raises the viscosity of blood and therefore also raises blood pressure. Note from equation 10.5 that an elevation in viscosity increases peripheral resistance; hence, to maintain a constant flow of blood to the tissues the pressure of blood in the tissues must be increased.

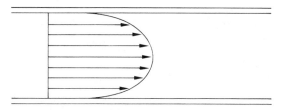

FIGURE 10–21
The velocities of concentric laminae of a fluid flowing in a tube (arrows indicate velocity of flow at different distances from the vessel walls)

Length The total distance through which the blood passes varies according to the physiological state of the animal. During exercise the number of capillary beds in the muscles which are open to blood flow increases. An increase in the local concentrations of carbon dioxide or hydrogen ions or both in the exercising muscle stimulates *vasodilation* and, subsequently, increases the number of open capillaries. Activity of the sympathetic nervous system also causes increased release of acetylcholine to the precapillary sphincters of skeletal muscle and thereby also increases the total number of open capillaries. But note that after exercise has ceased (or in other cases where there is an increased capillary perfusion without an elevation in venous return), blood pressure decreases. This decrease is due to the increased volume through which blood flows.

Radius If one compares the velocity with which blood moves, the fluid near the center of the vessel moves very rapidly compared to the fluid near the periphery (see Figure 10–21). This is apparently the result of interaction between the blood and the inner surface of the vessel wall. Thus, as vessel radius decreases, the *surface effect* (the relative action between the vessel endothelium and blood) increases. Therefore, in very small vessels ve-

locity should be very slow, simply because of increased interaction between blood and the vessel wall. In equation 10–5, note that resistance (R) is inversely affected by the radius (r) of the vessel. For example, constriction of a vessel to one-half its normal radius would actually cause resistance to increase by a factor of 16. Assuming for simplicity's sake that the numerator of the right side of equation 10.5 is equal to 1, the increase in resistance when the radius is halved is clear:

$$R = \frac{1}{r^4}$$

$$R = \frac{1}{(1/2)^4}$$

$$R = \frac{1}{1/16}$$

$$R = 16$$

And, as shown in equation 10.4, when resistance (R) is increased so too is pressure (P). Thus, the radius of blood vessels plays a critical role in the control of blood pressure. For instance, in a condition such as atherosclerosis where the radius of arterioles is severely reduced, blood pressure increases tremendously. On the other hand, where effective blood volume drops due to loss of blood or pooling (as in *anaphylaxis*), arteriole constriction can result in an elevation of blood pressure and return it to normal.

Effect of Exercise

Exercise is one of the principal causes of blood pressure alteration. When work is done by the muscles, there is a greater demand for oxygen by the tissues, a greater rate of venous return, an elevated tissue temperature, and an increased carbon dioxide content. In particular, increased plasma carbon dioxide stimulates breathing, which increases venous return by lowering thoracic pressure. The mechanical action of the diaphragm on the venae cavae also facilitates venous return. Both carbon dioxide and heat promote skeletal muscle capillary perfusion through their dilating effect on the precapillary sphincters of the metarterioles. This increase in vascular volume through which blood must be pumped during exercise causes a momentary fall in blood pressure, which is monitored by *baroreceptors* in the carotid sinus and wall of the aorta. As a result of this ephemeral drop in blood pressure in the major arteries, *tachycardia* (elevated heart rate) occurs along with increased cardiac output, and there is a consequent increase in blood pressure. During exercise, blood pressure increases significantly depending upon the physiological state of the animal. In the horse, for example, exercise results in an increase in left ventricular pressure from approximately 140 mm Hg at rest to 217 mm Hg during exercise.

Neurological Regulation

In addition to the methods already mentioned, blood pressure is also maintained by means of *reflex control* of cardiac output. From Poiseuille's equation (10.4), one can see that when peripheral resistance is constant, a change in flow rate or cardiac output results in a change in blood pressure. In order to maintain uniform tissue perfusion pressure when rapid changes in body position occur, reflex alterations in cardiac output must occur almost instantaneously. When an animal in the prone position stands up there is an instantaneous fall in arterial pressure in the carotid artery and in the aorta. This change in pressure results in a change in the activity of the carotid and aortic baroreceptors, which effects an immediate increase in heart rate. In other words, the so-called Marey and aortic reflexes have a definite homeostatic function in maintaining arterial blood pressure (see chapter 11, The Heart as a Pump). These reflexes operate very rapidly in comparison to other methods of blood pressure control.

It is probable that these receptors only respond to changes in pressure and are not responsive in the cases of long-term *hypotension* (low blood pressure) or *hypertension* (high blood pressure). When blood pressure is higher than normal due to excessive salt intake or from administration of hypertensive drugs, these reflexes act to maintain the acquired pressure that is perceived to be homeostatic at any particular time.

Hormonal Mechanisms

Three principal hormonal systems are involved in arterial pressure control. These are the *norepinephrine-epinephrine mechanism*, the *renin-angiotensin II vasoconstriction mechanism*, and the *vasopressin vasoconstriction mechanism*. These systems are activated differently but can function in a synergistic manner if evoked at the same time.

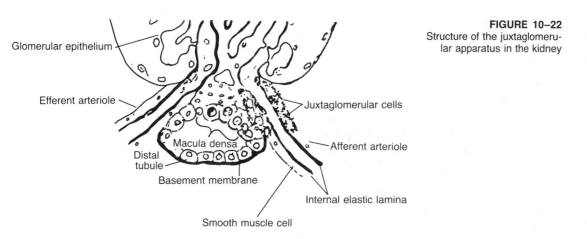

FIGURE 10-22
Structure of the juxtaglomerular apparatus in the kidney

Norepinephrine-epinephrine mechanism
When a mammal becomes excited or frightened there is normally an increase in sympathetic activity and, consequently, an increase in cardiac contractile force (the
inotropic effect) and rate (the *chronotropic
effect*), along with an increase in concentration of circulating epinephrine and norepinephrine. The net result is increased cardiac
output and increased vasoconstriction
throughout much of the circulatory system
and, in general, a rise in blood pressure. Constriction of parts of the metarterioles, which
lack innervation, is particularly effective here.
Also, venous return is increased as a result of
the reduced volume of vessels in the venous
circulation. Increased venous return results
in increased cardiac output, which further
enhances an elevation in arterial pressure.

**Renin-angiotensin II vasoconstriction
mechanism** When pressure in the renal arteries decreases, there is a point where hydrostatic pressure falls below colloidal-osmotic pressure in the *glomeruli* of the
kidney. At this point, filtration ceases and
kidney failure results. But before this point is
reached and when renal blood pressure is

sufficiently reduced to result in collapse of
the afferent arterioles which form part of the
juxtaglomerular apparatus in the kidney,
renin is released from the *juxtaglomerular
cells* (see Figure 10-22). *Renin*, an enzyme,
acts upon a peptide in the plasma called *angiotensinogen* to induce the formation of *angiotensin I* (see Figure 10-23). Renin persists
in the bloodstream and therefore has prolonged activity in promoting angiotensin I
formation. Angiotensin I is immediately converted to *angiotensin II* by a plasma enzyme.
Angiotensin II does not stay in the circulation very long and is deactivated by an enzyme called *angiotensinase*. Angiotensin II
carries out several reactions which result in

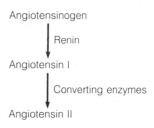

FIGURE 10-23
Formation of angiotensin II after release of renin into the
bloodstream

elevated arterial pressure. Its direct effect is to enhance vasoconstriction in the arteries, arterioles, and veins. Vasoconstriction in the arterial tree results directly in elevation of blood pressure. In addition, venous constriction increases the rate at which blood is returned to the heart. As a result, heart rate increases reflexly along with the stroke volume, and together they both increase cardiac output. In other words, increased return of blood to the heart causes cardiac output to increase as a result of the stretching effect on cardiac muscle *(Starling's law of the heart)*. It is suspected that the stretching action also activates the *Bainbridge reflex*, which promotes tachycardia and subsequent drainage of the venous system.

When blood pressure in the kidney falls, angiotensin II is formed, which (in addition to its vasoconstrictor effect) causes salt and water retention in the kidney. This elevates blood volume and therefore has a positive effect on blood pressure. The mechanism for this phenomenon is that angiotensin II acts on the adrenal cortex to promote the release of *aldosterone.* Aldosterone, in turn, enhances salt retention in the nephons. Increased salt retention promotes water retention, and the final result is an elevation in blood volume and, consequently, blood pressure. Angiotensin II in this case also stimulates drinking behavior and thereby aids indirectly in increasing blood volume.

Vasopressin vasoconstriction mechanism Control of total peripheral resistance is maintained by means of a hormone stored in the posterior pituitary. When blood pressure in the brain falls below normal levels, *vasopressin* is released from the *neurohypophysis* and acts directly upon arterial smooth muscles to cause vasoconstriction. Vasopressin release also results in increased permea-

bility of the collecting ducts of the kidney to water. Increased availability of this substance enhances water retention and acts synergistically with the salt retention activity of aldosterone. In other words, increased salt retention is able to promote water retention to a much greater level when vasopressin is secreted. The direct action of vasopressin on the arterial smooth muscles may be overshadowed by more rapid neural mechanisms, such as those associated with the baroreceptors (Marey and aortic reflexes) or the sympathetic nervous system. But the prolonged effects of vasopressin have been observed to last for as long as 48 hours in humans. By contrast, baroreceptor mechanisms usually only last for a few seconds or minutes, even though they can in some cases be used repeatedly to regulate blood pressure.

MEASUREMENT OF BLOOD PRESSURE

The technique used by the Reverend Stephen Hales to determine blood pressure in the horse is termed the *direct method.* This implies the insertion of a pipet or other device into the artery or vein and direct measurement of the force generated. An adaptation of this method which has been used for some time is illustrated in Figure 10–24. In this technique a vessel is *cannulated* (a needle, or *cannula*, is inserted into the vessel) and the blood is allowed to make contact with a saline solution in the manometer. As the mercury in the manometer is displaced, it moves a scribe which marks the oscillation on a chart. The movement of the scribe can be calibrated by means of a mercury manometer.

With the advent of polygraphs and electrical transducers other methods for directly

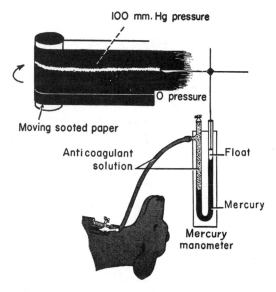

FIGURE 10–24
Direct measurement of arterial pressure in the dog.
From A. C. Guyton, *Textbook of Medical Physiology*,
6th edition (Philadelphia, Pa., 1981), 211, fig. 18–8. Reprinted by permission of W. B. Saunders Publishing Co.

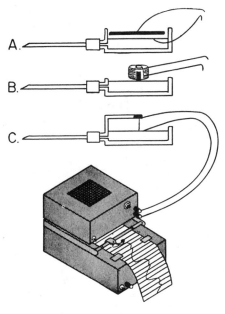

FIGURE 10–25
Measurement of blood pressure using three different
types of electronic transducers. For a description of A,
B, and C, see text. From A. C. Guyton, *Textbook of
Medical Physiology*, 6th edition (Philadelphia, Pa.,
1981), 211, fig. 18–9. Reprinted by permission of W. B.
Saunders Publishing Co.

measuring blood pressure have been devised.
In Figure 10–25, three methods are illustrated, all of which employ a direct introduction of a cannula into a vessel. Each fluid
chamber is enclosed on the top side by a
very thin, flexible piece of metal, which is in
turn connected to a recorder by means of a
preamplifier. In Figure 10–25A, a metal plate
placed above the membrane acts as the first
electrode. When the flexible plate of the
chamber is expanded by pressure, it moves
outward toward the other electrode. Changes
in the distance between the two electrodes
alter the capacitance, which is recorded on
the polygraph. In Figure 10–25B, the flexible
plate moves a metal core within a coil to alter
inductance. In Figure 10–25C, a resistance
wire connects the two electrodes. When the
wire is stretched, the resistance is changed,

allowing the resultant voltage change to be
recorded. In each case a change in the flow
of current is recorded on the polygraph. The
electrical change developed can be calibrated
with a mercury manometer to determine the
relationship between pressure and voltage
generated.

Most of us are familiar with the typical
routine of determining blood pressure by the
auscultatory method (see Figure 10–26). This
technique is frequently used by clinicians to
determine blood pressure in humans. In this
indirect and noninvasive method, pressure in
the *cuff* (the inflatable band) collapses the
brachial artery so that no blood is able to
pass through it. When pressure is gradually

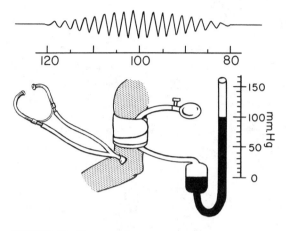

FIGURE 10–26
Measurement of arterial blood pressure by the auscultatory method. From A. C. Guyton, *Textbook of Medical Physiology*, 6th edition (Philadelphia, Pa., 1981), 247, fig. 21–2. Reprinted by permission of W. B. Saunders Publishing Co.

released in the cuff, sounds can be heard through a stethoscope as blood begins to pass through the artery in spurts. This signifies that maximum or systolic pressure of the arteries has reached a level equal to the pressure in the cuff. The pressure in the cuff is transferred to a mercury manometer, where it can be read in mm Hg. If the pressure in the cuff is allowed to decrease slowly, a point is finally reached where blood flows uniformly through the artery and no further sound is heard. This signifies minimum or diastolic pressure, which can also be read on the manometer. This indirect method has not been adequate, for the most part, for blood pressure determination in mammals other than humans. Also, because an experimental animal must be maintained in a steady position during the determination, the indirect method is difficult to employ under experimental conditions. Direct methods have been found to be more satisfactory.

SUMMARY

The circulatory system of mammals comprises arteries, veins, arterioles, metarterioles, venules, capillaries, and a four-chambered heart. In addition, the lymphatics drain the tissues and pass fluid back into the blood. The functions of the circulatory system are transportation, thermoregulation, and immunity (defense against disease). Of these the most important function is transportation. Nutrients, oxygen, heat, and blood cells are all transported through the blood, as are metabolic wastes.

Exchange between the blood and tissues only occurs when the blood is in the capillary beds. In the capillaries, only a single cell layer isolates the tissues from the blood, and it is for this reason that exchange of metabolites and other materials can occur. This phenomenon is, for the most part, explained by means of an equation developed by E. H. Starling in 1896. The exchange of materials between blood and the tissues is the result of passive movement controlled by a group of independent pressures. The algebraic sum of these pressures, the filtration pressure, is the primary driving force behind fluid exchange between blood and the tissues.

The volume of blood flow in different parts of the circulatory system is uniform, though the velocity of blood flow is not. Velocity is lowest through the capillaries as a result of increased cross-sectional area relative to the other parts of the circulatory system. This gives added efficiency to the filtration and diffusion processes, which occur between blood and tissues in the capillary beds.

Blood pressure varies widely among different portions of the circulatory system, but it is amazingly consistent among species. The factors which contribute to blood pressure are flow rate and resistance to flow. Peripheral resistance, the total resistance within the circulatory system, is a direct result of viscosity of blood and vessel length. Blood pressure is inversely proportional to the fourth power of the radius of the vessel.

Pressure in the system is controlled by several vasoactive hormones. The hormonal systems are activated by hydrostatic pressure changes or osmotic changes in the blood or both. Several neurological reflexes are essential to the maintenance of blood pressure. But these mechanisms respond to short-term blood pressure changes and are limited to stabilization of blood pressure following a change in body position or physical activity.

Blood pressure can be measured by direct or indirect methods. The direct method was first employed to determine blood pressure in the horse. This method has been aided tremendously in recent years by the development of modern electronic techniques. Later, indirect methods were developed and proved useful for clinical purposes in humans.

11

THE HEART AS A PUMP

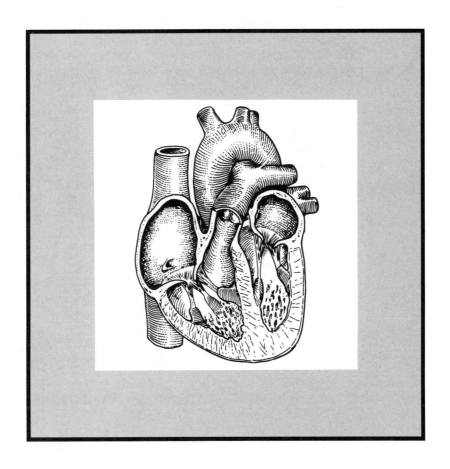

*T*he mammalian heart lies in the thoracic cavity, *usually slightly to the left of the midline. The* myocardium, *or muscular wall of the heart, is lined on the inside by a layer of epithelial tissue called the* endocardium. *The outer covering of the myocardium is called the* epicardium *(or visceral pericardium) (see Figure 11–1). The entire heart is covered by a sack of connective tissue, the* parietal pericardium.

The heart of mammals is a four-chambered structure which acts as a pump to force blood through the arteries, arterioles, and capillaries (see Figure 11–2). The four chambers are named the right *and* left atria *(or auricles) and the* right *and* left ventricles. Blood enters the heart from the* venae cavae *and passes through the right atrium and then into the right ventricle. From the right ventricle, blood is pumped through the* pulmonary trunk *to the lungs. After passing through the capillaries of the lungs, blood enters the left atrium and then the left ventricle before it is finally pumped through the* aorta *and into the systemic circulation.*

From this description it might seem that the heart acts in a sequence of four contractile intervals as blood passes through each of the four chambers. In fact, the heart contracts in a two-cycle sequence: both atria contract simultaneously and then both ventricles contract simultaneously. This two-cycle sequence is done with remarkable regularity throughout the life of the animal. The rhythm of the heart is maintained by an internal mechanism and does not require external stimulation. Because excitation of contractile events is generated internally, the heart is said to be myogenic. *The* neurogenic *heart of some invertebrates requires direct stimulation by efferent neurons from the brain in order to beat. In the mammals and other vertebrates, rhythm and rate of heartbeat are modified by the action of the autonomic nervous system, but the basic mechanism for generating heartbeat is completely intrinsic.*

FIGURE 11–1
Structure of the tissue layers
that constitute the heart wall

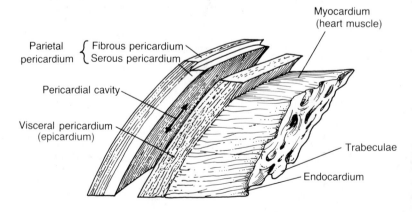

Myocardium
(heart muscle)

Parietal pericardium { Fibrous pericardium
Serous pericardium

Pericardial cavity

Visceral pericardium
(epicardium)

Trabeculae

Endocardium

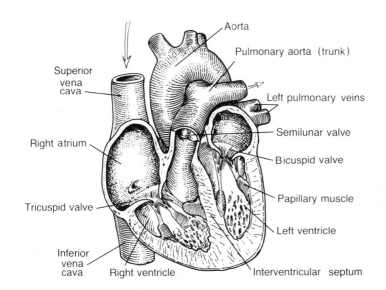

VALVES OF THE HEART

One-way flow of the blood through the heart is accomplished by two sets of valves. One set, the *atrioventricular valves (A-V valves)*, separates the ventricles from the atria. When the ventricles contract, the A-V valves prevent blood in the ventricles from entering the atria. The other set of valves, the *semilunar valves*, separates the aorta and pulmonary trunk from the left and right ventricles, respectively. When the ventricles are relaxed, the closure of the semilunar valves prevents blood from flowing from the aorta and pulmonary trunk back into the ventricles.

The A-V valves are composed of leaflike portions called *cusps* (points). On the right side of the heart three cusps are present which form the *tricuspid* or *mitral valve*. The *bicuspid valve* is located on the left side of the heart. The cusps open into the ventricles. When the valves are closed they fit together to form a uniform barrier to blood flow into the atria.

The A-V valves are attached to several strong cords called *chordae tendineae*, which

are in turn attached to the wall of the ventricles by the *papillary muscles* (see Figure 11–3). Papillary muscles are extensions of the myocardium but represent a specialized portion of the heart muscle. The valves close when force is exerted against them by blood inside of the ventricles. The papillary mus-

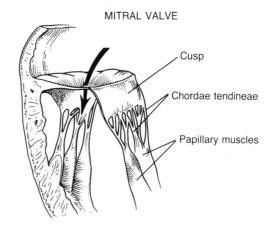

FIGURE 11-3
Section of the human heart showing chordae tendineae and papillary muscles

cles contract against the internal pressure, preventing the valve from opening into the atria and allowing backflow.

The semilunar valves prevent backflow of blood from the aorta and pulmonary artery when the ventricles are relaxed (see Figure 11–4). These valves, however, are not attached to an elaborate system of cords and muscles, as seen in the A-V valves. The pressure of blood in the aorta and pulmonary trunk tends to maintain the valves in the closed position. Minor scarring or thickening of the tissue of the heart valves reduces their ability to close tightly. Improperly closed valves allow blood to leak back into adjacent chambers. The sound made by blood movement through improperly fitted or damaged valves is one type of *heart murmur.*

The closure of the A-V valves separating the atria and ventricles results in the *first heart sound,* which can be described as a low-pitched "lub" sound. The *second heart sound,* caused by the closure of the semilunar valves, is sharper and gives a higher-pitched "dup" sound. The first sound occurs at the beginning of ventricular contraction; the second sound occurs shortly after the ventricles begin to relax.

THE CARDIAC CYCLE

As mentioned previously, a two-cycle beat is maintained in the heart, with both atria contracting in unison followed by the contraction of both ventricles. The *cardiac cycle,* the coordination of the two-cycle beat of the mammalian heart, is controlled by *nodal tissue,* which generates an intrinsic rhythm. A small amount of tissue called the *sinoatrial,* or *S-A node,* is located in the right atrium (see Figure 11–5). This tissue, called the *pacemaker,* develops from the sinus venosus in the embryo and has an intrinsic firing rate of 70 to 80 pulses per minute in the human. Nodal firing, which was described in an earlier chapter, has a continuous rhythm which is regulated by the potassium ion permeability

FIGURE 11–4
Transverse section of the heart between atria and ventricles showing valves which control blood flow

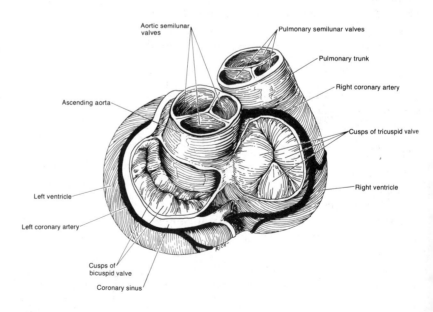

Aortic semilunar valves

Pulmonary semilunar valves

Pulmonary trunk

Right coronary artery

Ascending aorta

Cusps of tricuspid valve

Left ventricle

Right ventricle

Left coronary artery

Cusps of bicuspid valve

Coronary sinus

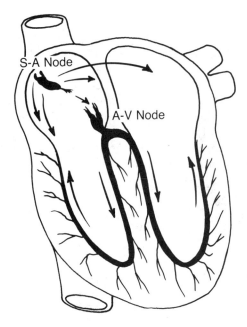

FIGURE 11–5
Pacemaker system in mammals. Impulses are generated in the S-A node, spread throughout the atria, and
activate the A-V node. Impulses generated in the A-V
node then spread throughout the myocardium via the
bundle of His and the Purkinje fibers.

of the nodal cells. The pulse generated at the
S-A node is able to set up action potentials
in the cells of adjacent myocardial tissue. Action potentials thus generated course
throughout the atrial myocardium by direct
electrical transfer between cells at the intercalated discs. The cells of the atria are arranged so that their action potentials im-
pinge upon the *atrioventricular*, or *A-V node*.
This collection of action potentials from adjacent cells induces an electrical impulse in
the A-V node which passes through the *bundle of His* to the *Purkinje cells*. The Purkinje
cells are uniformly dispersed throughout the
ventricular myocardium and generate action
potentials in the ventricular muscle. Contrac-

tion of the myocardium follows a wave pattern. In the ventricles contraction starts on
the *endocardial edge* near the *septum* and
proceeds through the ventricular myocardium. The contraction finally terminates at
the upper portion of the ventricles (see Figure 11–6).

The A-V node also has tonic activity, but
its pulse rate is slower than that of the S-A
node. Since the A-V node is stimulated by action potentials from the atria, its intrinsic
pulse rate is not expressed unless the pulse
of the S-A node is suppressed or otherwise
eradicated.

When ventricular contraction begins, increased blood pressure within the ventricles
causes both A-V valves to close. When ventricular pressure becomes equal to the pressure in the aorta and pulmonary trunk, the
semilunar valves open and blood flows from
the ventricles. Shortly after the beginning of
relaxation in the ventricles, pressure in the
aorta and pulmonary trunk is slightly higher
than the ventricular pressure. Currents generated by the slight movement of blood from
the aorta and pulmonary trunk back into the
ventricles force the semilunar valves to close.
Closure of the semilunar valves is accompanied by a minor, transient change in aortic
pressure (see Figure 11–7). The second heart
sound occurs simultaneously with this
change in pressure. Closure of the semilunar
valves ensures the elevated diastolic pressure
in the aorta and pulmonary trunk and allows
the ventricular pressure to return to 0.0 millimeters of mercury.

THE ELECTROCARDIOGRAM

The Dutch investigator Einthoven discovered
that electrical potentials could be recorded
on the surface of the skin of humans. For his

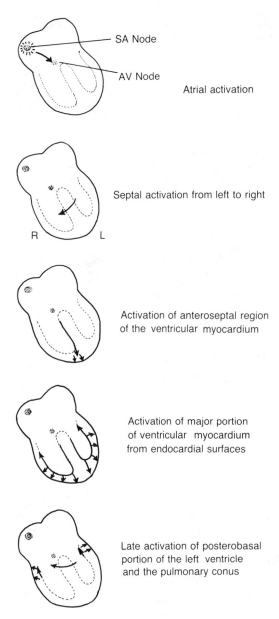

SA Node

AV Node

Atrial activation

Septal activation from left to right

R   L

Activation of anteroseptal region
of the ventricular myocardium

Activation of major portion
of ventricular myocardium
from endocardial surfaces

Late activation of posterobasal
portion of the left ventricle
and the pulmonary conus

FIGURE 11–6
Spread of electrical activity in the human heart. Reproduced with permission, from Goldman, MI: *Principles of Clinical Electrocardiography*, 11th ed. Copyright 1982 by Lange Medical Publications, Los Altos, California.

work he received the 1924 Nobel Prize in medicine and physiology. These basic recordings became known as an *electrocardiogram (ECG or EKG)*. The recording positions are typically termed *lead one* (recorded between the arms), *lead two* (recorded between the right arm and the left leg), and *lead three* (recorded between the left arm and the left leg). When the leads are connected to three limbs a triangle is formed with the heart in the middle (see Figure 11–8). The triangle thus formed is known as *Einthoven's triangle*. A number of additional leads have been developed by using chest electrodes in relation to the three limbs involved. The EKG has become a valuable tool for the clinician. In addition, it has become a desirable research tool for physiologists studying a variety of principles, ranging from diving physiology to hibernation. Many elaborate analyses of EKGs are possible, particularly in the area of medicine. The reader is referred to any of the current medical physiology texts for more information on this topic.

The typical EKG can be divided into three significant electrical events called *waves* (see Figure 11–9). The first wave, the *P wave*, occurs simultaneously with *atrial depolarization;* the last wave, the *T wave*, occurs as the ventricles are *repolarized*. The *QRS complex*, the second wave, signifies the repolarization of the atria and depolarization of the ventricles. The relationship between the EKG and various other cardiac events is given in Figure 11–7. Note that the first heart sound, closure of the A-V valves, immediately follows the QRS complex and results in ventricular contraction. The second heart sound, closure of the semilunar valves, occurs as ventricular pressure drops below aortic pressure.

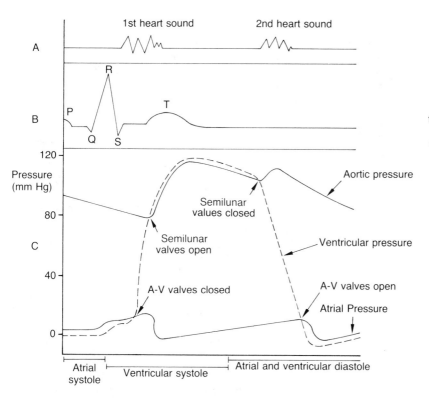

FIGURE 11–7
Cycle of events during cardiac cycle: (A) heart sounds
related to the cardiac cycle;
(B) deflections in the EKG as
related to the heart cycle; (C)
aortic, ventricular, and atrial
pressure changes along with
the opening and closing of the
atrioventricular (A-V) valves
and the semilunar valves during the cardiac cycle

INNERVATION OF THE HEART

The heart is innervated by the autonomic
nervous system. The system's parasympathetic branch affects the heart by releasing acetylcholine from the vagus nerve at both the
A-V and S-A nodes. The S-A node is innervated primarily by the right vagus nerve,
whereas the left vagus nerve primarily innervates the A-V node (see Figure 11–10). The
parasympathetic nervous system has the effect of reducing heart rate through delay of
the pulse rate at both nodes. The action of
acetylcholine is to maintain potassium ion
permeability at a high level, thus increasing
the time necessary for the prepotential to
reach threshold. By increasing the length of
the prepotential, heart rate is correspondingly reduced. This relationship of parasympathetic stimulation and heart rate seems
universal among the vertebrates.

The cardiac nerves of the sympathetic
branch form a perfuse network throughout
the myocardium and directly innervate the S-
A and A-V nodes. Application of epinephrine
reduces the length of the prepotential and
consequently increases the firing rate of the
nodes. The sympathetic nerves release norepinephrine and, to a lesser extent, epinephrine at a number of positions or *varicosities*
along the length of the individual nerve fibers. This arrangement, which is quite unlike
the typical one-to-one ratio found in myoneural junctions of skeletal muscle, reduces
the number of fibers necessary to innervate

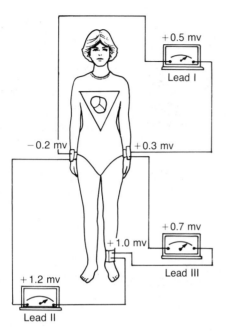

FIGURE 11–8
The typical leads used in obtaining the EKG from a human. Einthoven's triangle is superimposed on the chest.

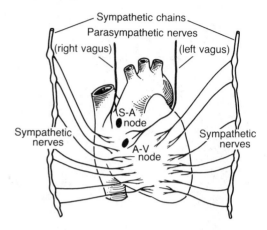

FIGURE 11–10
Autonomic innervation of the heart

the heart. Both of the catecholamines, norepinephrine and epinephrine, increase the activity of adenyl cyclase and therefore cause a greater conversion of ATP to cyclic AMP. This action enhances active transport and thus increases the rate of calcium ion re-

trieval from the sarcomeres, essential to relaxation and therefore repetitive muscle contraction. Unlike skeletal muscle, cardiac muscle depends upon both extracellular calcium and calcium stored in the terminal cisternae for contraction. It is essential that active transport occurs before each contraction to maintain both extracellular and terminal cisternae calcium ion levels. In addition to its role in ion homeostasis, the sympathetic nervous system is also essential to fatty acid mobilization and therefore is a primary factor in providing the energy sources for cardiac muscle.

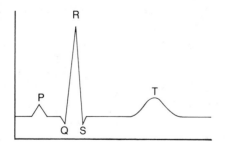

FIGURE 11–9
Recording of a typical electrocardiogram showing P wave, QRS complex, and T wave

CARDIAC OUTPUT

The quantity of blood pumped by the heart each minute, the *cardiac output*, is quite variable among different species and also varies according to the activity and the emotional state of the animal. In most mammals under resting conditions, the ventricles deliver about 70 percent of their total volume into the aorta and pulmonary trunk with each contraction. This is the *stroke volume* of the heart. In a human at rest the stroke volume is about 75 milliliters. With a heart rate of 72 beats per minute, a stroke volume of 75 milliliters results in 5.5 liters of blood being pumped per minute. Thus, the entire blood volume of a human is recycled through the heart each minute.

The transport of blood, and therefore the oxygen delivery to the tissue, seems to be the primary activating force behind cardiac output. But when cardiac output is expressed relative to body mass (i.e., liters per minute per gram), the relation is reversed. For example, small mammals, which have a high metabolic rate, have a much higher cardiac output relative to body weight than is found in large animals. The low metabolic rates of larger mammals place a lower demand on the tissues for oxygen consumption and waste removal. Cardiac output is not completely dependent upon body weight; there

are some species specific differences as well (see Table 11–1). Human males, for instance, have a cardiac output based on tissue weight of about 80 to 90 milliliters per kilogram per minute (ml/kg/min). *Citellus* (ground squirrel), when awake, has a cardiac output of 313 ml/kg/min. *Citellus* weighs approximately 250 grams (8.75 ounces) and thus pumps 69 milliliters of blood per minute. Since the total amount of blood in mammals is equal to approximately 7 percent of the total body weight, *Citellus* cycles its blood volume (about 21 milliliters) three times each minute. The blood volume of a 75-kilogram (165.3-pound) man is equal to approximately 5 liters and is only cycled about once each minute. In the cow, which weighs about 365 kilograms (804.7 pounds) and whose blood volume is approximately 22 liters, a cardiac output of 45.8 liters per minute is only about twice the blood volume. One could say that the cow's blood is completely recycled about twice

Species	Heart Rate (beats/min)	Cardiac Output (liters/min)	Wt. Specific Cardiac Output
Elephant	30–40		
Horse*			
at rest	35–40	38	79 ml/kg/min
exercising	190–200	241	506 ml/kg/min
Cow	45–60	45.8	113 ml/kg/min
Human (males)	75	5.5–6.0	80–90 ml/kg/min
Pig		4.5	146 ml/kg/min
Dog	90–100	2.0–3.0	
Rat	350		286 ml/kg/min
Bat			
at rest but awake	250–450		
excited	880		
House mouse**	500		
Grey shrew†	782 (588–1,320)		

TABLE 11–1

Heart rate, cardiac output, and weight specific cardiac output in a selected group of mammals

*Thomas and Fregin. 1981. Journal of Applied Physiology, 864–868.

**Irving *et al.*, 1941. Journal of Cellular Physiology, 17:145.

†Morrison *et al.*, 1953. Federal Proceedings 12:100.

each minute, which is still decidedly greater than that seen in humans.

Factors Affecting Cardiac Output

Cardiac output is affected by two independent factors: heart rate and stroke volume. Heart rate is affected by a number of environmental factors, by the concentration of dissolved gases in the blood, and by other physiological variables. Stroke volume is a function of the size of the heart, the degree of shortening of the heart muscle fibers, and the force of contraction. The maintenance of cardiac output adequate for tissue oxygen and nutrient demand requires the integration of a number of sensory and physical variables.

Heart rate Several external factors are known to affect heart rate. For instance, in the diving mammals the heart rate might decrease from 100 or so beats per minute to 4 or 5 beats per minute during a dive. In humans, the presence of a cold wind on the face causes a decrease in heart rate.

The rate at which the heart beats is also affected by the physiological state of the animal, emotional factors such as fear and anger, posture, age, and body size. Emotions expressed through actions of the autonomic nervous system have a marked impact on the rate of the heartbeat. When excited, mammals have an elevated heart rate; the rate decreases to one-half that value or less when quiescent. Remember, when the heart rate increases, the contraction time remains relatively constant and the relaxation time is reduced. Shorter relaxation time, therefore, allows for the increased rate of contraction. This decreases the total time that blood may flow through the coronary circulation.

Heart rate is greatly affected by the metabolic rate of the animal. Since the heart must pump enough blood to supply the tissues with adequate oxygen and nutrients, it is essential for the heart and metabolic rates to be closely correlated. But since the metabolic rate, or consumption of oxygen per gram of tissue per minute, is inversely proportional to body weight, one might expect the larger mammals to have lower heart rates than smaller ones. This is indeed the case. For example, the heart rate in the largest land mammal, the elephant, is approximately 35 beats per minute, whereas the heart rate of the mouse at rest is about 500 beats per minute (this equals eight complete cardiac cycles per second). In general, heart rate is closely tied to metabolic rate and therefore has an inverse relationship to body size (see Figure 11–11).

Exercise also causes heart rate to increase. The rate of increase in this case is a function of the elevated metabolic rate spurred by the exercise involved. In the horse, for instance, heart rate increases from about 38 to 40 beats

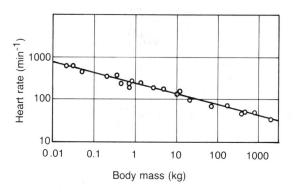

FIGURE 11–11
Relationship of heart rate to body size in mammals. From W. R. Stahl, Scaling of Respiratory Variables in Mammals, *J. Appl. Physiol.* 22(1967): 453–460. Reprinted by permission of The American Physiological Society, Bethesda, Md.

per minute at rest to about 190 to 200 beats per minute during exercise. This change in heart rate corresponds closely with the change in oxygen consumption of 38 l/min at rest to 241 l/min during exercise.

The age of the individual can also affect the heart rate (see Table 11–2). For the most part heart rate, like metabolic rate, is highest in young animals and continues to decrease throughout life.

An often overlooked factor which controls heart rate is posture. In the standing position, the force of blood from the head increases the work necessary for the heart to maintain a constant blood flow. The giraffe provides an excellent example of the effects of posture on heart rate. When the animal is lying down, heart rate is about 96 beats per minute as opposed to about 150 beats per minute when standing. It is important to note that the change in heart rate is not the result of a shift in metabolic rate but rather an alteration in the activity of the autonomic nervous system, which maintains the hom-

eostatic pressure levels in all parts of the circulation.

The contractile rate of the heart is modified primarily by the autonomic nervous system in conjunction with several reflexes triggered by pressure generated within the arteries and heart. The cardiac accelerator action of the sympathetic branch is known as the *chronotropic action;* the increased force of contraction due to sympathetic stimulation is known as the *inotropic action.* Factors that increase the strength of contraction are called *positive inotropic effects*, whereas those that decrease contractile force are said to be *negative inotropic effects.*

Two centers of the brain, known as the *cardiac inhibitory and cardiac excitatory centers*, are reputed to control heart rate. But only the cardiac inhibitory center can actually be demonstrated. Heart rate does accelerate as the activity of the inhibitory center decreases, but this is probably due to increased discharge in the sympathetic cardiac nerves and not to an increase in the activity of a cardiac excitatory center, as might be supposed.

Peripheral input to the cardiac inhibitory center originates from baroreceptors in the sinus of the internal carotid artery and in the wall of the aortic arch. The *glossopharyngeal nerve* innervates baroreceptors in the carotid sinus, and *vagal sensory fibers* innervate baroreceptors in the aorta. An increase in pressure in either the internal carotid or the aortic arch excites the cardiac inhibitory center and induces a decrease in heart rate. When blood pressure increases, the cardiac inhibitory center is stimulated and vagal activity increases. An increase in vagal firing rate decreases heart rate and reduces arterial pressure accordingly. Excitation of the baroreceptors in the carotid sinus with reflexive

TABLE 11–2
Effect of age on heart rate in several species of mammals

Species	Age	Heart Rate (beats/min)
Bos taurus	Newborn	141–160
(cattle)	Adult	46–53
Canis familiaris	Newborn	160–180
(dog)	Adult	72–200
Capra hircus	Newborn	145–240
(goat)	Adult	81
Equus caballus	Newborn	100–120
(horse)	Adult	34–55
Felis catus	Newborn	300
(cat)	Adult	110–240

Source: From P. L. Altman and D. S. Dittmer, *Biology Data Book* (Bethesda, Maryland: Federation of American Societies for Experimental Biology, 1964)

decrease in heart rate is referred to as the *Marey* or *carotid sinus reflex*. The similar reflex originating with baroreceptors in the aortic arch is called the *aortic reflex*. The aortic arch and carotid sinus reflexes are functionally similar and differ only in placement of the baroreceptors and the different nerves which innervate them (see Figure 11–12).

Another reflex believed to be effective in heart rate control is the *Bainbridge reflex*. In 1915, Bainbridge noticed that increased atrial pressure resulted in an increase in heart rate. The reflex tends to increase the rate at which blood is passed out of the heart when venous return is high. Thus, one function of the reflex is the prevention of excess accumulation of venous blood.

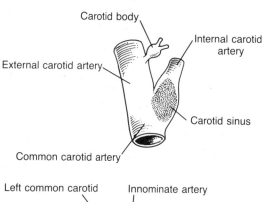

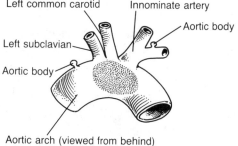

FIGURE 11–12
The baroreceptor areas in the carotid sinus and aortic arch (the shaded areas indicate receptor sites)

Stroke volume An essential part of the change in cardiac output during any state of physical activity depends in part on the stroke volume, or amount of blood which can be delivered to the tissues with each contraction of the heart. It has been shown in a variety of mammals that stroke volume increases with increased levels of exercise. In humans, stroke volume is 60 to 70 milliliters when standing. At maximum exercise, stroke volume increases to about 125 milliliters. In the horse, stroke volume increases from a little less than 1.0 liter at rest to 2.5 liters at maximum exercise. Similar changes have also been shown in the dog.

Two factors of principal importance in stroke volume are the percent of the cardiac contents emptied with each beat and the volume of blood filling the ventricles prior to each beat. Cardiac muscle develops maximum tension at resting length, which is identical to the response of skeletal muscle. The pressure developed in the ventricle is proportional to the degree of diastolic filling (see Figure 11–13). Thus, increased blood returned through the venae cavae can be more efficiently pumped into the arterial system. This phenomenon is known as *Starling's law of the heart*. An increased ventricular filling causes a stretching of the heart muscle, which increases the force of contraction. This type of control, in which force is a function of fiber length, is called *heterometric regulation*. Increased stretch can also be caused by increased arterial pressure. Increased cardiac output with increased myocardial stretch has been substantiated in dogs under moderate to severe exercise. This must also be true in other mammals, if one assumes that the stroke volume at rest is 70 percent of ventricular capacity. A doubling in the stroke volume during exercise must be

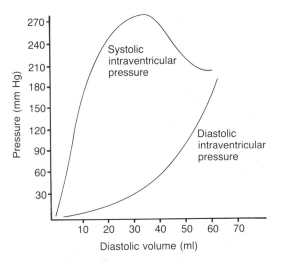

FIGURE 11–13
Length-tension relationship in heart muscle

associated with an increase in diastolic filling pressure.

The force of contraction can also be increased with drugs that increase calcium ion influx. Catecholamines cause an increase in the energy available for both ion transport and muscle contraction by increasing glucose absorption by the muscle cells. Because catecholamines increase the total available energy, they affect calcium ion release to the sarcomere, calcium ion removal from the sarcomere, and the amount of ATP for contraction. Calcium ions are chelated by troponin, and an increase in their availability at the filament level enhances the force of contraction. In fact, an excess amount of calcium ion, when applied directly to heart muscle, can cause it to remain in the contracted state for long periods of time. This condition is called *calcium rigor.*

It has also been demonstrated that increased stroke volume could be aided by increased emptying efficiency. The degree of

contraction of ventricular muscles is increased with increased sympathetic stimulation. Increased efficiency in the amount of blood pumped with each contraction is therefore in part due to the increased shortening associated with sympathetic stimulation during exercise. It is therefore probable that both factors, increased filling and increased contraction, enhance stroke volume.

When cardiac muscle contracts, the force generated must equal and then exceed the pressure in the aorta before flow can begin. The force necessary to reach this pressure is equivalent to *preload,* or the load added to muscle before its work actually begins (see Figure 11–14). During this phase of contraction, the *series elastic element* is stretched and no actual shortening of contractile fibers occurs. This phase of contractile cycle is therefore *isometric.* As cardiac fibers begin to shorten, blood begins to flow out of the heart and force remains constant. This phase of

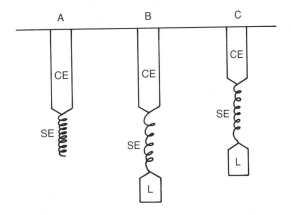

FIGURE 11–14
Effect of preloading on muscles: (A) resting tension; (B) preloaded with increased tension due to stretching of elastic element; (C) contraction under isotonic conditions (L. load; CE, contractile element; and SE, series elastic element)

the contractile process is *isotonic* because of the constant force generated.

Determination of Cardiac Output

Cardiac output can be measured by the *Fick* principle or by the *dye-slug method*. With the Fick principle, the oxygen consumption rate must be determined along with the oxygen concentration of the arterial and venous blood (see Figure 11–15). Cardiac output is then determined by means of the following equation:

$$CO \text{ (l/min)} = \frac{\text{ml } O_2 \text{ consumed/min}}{A_{O_2} - V_{O_2} \text{ (ml/l)}} \quad (11.1)$$

where,

CO = Cardiac output
A_{O_2} = Arterial oxygen concentration
V_{O_2} = Venous oxygen concentration

This method of analysis will allow the car-

diac output to be determined with a minimum amount of trauma to the experimental animal, since surgery is not needed to obtain blood samples.

Another method which works satisfactorily for the determination of cardiac output is the dye-slug method (see Figure 11–16). In this technique a known amount of dye is injected into the venous blood supply, and arterial blood samples are taken and analyzed as the dye passes through the heart and into the arteries. Cardiac output is then determined by the following equation:

$$CO \text{ (l/min)} = \frac{\text{(mg dye injected)} \times 60}{\text{(mg dye/l blood)} \times \text{(duration of the curve)}} \quad (11.2)$$

where,

CO = Cardiac output

In this case, duration of the curve represents the total time required for the total amount of dye injected to pass through the heart, usually less than a minute. To obtain cardiac output in terms of volume per minute, the duration (in seconds) must be divided into 60, which is part of the numerator in equation 11.2.

In order to use the Fick principle, one must be able to determine the oxygen consumption rate of the organism as well as the arterial and venous oxygen. The dye-slug method is simpler and more easily performed, because a known sample of dye is injected and the investigator need only analyze arterial plasma samples for dye concentration and measure the time required for the dye to be pumped through the heart.

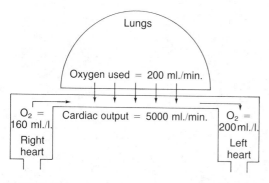

FIGURE 11–15
The Fick principle for determining cardiac output. From A. C. Guyton, *Textbook of Medical Physiology*, 6th edition (Philadelphia, Pa., 1981), 287, fig. 23–16. Reprinted by permission of W. B. Saunders Publishing Co.

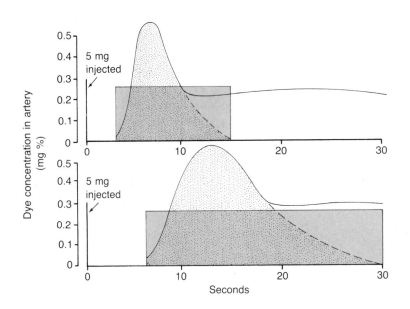

FIGURE 11–16
Concentration curves used to calculate the cardiac output by the dye-slug (dye dilution) method. Upper side of rectangle marks average concentrations for each curve. From A. C. Guyton, *Textbook of Medical Physiology,* 6th edition (Philadelphia, Pa., 1981), 309, fig. 23–17. Reprinted by permission of W. B. Saunders Publishing Co.

VENOUS RETURN

Blood is returned to the heart through the venous circulation, which has relatively low pressure. But the volume of blood returned to the heart must equal the amount forced through the arteries. This presents certain problems, since the venous flow of blood is by and large passive, whereas the heart actively forces blood throughout the arterial system. The problem of venous return is re-markable in some species because the distance over which the blood must travel is immense (see Figure 11–17). It is the function of the heart to force blood to the highest point in the animal; it is necessary for the venous system to return blood to the heart from the lowest part of the animal's body. In humans, it is known that pressure falls from about 35 mm Hg as the blood enters the capillary beds to about 15 mm Hg at the venous end. Blood pressure decreases throughout the venous

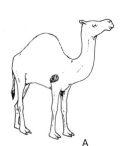

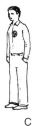

FIGURE 11–17
Heart in relation to stature of the animal: (A) camel, (B) dog, and (C) human

A

B

C

system and finally reaches nearly 0.0 mm Hg at the right atrium. This is true for other mammalian species as well.

How then is venous return accomplished? First, veins contain valves which establish a one-way flow of blood toward the heart. Second, muscular contraction in the legs generates pressure, which is exerted against the walls of the veins. The pressure generated by the muscles tends to collapse the veins and thus pushes the blood away from the site of muscular contraction. Because the one-way valves are present, blood pushed by muscular contraction must always travel toward the heart. In animals such as the giraffe, the pressure of a tight skin is also thought to be essential in the process of venous return, since the pressure generated by the muscles is greater if the enclosing membrane (the skin) is not easily stretched.

The circulatory system is similar to an open-ended U-tube and acts very much like the type used in a sump pump. In this type of continuous-fluid system, very little pressure needs to be exerted at the top of the U-tube to cause flow from the other end. The weight of the liquid in one half of the tube is balanced by the weight of the liquid in the other half of the tube. A slight difference in pressure on one side of the tube is instantly distributed to the opposite side.

In addition, the low pressure in the thorax resulting from expansion of the chest during inhalation must not be overlooked. As a result of breathing action, thoracic pressure in mammals drops below atmospheric pressure in order to draw air into the lungs. This same pressure change distends the flexible walls of the venous system of the thorax and thus influences the pressure differential necessary to cause blood to flow back to the heart.

In many hooved mammals, there is also a pump mechanism associated with the foot. In the horse, for example, the hoof provides a rigid outer surface through which the weight of the animal is applied via the *third phalanx*, or *coffin bone* (see Figure 11–18). This type of pumping action works so efficiently that it is sometimes said that the horse has five hearts. Actually, the coffin bone moves only slightly in the hoof because it is held in place by the laminae of the hoof wall, which interdigitate with the internal laminae firmly fixed to the coffin bone. The mechanism involved here is that the cartilagenous structure at the bottom of the hoof, the *frog*, is forced upward and outward by the weight of the horse (see Figure 11–19). Force on the frog is transferred to the collateral cartilages of the third phalanx, which expand outwardly. The force of the collateral cartilages is transferred to a large area of veins within the hoof, forcing blood toward the heart. Presumably, this mechanism also works in the giraffe (and most artiodactyls and perissodactyls). Certainly, it is part of the venous return of the horse, since almost no muscles exist below its knee. It is the absence of muscles which makes mus-

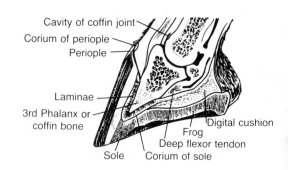

FIGURE 11–18
Section through the hoof of the horse showing structures involved in pumping action

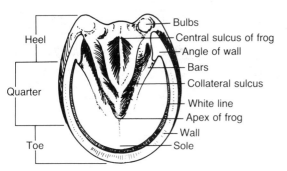

Heel

Quarter

Toe

— Bulbs
— Central sulcus of frog
— Angle of wall
— Bars
— Collateral sulcus
— White line
— Apex of frog
— Wall
— Sole

FIGURE 11–19
Bottom of horse's forefoot showing structures involved in support and blood pumping action. From O. R. Adams, *Lameness in Horses*, 3rd edition (Philadelphia, Pa., 1974), 26, fig. 1–38. Reprinted by permission of Lea and Febiger Publishers.

cular pumping action impossible in most artiodactyls and perissodactyls and forces them to rely on the pumping action of the hoof.

Venous return is also aided by venous constriction, which reduces the capacity of the veins. The control of venous diameter is a function of the vasomotor center of the medulla oblongata, which receives stimuli concerning blood pressure from several different areas of the body. One of its principal functions is to cause venous constriction when arterial pressure falls because of poor venous return. Constriction of the veins reduces the volume of the venous system, causing a massive transfer of blood from the venous to arterial side to increase oxygen delivery during a fall in blood pressure.

SUMMARY

The heart functions in mammals to propel blood through the arteries, arterioles, and capillaries. It consists of four chambers, two atria and two ventricles, and has a two-cycle

beat. Both atria contract at one time to force blood into the ventricles; then both ventricles contract to force blood into the aorta and pulmonary trunk.

The direction of flow of blood through the heart is controlled by the valves, which are closed and opened by pressure generated in the heart and arteries. The A-V valves prevent backflow of blood into the atria, and the semilunar valves prevent the flow of blood from the aorta and pulmonary trunk back into the ventricles.

The rate of heart contraction is internally controlled by a system of modified muscles generating tonic electrical impulses which initiate contraction. The S-A node is called the pacemaker of the heart because *in situ* it controls the rate of heartbeat. Its action is faster and therefore predominates over the pulse of the A-V node.

Activity of the nodes is regulated by both branches of the autonomic nervous system. The parasympathetic branch reduces the heart rate by release of acetylcholine through the vagus nerve. The sympathetic branch sends fibers through the cardiac nerves which innervate nodal tissue and the myocardium. The role of the sympathetic nervous system is to increase heart rate and contractile force by increasing active transport in cardiac muscle and the nodes. Increased active transport of potassium ion increases the rate of firing of nodal tissue, whereas increased calcium ion transport out of the cell increases its rate of relaxation. The sympathetic branch also makes energy reserves available to cardiac muscle by increasing fatty acid mobilization.

The rate at which blood is pumped, termed cardiac output, can be modified by the degree of stretch applied to cardiac muscle cells, by the size of the heart, and by autonomic stimulation. Cardiac muscle contracts with greater force when stretched or when stimulated by the sympathetic nervous system. Increased force of contraction results in greater emptying action by the heart and therefore increased cardiac output.

Cardiac output is measured by the Fick principle and the dye-slug method. Accuracy is equal for both methods, though less laboratory equipment is necessary for determination by the dye-slug method.

12

FEEDING AND DIGESTION

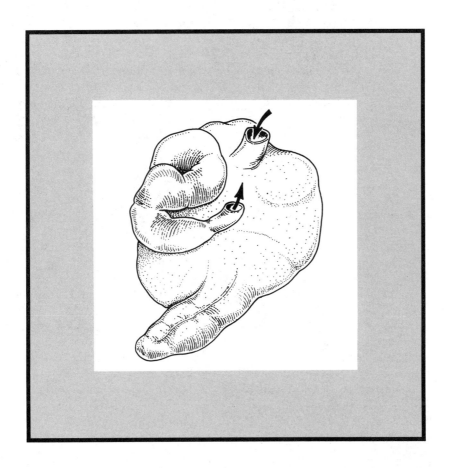

*F*ood consumption by animals provides a source of energy and a source of structural materials needed for growth and maintenance of the body. With only a few exceptions, adult mammals consume particulate food and therefore have characteristic dentition, which is usually modified through evolution to conform to a specific eating style or food source. Since most mammals take in particulate food, they are referred to as macrophages (macro, large; phage, to eat). The macrophagic condition has been instrumental in the acquisition of a terrestrial habitat and has allowed for a reduction in time spent in food gathering. A comparison with the microphages might make the advantages of macrophagic feeding clear. Microphages must consume food that is suspended or dissolved in a fluid medium or that has collected in sediments from an aquatic medium. Since the food for these animals is less dense than that available to particulate feeders, the animal must spend a large part, if not most, of its time feeding.

Subadult or juvenile mammals are microphages since their food must be taken in as milk, through nursing. In many other species, food for the juvenile is received after being masticated and partially digested by an adult. An example of the latter case is seen in many of the canids, such as the wolf, which feed on meat from prey and later regurgitate it for consumption by the young. The food is thereby made more soluble through mastication and stomach action so that only part of the food is particulate in nature.

FEEDING GROUPS

Mammals can be divided into specific groups based upon the type of food materials relied upon for basic sustenance. The type of food eaten by a species is generally associated with a particular habitat and specifies a mammal's role in the food chain. The *herbivore*, the feeding group that consumes plant material exclusively, is the most numerous and widespread. Many variations of digestive and feeding mechanisms have evolved among the herbivores, which are represented in many mammalian orders. A second feeding type is the *carnivore*, or meat eater. Carnivore digestive tracts are usually simple because meat eaters consume other organisms which contain most of the dietary essentials in the required orders of magnitude. Specialization in this feeding group is usually limited to variations in the mode of acquiring food and to minor variations in the digestive system based upon the relative amounts of fat and protein acquired from the organisms consumed.

The *omnivore* is the feeding group with the greatest variety of dietary sources, since mammals of this group consume both animal and plant material. Because of their ability to survive on both kinds of food, omnivores are usually *opportunistic* in their feeding habits. The digestive tract of most of these species conforms with that of the true carnivores: few specializations for consumption of plant materials have evolved.

There are certain groups of mammals which have narrowly specialized feeding habits. The vampire bats and such insectivores as the spiny anteater consume a diet restricted to a specific food source. Vampire bats, found predominately in Mexico and South America, bite into the backs of unprotected animals like horses and cattle and lap up the blood from the wound. The spiny anteater feeds exclusively on ants and other small insects even though many plant and animal food types are readily available in its habitat. Another feeding group is represented by the baleen whale, which filters crustaceans from ocean water as its sole food source.

Herbivores

Most herbivores consume large quantities of *cellulose,* which forms the basic and most abundant carbohydrate in their diet. Mammals are not, however, equipped to digest cellulose and have evolved some fairly elaborate relationships with symbiotic microorganisms capable of enzymatically breaking the β-1,6-linkage of the consecutive glucose units which constitute the cellulose molecule.

Ruminants Microorganisms in the ruminant digestive tract are maintained in a specialized compartment. The *ruminants* possess a large stomach pouch, or *rumen,* which provides an ideal environment for cultures of bacteria and protozoa, which digest the huge amounts of ingested cellulose (see Figure 12–1). Domesticated cattle usually harbor at least 30 species of microorganisms capable of breaking down cellulose and fixing nitrogen, though that number varies. *Nitrogen fixation*

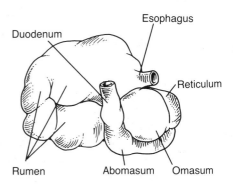

FIGURE 12–1
Bovine stomach viewed from the right side

by ruminant microorganisms is essential because the plant material consumed by ruminants is low in protein and essential amino acids. Thus, through the use of its own *microflora,* the ruminant makes available a relatively insoluble carbohydrate, cellulose, and also produces its own source of amino acids. The nitrogen utilized in the recycling process is obtained from *urea,* which is present in the saliva of ruminants.

The digestive process in ruminants originates with *mastication* of plant materials, which mix with saliva in the mouth. Next, the ruminant swallows a portion of the ingested material, called a *bolus,* which passes through the esophagus into the rumen. When feeding has ceased, the ruminant usually relaxes and proceeds to rechew the plant material previously consumed. It does this by reforming the ingesta into boluses in the reticulum and eructating them one at a time into the mouth for further chewing. By repeatedly chewing the *cud,* or eructated boluses, ruminants are able to increase the available surface area of the ingesta for more effective enzyme action.

In the rumen, microbial *glycosidases* break down cellulose to form glucose. The sugar thus formed is utilized by the microflora in an anaerobic state to produce volatile fatty acids such as *acetic, propionic, butyric,* and *valeric acids.* Acetic acid seems to be the most abundant. The fatty acids thus formed become the primary carbon source for ruminant metabolism. Because of the microorganisms, very little hexose remains for absorption by the ruminant. Consequently, blood sugar levels in these animals seldom rise above 50 mg percent (i.e., 50 mg/100 ml plasma), as opposed to approximately 100 mg percent in most nonruminant mammals.

The ruminants also benefit from the symbiotic microorganisms through their action on ingested proteins. The microorganisms produce *proteolytic enzymes,* which convert proteins to constituent amino acids that can be absorbed in the small intestine of the ruminant. Most of the protein, however, is incorporated into the microorganisms, which later enter further portions of the digestive tract and are digested by proteolytic enzymes secreted by the host. The recycling process of microorganisms has an additional advantage in that ruminants can ingest protein which has poor biological value (i.e., does not consist of an adequate ratio of various amino acids to form mammalian protein) with few ill effects. The ingested protein, though not readily utilizable by the ruminant, can be subsequently converted to bacterial protein, which is of high biological value to the ruminant.

Another advantageous characteristic of the ruminants' symbiotic relationship with the microorganisms is that the mammals are able to recycle *urea nitrogen.* With a low nitrogen or protein diet, urine contains almost no nitrogen. The urea produced in the liver is carried by the bloodstream to the salivary glands, where it is released into the digestive tract. In the rumen the urea is broken down by the microorganisms, which utilize urea nitrogen to aminate alpha keto acids derived from the carbohydrates ingested by the host. In this way ruminant microorganisms are able to supply the necessary amino acids for the diet of the host. This process frees the ruminant from the external protein source and allows adult animals to survive on a high carbohydrate diet.

When the ingesta have been converted to a uniform mass of well-masticated material, they pass into the *omasum* and finally to the *abomasum,* or *true stomach,* of the ruminant. In the abomasum, gastric acids kill the microorganisms, which are sensitive to low pH. In the rumen, microorganisms flourish because the pH is held near neutrality through bicarbonate from the saliva. Most of the material from the abomasum is further digested by enzyme action in the *duodenum.* Most absorption of digested products occurs in the small intestine.

Cecants Several domesticated herbivores which lack a rumen are still able to profit from the fermentation of ingesta by microorganisms. These mammals usually have a large fermentation pouch, called a *cecum,* attached to the colon. The cecum harbors a variety of bacteria as well as protozoans, which are capable of breaking down cellulose and converting the resultant sugars to short-chain fatty acids. Although this process is very similar to rumination, the cecants are at a disadvantage because fermentation follows rather than precedes the small intestine, where most absorption usually occurs. This problem is solved in the rabbit, which has adopted the process of *coprophagy,* or eating its own feces directly out of the anus. This allows materials produced from microbial fermentations to enter the small intestine where they can be absorbed. But not all of the pellets produced by the rabbit are formed in the cecum. Pellets from the cecum are beneficial because of their high fatty acid and protein content; thus, the rabbit must differentiate between pellets formed in the cecum and those formed in the large intestine. It does so by producing and eating cecal pellets during the night. The typical feces produced in the large intestine during the day are not eaten. The horse, another typical cecant, employs coprophagy only to a limited extent and derives much less benefit from the cecum than would otherwise be possible.

Ruminants and cecants compared Although the rumen provides many nutritional benefits and many water-soluble vitamins, it reduces the mobility of some mammals because of its enormous size. In cattle the rumen contents occupy about 15 percent of total body weight. The human stomach contents, for example, may occupy only as much as 2.5 percent of body weight. In addition, rumen material in cattle is not evacuated rapidly and may be retained for as long as five days. In fact, experiments in which cattle were fed sporadically on alternate days have shown that steady intake of food is not essential in these animals.

Because of the large volume of saliva which must be secreted by ruminants, most are not usually able to go for long periods without water. The camel, by contrast, is a ruminant which can survive for some eight days without consuming water. The stomach of camels possesses numerous *water cells* or *pouches* which are filled with water and released as needed into the stomach. These pouches are apparently the source of rumors about water storage in camels. It appears, though, that the water in the stomach pouches is not obtained externally but is secreted by the mucosal lining as a means of maintaining adequate digestive supplies. In this sense, water in the pouches is not unneeded water stored for later use.

There are several very distinct advantages bestowed by herbivores' rumen. Rechewing of the food and nitrogen recycling have been previously mentioned. A third advantage is that fermentation occurs prior to the passage of the food into the small intestine. Cecants, on the other hand, realize these advantages to a lesser degree unless they have developed the coprophagic habit. Cecants do not profit in an appreciable way from recycling nitrogen through saliva, as is the case in ruminants, though volatile fatty acids and water-soluble vitamins are absorbed from the colon of the cecant animals. On the other hand, mobility is usually greater in cecants than in ruminants, primarily because a smaller volume of the body is being occupied by the digestive tract. As a result of the reduced size of storage volume in the cecum, these animals must eat more or less continually to maintain a normal nutritive state.

Other types of herbivores The existence of a rumen or rumenlike structure is by no means limited to domesticated bovines. A rumenlike structure has evolved in the marsupials, which consume plant material (see Figure 12–2). An enlarged stomach pouch is present in the platypus (see Figure 12–3). The platypus's pouch is believed to be used for food storage and does not represent a fermentation pouch similar to the rumen.

Several species of the subclass Eutheria (the placental mammals) have modified storage pouches which appear similar to the rumen in artiodactyls. The whales and hippopotomi have a stomach divided into several compartments. In humans the stomach is sometimes abnormally divided into *cardiac* and *pyloric* portions to form an hourglass

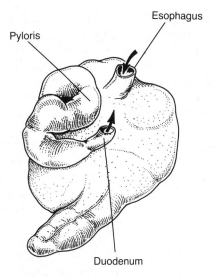

FIGURE 12–2
The stomach of the sloth (*Bradypus tridactylus*). Its numerous diverticula are reminiscent of the rumen.

shape. In the vampire bat *(Desmodus)* the pyloric portion of the stomach forms an elongated pouch for blood storage.

Almost all mammals have an extension of the large intestine which can be called a cecum. In the human the cecum is rarely

over a couple of inches long, though most have a *vermiform appendix* which forms in place of the true cecum (see Figure 12–4). The cecum is small or reduced in size in most carnivores. Some edentates (e.g., sloths, anteaters) have two cecae which are reduced in size. Likewise, a number of species have enlarged cecae even though they are not considered to be cecants. In most marsupials and rodents the cecum is enlarged and may exceed the length of the entire body.

Carnivores

Most of the mammals which exhibit carnivorous feeding habits belong to the order Carnivora. But the name of the order in this case can be quite misleading. Many species in this order are omnivorous and can in no way be described as strict carnivores. Members of the order Carnivora that are actually omnivorous include the genus *Ursula* (bears) and the genus *Canis* (dogs, wolves, and coyotes). A number of species belonging to other orders are indeed strict carnivores. Examples of these are shrews (order Insectivora), dolphins and certain whales (order Cetacea), and a number of marsupial species (subclass Metatheria). In fact, certain human popula-

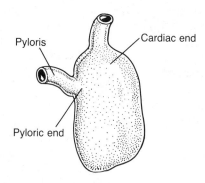

FIGURE 12–3
Platypus stomach. Although a large storage capacity is present, microbial fermentation is not believed to occur.

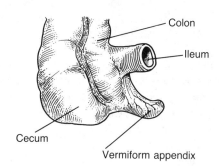

FIGURE 12–4
Human appendix and almost nonexistent cecum

tions, such as the Masais of Africa and the Eskimos of the Arctic, were at one time restricted to a pure meat or meat-product diet before the intrusion of "civilization."

Because a pure meat or carnivorous diet contains all of the essentials for survival in approximately the correct proportions, the *alimentary tract* of carnivores is correspondingly simple. The major digestive modifications seen in carnivores are the ability to secrete copious volumes of bile salts for fat emulsification and the absence of many of the enzymes necessary to digest simple carbohydrates. For instance, the secretion of *ptyalin*, an amylase found in the saliva, is reduced in these species, and the pH of the saliva is less basic than that of herbivores, thus enhancing ptyalin activity. This is particularly true when the carnivores are compared to the ruminants, since the latter must produce copious amounts of bicarbonate in saliva. The bicarbonate is necessary to maintain a high pH for sustained activity of salivary amylase and for survival of symbiotic microflora.

The ability of carnivores to hydrolyze the *peptide bond* is exceptional. They produce larger quantities of *proteases* and have a great capacity for deamination (removal of amino acids) in the liver. As a result of their protein intake, carnivores must produce large volumes of urea and for that reason do not endure dehydration well. Clearance of urea through the kidneys results in large quantities of water being lost in the urine.

It is worthy of mention that at one time the northernmost Eskimo populations did not have an obvious source of vitamin C, which is thought essential to human survival. Some authors have claimed that vitamin C can be obtained by consuming the intestines of herbivores, which are rich in this substance. This is probably a false assumption, though the consumption of internal organs was no doubt common under certain circumstances. Modern Eskimos at Point Barrow and Wainwright, Alaska, store large quantities of whale and caribou in permafrost cellars. In no case does their storage include intestines, and it seems that recipes of delicacies inherent in their bygone culture do not allude to the preparation of tripe for human consumption. Along these lines, the arctic explorer V. Stefansson once consumed a pure meat diet for one year without ill effects, which demonstrates the lack of importance of vegetable sources of vitamin C to humans.

Omnivores

The digestive system of most omnivores is very similar to that of carnivores, in that it consists of a simple stomach and intestines with no complicated *diverticula* (pockets) for microbial fermentation. In fact, many omnivores, such as bears and dogs, belonging to the order Carnivora seem to have acquired the omnivorous trait secondarily.

The opportunistic behavior of omnivores would necessitate a fairly simple digestive system. For these animals to evolve elaborate ruminant or cecal systems would be prohibitive, since they are not restricted to a plant diet. Some omnivores, such as domesticated pigs, have evolved bacterial fermentation mechanisms to a limited extent. In fact, some fermentation in the large intestine is common to almost all omnivores. There seems to be little congruence among the digestive tracts of different omnivores. Most have well-developed gall bladders and can produce large amounts of bile salts for lipid digestion. But some omnivores, such as the Norway rat, lack a gall bladder altogether and seem to have a limited ability to digest fats.

DIGESTION

Fundamental elements of food are universally similar in mammals. Major differences lie only in the methods of acquiring and consuming food, which do not constitute differences in the elements necessary for growth or existence of mammals. Three substances are universal and provide most of the fuel utilized in mammalian metabolism. The *carbohydrates* are used as energy sources except for their role in the formation of certain glycoproteins. The *lipids* function primarily as energy sources but also have other functions, such as insulation, steroid hormone synthesis, and cell membrane constitution. The *proteins* provide enzymes and structural elements and function as a significant energy source only when the quantities of carbohydrates and lipids are insufficient to meet a mammal's energy requirements. All of these materials must be *masticated,* or broken down into smaller particles by the teeth, and *digested,* or converted to soluble compounds by enzyme action. Digested material must be absorbed and transferred to cells where *internal* (or *intermediary*) *metabolism* converts them into usable energy sources, structural parts of the cell, or enzymes and hormones that can be used in metabolism.

External digestion in the mammal occurs in a specific tract designed for hydrolysis and absorption of food and in the presence of enzymes which are secreted into the tract. By contrast, *internal digestion* occurs in cellular inclusions and is so named because the raw materials are taken directly into the cell, where digestion as well as utilization occurs. External digestion is an essential mechanism.

In this system, particulate food passes into the *digestive tract* in fairly large pieces, to be digested gradually over a considerable period of time. This leaves the animal free to perform other functions.

The complex digestive tract of mammals is divided into concise units where food may be treated in a specific manner. For example, fluid may be basic in one portion, acidic in another, and neutral in a third area. Enzymes or other substances used in the digestive process are secreted into specific units of the digestive system where pH and other environmental conditions are ideal. For example, pancreatic secretions pass into the small intestine, where pH is maintained near the optimum for pancreatic and other enzymes which require a basic medium. Similarly, enzymes functional in the stomach have their maximum effect in an acidic medium. Even in ruminants, whose initial digestion is performed by symbiotic microorganisms, the pH of the *anterior chamber* of the stomach is maintained at a level easily tolerated by the exoenzymes produced by the microorganisms. The individual chambers or units of the digestive tract, such as the stomach and small intestine, are isolated by *sphincter valves,* which aid in controlling the movement of ingesta. In this way, specific environments can be maintained. Thus, the entire digestive tract does not function as a single unit.

The overall function and coordination of specific parts of the digestive system are monitored and controlled by the autonomic nervous system and a system of hormones which are produced by the digestive tract, or *gastrointestinal (GI) tract.* The gastrointestinal hormones are usually produced by the intestinal lining and transmitted through the bloodstream, but they may have a direct and exclusive effect on another part of the digestive system. The digestive tract also contains numerous glands and secretory cells for the production of enzymes and emollients. Several glands are also coordinated with the digestive tract so that additional enzymes may be secreted to aid in the digestive process. Secretory cells are part of the mucosa of the intestines and the internal lining of the stomach. All of the enzymes are protein in nature and contain amino acid sequences which make them distinct. Therefore, differentiation has led to the distribution of cell types capable of producing different enzymes according to the intestinal chamber in which they are located.

Gastrointestinal tracts have increased surface areas as a result of the development of *villi* and diverticula. Portions of the digestive tract whose primary function is absorption have the greatest surface area. The number of villi and *microvilli*, as well as the blood and lymph vessels present in the small intestine, is astounding when compared to other parts of the digestive tract.

Parts of the Digestive System

The digestive process involves a series of enzymatic reactions which are segregated into separate compartments where specific chemical environments are maintained. Individual compartments are: the *mouth* and *pharynx*, which together constitute the *oral cavity;* the *stomach* (in the case of polygastric animals there may be several additional stomach compartments); the *small intestine;* the cecum; the *large intestine*; and the *rectum*. The enzymes involved in digestion are usually named for the substrate upon which they act and for the specific type of reaction carried out. For instance, enzymes involved in the breakdown of proteins are called *proteases*, those which lyse sugars are referred to as *amylases*, and those which break down lipids are called *lipases*. The release of the enzymes and the fluids which carry them is controlled by means of the autonomic nervous system and various intestinal hormones.

Structure of the digestive tract The structure found among digestive tracts of different species of domesticated mammals varies considerably and reflects the nature of the food consumed. Such specialization is reflected not only in the compartmentalization of the units of the digestive system but also in the order and arrangement of the teeth. For instance, the carnivores possess large *canines* frequently absent in herbivores. The herbivores, on the other hand, are usually endowed with well-developed *incisors* for cropping vegetation and flattened *molars* for crushing plant material. The molars of carnivores are more suited for shearing or slicing meat of the prey, which is less easily crushed and pulverized than the plant material taken in by herbivores.

The mouth and pharynx The oral cavity produces saliva from the *parotid* and *sublingual salivary glands* that is released as the result of parasympathetic action directly upon the salivary glands. As mentioned earlier, saliva contains an alpha amylase called ptyalin. Ptyalin splits starch and glycogen to form *dextrins* (polysaccharides of intermediate chain lengths) and *maltose* (a disaccharide). The enzyme hydrolyzes internal α-*1,4-glucoside* bonds and is therefore referred to as an *endoamylase*. Ptyalin functions in a neutral-to-basic medium and is quickly denatured by most mammals when it reaches the stomach. In monogastric animals, ptyalin functions only for a few seconds to a few minutes and is therefore not a very effective enzyme. In the case of ruminants, in which large volumes of a saliva that contains bicarbonate as a buffer are carried to the stomach, ptyalin acts over a longer period of time. In cattle, as much as 160 liters of saliva may be secreted each day.

The stomach When ingesta reach the stomach, they are subjected in most cases to a highly acidic medium. *Hydrochloric acid* is provided by the *parietal cells*, which form part of the stomach lining. A proteolytic enzyme called *pepsin* is secreted by the *chief cells*, which are also part of the stomach epithelium. Pepsin is produced by the abomasum of ruminants. Pepsin is an *endopeptidase*, which splits proteins into shorter peptides. Specifically, the endopeptidase hydrolyses nonterminal peptide bonds adjacent to aromatic or dicarboxylic amino acids. Another proteolytic enzyme, *rennin*, whose action is similar to that of pepsin, is present in juvenile mammals and is usually not secreted in the adult. Its function is presumably directed toward the hydrolysis of milk proteins.

The small intestine By the time the ingesta leave the stomach, they are for the most part in a semiliquid form. As they enter the duodenum of the small intestine the ingesta are exposed to a basic medium, part of which is due to bicarbonate from the pancreatic juices. The pancreatic secretions contain enzymes which function maximally in a neutral-to-basic medium. Several enzymes are also produced by the *intestinal mucosa*, or inner lining of the intestine. In some cases these enzymes duplicate the function of the pancreatic enzymes. Most digestion and absorption occurs in the small intestine in monogastric mammals.

The principal lipids entering the small intestine of monogastric mammals are *triglycerides*. Triglycerides are converted to fatty acids, diglycerides, monoglycerides, and glycerol by lipase. Lipids present a special problem, since they are not water soluble and therefore not readily accessible to the water-soluble enzymes present in the digestive tract. In order to become available to lipases, lipids must be *emulsified*. Emulsification is brought about by *bile* released from the *gallbladder*. Bile contains various pigments as well as bile salts, which are primarily salts of cholesterol. Bile salts act as a soap and therefore have water-soluble and water-insoluble portions. These portions of the bile salt molecule are sometimes referred to as *hydrophilic* and *hydrophobic*, respectively. When lipids are present in the gut, bile salts emulsify them by forming a water-lipid *interphase* with the hydrophobic portion of the salt dissolved in lipid and the hydrophilic portion dissolved in the surrounding aquatic medium. This emulsification allows contact between the lipase and the lipid and reduces the larger lipid droplets to smaller sized droplets called *micelles*. The reduction in size of ingested lipids to small droplets increases the total surface area of the lipids and further increases the rate of enzyme hydrolysis. Lipases are produced by the gastric mucosa as well as the intestinal mucosa and pancreas in most mammals. But since bile is only present in the small intestine, the function of gastric lipase is considered negligible.

A series of enzymes reduces the carbohydrates in the intestine to simple sugars which can be taken up by the circulation in the intestinal mucosa. Polysaccharides such as glycogen and starch are broken down by α-*amylase*, which hydrolyzes nonterminal α-*1,4-glucoside* bonds. The net result is the formation of disaccharides and some small polysaccharides. Additional amylases such as α-*glucosidase*, a disaccharidase, hydrolze α-D-*glucosides* such as maltose and sucrose to simple sugars. The α-*1,6-glucosidic* bonds which are present in dextrins, derived from amylopectin moieties of starch and glycogen, are cleaved by *oligo-1,6-glucosidases* into smaller subunits (glucose and a smaller polysaccharide). Such α-D-*galactosides* as lactose are cleaved by α-*galactosidase* to form galactose and glucose. The most common sugar consumed by humans is *sucrose*, which is hydrolyzed by *sucrase* to form *fructose* and glucose. A third disaccharide, *maltose*, is hydrolyzed to form two molecules of glucose.

Proteins which enter the small intestine are hydrolyzed to form amino acids, which can be taken into the bloodstream. In infants, some proteins are absorbed intact, but this does not occur in the adult mammal under normal circumstances. In fact, a possible function of the digestive process is the reduction of complex proteins that might be allergenic to smaller subunits not recognized as antigens by the immune system. Several of the peptidases hydrolyze large proteins to form smaller peptides. *Trypsin* hydrolyzes nonterminal peptide bonds involving carboxyl groups of basic amino acids to form smaller peptides. As a result of trypsin's action on nonterminal amino acids (amino acids within the polypeptide chain), trypsin is said to be an endopeptidase (see Figure 12–5). Another endopeptidase, *chymotrypsin*, splits proteins into smaller polypeptides by hydrolyzing the peptide bonds adjacent to aromatic amino acids.

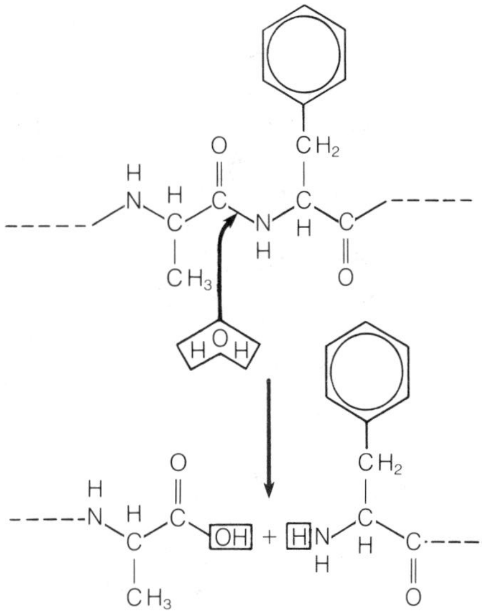

Several peptidases are termed *exopeptidases* because they hydrolyze peptide bonds adjacent to terminal amino acids. Exopeptidases are usually specific for a particular ter-

FIGURE 12–5
Hydrolysis of peptide bond by endopeptidase. Note that hydrolysis occurs not at terminal amino acids but at adjacent aromatic amino acids.

minal radical (i.e., a carboxyl group or an amino group). *Carboxypeptidases A* and *B*, examples of this type of peptidase, act upon the carboxyl terminal end of the peptide chain to form free amino acids and a polypeptide. Several exopeptidases called *aminopeptidases* hydrolyze peptide bonds at the amino terminal end of the peptide chain. Aminopeptidases split polypeptides into free amino acids and polypeptides. Several peptidases are present which hydrolyze specific dipeptides to form free amino acids. In the adult, all digestible polypeptides must ultimately be broken down into smaller units and finally into individual amino acids. As stated earlier, only amino acids can be utilized in the adult under normal conditions. Therefore, the ultimate product of protein digestion must be the formation of free amino acids from ingested polypeptides.

In addition to the groups of enzymes mentioned (i.e., lipases, amylases, and proteases), enzymes are also present which hydrolyze nucleic acids to form nucleotides. Both *ribonucleases* and *deoxyribonucleases* are present in the small intestine.

An unusual enzyme is present in insectivorous bats which allows them to digest chitin which forms the exoskeleton of their prey. *Chitin* is a polymer of *β-1,4-glucose* with an acetylamine group attached to the number-two carbon of each glucose subunit. The enzyme *chitinase* hydrolyzes chitin to form *N-acetyl-D-glucosamine* residues which can be absorbed from the intestinal lumen. This is the only instance in the class Mammalia in which the enzyme is known to occur.

The large intestine The large intestine in mammals extends from the distal end of the small intestine to the rectum and is one of the major sources of several water-soluble vitamins. It is also utilized as an organ of water balance and serves as a reservoir for the material not absorbed in the small intestine. In the latter function, it provides a delay period for final absorption of water and vitamins. The final product of the large intestine is the *feces*, which are retained in the rectum until defecated.

In most mammals the cecum provides a diverticulum to the large intestine. In such species as the human that do not profit extensively from fermentation, the cecum is insignificant in size as well as function. In other noncecant mammals, such as the Norway rat, the cecum is quite long and extensive even though these animals do not rely on cecal fermentation as a major source of nutrients. Microbial fermentation in the large intestine, similar to that of the cecum, is probably a universal condition in mammals.

It has been reported in dogs, rats, and pigs as a beneficial phenomenon. The production of vitamin B_{12} is the result of beneficial intestinal fermentation in humans. Intestinal fermentation is anaerobic, and its gaseous product is primarily *methane*. Methane is a major by-product of ruminant fermentation as well.

Absorption of Digested Materials

Most absorption of digested materials in mammals occurs in the small intestine. But the large intestine also plays a major role in substrate absorption. For example, volatile fatty acids and certain water-soluble vitamins are absorbed through mucosa of the large intestine. This is particularly true of cecants, but has been noted in other mammals as well. The role of the large intestine in vitamin-K and vitamin-B_{12} production and absorption is of critical importance. The inner lining of the intestinal wall in both the small and large intestines, called the *mucosa*, is composed of one cell layer of epithelial tissue. The cells of the mucosa are constantly being sloughed off and replaced by new cells. The inner surface of the small intestine is folded and possesses fingerlike projections on the surface of the folds called *villi* (see Figure 12–6). The surface area of the intestinal mucosa is tremendous when compared to the area of the inner surface of a cylinder of like dimensions. In addition to the villi, *microvilli* project from the epithelial cells of the intestine, giving the absorptive area of the intestinal mucosa an immense proportion. The villi are adequately supplied with blood and lymph vessels to aid in the removal of absorbed materials. Vessels and nerves inside the villi compose part of the *submucosa*.

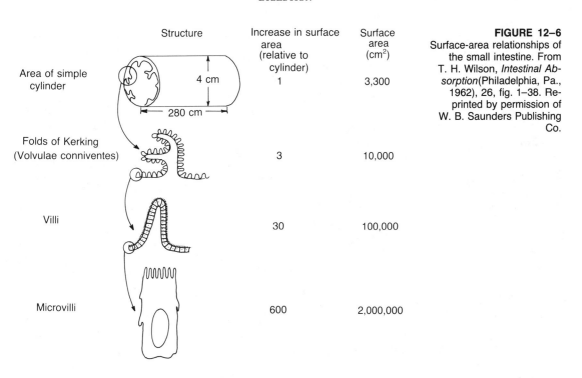

Structure	Increase in surface area (relative to cylinder)	Surface area (cm²)
Area of simple cylinder	1	3,300
Folds of Kerking (Volvulae conniventes)	3	10,000
Villi	30	100,000
Microvilli	600	2,000,000

FIGURE 12–6
Surface-area relationships of the small intestine. From T. H. Wilson, *Intestinal Absorption* (Philadelphia, Pa., 1962), 26, fig. 1–38. Reprinted by permission of W. B. Saunders Publishing Co.

Carbohydrate absorption The carbohydrates absorbed in the mammalian intestine are primarily simple sugars. But in some cases disaccharides are absorbed by the epithelial cells, with further digestion occurring internally. Evidence indicates that all sugars are associated with carrier molecules when absorbed, and therefore absorption is not carried out by simple diffusion. The hypothesis that absorption is an active process is enforced by the action of *ouabain*, which poisons the active transport of sodium ion in the gut and also inhibits sugar absorption. It appears that the absorption of sugars is in some way dependent upon the active transport of sodium and is not an active process per se but rather a type of carrier-mediated transport facilitated by the transport of sodium.

Protein absorption Proteins which enter the digestive tract are usually large in terms of numbers of amino acids and frequently have a very complex tertiary and perhaps quaternary structure. If polymers of this type were to enter the bloodstream, they would in many cases induce massive immune responses which could result in death of the animal. But infants are able to take in large proteins without first digesting them, since the *colostrum* (first milk from the mother) is heavily endowed with antibodies, which are absorbed intact through the intestinal mucosa. The mother is thus able to impart immunity to the newborn which could not have been present at birth. In most species the inability to obtain colostrum at birth leads to immunodeficiencies and frequently results in contraction of diseases that may result in early death. In the human, babies unable to obtain colostrum are sometimes later found to be hypersensitive to environmentally contracted diseases. When cases of this type have been followed to adulthood, certain hypersensitivity diseases, such as asthma, hay fever, and food allergies, have been found to be more common in the colostrum-deprived individuals than in control groups. The absorption of larger proteins in infants seems to result from an ability to take in large molecules by the process of pinocytosis. This ability to utilize pinocytosis for absorption in the intestine is usually lost within a few months after birth.

The adult mammal can absorb dipeptides as well as single amino acids. But in the same manner as previously described for disaccharides, dipeptides are hydrolyzed in the mucosal cells. Therefore, only amino acids enter the bloodstream in the normal condition.

Certain amino acids diffuse passively through the intestinal wall. This seems to be the case for such acidic amino acids as *glutamic* and *aspartic acid*. The other amino acids appear to be absorbed by means of active transport, though evidence indicates that each amino acid does not have a distinct transport system. The neutral amino acids are transported by one enzyme system and the basic amino acids are transported by another.

Lipid absorption Considerable interest has arisen over the years concerning lipid absorption and its variation among different species and individuals within a species. Most lipids entering the digestive tracts of carnivores are *triglycerides* (neutral fats). Triglycerides are broken down to free fatty acids and glycerol as a result of enzyme hydrolysis in the small intestine. Fat absorption occurs

in sections of the small intestine called the *duodenum* and *jejunum*. Bile salts are recycled by being absorbed through the mucosa of the jejunum. Fatty acids which contain ten or more carbons are used to resynthesize triglycerides inside mucosal cells and are transported as triglycerides through the lacteals of the lymphatic system into the bloodstream. Short-to-medium-chain fatty acids are transported through the portal system of the liver.

Lipids entering the digestive tract of herbivores are usually oils (e.g., cottonseed oil, linseed oil, and sunflower seed oil) and are composed of fatty acids rather than glycerol salts of fatty acids. Such oils are not typical: most oils are *unsaturated* or *polyunsaturated* and are liquid at room temperature. Carnivores and other mammals with gallbladders have the ability to unload large quantities of bile after consuming a meal rich in fat and thus facilitate lipid absorption by the formation of lipid-bile emulsions. Herbivorous monogastric mammals usually lack a gallbladder but are still able to absorb oils, apparently without the formation of bile emulsions. Mammals which lack gallbladders include certain rodents, whales, hyraxes, some artiodactyls, and all perissodactyls. Fat or oil consumed by ruminants almost never reaches the intestine in the form in which it is ingested. Oils contained in the diet of ruminants are metabolized by the intestinal microflora and are converted to other products. In most cases, the oils are hydrogenated to form saturated fatty acids.

Among the domesticated species, a large variation in quantity of *volatile fatty acids* in the gastrointestinal tract has been noted (see Figure 12–7). In such ruminants as the cow, sheep, and deer, volatile fatty acid concentrations are high in the anterior portion of the gastrointestinal tract; in other species, they

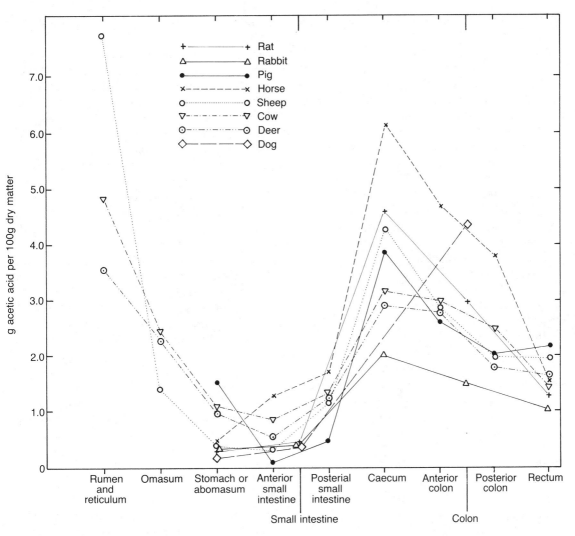

FIGURE 12–7
Average concentrations of volatile fatty acids in specific portions of the gastrointestinal tract in several mammalian species. From Andrew T. Phillipson, "Ruminant Digestion," in *Duke's Physiology of Domestic Animals, Ninth Edition*, edited by Melvin J. Swenson, pages 250–286. Copyright © 1977 by Cornell University. Used by permission of the publisher, Cornell University Press.

are fairly low. Volatile fatty acids fall to a low level in the anterior small intestine of all domesticated species studied and subsequently rise in the posterior regions of the gut. The content of volatile substances is noticeably higher in the posterior gut of those species which maintain a viable cecum for bacterial fermentation.

The *protected fats* that form part of the diet of cattle have evoked considerable interest among cardiologists and nutritionists in view of the suspected role of saturated fatty acids in coronary diseases. Protected fats are fats that have been encapsulated in formaldehyde-treated *casein*, which cannot be hydrogenated by microorganisms of the rumen. When fed to cattle they pass into the abomasum, where the acid conditions permit the capsule to be hydrolyzed. The fatty acids thus released can then be absorbed in the small intestine and carried to depot sites in the body. By feeding encapsulated polyunsaturated fats such as linseed oil or corn oil, the proportion of unsaturated fat in milk can be changed from a normal level of 2 to 3 percent to 20 to 30 percent in a matter of a few days. This change is beneficial because it provides a technique for producing milk that contains unsaturated fats rather than saturated ones. Since depot fat is not static but has a steady rate of turnover in the adipose cells, an increase in unsaturated lipids in meat products also occurs when beef animals are fed protected fats. Another advantage of dietary treatment of oils in this way is that much more fat than normal can be included in the diet, which allows beef animals to make substantial weight gains.

The Role of the Liver in Digestion

The primary functions of the liver are associated with its role in digestion. These functions and the liver's relationship to the circulatory system make it virtually impossible to find an organ or organ system which is not dependent upon the liver in some fashion. With the exception of long-chain fatty acids, all substances absorbed in the intestine are carried to the liver by means of the hepatic portal system.

The liver in carbohydrate metabolism
Carbohydrates are transported to the liver from the intestine as simple sugars. Most of these sugars are in the form of glucose, which can readily be converted to glycogen in the liver, where glycogen is stored. Glucose is also stored in other tissues as glycogen, the greatest amount being stored in muscle. The liver is also capable of converting glucose to fatty acids, which can then be converted to triglycerides and carried by the blood to other tissues. Blood levels of glucose are maintained at a fairly constant level through the interaction of the liver and the hormones produced by the pancreas. When plasma glucose levels fall below the homeostatic level (about 100 mg percent in most species), the hormone glucagon is released, which induces *glycogenolysis* (see Figure 12–8). Above normal plasma levels of glucose stimulate insulin release, which is followed by *glycogenesis* in the liver (see Figure 12–8). Insulin also enhances glucose absorption by other tissues. Whenever glycogen levels are depleted, the liver is able to resynthesize glucose and intermediate compounds in its synthetic pathway from alpha keto acids. This process, called *gluconeogenesis*, results in *de novo* production of carbohydrates.

The liver in protein utilization The liver is responsible for the synthesis of approximately 85 percent of the plasma proteins. The principal protein product found in the blood is the *albumin fraction*. Most substances, such as free fatty acids, amino acids, and various hormones, are loosely bound to the plasma albumins. In this way most substances transported in the blood are loosely bound to the protein fraction and are not unencumbered as are unbound molecules in true solution. The liver also produces specific clotting factors which are carried in the pro-

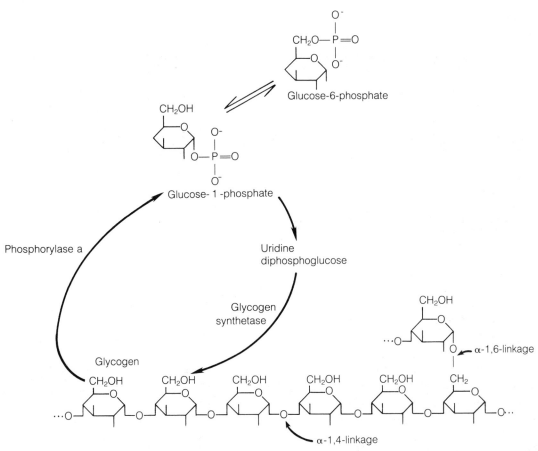

FIGURE 12–8
Glycogenolysis and glycogenesis. These processes occur in both liver and muscle tissue.

tein fraction of the blood. Another protein synthesized by the liver, *angiotensinogen,* is essential to the formation of angiotensin when blood pressure decreases. The remainder of the plasma proteins is produced from white blood cells (plasma cells) and form the gamma-globulin fraction of blood.

The liver must also deaminate amino acids from digested proteins to form ketone bodies during gluconeogenesis. This process along with deamination of amino acids in the gut by the intestinal microflora results in the production of *ammonia,* which is highly toxic to mammalian tissue. The liver is responsible for the subsequent production from free ammonia of *urea,* which can be voided from the body through the kidneys and skin.

In addition to deamination, the *nonessential* amino acids are synthesized in the liver from appropriate keto acids (see Figure 12–9). The *essential* amino acids are those which cannot be resynthesized and therefore must

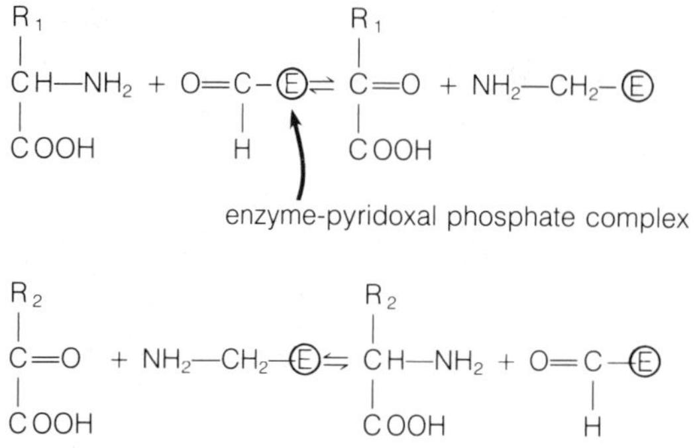

FIGURE 12–9
Transamination of amino acids to form ketone bodies and amination of ketone bodies to form amino acids are reciprocal processes requiring pyridoxal phosphate

be obtained from the diet. Mammalian species differ remarkably in their abilities to synthesize specific amino acids and as a result also differ markedly in the specific amino acids essential in the diet.

Storage functions of the liver The liver is able to break down fatty acids to form *acetyl CoA* and, subsequently, *acetoacetic acid*. It also synthesizes glucose intermediates from fatty acids, which constitutes a mechanism for gluconeogenesis. Fat is synthesized from carbohydrate and protein in the liver through the *malonyl-CoA pathway* (see Figure 12–10). Lipids synthesized in the liver are usually not stored there but instead are carried to adipose and muscle tissue for storage. In addition, phospholipids, cholesterol esters, and triglycerides (all synthesized in the liver) form a major part of cell membranes and thus are transferred throughout the body for membrane synthesis. Cholesterol is converted to bile salts in the liver and passed into the gallbladder. Also, cholesterol can be removed from the blood by the liver for the production of bile. This is considered to be one of the excretory functions of the liver.

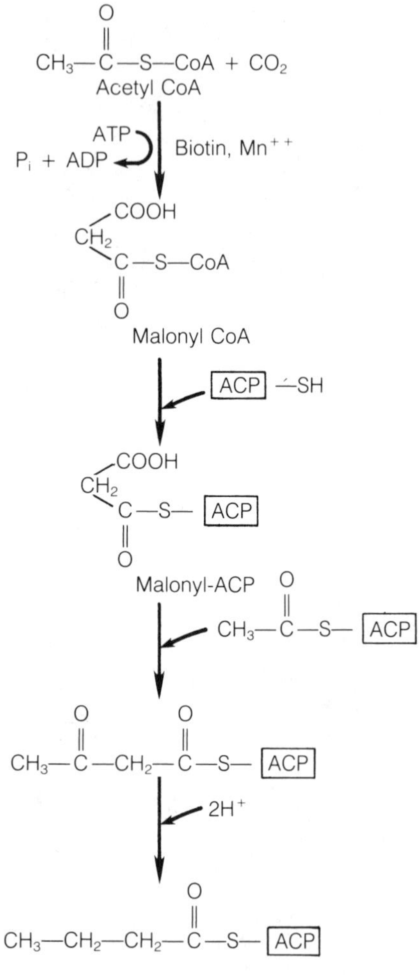

FIGURE 12–10
Fatty acid synthesis through the malonyl-CoA pathway. ACP designates acyl-carrier protein, a protein which is part of the enzyme complex to which acyl residues are attached as fatty acid synthesis proceeds.

The liver is the principal storage organ for vitamins A, D, and B_{12}. Vitamin A is stored in large quantities in the liver and in such Arctic mammals as the polar bear, which take in large amounts of this vitamin in their diet, liver storage of vitamin A takes on an elimination function. In other words, plasma vitamin A in the polar bear might be excessive if liver storage did not occur. The liver content of vitamin A is so high in polar bears that consumption of the liver is believed to be toxic by some Arctic peoples.

Both iron from the intestinal tract and re-cycled iron from hemoglobin is stored in the liver in the form of *ferritin*. In fact, the liver of human males usually stores enough iron by the time the individual reaches adolescence to last throughout life. This is not true of the human female since menstruation results in a regular loss of iron from the body.

The formation and storage of bile. The gall-bladder contains pigments formed from he-moglobin and bile salts along with some cholesterol from the liver. *Bile pigments* are produced from the porphyrin portion of hemoglobin, which is broken down by the liver to release iron and four interconnected pyrol rings. The first compound formed from porphyrin is called *biliverdin*, or *green bile*, and is quickly converted to *bilirubin*, or *red bile*, before storage in the gallbladder (see Figure 12–11).

Liver cells form certain compounds by the reaction of *cholic acid* with *glycine* and to a lesser extent with *taurine* (see Figure 12–12). The cholic acid used in these reactions is an oxidized derivative of *cholesterol*, also produced in the liver. The salts formed in this manner, called *bile salts*, are necessary in the small intestine for fat emulsion.

The bile salts and bile pigments formed in the liver cells are filtered into the *bile canal-culi*, which traverse the liver tissue. Material in the canalculi is passed into the *bile duct*, then into the *right* and *left hepatic ducts*, and finally through the *cystic duct* into the gall-bladder (see Figure 12–13). Between meals the *sphincter of Oddi*, which is located in the

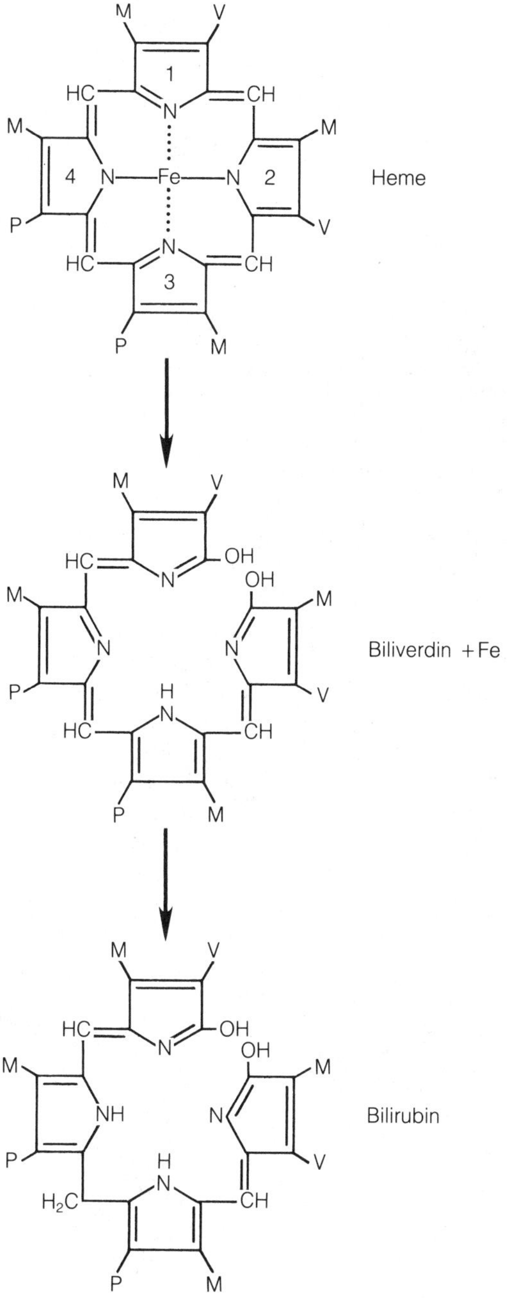

FIGURE 12–11

Formation of biliverdin and bilirubin from the porphyrin (heme) portion of hemoglobin

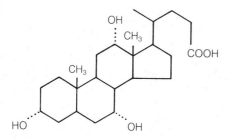

FIGURE 12–12
Cholic acid, one of the principal bile salts formed from cholesterol. Note that the hydrophilic portion is represented by the carboxyl group; the opposite end of the molecule is hydrophobic and therefore insoluble in water.

common bile duct, is closed which allows pressure in the hepatic duct to force the bile fluid, which is quite low in viscosity at this time, into the gallbladder. After entering the gallbladder, water is reabsorbed, leaving an even more viscous mass known as *bile*. Under proper stimulation the gallbladder is evacuated into the small intestine to perform its emulsification function.

Coordination of Activity of the Gastrointestinal Tract

Activity of the esophagus, stomach, and intestines is modified by actions of the autonomic nervous system. The smooth muscle surrounding the GI tract lie in two layers and can cause the intestines to constrict as well as to shorten (see Figure 12–14). Muscular activity within the GI tract usually results from a combination of stimuli from the autonomic nervous system, two internal nerve nets, and several hormones. The internal nerve nets which assist in the integration of these muscles are called *Auerbach's plexus* and *Meissner's plexus*. Meissner's plexus is thought to be primarily sensory. Auerbach's plexus consists of motor neurons which provide stimuli to the smooth muscle layers. In addition to the stimulating activities of nerves and hormones, smooth muscles respond readily to stretch and are never completely stretched

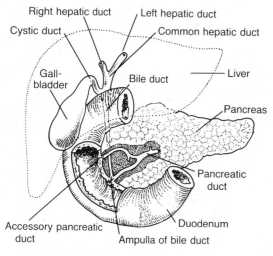

FIGURE 12–13
Relation of gallbladder, liver, and pancreas to the duodenum in the human

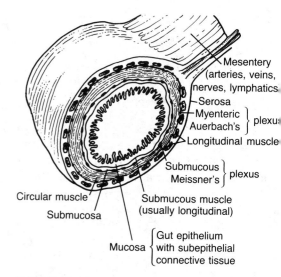

FIGURE 12–14
Cross section of intestine showing muscle layers and nerve nets

or completely relaxed under normal conditions.

The parasympathetic nervous system via the vagus nerve does not directly induce contraction of gastric or intestinal smooth muscle, but such stimulation enhances the rate and intensity of muscle contractions. In addition to its effect on smooth muscle, the parasympathetic nervous system enhances the production of both *gastrin* by the G cells and *hydrochloric acid* by the parietal cells of the gastric mucosa. Hydrochloric acid production by the parietal cells is enhanced in the presence of gastrin. Gastrin, in addition, increases the rate and force of smooth muscle action in the stomach.

When food passes through the pyloric sphincter into the small intestine it alters the pH in the gut as a result of the high acidity of the stomach contents. The resultant pH change triggers the release of the hormone *enterogastrone*, which is absorbed into the bloodstream. At contact with enterogastrone, the gastric smooth muscle relaxes. Enterogastrone thus is an antagonist to gastrin. The increased hydrogen ion content of the duodenum, which ensues when stomach contents enter, enhances two other hormones, *secretin* and *pancreozymogen*. Secretin induces pancreatic flow, whereas pancreozymogen enhances the production of pancreatic enzymes. At one time *choleocystokinin (CCK)* was thought to be produced by the intestinal mucosa when fat entered the small intestine, but it was later found that CCK and pancreozymogen are one and the same. Pancreozymogen (or CCK) thus induces the release of bile into the duodenum by causing two apparently opposite reactions: the relaxation of the sphincter muscle of Oddi and contraction of the smooth muscles of the gallbladder. Along with secretin, it probably induces closure of the pyloric sphincter, thus preventing additional stomach contents from being emptied into the duodenum at that time.

The smooth muscles of the GI tract Several very regular actions in the GI tract can be determined. The best known of the muscular actions of the GI tract is *peristalsis*, which is necessary for the movement of food in a regular fashion during swallowing. *Eructation*, or regurgitation, is the reverse of peristalsis and can be performed at will in ruminants. *Vomiting*, the reverse of the swallowing process, is caused by nausea and thus is generally involuntary in nature.

The amount of striated versus smooth muscle in the esophagus is quite variable among species and greatly affects the ability of mammals to eructate willfully. In sheep and cattle, striated fibers occur along the entire length of the esophagus. This is presumably necessary to allow repeated eructation of the ingesta from the rumen in order to chew the cud. Striated fibers also occur along the entire length of the esophagus in the rat. In the pig and the domesticated dog (and presumably wild species of the genus *Canis*), the circular layer of muscle is striated, except for a short portion near the cardiac end of the stomach, as is the entire length of the longitudinal layer. This allows these species to regurgitate food with a process very much like eructation in ruminants. An example of the utility of this striation can be seen in wolves, which regurgitate chewed and partially digested meat for their pups. In humans and at least some of the marsupials, only about the upper one-fourth to one-third of the length of the esophagus contains striated muscle fibers.

The mechanism for peristalsis involves integration of both Auerbach's and Meissner's plexi. The sensory neurons of Meissner's

TABLE 12–1
Essential vitamins: their function and deficiency symptoms in domesticated mammals

Vitamin	Function	Deficiency Symptoms
A	Visual cycle, formation of rhodopsin	Cattle: Night blindness, convulsions, kidney degeneration, elevated cerebrospinal fluid pressure Horses: Night blindness, keratinization of the cornea Sheep: Night blindness Hogs: Paralysis, incoordination
D	Calcium absorption	Rickets in young animals, calcium deficiency in adults
E (tocopheral)	Antioxidant, unknown relationship involving selenium metabolism	Embryo resorption, testicular germinal epithelium degeneration, muscular dystrophy (skeletal and cardiac muscle)
K	Production of prothrombin necessary for blood coagulation	Hemorrhage
Thiamine	Decarboxylation of alpha keto acids	Severe anorexia, bradycardia, lesions of heart muscle, peripheral nerves and the central nervous system
Riboflavin	Hydrogen transport	Dermatitis, opacity of the lens, atrophy of sebaceous glands and hair follicles, cleft palate
Niacin	Hydrogen transport	Pellagra in humans, dermatitis, diarrhea, delerium, lesions of the mouth and gastrointestinal tract, black tongue in dogs
B_6 (pyridoxine)	Decarboxylation of amino acids, transamination of amino acids, metabolism of tryptophane	Lesions of the skin, anemia, hyperexcitability, convulsions, microscopic lesions of the nervous system

plexus respond to pressure generated by the bolus in the esophagus and transmit the information through the excitatory impulse to the neurons of Auerbach's plexus several millimeters behind the bolus. This induces a *contractile ring* in the circular muscle behind the bolus, thus pushing the food further into the GI tract.

Another action of the GI tract is called *segmentation* (see Figure 12–15). By this process, which seems to be spontaneous, the small

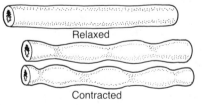

Relaxed

Contracted

FIGURE 12–15
Segmentation in the intestine is caused by alternately contracting rings, which cause the chyme to mix

TABLE 12–1
(continued)

Vitamin	Function	Deficiency Symptoms
Pantothenic acid	Component of the coenzyme A	Rat and fox: graying of the hair Swine: Ulceration of the gastrointestinal tract, degeneration of dorsal root ganglia, reproductive failure, characteristic gait known as "goose step"
B₁₂	Metabolism of propionic acid	Humans: Pernicious anemia Rats, guinea pigs, and swine: Reduced growth rates Ruminants: Anorexia, depressed growth, anemia
Folacin	Erythrocyte formation, coenzyme in the formation of tetrahydrafolic acid (which is important in amino acid choline, thymine and purine synthesis)	Anemia
Biotin	Carbon dioxide fixation i.e. methylmalonate fixation, transcarboxylation, aspartic acid formation, amino acid deamination	Rats and swine: Dermatitis and scaly skin accompanied by alopecia Mice: Depigmentation of the hair
Choline	Transmethylation	Fatty livers
C (ascorbic acid)	Hydroxylate proteins necessary for collagen, osteoid and dentine production, antioxidant, incorporation of plasma iron into ferritin, normal tyrosine oxidation maintenance	Humans: Capillary fragility, weak bones, anemia Essential only to primates, guinea pigs, fruit bats and flying fox

intestine becomes divided into segments by contractile rings, which occur at different positions along its length. This action tends to force the intestinal contents back and forth and provides a mechanism for mixing the ingesta and intestinal secretions during digestion.

The *defecation reflex* is initiated by pressure created by the feces in the colon and rectum. Pressure receptors, which are part of the sympathetic nervous system, receive the stimuli caused by increased pressure in the intestine. The stimuli are carried to the spinal cord and back to the smooth muscles which form the *rectal sphincter*. Thus, pressure in the rectum results in relaxation of the rectal sphincter (smooth muscle) and defecation occurs. But there is a second anal sphincter which lies external to the smooth muscle sphincter. This *second* or *external anal sphincter* is composed of striated muscle and is therefore under conscious control.

Defecation therefore usually involves both autonomic and somatic nervous control.

Vitamins and Minerals in Nutrition

The word vitamin was first formulated from the term "vital amines," which were believed to be essential to the health of the animal. Since that time many types of vitamins have been described, some of which are amines, though most are not. In general, vitamins are chemically unrelated and serve primarily as coenzymes in metabolic reactions. The fact that they are essential for the diet of a particular species indicates that they are necessary for metabolism but must be obtained through the diet.

Based upon solubility, two classes of vitamins are found. One class comprises the water-soluble vitamins: *thiamine, riboflavin, niacin, pyridoxine, pantothenic acid, vitamin B_{12}, folacin, biotin, choline,* and *ascorbic acid.* The other class comprises the fat-soluble vitamins: vitamins *A, D, E* and *K.* The water-soluble vitamins are usually absorbed with ease in the small intestine, whereas the fat-soluble vitamins are taken into the circulation along with other lipids and are usually emulsified in the gut by bile from the liver. A list of the vitamins, their functions, and deficiency symptoms is given in Table 12–1. (See pages 258–259.)

In the mammals, inorganic elements play an integral role in all organ systems. For instance, the role of sodium in blood, iodine in the thyroid gland, and calcium and phosphorus in bone have been discussed elsewhere in this text. Normal levels of various minerals are essential for the health of mammals, though in many cases an excess of a particular mineral results in toxicity. A deficiency can be related to abnormalities and even death. It has been shown that mammals utilize, in one form or another, calcium, phosphorus, magnesium, sodium, potassium, sulfur, chlorine, iron, copper, cobalt, iodine, manganese, selenium, zinc, fluorine, nickel, chromium, molybdenum, silicon, tin, and vanadium. Other elements, such as aluminum and arsenic, are found in mammalian tissue, though their significance is unknown.

The minerals obtained by nondomesticated mammals cannot be regulated by humans and, in the case of herbivores, generally reflect the mineral balance of the forage. Depending upon the geographic area, this can result in serious depletion of certain minerals or excess of others. Carnivorous mammals are not normally limited in this way because they receive a more balanced mineral intake from the prey consumed. But when excesses of nonessential minerals are present, they sometimes work their way through the food chain and become concentrated in the top carnivores of a particular region.

In domesticated mammals control of dietary minerals is essential, and numerous data have been accumulated on the effects of mineral deficiencies and excesses. Dietary mineral requirements in several domesticated mammals are listed in Table 12–2. This is by no means an exhaustive treatment of the *essential elements.* Numerous diseases and abnormal conditions are related to *trace elements* in the diets of domesticated species. It should be pointed out that essential dietary requirements have not been quantified in the case of many of the trace elements. Requirements are clouded to some degree by the interrelationships of many minerals. For instance, the dietary requirement for copper is increased in ruminants by excessive molybdenum, and high levels of phosphates in the diet interfere with the rate of iron absorption. Other factors, such as the requirement for cobalt, are affected by the

TABLE 12-2
Elements essential in the diets of domesticated species, and the effects of excesses and deficiencies in the diet

Mineral	Species	Dietary Requirement (ppm)	Abnormal Effects	
			Excess	Deficiency
Magnesium	Rats	—	—	Vasodilation, erythema, hyperemia, neuromuscular hyperemia
	Cattle	500–750	—	Grass tetany
	Swine	400	—	—
Iodine	All species studied	—	—	Goiter, lethargy, reduced metabolic rate
Fluorine	Cattle	0.2–0.3	—	Decreased bone density, dental caries, retarded growth rate, reduced fertility
	All species studied	—	Metabolic disturbances, reduced food intake, starvation, exostosis of the jaw and long bones	
Selenium	All species studied	0.1	Loss of hair	White muscle disease
	Cattle and sheep	—	Blind staggers, loss of hair, sloughing of hooves	—
	Horses	—		
Copper	Rats	—	—	Liver necrosis
	All species studied	—	—	Anemia, bone disorders, neonatal ataxia (except in pigs and dogs), depigmentation and abnormal growth of hair or wool, impaired growth and reproductive performance, heart failure, gastrointestinal disturbances, osteoporosis

TABLE 12-2
(continued)

Mineral	Species	Dietary Requirement (ppm)	Abnormal Effects	
			Excess	Deficiency
Cobalt	All species studied	—	Polycytemia	Anorexia, fatty liver, anemia, wasting of skeletal muscles
	Cattle and sheep	0.07–0.1		
	Swine	0.0005–0.001		
Zinc	All species studied	—	—	Depressed food consumption, growth rate, hemoglobin formation, rough and scaly skin, breaks in the skin around the hooves
	Swine	3–4		
Manganese	All species studied	—	—	Ataxia, skeletal abnormalities, impairment of growth and reproduction, blood clotting
	Swine	—	—	Enlarged hock joints, leg deformities, shortened legs, inhibition of estrous cycle

quantities of vitamin B_{12} in the diet and, in the case of some species, by the amount of vitamin B_{12} produced by the intestinal flora.

SUMMARY

Mammals are frequently specialized in their feeding types. Some are strict herbivores and feed exclusively on plant material, whereas others are carnivores and feed on other animals. A third type, the omnivore, consumes both plant and animal material. The herbivores show a number of specialized adaptations which are reflected in the anatomy and physiology of their digestive tracts. Two very specialized groups, the ruminants and the cecants, utilize enzymes contributed by symbiotic microorganisms to break down cellulose to form glucose. The ruminant species also profit from the amino acids contributed by the protein of the microorganism and are able to recycle urea nitrogen to form additional microbial protein.

Digestion is a complex process involving several very distinct chambers in the alimentary tract. Integration between these chambers or areas is made possible by means of the autonomic nervous system and several very specific hormones. Movement by means of smooth muscle contraction as well as secretion from the intestinal mucosa and digestive glands are mediated by the autonomic nervous system and the gastrointestinal hormones.

Digestion, or hydrolysis of food materials to form compounds which can be readily utilized, occurs in all portions of the digestive system. But in the monogastric mammals most digestion and absorption occur in the small intestine. Even in ruminants and cecants absorption prevails in the small intestine.

The liver acts as a clearinghouse for absorbed materials and also produces bile for lipid emulsion. Most of the plasma proteins are synthesized in the liver from absorbed amino acids. The liver also functions in the storage of glycogen and is primarily responsible, along with insulin and glucagon, for control of plasma glucose levels. Short-chain fatty acids are carried to the liver from their site of absorption in the small intestine, where they are converted to triglycerides. The storage of lipid in the liver is limited. But synthesis of saturated fatty acids from carbohydrates occurs in the liver. Also, the liver is primarily responsible for gluconeogenesis from both lipid and amino acid sources.

13

METABOLISM

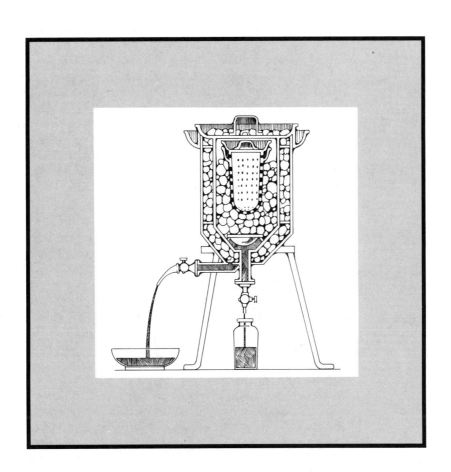

*M*etabolism in mammals provides the energy necessary to carry out all life functions and to maintain a relatively stable body temperature in both cold and hot climates. Metabolism can be divided into two major categories: anabolism and catabolism. Anabolism is the process of building complex cellular molecules and requires that energy be expended by the cell. Construction of cellular components is accomplished through anabolic reactions. Some of these cellular components provide the framework and environment for a controlled catabolism. Catabolism is the breakdown of complex molecules into simpler ones with the release of energy. Chemical energy from catabolism is retained in energy-rich compounds which can be used by the cell. Note that heretofore this text has assessed the physiology of the mammal from a whole-body or systems perspective; at this point attention is turned to events at the cellular level.

Metabolism involves the exchange of energy and in that sense always follows the second law of thermodynamics. Thus, in all metabolic reactions, anabolic and catabolic, there is a loss of usable energy. Yet the approach toward life taken by homeotherms (i.e., warm-blooded animals) is efficient in that the heat produced in metabolic reactions is not wasted on the environment but is instead retained to some degree by the organism to maintain a suitable internal climate for its metabolic reactions. In other words, homeotherm "strategy" has been to take advantage of the second law of thermodynamics such that they profit from their losses. As a result of achieving a near stable body temperature, mammals are essentially autonomous in their environment, within specific limits, and can inhabit almost every portion of the globe in any season.

The materials used by mammals to release chemical energy are carbohydrates, lipids, and proteins. Carbohydrates are basic to energy release and provide a direct source of energy for mammals. The most prevalent form of carbohydrates involved in mammalian metabolism is glucose. Dietary glucose is ready for use after phosphorylation, which means that only a one-step reaction is necessary to prepare glucose for energy release. In an oxygen-free or anaerobic environment, glucose can be catabolized with the release of several moles of ATP. This is accomplished through the Embden-Meyerhoff pathway, or anaerobic glycolysis (see Figure 13–1). If oxygen is available, pyruvic acid, which is the final product of anaerobic glycolysis, is oxidized in the presence of coenzyme A (CoA) to form acetyl CoA. Acetyl CoA can subsequently be used as an energy source in the tricarboxylic acid cycle (TCA), or Krebs cycle (see Figure 13–2). This cycle is referred to as aerobic glycolysis because it only occurs in the presence of oxygen.

Lipids contribute directly to the energy-yielding reactions of the Krebs cycle. The principal lipid used as an energy source is free fatty acid (FFA), which contributes an acetate fraction to oxaloacetic acid to form citrate. It is important to note that, unlike for carbohydrates, oxygen is necessary to metabolize lipids. Proteins are the least useful energy source since they contain nitrogen. For proteins or their amino acid constituents to be used in energy production, they must first be deaminated. Extra energy is required for this process. An additional energy expenditure results from urea synthesis, which is necessary to remove ammonium produced by deamination from the circulation. Also, proteins have such a great role in structure that most are normally not available for energy consumption unless carbohydrates and fats are depleted.

OXYGEN DEBT

When oxygen is unavailable some energy may continue to be formed, resulting in a condition known as *oxygen debt.* Oxygen debt occurs in mammals which are exercising vigorously and are unable to take in sufficient oxygen to complete *oxidative metabolism.* This condition also occurs in diving mammals which are unable to breathe underwater and consequently must rely upon anaerobic glycolysis for energy production.

In oxygen debt, pyruvic acid is used as a hydrogen acceptor and *lactic acid* (or *lactate*) is formed (see Figure 13–1). Most terrestrial mammals have little tolerance for acidic substances. Consequently, the buildup of lactate in the blood and other tissues presents certain problems as a result of the pH changes incurred. On the other hand, diving mammals have evolved a tolerance for the pH changes associated with lactate accumulation and are able to build up a sizable oxygen debt. The tolerance of diving mammals for oxygen debt allows them to remain submerged for long periods of time without attempting to breathe or surface. If terrestrial mammals are subjected to the same conditions endured by divers, the action of hydrogen ions from lactate places a tremendous stimulus on respiratory chemoreceptors. In such a situation, nondiving mammals are forced to follow the breathing reflex and consequently drown (see chapter 15, Respiration).

Oxygen debt then results in the buildup of lactate in the tissues. In terrestrial mammals the lactate from muscle is released into the circulation, where obvious pH changes occur. In the diving mammal circulation to the muscles is restricted by arterial constriction, and as a result little lactate enters the blood until the dive is completed (see chapter 19, Physiology of Some Specialized Mammalian Adaptations).

When the oxygen debt is "repaid" (when sufficient oxygen is taken into the blood), lactate is converted back to pyruvate and aerobic glycolysis proceeds. In other words, the oxygen debt is repaid by providing enough oxygen to the tissues to convert excess lactate to pyruvate, which is utilized in the aerobic catabolic process, or Krebs cycle.

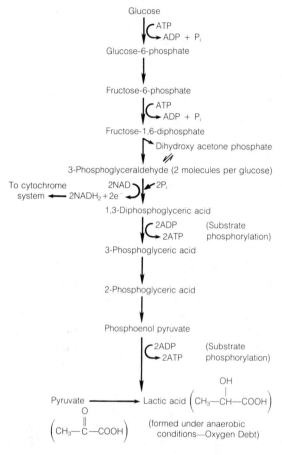

FIGURE 13–1
The Embden-Meyerhoff pathway of glucose degradation (anaerobic glycolysis)

PRODUCTION OF HIGH-ENERGY PHOSPHATES

Carbohydrate Catabolism

For chemical energy from carbohydrate to be of benefit to mammals, it must be trapped and retained by compounds which can be readily utilized in the metabolic mill. The energy of a fuel source such as carbohydrate can be obtained in usable form in two ways, both of which yield high-energy phosphate molecules, predominately *adenosine triphosphate (ATP)*. ATP is formed by two principal metabolic mechanisms: *substrate phosphorylation* and *oxidative phosphorylation*. In substrate phosphorylation the carbohydrate is converted into a compound with high-bond energy. An example of such is *phosphoenolpyruvate*. In this case the bond energy of phosphoenolpyruvate can be transferred directly to *adenosine diphosphate (ADP)* to form ATP. The energy of phosphoenolpyruvate, the *substrate* of the reaction, has been transferred directly to ATP and is retained in the phosphate bond, hence the name substrate phophorlyation. Bond energy can be looked upon as internal tension or pressure which results from restriction of the compound to one of its resonant forms.

Most of the energy obtained from carbohydrates is derived from oxidative phosphorylation, in which hydrogen is removed from the substrate by a hydrogen transport substance in the presence of the appropriate enzyme. The hydrogen transport substances in mammals are *flavin adenine dinucleotide (FAD)*, *nicotinamide adenine dinucleotide (NAD)*, and *nicotinamide adenine dinucleotide phosphate (NADP)*. Each of these substances is specific in the removal of hydrogen from certain substrates. Specifically, NAD and NADP can remove hydrogen from substrate molecules which have adjacent aliphatic and hydroxyl groups. FAD can remove hydrogen from adjacent aliphatic carbons (see Figure 13–3). These hydrogens and their electrons are essential to oxidative phosphorylation. Thus both the Krebs cycle and the Embden-Meyerhoff pathway are mechanisms by which substrate hydrogen is organized into the configuration acceptable to the hydrogen transport substances. It is further apparent that, regardless of the complex pro-

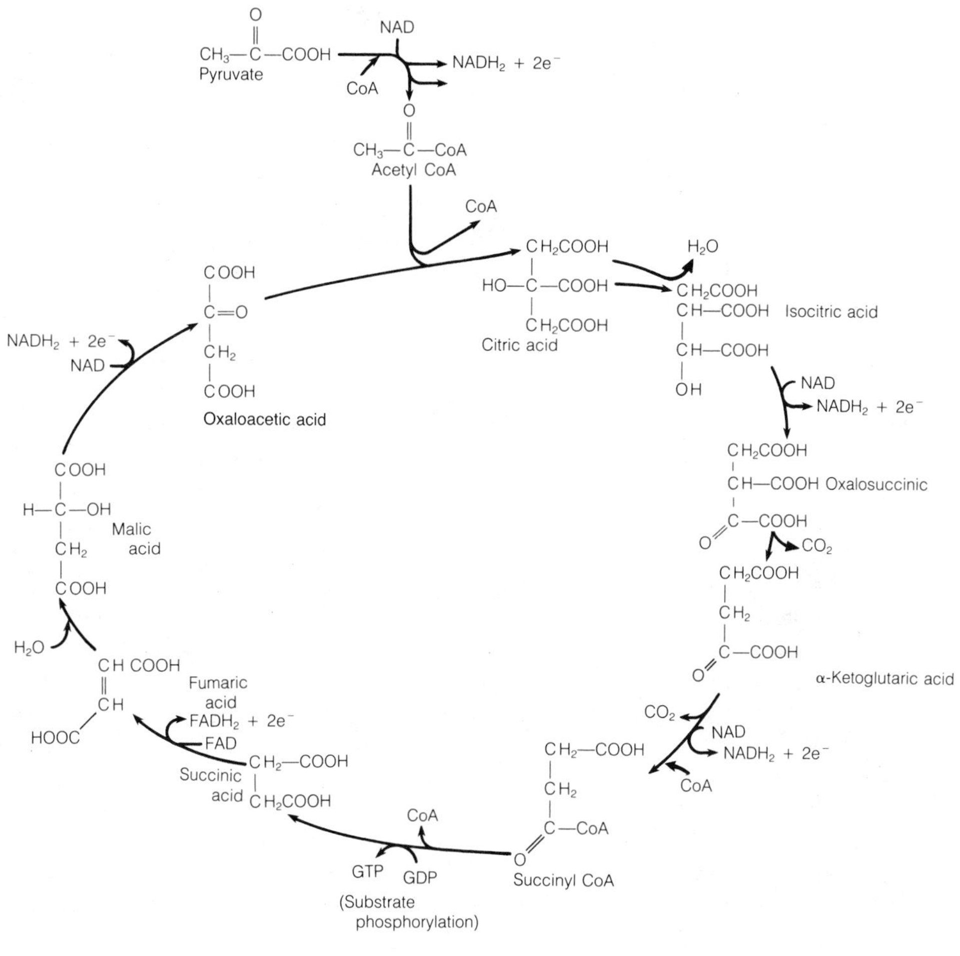

FIGURE 13–2
The Krebs cycle (tricarboxylic acid cycle) or aerobic cycle of catabolism

teins, carbohydrates, and lipids consumed, mammals as well as most other animals essentially live by "burning" hydrogen.

Hydrogens are transferred to the *cytochrome* or *electron transport system*, which is located inside the mitochondria. Since most of the phosphorylation is oxidative and occurs within mitochondria, they are sometimes called the "powerhouses" of the cell. The cytochrome system consists of a series of enzymes and related compounds which

are oxidized in sequence as the electron from hydrogen is transferred between compounds (see Figure 13–4). Each cytochrome enzyme is linked to a subsequent enzyme by a coupled reaction. It is interesting that these enzymes are not free in solution, but instead are attached to the cristae of the mitochondria in a very regular and orderly fashion. Therefore, when an electron is received by the first enzyme in the sequence it must be transferred to a second enzyme in the se-

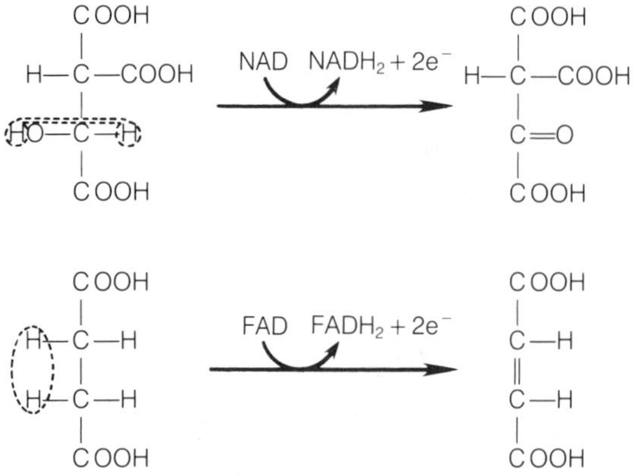

FIGURE 13–3
NAD and FAD are involved in removal of hydrogens from substrate molecules having specific hydroxyl or aliphatic arrangements

quence, which has previously been positioned adjacent to the first enzyme. It should be realized that this is not a random series of reactions and is therefore entirely different from an enzyme-substrate-type reaction which might be carried out *in vitro*. The organized structure of the cytochrome system in the mitochondria enhances metabolic efficiency of cellular metabolism.

The principle whereby energy is made usable by the electron transport system is governed by the driving forces behind coupled reactions. The cytochrome enzymes contain a *porphyrin subunit* which is very similar to the heme portion of hemoglobin. The iron in the cytochrome enzymes can be reduced

(ferrous state) or oxidized *(ferric state)*. When the porphyrin molecule accepts an electron from hydrogen, the electron becomes associated with iron, which assumes the reduced state. When iron is in the ferrous state, the cytochrome enzyme has a higher energy content relative to the energy contained in the ferric state. One might think of the molecule as being energy enriched. At this time the reduced molecule is relatively unstable and is able to give up or release energy and return the iron to its oxidized condition. When this return occurs, the electron is transferred to an adjacent molecule which is then reduced. At the time of its oxidation, the first compound yields energy which can be taken up by another substance (such as ATP) or released as heat.

The tendency of a molecule to convert spontaneously to its oxidized state is a function which can be measured. The measurement can be accomplished in terms of the *electromotive force (EMF)* produced. Stated another way, the tendency for a reaction of this type to take place is a function of its instability and the energy released as it attains the stable form can be measured as the voltage generated by its change in electrical status. The tendency for a compound in the cytochrome system to assume its oxidized form is called the *reduction-oxidation (redox) potential* (see Table 13–1). Different redox potentials are characteristic of specific reaction systems.

FIGURE 13–4
The electron transport system (cytochrome system), which results in oxidative phosphorylation to form ATP

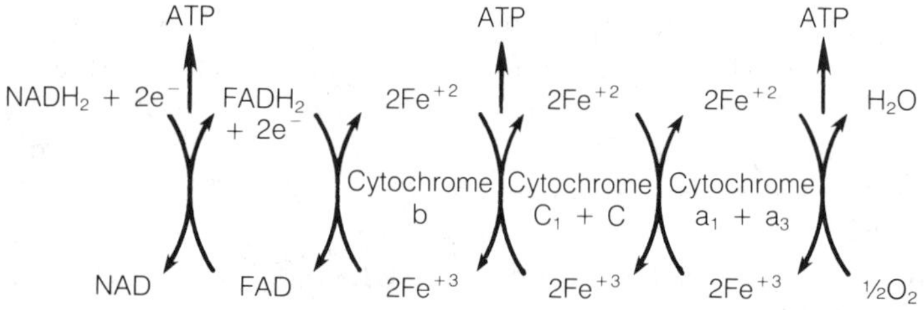

TABLE 13–1
Normal reduction-oxidation potentials of some biological reactions at pH 7.0

System	E'_0	T in °C.
Ketoglutarate $\rightleftharpoons$ succinate + CO_2 + $2H^+$ + 2e	−0.68	—‡
Ferredoxin	−0.432	—§
Formate $\rightleftharpoons$ CO_2 + H_2	−0.420	38
$H_2 \rightleftharpoons 2H^+$ + 2e	−0.414	25
NADH + $H^+ \rightleftharpoons NAD^+$ + $2H^+$ + 2e	−0.317	30†
NADPH + $H^+ \rightleftharpoons NADP^+$ + $2H^+$ + 2e	−0.316	30†
Horseradish oxidase	−0.27	—†
$FADH_2 \rightleftharpoons FAD + 2H^+$ + 2e	−0.219	30†
$FMNH_2 \rightleftharpoons FMM + 2H^+$ + 2e	−0.219	30†
Lactate $\rightleftharpoons$ pyruvate + $2H^+$ + 2e	−0.180	35
Malate $\rightleftharpoons$ oxaloacetate + $2H^+$ + 2e	−0.102	37
Reduced flavin enzyme $\rightleftharpoons$ flavin enzyme + $2H^+$ + 2e	−0.063	38
Luciferin* $\rightleftharpoons$ oxyluciferin + $2H^+$ + 2e	−0.050	?*
Ferrocytochrome B $\rightleftharpoons$ ferricytochrome B + e	−0.04	25
Succinate $\rightleftharpoons$ fumarate + $2H^+$ + 2e	−0.015	30
Decarboxylase	+0.19	—†
Ferrocytochrome C $\rightleftharpoons$ ferricytochrome C + e	+0.26	25
Ferrocytochrome A $\rightleftharpoons$ ferricytochrome A + e	+0.29	25
Ferrocytochrome $A_3 \rightleftharpoons$ ferricytochrome A_3 + e	?	—‡
$H_2O \rightleftharpoons \frac{1}{2}O_2 + 2H^+$ + 2e	+0.815	25

Source: From *Cell Physiology* by A. C. Giese. Copyright © 1968 by W. B. Saunders Co. Reprinted by permission of W. B. Saunders, CBS College Publishing.
Data from Goddard. 1945. Potentials in all cases are at or near neutrality.
*From McElroy and Strehler. 1954: Bact. Rev. *18*.
†From Clark. 1960.
‡From Goddard and Bonner. 1960: *In* Plant Physiology, a Treatise. Steward, ed. Academic Press, New York.
Goddard and Bonner give the NADPH NADP$^+$ system as −0.324, and NADH/NAD$^+$ as −0.320.
§From Tagawa and Arnon. 1962: Nature 195:537–543. The value cited is for spinach ferredoxin.

The energy released when a cytochrome enzyme goes from the ferrous to the ferric state (i.e., reduced to oxidized) can be trapped by a second coupled reaction to form ATP from ADP and inorganic phosphate. Some of the energy escapes the coupled reaction and is given off as heat. All of the energy obtained from the carbohydrate substrate will ultimately be released to the environment as heat.

As the cytochrome reactions progress, energy is released at each coupled reaction, but only certain steps result in ATP formation.

The total energy involved from the cellular metabolism of one gram of glucose is 4.1 kilocalories, or the amount of heat derived from burning (complete oxidation) of an equivalent quantity of glucose. The metabolic process has a basic advantage over burning: during metabolism energy is gradually released in small amounts and can be trapped in coupled reactions. Burning involves the sudden oxidation of a substance with all of the energy being released in a relatively short period of time (see Figure 13–5). That the energy released from metabolism is identical to

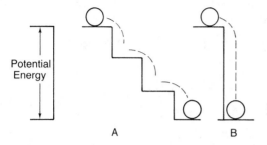

FIGURE 13–5
The total potential energy in A and B are equal. But in A the energy is lost in smaller units, or in stepwise fashion. In B the entire potential energy is lost at once. A is analogous to the oxidation processes of metabolism; B is analogous to oxidation that occurs during simple combustion.

free fatty acids by the cells is a purely passive process. It is for this reason that utilization of free fatty acids is a function of their concentration in the plasma and is not dependent upon selection mechanisms within the cell. But transport of the free fatty acids from cytoplasm to the mitochondria is dependent upon the presence of carrier molecules. The concentration of the carrier substance limits the amount of free fatty acid utilization.

Once a free fatty acid enters a cell it forms a derivative of coenzyme A (see Figure 13–6). Oxidation of the coenzyme A derivative proceeds through oxidation of the aliphatic

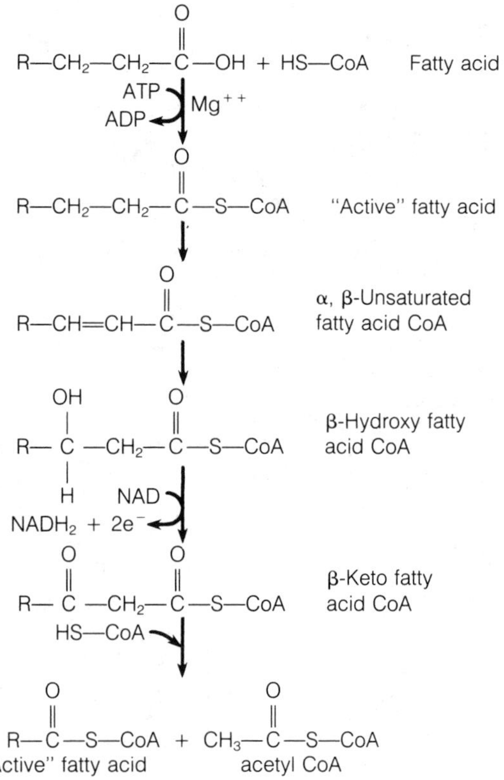

the heat released from combustion was discovered by Lavoisier in 1777.

In the electron transport system of mammals, the ultimate electron acceptor is oxygen. When free oxygen accepts an electron, an oxygen ion is formed. Hydrogen ions react immediately with the reduced oxygen to form metabolic water. In some desert species, water retention is very efficient and metabolic water formed in this way can be the animal's sole source of water. Mammals of this type require a diet high in lipids. A great deal of water for digestion or absorption is then unnecessary, since a high lipid diet produces a great deal of water per gram ingested.

Lipid Catabolism

As mentioned earlier, most of the lipids are stored in mammals by the adipose cells as triglycerides. When mobilized they are hydrolyzed by cellular enzymes to form free fatty acids and glycerol. Free fatty acids are loosely bound to the albumin fraction of plasma proteins and transported to the cells, where they are oxidized. The absorption of

$$R-CH_2-CH_2-\overset{\overset{\displaystyle O}{\|}}{C}-OH + HS-CoA \qquad \text{Fatty acid}$$

$$\text{ATP} \searrow \quad Mg^{++}$$
$$\text{ADP} \nearrow$$

$$R-CH_2-CH_2-\overset{\overset{\displaystyle O}{\|}}{C}-S-CoA \qquad \text{"Active" fatty acid}$$

$$R-CH=CH-\overset{\overset{\displaystyle O}{\|}}{C}-S-CoA \qquad \begin{array}{l}\alpha, \beta\text{-Unsaturated} \\ \text{fatty acid CoA}\end{array}$$

$$R-\overset{\overset{\displaystyle OH}{|}}{\underset{\underset{\displaystyle H}{|}}{C}}-CH_2-\overset{\overset{\displaystyle O}{\|}}{C}-S-CoA \qquad \begin{array}{l}\beta\text{-Hydroxy fatty} \\ \text{acid CoA}\end{array}$$

$$\text{NAD} \searrow$$
$$\text{NADH}_2 + 2e^-$$

$$R-\overset{\overset{\displaystyle O}{\|}}{C}-CH_2-\overset{\overset{\displaystyle O}{\|}}{C}-S-CoA \qquad \begin{array}{l}\beta\text{-Keto fatty} \\ \text{acid CoA}\end{array}$$

$$\text{HS-CoA} \searrow$$

$$R-\overset{\overset{\displaystyle O}{\|}}{C}-S-CoA \; + \; CH_3-\overset{\overset{\displaystyle O}{\|}}{C}-S-CoA$$
"Active" fatty acid   acetyl CoA

FIGURE 13–6
Beta oxidation or degradation of fatty acids to form acetyl CoA, which enters the Krebs cycle

chain of the fatty acid at the beta position. The ultimate result of such *beta oxidation* is the formation of acetyl CoA and a coenzyme A derivative of the original fatty acid minus the acetyl group. The acetyl CoA fraction is passed into the Krebs cycle (refer back to Figure 13–2).

By reason of their point of entry into the glycolytic cycle and their aliphatic nature, fatty acids produce a very high proportion of energy per unit mass. Since they also form neutral esters with glycerol, fatty acids are ideal for storage in mammals. Indeed, in most mammals the majority of stored chemical energy is in the form of triglycerides. This provides a light, energy-rich, neu-

tral substance which can release a maximum volume of metabolic water per mole of ATP formed.

Protein Catabolism

Proteins are brought into the metabolic pathway by hydrolysis of peptide bonds to form amino acids and subsequent deamination of amino acids to form α-*keto acids*. Amino acids form specific α-keto acids that enter aerobic catabolism at specific sites of the Krebs cycle, sites of necessity because of the various molecular structures involved (see Figure 13–7). As a result of the size of the molecules and the different points of entry into

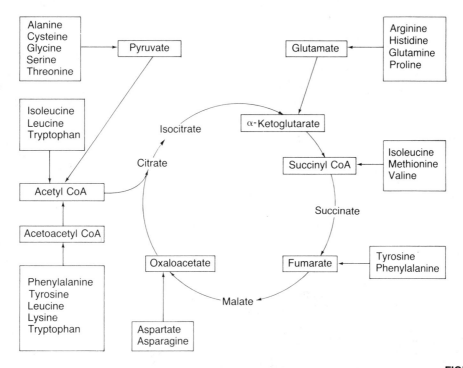

FIGURE 13–7

Point of entry of amino acids into the Krebs cycle. From A. L. Lehninger, *Short Course in Biochemistry* (New York, N.Y., 1973), 14-5. Reprinted by permission of Worth Publishers, Inc.

Krebs cycle, specific amino acids vary in their contribution of total amounts of energy to the cell. In other words, when glutamine is deaminated to form α-*ketoglutaric acid*, it contributes more hydrogens for the formation of ATP than does *tyrosine*, which enters the Krebs cycle by being converted to *fumarate*.

The nitrogen produced from deamination of amino acids is combined with carbon dioxide to form urea through a series of chemical reactions called the *urea cycle*. Amino acid nitrogen produced by deamination is lost through the urine. By this system of reactions, ammonia is not permitted to build up in mammalian tissues. Urea is more soluble in plasma than *uric acid*, which is produced from protein catabolism in the reptile and avian vertebrate classes. In these vertebrates a relatively insoluble substance is needed because the products of protein catabolism are stored in the *cloaca* until defecation rather than being passed out of the body through a separate opening, as is the case in most mammals. The monotremes (egg-laying mammals) retain the cloaca, and in males urinary products are passed directly into it by a separate opening in the urethra. In the female monotremes the urethra opens directly into the cloaca.

METABOLIC RATE

When an animal is completely at rest, has not been fed for approximately twelve hours, and is not under thermal stress (i.e., oxygen consumption is at its lowest point in the awakened state and heat loss is equal to heat production), metabolism is maintained at a minimal level called the *basal metabolic rate*. It should be pointed out that basal metabolic rate is a term most frequently used in human biology. A more appropriate term used in investigations of metabolic rate in nonhuman species is *resting* or *standard metabolic rate*. The metabolic rates of mammals vary according to species and physiological conditions, but each species has a characteristic resting metabolic rate under thermoneutral conditions. For further discussion of metabolic rate and temperature, see chapter 16, Thermoregulation.

Respiratory Quotient

The complete catabolism of carbohydrates and lipids yields a characteristic quantity of carbon dioxide and water and, depending upon the type of substrate being metabolized, utilizes a specific quantity of oxygen (see Figure 13–8). Protein catabolism yields ammonium ions, carbon dioxide, and water. The ammonium produced in this process is converted to urea and passes into the urine unless it is recycled, as in ruminants. The amount of carbon dioxide and water yielded

Carbohydrate
$$C_6H_{12}O_6 + 6O_2 \rightarrow 6CO_2 + 6H_2O$$
$$RQ = 6/6 = 1.0$$

Fat
$$2C_{51}H_{98}O_6 + 145\,O_2 \rightarrow 102\,CO_2 + 98\,H_2O$$
$$RQ = 102/145 = 0.703$$

Protein
$$2C_3H_7O_2N + 6O_2 \rightarrow (NH_2)_2\,CO + 5CO_2 + 5H_2O$$
$$RQ = 5/6 = 0.83$$

FIGURE 13–8
Respiratory quotients (RQ) for three principal dietary energy sources. Note that the RQ for fats and protein vary slightly depending upon which fatty acid or which amino acids are involved.

by proteins is also characteristic. The ratio of carbon dioxide produced to oxygen consumed in the catabolism of a specific substance has been termed the *respiratory quotient (RQ)* or *respiratory exchange ratio*. The respiratory quotient for carbohydrate is 1.0, for lipids approximately 0.7, and for proteins approximately 0.83. If the ratio of carbon dioxide released to oxygen consumed is determined, the determination of the metabolic fuel being utilized by a mammal at any particular time may then be obtained. If the RQ is 1.0, it can be assumed that the animal is metabolizing pure carbohydrate. If the metabolic fuel is lipid, the RQ should be near 0.7. But, since there are three substrates, any number between 0.7 and 1.0 could be caused by metabolism of various combinations of the three fuels. Thus, RQ data does not reveal anything about the probable fuel source as long as there are three unknown fuel materials. But if a *nonprotein respiratory quotient (NPRQ)* can be determined, the fuel being used and the relative proportions metabolized by the animal can also be determined. By collecting the urea formed from amino nitrogen in a nonruminant, the amount of protein metabolized can be deduced. It has been shown that the quantity of protein that is catabolized by a mammal is equal to grams of urinary nitrogen times 6.25. This is an accurate determination that can be made by simply collecting the urine of a mammal and analyzing it to determine the quantity of urinary nitrogen present. During the catabolism of protein, a very regular amount of carbon dioxide is given off in relation to oxygen consumed. This bears a direct relationship to the quantity of urinary nitrogen produced. This figure has been found to be 0.78 liters per gram for carbon dioxide released and 0.97 liters per gram for oxygen consumed.

Since the amount of carbon dioxide produced and the amount of oxygen consumed in excess of the quantity of these gases involved with protein catabolism are derived from fat and carbohydrate, the formula to calculate the nonprotein respiratory quotient (NPRQ) is the following:

$$NPRQ = \frac{Total\ CO_2 - Protein\ CO_2}{Total\ O_2 - Protein\ O_2} \quad (13.1)$$

In other words, the total carbon dioxide minus the carbon dioxide released in protein catabolism equals the carbon dioxide evolved from carbohydrate and lipid catabolism. Also, the oxygen utilized in carbohydrate and lipid catabolism is equal to the total oxygen used minus the oxygen necessary for protein catabolism. The ratio of the nonprotein carbon dioxide and nonprotein oxygen (i.e., NPRQ) is some number between 1.0 and 0.7. By interpolation this value yields approximate quantities of carbohydrate and lipid utilized by the mammal as metabolic fuel.

The NPRQ is useful in determining the relative quantities of different fuels which are used by mammals for different activities and under different environmental conditions. For instance, it has been found that when mammals are forced to increase their metabolic rate in order to maintain body temperature, the RQ is near 0.7. This would indicate that lipid is being used when a mammal is exposed to cold. During maximum exertion for short periods of time, NPRQ is near 1.0, which indicates that pure carbohydrate is being used as the primary metabolic fuel. When fasting for short periods of time, humans usually have a NPRQ near 0.82, which indicates that both carbohydrates and lipids are being metabolized in approximately equal amounts.

Measurement of Metabolism

Calorimetry is the measurement of heat generated by metabolism of an animal or by combustion of any inanimate object or substance. Two types of calorimetry are used in physiology: *direct* and *indirect*. Direct calorimetry is a method whereby the heat from a body or object is measured; indirect calorimetry is a measurement of heat generated in metabolism, as calculated from the volume of oxygen consumed. Indirect calorimetry gives only an approximation of heat generated since the amount of oxygen consumed is dependent upon the specific fuel source used by the animal. In such calculation, NPRQ usually is taken to be 0.82, or that of a resting animal in the *postabsorptive state* (i.e., state at which intestinal absorption is complete and plasma metabolite levels do not reflect materials from the previous meal).

In 1780, Lavoisier constructed a crude but accurate calorimeter that was large enough to contain a rat (see Figure 13–9). The principle behind Lavoisier's calorimeter was based upon the *specific heat of fusion of water*, or the heat necessary to melt one gram of ice to form water. An internal jacket containing ice was insulated from the environment, so ambient heat had little effect on it. An animal could be placed inside the inner compartment so that its body heat could be directly absorbed by the ice. The water from the melting ice was caught in a cup underneath the calorimeter and weighed. The total heat produced by the animal was then determined by multiplying grams of ice melted times the specific heat of fusion for water. Since the specific heat of fusion for water is 80 calories, this was indeed a very easy and accurate calculation. Lavoisier's was one of the first published accounts of direct calori-

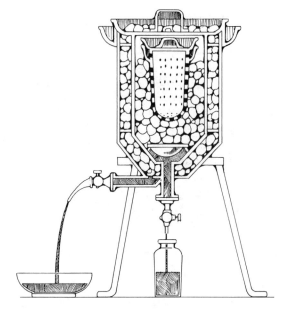

FIGURE 13–9
The calorimeter used by Lavoisier. Water formed from the ice in the inner jacket was collected to determine calories generated in the central chamber. From K. E. Rothschuh, *History of Physiology* (Melbourne, Fla., 1973). Reprinted by permission of Robert E. Krieger Publishing Co.

metry. Modern whole-body calorimeters have been constructed which are large enough to contain humans, and the more elaborate ones are large enough to contain both a human and the equipment necessary to perform specific physical tasks (see Figure 13–10). An ice jacket is no longer used in this type of calorimeter to measure heat generated. In modern calorimeters, water flowing through a radiator, or a similar device which can be placed in or around the chamber, absorbs heat given off by the animal. The number of calories generated can be calculated by means of the following formula:

$$N = Ftc\,(T_e - T_i) \qquad (13.2)$$

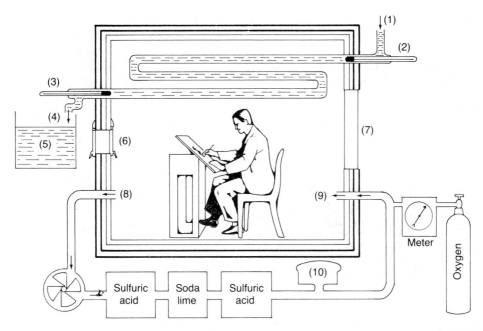

FIGURE 13–10

View of Atwater-Benedict respiration calorimeter. Water flows from (1) to (4), and its temperature is measured at the inlet and outlet. Air enters at (9) and leaves at (8). Water is removed from it by means of sulfuric acid, and carbon dioxide is absorbed by the soda lime. Water enters at (1), and its temperature is measured at (2) and (3). A porthole is provided at (6) and a window at (7). An air cushion is present at (10). From G. H. Bell et al, *Textbook of Physiology and Biochemistry,* 9th edition (New York, N.Y.: Livingstone, 1976). Reprinted by permission of Churchill-Livingstone, Inc.

where,

N = number of calories generated
F = rate of water flow through the calorimeter (ml/min)
t = total time inside the calorimeter (min)
c = specific heat of water (1.0 cal/°C/ml)
T_e = temperature of water in excurrent flow (°C)
T_i = temperature of water in incurrent flow (°C)

Bomb calorimeters have been developed to measure the heat generated as the result of combustion of food materials by the direct method. In this process materials are placed in an inner chamber, which is surrounded by a water jacket. The water jacket is insulated on the outside so as to impede the influence of external heat. An electric spark ignites the materials in the inner chamber and the combustion of the material generates heat, which is absorbed by the water in the surrounding jacket. The total calories generated are determined by multiplying the volume of water (in milliliters) by the change in water temperature (°C) by the specific heat of water. The data derived from this method of caloric analysis of specific foods or dietary substances have been very useful, since the exact caloric values of fats, carbohydrates, and proteins have been so determined. These values can be compared to the caloric production of substances in the intact organism.

Recently ingested food sometimes increases the metabolic rate above what is expected. The extra metabolism required to assimilate foods is called the *specific dynamic action (SDA)*. Although the cause of the SDA is still uncertain, it is associated with assimilation of a food into the body. For instance, protein, the food substance with the highest SDA, must be deaminated, and urea must be produced in order for the protein to contribute to the production of energy. The chemical reactions necessary to carry out these actions generate heat, which is reflected in calorimetry as heat generated during protein metabolism. All substances show some SDA. For instance, fatty acids must be oxidized (beta oxidation) before an acetyl group is free to perform its function in aerobic glycolysis. Glucose, which has the lowest SDA of all the substances eaten by mammals, must be phosphorylated prior to catabolism.

Indirect calorimetry is less costly but probably also less accurate than direct calorimetry. An accurate whole-body calorimeter is difficult to build for large animals because of space limitations and the cost of constructing a well-insulated chamber large enough to contain an animal 75 kilograms or more. Therefore, most calorimetric measurements reported for large animals have been determined by the indirect method. In measuring the heat produced by metabolism in large animals, a mask is fitted to the face of the animal so that only air coming through the mask can be inhaled. A gas of known oxygen content, usually ambient air, is forced through the mask, and the oxygen content of the *excurrent* (exhaled) *air* is measured to determine the total oxygen consumption by the animal. The total calories generated are determined by multiplying the amount of oxygen consumed by the caloric equivalent of oxygen where the NPRQ is 0.82. This method is limited because of the many possible variations in the physiological state of the mammal used in the determination. If for some reason the animal is using fat or carbohydrate exclusively as a body fuel, the indirect calculations will not be accurate. As an extreme example, suppose that the mammal is diabetic. In this case, little if any carbohydrate will be used in the metabolism and the NPRQ will be considerably lower than 0.82. Thus, the caloric equivalent of oxygen would be lower than expected, and the results would not be accurate (see Table 13–2). If the

TABLE 13–2
Thermal equivalents of oxygen for the principal classes of food materials

| | O_2 Required | | CO_2 Produced | | Thermal Equivalent |
	(Kcal/gm)	(l/gm)	(l/gm)	(RQ)	(Kcal/l O_2)
Carbohydrates	4.1	0.81	0.81	1.00	5.061
Fats	9.3	1.98	1.40	0.70	4.696
Proteins	4.3	0.97	0.78	0.80	4.432

animal being tested is a ruminant that has blood glucose content of 50 mg/100 ml blood glucose or less, the NPRQ is expected to reflect fat metabolism, and the results would be erroneous again, provided that 0.82 is used again as the resting NPRQ. Also, exhaled air of ruminants contains methane and perhaps other gases from microbial fermentation. This makes indirect measurement of metabolic rate difficult in these animals because the percent of oxygen in the excurrent air varies with the metabolic rates of ruminant microorganisms. The indirect method, however, can be accurate when used for monogastric mammals if the NPRQ is determined at the same time as the calories produced are determined using the indirect method. In order to do this, one needs to determine the quantity of carbon dioxide evolved along with oxygen consumed and the urinary nitrogen produced. If these measurements are carried out, indirect calorimetry becomes very accurate, and calories generated under different circumstances such as exercise and exposure to cold can be measured.

An excellent method of making this determination in humans is carried out by the use of a *Douglas bag*. The Douglas bag can be worn while performing a number of different exercises in various types of terrain or under different environmental conditions. By this method, calories generated can be determined while walking, jogging, running, climbing stairs, going to class, or carrying out other daily activities.

As a result of modern techniques essential to indirect calorimetry, many very useful bits of data have been derived which give insight into the metabolic costs of various activities, diets, and body sizes. Some of the more useful devices have been *gas analyzers*, which can measure the oxygen and carbon dioxide

content in excurrent air as it flows from a mask. In this way, oxygen consumption can be determined continuously in a variety of mammals of different sizes, activities, and environmental conditions. Frequently, this type of data is reported simply as oxygen consumption rate rather than as calories produced. This is useful information as long as proper controls and sample sizes are maintained. Such a statement might well apply to all experiments.

It is interesting to compare metabolic rates among species and among individuals of different size and age classes. But this is difficult because metabolic rates of mammals of widely differing body sizes are extremely different when compared on a gram-weight basis. If the energy utilization of a 441-kg horse (4,983 Kcals/hour) is compared to that of a 15.2-kg dog (782 Kcals/hour), the data show that the rate at which one gram of horse tissue uses energy is extremely slow when compared to one gram of dog tissue. To put it another way, 29 dogs have a body mass equivalent to one horse. What is the metabolic cost of maintaining this many dogs as opposed to one horse? The answer for one day is 22,701 Kcals consumed by 29 dogs as opposed to 4,983 Kcals consumed by a single horse. It can readily be deduced that one gram of dog tissue is much more metabolically active than one gram of horse tissue.

If mammals are compared on the basis of metabolism per unit weight, energy utilization per gram is inversely proportional to body size. But when comparison is made among metabolic rates of mammals based upon surface area, a much more uniform picture is produced (see Table 13–3). These data indicate that mammals with greater surface-to-body-weight ratios have greater metabolic rates. Note that the ratio of surface to

TABLE 13–3
Heat produced by resting mammals as a function of body weight and body surface area

Species	Weight (kg)	Heat Produced in 24 Hours (Kcals)	
		Per kg Weight	Per sq Meter of Surface
Horse	441	11.3	948
Pig	128	19.1	1,078
Human	64.3	32.1	1,042
Dog	15.2	51.5	1,037

Source: From *Fundamentals of Nutrition* by L. E. Lloyd et al. Copyright © 1978 by W. H. Freeman and Company. All rights reserved.

body weight of a mammal is inversely proportional to size. The significance of this phenomenon has been argued intensively, and several conclusions have been drawn. First, it would appear that since mammals lose heat through the body surface, large surface-to-mass ratios would require high metabolic rates in order to balance the heat lost and the maintenance of a stable body temperature. But even though surface-to-body-mass ratios are a function of body size, heat loss is also affected by insulation. The degree to which skin is insulated in mammals cannot be assumed from body size. From these data it would appear that though metabolic rate is correlated with body size, to say that this phenomenon is based entirely on ratios of surface to body mass would certainly be naive. If body mass (M_b) is compared to oxygen consumed $(V_{O_2}$, in liters oxygen per hour), a line of best fit whose equation is obtained as follows:

$$V_{O_2} = 0.676 \times M_b^{0.75} \qquad (13.3)$$

The slope of the line graphed is 0.75 (see Figure 13–11). Thus, the primary factor or factors controlling metabolic rate must be some physical parameter which bears this same relationship to body size. Such factors as surface area, insulation, and metabolic tissue content are known to affect metabolic rate, which probably results from a number of

causative factors rather than a single variable that can easily be determined.

METABOLIC COST OF LOCOMOTION

Mammals move in three very distinct ways. The most typical is *terrestrial locomotion*, which involves walking and running. In this manner of movement the animal must support the body as well as exert energy to propel it forward. The atmosphere provides little

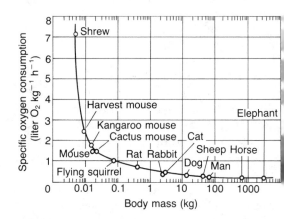

FIGURE 13–11
Oxygen consumption rate per unit body mass of several mammalian species plotted against total body mass. From K. Schmidt-Nielsen, *Animal Physiology: Adaptations and Environment*, 2nd edition (New York, N.Y., 1979). Reprinted by permission of Cambridge University Press.

resistance to terrestrial movement. When terrestrial animals move in still air, the principal energy required is for resisting the force of gravity and propelling the mass horizontally on a level plane. Obviously, it makes a difference if the animal is moving against a wind or with a wind. But if different modes of movement by mammals are compared when movement of the surrounding medium (i.e., air or water) is held at an insignificant level, some very interesting data can be derived.

The second type of movement is *aquatic locomotion*, which involves swimming. Some mammals, such as the cetaceans, are completely aquatic, whereas others (such as seals and walruses) move poorly on land and have evolved mechanisms of movement which function primarily in water. Aquatic mammals move in an entirely different medium than terrestrial mammals and have evolved appropriate body form and musculature for this type of movement. For instance, water is more viscous than air and therefore acts to retard movement. Resistance to movement in an aquatic environment is great even at moderate speeds. For this reason aquatic mammals usually have streamlined bodies which function to reduce the resistance exerted by the water in which they swim. On the other hand, water is more buoyant than air and therefore removes most of the necessity of aquatic organisms to exert energy for support. Because they are supported by water, almost all of their energy can be exerted to propel the body.

The third type of movement, *aerial locomotion*, involves the members of only one order of mammals, though it comprises many species. These are the *chiropterans* (bats), which are the only mammals capable of independent flight, as opposed to the gliding seen in flying squirrels and perhaps other mammals. Bats move through the air, a situation very similar to water as far as movement is concerned. Essentially, a mechanism has evolved which allows bats to support themselves in air. But like the animal moving on land, the bat must constantly exert energy in supporting the body. The resistance of air to movement is quite low, and the energetic cost of locomotion is still lower than terrestrial locomotion. *Cost of locomotion* (i.e., the energy necessary to move one unit of body mass over one unit of distance) is especially low when an animal soars or rides an air current with wings outstretched, as seen in a number of birds of prey. This is typically more characteristic of birds but has also been noted in bats. When soaring, the animal is supported in air with almost the same ease as aquatic mammals are supported. Such support contributes tremendously to the economy of movement. Also, the resistance to forward motion in air is almost negligible at the moderate speeds exhibited by bats, thus negating the lack of streamlined bodies of these mammals.

When aquatic, terrestrial, and aerial locomotion are compared it is obvious that terrestrial mammals exert a great deal of energy in resisting the force of gravity. The aquatic and aerial modes of locomotion are much more economical from an energy standpoint than is terrestrial locomotion (see Figure 13–12). But these data should be treated with some reservation because such experiments with chiropterans and cetaceans are scarce.

Since most mammals are terrestrial, questions about the energetics of terrestrial movement arise. First, which mode of travel (walking, trotting, running) is most economical in terms of weight moved as a function of energy expended? Second, since a wide variety of sizes occurs in mammals, what is the role of body size in mammalian locomotion? Also, body structure and muscle attachment vary

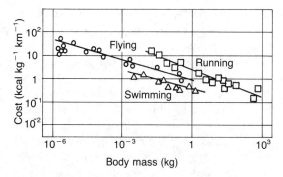

FIGURE 13–12
Comparison of economy of terrestrial, aerial and aquatic modes of locomotion. From K. Schmidt-Nielsen, Energy Cost of Swimming, Flying and Running, *Science* 177(1972):222–228. Reprinted with permission. Copyright 1972 by the American Association for the Advancement of Science.

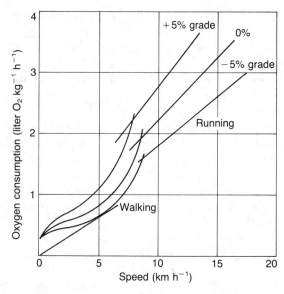

FIGURE 13–13
Energy expenditures of a human while walking and running at three different grades. Line drawn from origin tangent to curve produced from oxygen consumption while walking represents maximum economy. From R. Margaria et al, Energy Cost of Running, *J. Appl. Physiol.* 18(1963):367–370. Reprinted by permission of the American Physiological Society, Bethesda, Md.

tremendously among individuals of different species and perhaps among individuals of the same species as well, but little data about the role of structure and muscle attachment in economy of locomotion exist. If an attempt is made to discover which mode of terrestrial locomotion is most economical, some very good examples can be found. It has been observed that walking and running in humans produce decidedly different energetic results (see Figure 13–13). When running, oxygen consumption increases with a very regular relationship to velocity, whereas walking produces a curvilinear relationship of oxygen consumption to velocity. In this case, walking causes an accelerated consumption of oxygen as the maximum rate is approached. Running does not have this effect, though maximum running speed is not reached in the graph of Figure 13–13. If these data were continued until a maximum sprint was reached, the curve for running might eventually have a shape similar to the curve expressing the energetic costs of walking. It has been shown that the most economical cost

of flying in birds can be calculated graphically by drawing a line from the origin tangent to the curve showing oxygen consumption as a function of flight speed (see Figure 13–14). If the same type of calculation is carried out with humans when walking, it can be shown that efficiency on flat ground is greatest at about 5 km/hour (see Figure 13–13).

If the cost of locomotion among species which differ in size is compared (in some cases the mode of locomotion as well), the larger species are much more efficient than the smaller ones for moving a given amount of mass a given distance (see Figure 13–15). In other words, on an energy-cost basis a dog consumes much less energy per unit body

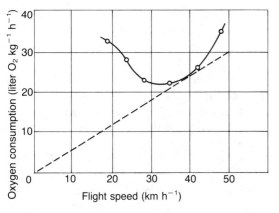

FIGURE 13–14
Oxygen consumption of a budgerigar (parakeet) in flight.
The lowest metabolic cost of flying occurs at about 40
km/hour. From K. Schmidt-Nielsen, *How Animals Work*
(London, U.K., 1972). Reprinted by permission of Cambridge University Press.

weight in locomotion at any speed than is consumed by a white mouse. The size factor holds true even for animals larger than the dog (see Figure 13–16). At 8 km/hour on an 11.5-percent grade the horse uses about 45 ml O_2/kg/min, whereas at the same speed a 2.6 kg dog on a flat surface uses about 58.4 ml O_2/kg/min.

Strangely, the difference in economy between walking and running observed in humans is not seen in other species. If the data of Figure 13–16 are considered, it should be obvious that a speed of 4 km/hour is less than an average walk for a horse, whereas 8 km/hour is certainly no more than a slow trot. The point is that if economy of locomotion at the same speed among species is compared, moderate speed for one species would be maximum speed for smaller spe-

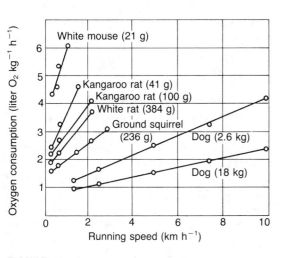

FIGURE 13–15
Oxygen consumption of mammals of different sizes
while running. From R. Taylor et al, Scaling the Energy
Costs of Running to Body Size in Mammals, *Am. J.
Physiol.* 219(1970):1104–1107. Reprinted by permission
of the American Physiological Society, Bethesda, Md.

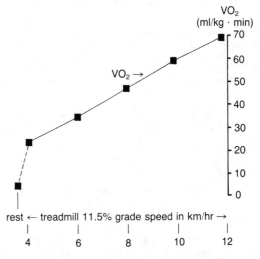

FIGURE 13–16
Cost of locomotion at different speeds in the horse. Data
represent five animals. Oxygen uptake is indicated by
VO_2. From D. P. Thomas and G. F. Fregin, Cardiorespiratory and Metabolic Responses to Treadmill Exercises in the Horse, *Am. J. Physiol.* 50(1981):864–868.
Reprinted by permission of the American Physiological
Society, Bethesda, Md.

cies. When velocity is maintained at a constant speed for different species, data showing energy consumed per kilogram body weight are meaningless. But based on the original definition of cost of locomotion (i.e. the energy necessary to move one unit of body mass over one unit of distance), such data have both ecological as well as evolutionary significance.

SUMMARY

Mammals consume food as an energy source as well as a source of structural elements. The breakdown of substances to release chemical energy is called catabolism, and the synthesis of compounds in the cell is called anabolism. Metabolism comprises all of the catabolic and anabolic reactions.

Adenosine triphosphate (ATP) is the substance most often used as a direct energy source in mammals. The catabolism of glucose to yield ATP can be separated into an anaerobic pathway (the Embden-Meyerhoff pathway) and an aerobic pathway (the Krebs or tricarboxylic acid cycle). The production of ATP from ADP occurs by means of direct intermolecular transfer of a high-energy phosphate (substrate phosphorylation) and an exchange of energy between coupled reactions in the cytochrome or electron transport system (oxidative phosphorylation). Substrate phosphorylation occurs in both the Embden-Meyerhoff pathway and the Krebs cycle and can occur in the absence of oxygen through the buildup of lactic acid, or oxygen debt. Oxidative phosphorylation involves hydrogen and electron transfer in order for ATP to be synthesized. Three hydrogen transport substances pick up hydrogen along with its electron and transport them to the cytochrome system. Coupled reactions in the electron transport chain lead to the formation of high-energy phosphates.

Fatty acids, the principal lipid fuel source, are catabolized by beta oxidation within the cells to yield acetyl groups in combination with coenzyme A. Acetyl CoA is then catabolized to form carbon dioxide and yield hydrogens by the Krebs cycle. Because of the aliphatic nature of fatty acids, these lipids yield more energy per gram than do other fuel sources. The net result of fatty acid catabolism also yields a greater quantity of metabolic water per unit weight than do the other sources of chemical energy metabolized by mammals.

Protein catabolism for the production of ATP must accompany deamination followed by urea synthesis. The net production of energy by protein is less than that obtained from the metabolism of other fuel sources because some energy must be used in the production of urea. In addition to its reduced energy yield, protein catabolism results in a net loss of water. Urea, which is voided through the kidneys, is accompanied by the loss of more water molecules than can be synthesized from an amino acid substrate.

More heat is generated when each of the fuel substances is catabolized in excess of the heat content of the substrate. This heat, which is greatest when proteins are being used for energy, must be derived from other substances in the cell that are undergoing reactions pertinent to catabolism of the fuel substrate. The processes which contribute to this additional heat are said to result from specific dynamic actions (SDA) of the substrate.

Each substance metabolized produces a specific volume of carbon dioxide and uses a specific amount of oxygen. The ratio of carbon dioxide produced to oxygen consumed is called the respiratory quotient (RQ) for the substance. When the carbon dioxide and oxygen associated with protein catabolism are accounted for, the ratio of remaining carbon dioxide and oxygen is called the nonprotein respiratory quotient (NPRQ).

Heat produced by the metabolism can be measured directly by means of a calorimeter or indirectly through analysis of oxygen consumption rates. The total heat generated from the combustion of food sources can be measured by a bomb calorimeter.

Basal metabolic rate can be measured when an animal is at rest and at ambient temperatures which do not cause above normal heat production. This is considered to be the metabolic rate necessary for minimum maintenance. It has been known for some time that basal metabolic rate on a gram-weight basis is greater in small mammals than it is in large mammals. Heat production of members of different species becomes more uniform when compared as a function of the percentage of the total weight of the animal represented by metabolic tissue.

When energy expenditures by mammals of differing body size are compared, it is obvious that larger mammals have a greater economy of locomotion. In addition, flying mammals have been found to show greater economy over those species restricted to terrestrial locomotion. The greatest economy of all, however, is found in aquatic animals, since the buoyancy provided by water almost completely negates the need for support against gravity.

14

THE EXCRETORY SYSTEM
AND WATER BALANCE

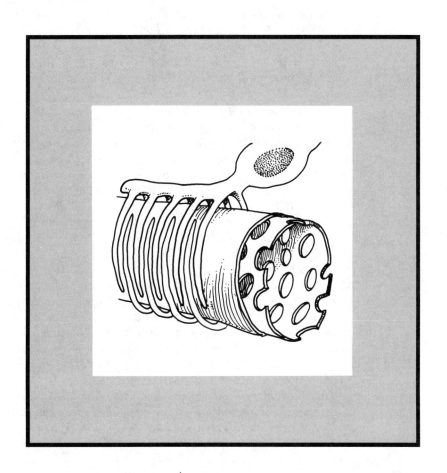

*T*he kidney of the mammal develops from embryonic mesodermal tissue and consists of two principal portions, as shown in longitudinal section (see Figure 14–1). The outer portion, or cortex, is extremely well vascularized and delicate and is contained within a tough membrane called the capsule. In many mammals, such as cattle and goats, the cortex is divided into lobes. In humans and dogs, the cortex is smooth in appearance and is not lobular. The inner portion, the medulla, is lighter in color, contains fewer capillaries, and is tougher and more coarsely textured.

The entire kidney is well vascularized by a branch of the dorsal aorta called the renal artery, which further divides into smaller branches to form the interlobar arteries (see Figure 14–2). These, in turn, form arcuate arteries. The arcuate arteries divide into smaller vessels called interlobular arteries. These give rise to afferent arterioles, which enter the densely coiled small vessels of the glomeruli. Blood passing through the glomeruli enters the efferent arterioles, passes through the peritubular capillaries and then into the interlobular vein. It then enters the arcuate vein, which anastomoses with other arcuate veins to form interlobar veins. The interlobar veins ultimately converge to form the renal vein, which drains into the vena cava.

The functional unit of the kidney is called the nephron (see Figure 14–3). The bulbular part of the nephron, Bowman's capsule, surrounds the glomerulus, where plasma filtration occurs. Mention should be made here of the anatomical relationship between Bowman's capsule and the glomerulus, which allows plasma filtration to take place. There are three distinct layers through which plasma must be filtered: (1) the capillary endothelium; (2) the basal lamina, which lies between the capillary and the epithelial cells of the kidney; and (3) the slits formed by these epithelial cells, or podocytes (see Figure 14–4). The pores of the endothelium are approximately 100 nanometers (nm) in diameter in the human, and the pseudopodia of the epithelial cells form slits along the capillary wall that are approximately 25 nm wide. No pores or gaps are apparent in the basal lamina. The upper limit in size of filtered substances is about 8.0 nm; therefore, the basal lamina or some other factor, such as surface charge, must limit the size of the particles which are filtered. From the size of the endothelial pores and the gap width between podocytes, one would expect much larger particles to pass.

The remainder of the nephron consists of the proximal and distal convoluted tubules and the ascending and descending portions of the loops of Henle, which are all involved in the exchange of materi-

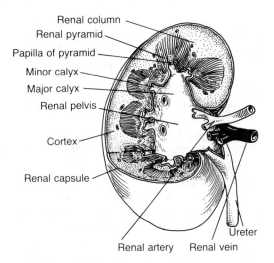

FIGURE 14–1
Longitudinal section through the kidney illustrating gross internal anatomy

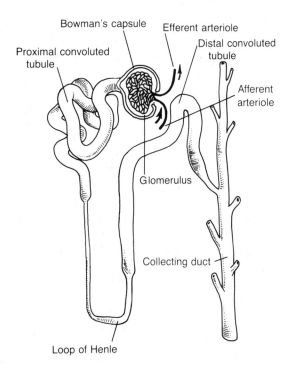

FIGURE 14–3
A typical nephron found in the mammalian kidney

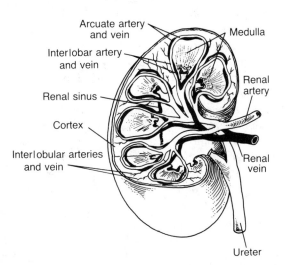

FIGURE 14–2
Arterial circulation of the kidney as seen in cross-sectional view. Veins closely parallel the arteries.

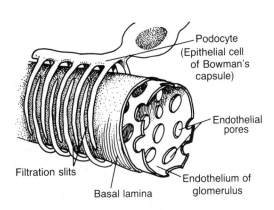

FIGURE 14–4
Membranes of the glomerulus and Bowman's capsule through which plasma filtrate must pass

als between the plasma and the filtrate by diffusion and active transport. Plasma is filtered from the glomerular blood into the cavity of Bowman's capsule and passes into the proximal convoluted tubule, which enters a relatively long, thin-walled portion of the nephron called the loop of Henle. The convoluted tubules and the loop of Henle are closely followed along their entire lengths by the peritubular capillary, which with the glomerulus allows for close contact between the nephron and the circulatory system. The distal convoluted tubules coalesce to form the collecting ducts. A number of collecting ducts converge to form the renal pyramids, which empty into the primary cavity of the kidney, the renal pelvis. Once the filtrate enters the renal pelvis it can be called urine. It then flows from the pelvis through the ureters into the bladder for storage. As urine builds up in the bladder, increased pressure activates stretch receptors in the smooth muscles which form its walls. At a critical pressure, these stretch receptors induce relaxation of the sphincter valve at the juncture of the bladder and its externally directed tube, the urethra. Subsequent contraction of the bladder muscles increases the urine flow and micturition (urination) follows. In the male the urethra exits the body through the penis, and in the female the urethra leads to the vulva.

Two relatively distinct types of nephrons are found in the mammalian kidney (see Figure 14–5). In mammals inhabiting a moist or aquatic environment, most of the nephrons are located in the cortex and adjacent to the outer zone of the medulla. By reason of their location these are known as cortical nephrons. Mammalian species well adapted to arid regions have an abundance of nephrons with elongated loops of Henle, which are known as juxtamedullary nephrons. The degree of adaptation of a species to xeric (dry) conditions is reflected in the relative number of juxtamedullary nephrons and the length of the loops of Henle. Desert animals such as the kangaroo rat have extremely long loops of Henle and can survive on metabolic water alone. Some mammals are able to retain water and excrete a urine of such great osmotic concentration that they can successfully consume marine or brackish water without noticeable discomfort.

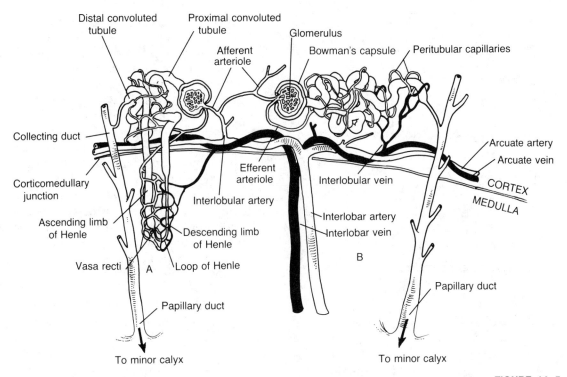

FIGURE 14–5

Contrasting positions of cortical and juxtamedullary nephrons in the mammalian kidney. Note the loop of Henle of the juxtamedullary nephron and its position relative to the kidney medulla.

EVOLUTION AND DEVELOPMENT

Primitive vertebrates have evolved from organisms which originally inhabited fresh water, and thus, survived in an environment hypotonic to their cellular fluids. Thus, the first vestiges of the vertebrate kidney functioned primarily to remove excess water from the organism while retaining the essential ions. These primitive structures were probably similar to the *nephridia* of modern invertebrates, which take on a segmented arrangement in the *coelom* rather than being collected into the paired organs which form the renal system of modern vertebrates (see Figure 14–6A). In these primitive organisms, the glomerulus or adjacent capillaries functioned only as a means of exchanging materials between the blood and the coelomic fluid. In later adaptations, the glomerulus was closely attached to the nephron, but the connection with the coelomic cavity still existed (see Figure 14–6B). Finally, all connection with the coelom was lost, and a typical nephron evolved which was capable of both exchanging materials with the bloodstream and reducing water loss, traits necessary for terrestrial survival (see Figure 14–6C). In this manner basic evolution of the nephridia probably preceded the kidney as an organ of excretion.

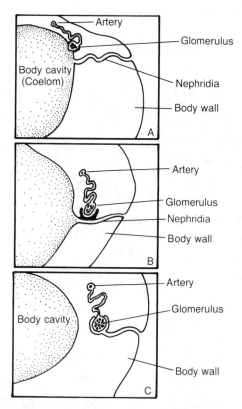

FIGURE 14-6
Possible evolutionary stages (A to C) in the development of the mammalian nephron

The mammalian kidney provides numerous advantages over the primitive excretory system of evolutionary predecessors. It does not retain direct (open) connection with the coelom; therefore, fluid removal need not be constant and can be regulated through pressure and quantity of blood flow to the nephron. Mammals can maintain a high pressure filtration system and more efficiently regulate ions through active transport. The mammalian kidney therefore frees its bearer from a constant source of water because its easily modified regulatory system is able to control the rate of water loss.

Embryological development of the mammalian kidney shows a series of changes in the development of the excretory system which terminates in the formation of a kidney. The first kidney in mammals is called the *pronephros*. This usually consists of a series of cell masses between the fourth and fourteenth somites. Glomeruli form with the pronephros which protrude into the coelom. The *pronephric duct*, formed by the lateral ends of the pronephric tubes, grows back to the *cloaca*. It is not known if excretory products are formed by the pronephric kidney. The pronephric duct leads to the development of the *mesonephros* and the *metanephros*. The mesonephros forms a prominent ridge behind the pronephros and contains a number of tubules with invaginated walls to accent the glomeruli. The mesonephric tubules also open into the pronephric duct and in some cases probably excrete urine.

The pronephros disappears completely in mammals. The mesonephros forms the *vasa efferentia* and the *paradidymis* in the male of the species and the *epoopheron* in the female of the species. Consequently, in early development both the urinary and genital systems are closely intertwined, as they are in adults of the more primitive vertebrates. For example, in lampreys genital products of both sexes are shed into the main coelomic cavity, which in this case can be considered an expanded genital sac. In the adult mammal, the kidney is formed from the metanephros, which was in turn formed from the mesoderm. All elements of a well-developed glomerulus are present, with the collecting tubules opening into a central pelvis of the kidney rather than a duct which runs the length of the body cavity. The only true link in the adult with the pro- and mesonephros of the embryo is the connection of the ureter to the posterior end of the pronephric duct, which in the adult is called the Wolffian duct.

KIDNEY FUNCTION

Filtration

The removal of proteins and large blood-borne particles by screening the plasma through microscopic pores in the glomerulus is known as *filtration*. This process is the result of several individual forces giving rise to a net force called the *filtration pressure* or *net pressure*. The causative factors of filtration pressure are: (1) *hydrostatic pressure*, which results from the pressure of the blood as it enters the glomerulus; (2) hydrostatic pressure in Bowman's capsule, which opposes the hydrostatic pressure of the blood; and (3) *colloidal-osmotic pressure*, which results from the protein molecules such as albumins and globulins in the plasma which are stopped by the glomerular membrane. An example of net pressure determination and its relationship to individual pressures with Bowman's capsule is given in Figure 14–7. Since filtration only leaves behind such large molecules as the plasma proteins, the osmotic concentration of the filtrate in the normal kidney is essentially equivalent to the osmotic pressure of the blood plasma minus its proteins.

The rate at which plasma is filtered in the glomerulus is defined as the *glomerular filtration rate (GFR)*. In the human the glomerular filtrate is produced at an average rate of 125 milliliters per minute, or about 200 liters per day. If this average rate is compared to the normal intake of fluids, it is evident that the body would be rapidly dehydrated if some mechanism for returning most of the

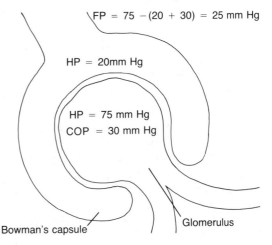

FP = 75 − (20 + 30) = 25 mm Hg

HP = 20mm Hg

HP = 75 mm Hg
COP = 30 mm Hg

Bowman's capsule

Glomerulus

FIGURE 14–7
Diagrammatic illustration of pressure relationships in the kidney (HP, hydrostatic pressure; COP, colloidal-osmotic pressure; and, FP, filtration pressure, net pressure). The filtration pressure is equal to the capillary hydrostatic pressure minus the capsule hydrostatic pressure plus the colloidal-osmotic pressure of the capillary.

filtrate back into the plasma did not exist. In most mammals, returning fluid is ultimately a function of the anatomical and functional relationship which exists among the collecting duct, parts of the convoluted tubules, and the loop of Henle. This relationship will be taken up in detail later, especially in relation to its importance in adaptation of mammals to habitats of varying water conditions.

Measurement of the glomerular filtration rate was very difficult prior to the discovery of an organic substance called *inulin* which passes freely from the blood into Bowman's capsule during the formation of the glomerular filtrate. Inulin is subsequently neither secreted nor absorbed by the nephron and remains in rather constant concentration after it is filtered. Thus, the plasma is cleared of this substance at a rate equal to the rate at which it is filtered and subsequently excreted in the urine. By definition the *renal*

clearance or plasma clearance rate is equal
to the volume of plasma completely cleared
of a substance or from which the substance
is completely removed per unit time (usually
one minute). The filtration rate is simply the
volume of plasma filtered through the membranes of Bowman's capsule each minute. In
humans one-fourth of the renal plasma flow
is filtered each minute, which amounts to
about one-twentieth of the total cardiac output (5 liters/min). In the case of inulin, both
filtration rate and clearance rate are equal
since the substance is neither secreted into
nor actively absorbed from the lumen of the
nephron.

Quantitatively, this can be determined in
terms of milliliters of plasma cleared each
minute. The glomerular filtration rate of inulin can be determined by the following equation:

$$GFR = \frac{UV}{P} \qquad (14.1)$$

where,

GFR = glomerular filtration rate (ml/min)
 U = concentration of inulin in the urine
  (mg/ml)
 V = volume of urine (ml/min)
 P = plasma concentration of inulin (mg/ml)

In determining the glomerular filtration
rate in an experimental animal or a clinical
patient, the subject is first injected with a
known amount of inulin, which is allowed to
mix uniformly throughout the plasma. Then
a sample of blood is removed and the concentration of inulin is determined. The rates
of urine production and urine inulin concentration are then determined and the values
are plugged into equation 14.1.

If the clearance rate of a substance is
greater than the glomerular filtration rate, it

must be assumed that, in addition to being
filtered, the substance must also be actively
secreted from the blood into the lumen of
the nephron. On the other hand, if the clearance rate is less than the filtration rate, the
substance must be actively absorbed from
the nephron and taken back into the blood.
If plasma is completely cleared of a substance as it passes through the kidney, the
clearance rate must be equal to the renal
plasma flow. In the average human this is approximately 500 milliliters per minute. Para-
aminohippuric acid (PAH) is a substance
which is almost completely cleared as blood
flows through the kidney. This phenomenon
is useful to both researchers and clinicians,
since by determining the rate of clearance of
PAH total renal plasma flow can be determined. When this value is divided by the hematocrit (percent of whole blood occupied
by the red blood cells, which is usually 42 to
48 percent for mammals), the renal blood
flow can be determined.

Ion Regulation: Secretion and Absorption

Ions obtained through the food or drinking
water of mammals are usually of different relative concentrations in comparison to the
concentrations in the blood. The water consumed is usually hypotonic to mammalian
blood, and ions must be absorbed as water is
removed by the kidney. When large quantities of ions are consumed, water must be retained and salts must be lost through the
urine in order to maintain the proper ionic
balance. For instance, herbivorous animals
consume food high in potassium, but their
blood and extracellular fluids rely principally
on sodium ions as the primary cation for
maintaining a favorable osmotic distribution.
As a result, herbivores must excrete a rela-

tively high amount of potassium and must absorb sodium in order to maintain a favorable salt concentration in the blood and other tissues. Mammals must maintain stable plasma concentrations of calcium and glucose, albeit these substances are also filtered and must constantly be reabsorbed to maintain adequate plasma levels.

Techniques developed in the mid-twentieth century allow researchers to study the concentration of dissolved materials in the filtrate as it passes through the nephron toward the collecting duct. By means of a *micropuncture technique,* using very small glass pipets only a few micrometers in diameter, the concentrations of fluids within the *lumen* (cavity) of the nephron and the fluid surrounding it can be determined. If an ion is being absorbed within the tubule, its concentration in the filtrate will be less than its concentration in the blood plasma or the surrounding interstitial fluid. The opposite, of course, is true where a substance is actively secreted within the kidney. In either secretion or absorption, energy must be expended in order to pump ions against their concentration gradients.

Several segments of the nephron can be distinguished morphologically, and the structures of these regions seem to be adapted for specific functions. For example, in the proximal convoluted tubule, microvilli are abundant on the *mucosal* (lumen) side. These microvilli enormously increase the to-

tal surface area. The increased numbers of microvilli enhance active transport from the lumen of the nephron by providing greater surface area for interaction between solutes and specific membrane sites, where the solutes must be bound before active transport can take place. Where surface areas are greater, active transport can also be greater; in other words, specific solutes can be removed from the filtrate more rapidly. Mitochondria, which supply energy in the form of ATP for active transport, are grouped on the serosal side (exterior portion of the organ). Due to the rapid metabolism of the mammalian kidney, a large oxygen demand exists. For example, this rate in the human kidney is 6.0 milliliters per 100 grams of tissue per minute, compared to 3.3 milliliters per 100 grams per minute in the human brain.

In the case of most terrestrial mammals, water is readily available and the primary role of the nephron becomes that of *ion regulation,* or maintaining very accurately the specific levels of ions within the blood. Thus, active transport of certain ions from the filtrate back into the plasma to avoid depletion becomes essential (see Figure 14–8). Each dissolved substance retained by the body has a *maximum reabsorption concentration.* Any concentration above this maximum amount is lost through the urine. This can be explained through a closer look at active transport.

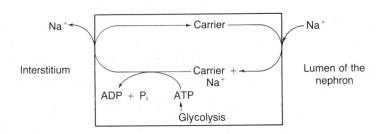

FIGURE 14–8

Active transport is an energy-requiring mechanism which is essential in reabsorption of essential ions filtered through the glomerulus

There are very specific enzymes for each substance removed from the filtrate. These enzymes, which act as carrier molecules, occupy a finite number of receptor sites or positions on the mucosal wall of the nephron. In order to be transported, a substance must make contact with its specific transport enzyme, which binds it and then transports it to the serosal side of the nephron. In other words, there is a fixed number of enzymes present in the tubules which bind specifically with a given substance. Consequently, each ion or substance retained has its own maximum absorption (measured in mg/liter or mg percent) called the *tubular max (T max* or *transport maximum)*. Specific carrier molecules exist for each substance absorbed from the tubule. When concentration of a substance is high enough to exceed the number of available transport enzymes, it has exceeded its transport maximum and appears in the urine. An example of this phenomenon would be glucose with a T max of approximately 100 mg percent. Any abnormal condition, such as diabetes mellitus, that would cause plasma glucose concentrations to exceed this value would also cause the excess sugar to spill over into the urine.

In many cases, substances are taken into the bloodstream in much greater concentrations than they are utilized; in other cases, constituents in the food of the organism may not be utilized by the metabolism at all. Thus, active secretion into the renal tubules is desirable, and many substances are readily cleared from the plasma by renal secretion. A prime example of this can be seen in herbivores, which consume plant material high in potassium that is absorbed into the bloodstream via the intestine. Potassium thus acquired is actively secreted in the kidney to avoid *hyperkalemia* (i.e., excess blood potassium levels), which results in weakness and flaccid paralysis. Calcium ions, on the other hand, are absorbed in the kidney and thus can be maintained in ample supply for muscle contraction, synapse stability, blood clotting, and bone formation, as well as numerous other processes.

Composition of the Urine and Body Fluids

Mammals have been able to survive in very unfavorable conditions of water and solute concentrations, such as the deserts and oceans, where little if any free water is available. The ability of mammals to survive in these situations is largely dependent upon their ability to regulate the concentration of their internal body fluids. This stable internal osmotic condition was referred to by Claude Bernard as the constancy of the *internal milieu*, or internal mixture. Walter Cannon later coined the term *homeostasis* to describe the steady-state conditions which allow life to exist in the face of a changing external environment.

Not only must the tonicity of body fluids be regulated by mammals, but a careful regulation of individual ions to provide a favorable balance is also required. Toxic wastes which must also be eliminated from the body fluids are produced by metabolism. Hence, the kidney serves as an excretory organ as well as an ion and osmotic regulator.

Body fluid compartments within a mammal may be divided into *plasma* (the fluid portion of blood), · *interstitial fluid* (fluid which bathes the outside of the cells), and *intracellular fluid*. The comparative volumes occupied by the body fluids are shown in Figure 14–9. Inside the cells, fluid content varies considerably from tissue to tissue but

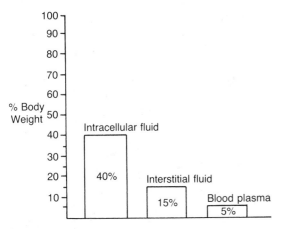

FIGURE 14–9
Body fluid compartments as percent of total body weight in humans

remains fairly constant in any particular cell type.

In some species of desert mammals, such as the camel and donkey, the tonicity of body fluids may vary considerably. These animals are able to survive the loss of large volumes of water from the body fluids which would be intolerable to many species. Relative ion composition is slightly variable from species to species but is quite stable within a species, except where adapted to desert or marine environments.

In essence the kidney functions to regulate ions, water content, pH, and other materials in the plasma. The concentrations of substances found in urine often reflect the rate at which they are taken into the body or the rate at which their precursors are utilized in metabolism. *Urea*, one of the principal products of protein metabolism, is voided through the skin by some mammalian species but is removed through the kidney in most species. Urea is toxic in high concentrations; and in conditions where protein is being rapidly metabolized (i.e., starvation), urea must be cleared from the blood almost as fast as it is formed. This basic homeostatic function is one of the kidneys' most important and essential roles as a life support system.

Water Balance

Most mammals live in areas adequately supplied with fresh water. But both marine and desert mammals must conserve water in order to survive. Unlike reptiles and birds, which sometimes have specialized salt-secreting glands, regulatory mechanisms of mammals are limited to the skin, respiratory system, digestive tract, and kidneys.

One of the most successful methods of water conservation employed by mammals has been the *countercurrent multiplier system*, which enables them to produce concentrated urine with a minimum gradient of active transport. Since concentration is usually measured as particle concentration regardless of ion or molecular species, the term osmolar as opposed to molar is used here. Two types of countercurrent systems will be described here: the countercurrent multiplier and the countercurrent exchanger. Both are extremely important in thermoregulation as well as water balance. In all countercurrent systems, fluids must move in opposite directions (as the term implies) and favorable situations for diffusion of the substances to be exchanged must be available. In the countercurrent exchanger, fluids must move past each other in opposite directions in closely aligned vessels (see Figure 14–10). In the countercurrent multiplier, it is essential that a hairpin or short loop be incorporated and that only one system of flow be involved (see Figure 14–11). The kidney of desert and semi-

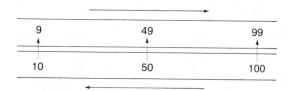

FIGURE 14-10
Countercurrent exchanger. Flow directions are indicated
by solid lines with arrows. Materials and direction of exchange are indicated by dashed lines with arrows.

desert mammals, which is adapted to xeric
conditions, has an abundance of nephrons
that act as countercurrent multipliers. In addition, parts of the nephron act as countercurrent exchangers.

The nephron in Figure 14–12 represents a
countercurrent multiplier which is able to increase the ion concentration filtered from the
plasma to create a steady state of increasing
concentrations from cortex to pyramid in the
kidney. In this system water diffuses from the
collecting ducts into the fluid surrounding
the nephron and is therefore not lost in the
urine. This type of concentrating mechanism
depends upon: (1) a permeable proximal
convoluted tubule and a permeable descending portion of the loop of Henle that allows
water to diffuse out and ions to diffuse in; (2)
an impermeable distal convoluted tubule

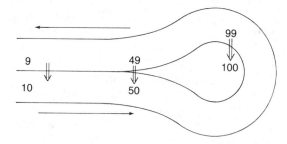

FIGURE 14-11
Countercurrent multiplier with one system of flow involving a hairpin loop. Direction of flow is indicated by solid
lines with arrows. ⇒ indicate active transport. Note that
the gradient for active transport is kept at a minimum.

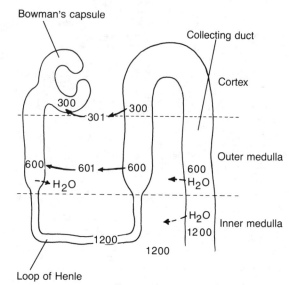

FIGURE 14-12
Countercurrent multiplier system created in the nephron
of the kidney. Solid → indicate active transport of chloride; dashed → indicate diffusion of water. The countercurrent multiplier of the nephron concentrates solutes
maximally at the bottom of the loop of Henle and the
collecting duct. Water follows its concentration gradient
as it exits the collecting duct.

and an impermeable ascending portion of
the loop of Henle that are able to remove
salts from the filtrate by active transport; and
(3) a permeable collecting duct that allows
water to diffuse into the interstitial (surrounding) fluid. Specifically, in mammals a
dilute fluid (the filtrate) is filtered and passes
by means of the descending convoluted tubule and the loop of Henle through an interstitial fluid of *increasing concentration*. Since
the descending tubules are permeable to
both water and ions, salts diffuse into the filtrate and water diffuses into the more concentrated surrounding fluid. The ascending
convoluted tubules are essentially impermeable to water; chloride ions are pumped out
by active transport, thus creating increasing
concentrations as the apex of the pyramid is

reached. The chloride ions are followed passively by sodium ions to maintain electric neutrality. Urea is also removed from the nephron by active transport and contributes to the osmotic gradient developed by sodium and chloride ions.

The principal economic value of the countercurrent multiplier system in the mammalian kidney from an energy standpoint is that a constant gradient, well within the realm of efficiency for active transport, can be maintained while the absolute concentration is increased. In this situation, the basic difference in concentration between the fluid of the nephron and the surrounding fluid is very slight, making the total gradient for active transport achievable. In other words, the relative difference between the two concentrations is slight, but the absolute concentration of the filtrate becomes greater as it reaches the apex of the loop of Henle. Since the collecting duct passes in a direction counter to the ascending tubules, water is free to diffuse out, leaving a concentrated urine within the lumen. It should be emphasized that adequate permeability of the collecting duct only occurs in the presence of sufficient *vasopressin*, or *antidiuretic hormone (ADH)*, which is released from the posterior lobe of the pituitary. Vasopressin is released as the result of an increase in plasma *osmolarity* (osmotic concentration), which is detected by *osmoreceptor cells* in the hypothalamus. This hormone circulates in the blood and binds specific proteins on the cell membranes of the collecting ducts, which increases their permeability to water. If enough water can be reabsorbed to reduce plasma osmotic concentration to its normal level, vasopressin release will be reduced and reabsorption in the kidney will likewise decrease.

Most mammals cannot concentrate urine or otherwise regulate water loss with great enough efficiency to avoid drinking water. When plasma osmotic concentration is high, a sensation of thirst is generated as the result of stimulation of osmoreceptor cells in the hypothalamus, and the animal seeks water. After the intake of water, vasopressin decreases and excess water may be lost through the urine *(diuresis)*.

The ability of mammals to conserve water is reflected in their ecological distribution. In some desert animals, the urine has a pasty, thick consistency due to the high solute concentration. Obviously, all desert animals lose some water through respiration, urination, or defecation, and, in some cases, water is lost through the skin as well. Essential water lost by any means must be replaced. In those mammals which do not drink water, survival depends upon the production of metabolic water, which is produced as a by-product of oxidative metabolism (see chapter 13, Metabolism).

Mammals which are better adapted to xeric conditions have longer loops of Henle and a greater percentage of juxtamedullary nephrons when compared to the number of nephrons limited to the cortex. A mammal such as the kangaroo rat, which can survive without drinking water, has very long nephrons with loops of Henle so long that they extend into the pelvis of the kidney. It should be obvious that the longer the length of the countercurrent system, the greater will be the efficiency for the active transport of substance, because a lower gradient for active transport can be established. Likewise, the greater the percent of juxtamedullary nephrons, the greater the volume of filtrate that can be concentrated. In order to better visualize the job performed, consider the structure in Figure 14–13, where a gradient is reached that makes active transport impossible. In this system each successive cell has

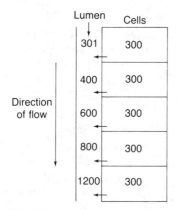

FIGURE 14–13
Hypothetical situation with cellular tonicity fixed at 300 milliosmoles with maximum concentration for urine reaching 1200 milliosmoles. This would be an impossible gradient, over which active transport could not function. Solid lines indicate theoretical direction of active transport.

a greater osmotic gradient than the preceding cell to move or pump ions against. In this situation where the ratio finally reaches four to one, a seemingly impossible gradient exists for active transport and urine concentration.

Control of Blood Pressure and Ion Exchange by the Kidney

Many of the nephrons, approximately one-third in the human kidney, pass through a very densely packed group of cells known as the *juxtaglomerular apparatus*. In those nephrons associated with the apparatus, the smooth muscles of the afferent and efferent arterioles are modified so that their function is secretory rather than contractile. When pressure in the arterioles decreases, their walls tend to collapse against the rather rigid juxtaglomerular cells, causing the physical deformation of the modified smooth muscle, which triggers the release of renin. Renin

acts indirectly to affect blood-hydrostatic pressure and colloidal-osmotic pressure.

The primary role of renin in controlling hydrostatic pressure is to act as a catalyst in the conversion of a plasma peptide, angiotensinogen to angiotensin I. The final product, angiotensin II, is formed automatically from angiotensin I due to the presence of a plasma factor already present. Angiotensin II is the active peptide of the series and acts directly upon vascular smooth muscle to induce vasoconstriction and thus cause increased peripheral resistance. After blood pressure returns to normal, renin secretion ceases due to distention of the arterioles in the juxtaglomerular apparatus (see chapter 10, The Circulatory System and Blood Pressure).

In addition to the direct effects of angiotensin II upon smooth muscle, when it is carried to the *adrenal gland*, it induces the release of the steroid hormone *aldosterone* from the *zona glomerulosa* of the *adrenal cortex*. Aldosterone is the principal *mineralocorticoid*, or steroid hormone, important to mineral reabsorption in the nephron. As a result of the action of aldosterone, more sodium and chloride ions are reabsorbed from the filtrate, resulting in higher osmotic pressure of the plasma. As more ions are reabsorbed and osmotic pressure of the plasma increases, more water is retained in the blood and blood pressure increases. Thus, through the vasoconstriction effects and the promotion of aldosterone production from the adrenal cortex, the production of angiotensin II in the plasma has a net effect of increasing systemic blood pressure.

Control of Plasma and Urine pH

Urine varies widely in pH, but plasma must be maintained at a relatively constant pH in the normal animal. The accomplishment of this difference is the result primarily of the effective job performed by the kidney in maintaining the pH of the blood. The mechanisms by which plasma pH is maintained are closely associated with cellular respiration and the sodium level in the plasma. In the tissues, *carbon dioxide* is produced as a by-product of the oxidation of carbon compounds. Later, carbon dioxide passes into the red blood cells, and it is converted to *carbonic acid* in the presence of water and the enzyme *carbonic anhydrase.* Carbonic acid thus produced forms *sodium bicarbonate* upon ionization. This is filtered with the plasma into Bowman's capsule. In the tubules, sodium ion is actively reabsorbed, allowing the bicarbonate ion to react with hydrogen ions to form carbonic acid again. Carbonic acid is not a strong acid and therefore does not readily ionize. Hydrogen ions, by being bound to the bicarbonate ion in the filtrate, can be removed from the plasma and carried out of the body as carbonic acid.

Much of the carbon dioxide produced by the catabolism of carbon compounds is the result of kidney metabolism during reabsorption of sodium ions. Mammals normally maintain fairly high levels of sodium ions in the blood but excrete a large portion of the potassium ions taken into the body. In order to excrete potassium ions and retain sodium ions from the plasma, energy is required; and thus carbon dioxide is produced from metabolism in the tubular cells. Carbon dioxide is then converted by the kidney cells, in the presence of carbonic anhydrase, to carbonic acid, which is removed through the urine. Another salt of sodium found in the filtrate that is important to hydrogen ion removal is the *biphosphate ion,* which is available to combine with hydrogen ions in the same manner as described for bicarbonate (see Figure 14–14). The acid form of biphosphate is similar to carbonic acid, in that it has a low *dissociation constant* and the hydrogen ions which react with it are thus retained in the filtrate and pass into the urine.

In addition to the previously mentioned buffers, a third mechanism is essential for urine pH control. When the urine becomes acidic, as in the case of prolonged *acidosis,* the kidney cells secrete ammonia, which accepts hydrogen ions and allows for further sodium ion retention. Ammonia produced by the tubular cells is derived exclusively from *glutamine* in the presence of kidney *glutaminase* through the following reaction:

$$glutamine \xrightarrow{\text{glutaminase}} glutamic\ acid + NH_3$$

The ammonia thus produced combines with hydrogen ions to increase the pH of the urine. This process of ammonia production

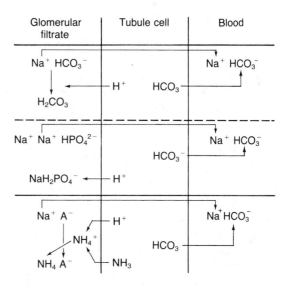

FIGURE 14–14
Buffering action in the kidney showing role of bicarbonate, biphosphate and ammonia

by the cells of the kidney tubules is relative to the acidity of the urine and has a sparing effect on sodium ions, which can be absorbed. The mechanism by which the production of ammonia is induced is unknown.

FACTORS AFFECTING URINE FORMATION

Plasma Solute Concentrations

When the osmotic pressure of the plasma increases due to excessive salt intake or water loss, certain cells of the hypothalamus sensitive to osmotic changes in the blood are stimulated. Stimulation of these cells of the so-called *osmotic center* of the brain results in increased ADH release. Antidiuretic hormone in turn increases the permeability of the collecting ducts to water and thus increases the retention of water by the kidney. At the same time salt is lost through the urine, and osmotic pressure of the plasma approaches normal. This is an opposite or antagonistic action to the role played by the adrenal gland and aldosterone.

Aldosterone functions to increase the sodium ion retention, causing an increase in plasma osmotic concentration. Aldosterone secretion is enhanced by several factors: (1) *adrenocorticotropic hormone (ACTH)* release from the pituitary (a transitory release), (2) release of renin by the kidney, and (3) a direct effect of increased levels of plasma potassium ion concentration. A sudden decrease in plasma sodium also seems to have a direct effect on the renal cortex to cause aldosterone release. Most of the changes of plasma electrolytes must be quite large before aldosterone secretion is effected. It is not likely that such changes play an important role in plasma electrolyte balance.

Diuretics

Substances which increase the flow of water from the body are referred to as *diuretics*. In most organisms substances such as caffeine and alcohol act directly upon the osmoreceptor cells of the hypothalamus to reduce their response to changing plasma osmolarity. The net result of this type of diuretic is to increase water loss from the body as the result of decreased vasopressin secretion from the posterior pituitary. An increased loss of water caused by these substances is usually followed by increased thirst after their effects have worn off because the net loss of water is greater than the amount consumed.

Other diuretics act directly upon the kidney to reduce active transport and thus reabsorption of solutes from the filtrate. Heavy metals, such as mercury and lead, are known to have this effect since they bind irreversibly to enzymes necessary for active reabsorption of sodium and other plasma solutes. Consequently, there is a loss of both salts and water, since loss of dissolved substances results in a corresponding loss of water.

When plasma solutes are increased to such a magnitude that further absorption is impossible, they begin to appear in greater quantities in the urine. Because of the *osmotic effect* (the attraction of water) by these substances, an increased urine flow is observed. Such a situation is referred to as *saline* or *osmotic diuresis*. Mammals which consume food or water of very high salt content must excrete the salt through the urine and thus, in the process, also lose a certain amount of water. The increase of urine when salt is consumed is one of the reasons that seawater consumption is out of the question for the survival of most mammals. Since seawater has a higher osmotic concentration than normal mammalian plasma, the net result of drinking it is the loss of body water through the kidneys due to saline diuresis. The consumption of fluids of high salt content, therefore, causes a greater loss of water than can be consumed and results in a negative water balance. But, some mammals, such as the kangaroo rat, can excrete urine which is more concentrated than seawater and can therefore extract water from saline solutions and retain it in the tissues. In other words, if the saline content of the urine maintained by means of the countercurrent mechanism is greater than the concentration of the salt in the filtrate, water can still be reabsorbed and thus utilized by the animal. This type of efficiency is found in only the few mammals that are adapted to desert habitats. No marine mammal investigated has been found to concentrate salts in great enough quantity to allow it to consume seawater for survival. It is assumed that water for these organisms must come from their food. Marine mammals that survive on marine invertebrates, which are often isosmotic with seawater (i.e., of the same salt concentration), present an especially difficult problem to explain. Further research in this area may lead to some exciting discoveries.

DISEASES THAT AFFECT KIDNEY FUNCTION

Some diseases common to humans and other mammals affect the kidney so predictably that the altered function of the kidney becomes the symptom of the disease. For instance, malfunction or decreased production of insulin by the *islets of Langerhans* results in a greater than normal blood sugar level. This condition is named *diabetes mellitus* ("honey-sweet" diabetes) because the suffer-

ers produce an excessive amount of urine which is sweet to the taste. The physiological explanation for the excessive fluid losses resulting from this disease is based upon two well-known principles. First, sugar appears in the urine because the transport maximum for sugar is exceeded in the plasma. Second, excessive water is lost by the diabetic because the excess sugar in the urine increases the fluid's osmolarity.

In another endocrine-related condition, an increase in urine flow occurs without the presence of sugar and with very low solute content. This is known as *diabetes insipidus*, which is characterized by an increased flow of tasteless urine. In this form of diabetes the posterior pituitary releases insufficient amounts of vasopressin and the collecting ducts become impermeable; water absorption is thus effectively blocked. Without the ability to absorb water in the collecting duct, a large volume of urine is lost that has relatively few solutes.

Another condition in which kidney function is impaired occurs when the glomerular membrane is damaged so that protein (and, in severe cases, red blood cells) that is normally filtered out appears in the urine. This condition, known as *glomerular nephritis*, can result from several conditions which cause increased porosity, or breakdown of the membrane of Bowman's capsule.

SUMMARY

The kidney is structurally designed to receive 20 to 25 percent of the cardiac output and is equipped with nephrons for filtering plasma, exchanging ions with the plasma, and concentrating urine. It has evolved from an organ whose primary function was ion regulation to one that is part of the numerous regulatory mechanisms which maintain blood homeostasis. It functions in the regulation of blood tonicity, pH, and pressure. In addition, it provides a major route of excretion of nitrogenous wastes and excess inorganic ions.

The basic unit of function of the kidney is the nephron, which consists of Bowman's capsule for filtration as well as the ascending and descending convoluted tubules and the loops of Henle for secretion and absorption. Through the action of salt accumulation in the extracellular fluid, the nephron is able to produce a hypertonic urine without an exceptionally great concentration gradient for active transport. To aid in the concentration of urine, vasopressin is secreted by the posterior pituitary in response to several internal stimuli. Vasopressin increases the permeability of the collecting ducts so that water may be extracted from the filtrate to form urine.

Several factors affect kidney function, such as the intake of fluids through the gastrointestinal tract, diuretics, and a variety of diseases. If any factor upsets the ability of the kidney to carry out its homeostatic role, the results are seen as blood pressure changes, ion imbalance, and problems of water balance. Without completely normal kidney function, survival of the organism becomes impossible in many cases.

15

RESPIRATION

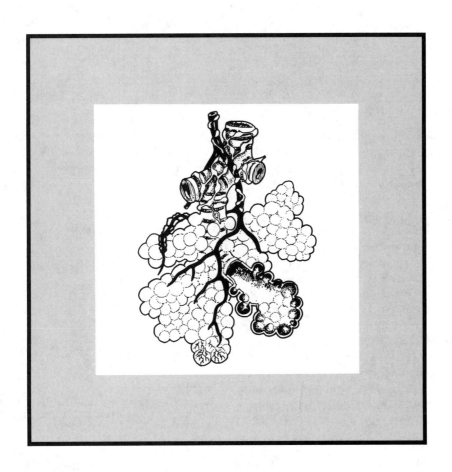

*R*espiration is the exchange of gases between metabolic tissues and the atmosphere. That exchange is sometimes called external respiration as opposed to internal respiration, which occurs within the cells where oxygen is utilized as an electron acceptor. Respiration in total is dependent upon diffusion of oxygen into the blood from the air within the lung, transport by the blood to the tissues, and diffusion from the blood into the tissues. The removal of carbon dioxide from the tissues follows this path in a reverse direction. Carbon dioxide, formed in the cells as a result of metabolism, diffuses into the blood and is carried to the lungs by the blood, where it diffuses out of the blood and into the air of the lungs.

Respiration is also dependent upon two vital processes which regulate gaseous exchange. In order for a favorable gradient of oxygen and carbon dioxide to exist, the lungs must be flushed regularly (breathing), and the transport substance (blood) must be circulated so that transfer to and from even the most distant tissues is a regular occurrence. In order for these two functions to be carried out efficiently, both breathing rate and blood flow must be regulated and coordinated.

CHARACTERISTICS OF AIR

Air is a mixture of gases containing approximately 78 percent nitrogen, 21 percent oxygen, 0.03 percent carbon dioxide, and a fraction of a percent of rare gases. At sea level the force of weight of these gases is approximately 760 millimeters of mercury (mm Hg), or pressure sufficient to support a column of mercury 760 mm in height (see Figure 15–1). The pressure of air at sea level is referred to as *one atmosphere*. That fraction of pressure exerted by a particular gas in a mixture such as air is known as its *partial pressure*. Every gas in a mixture expresses its own partial pressure irrespective of the other gases present. Thus, if air is 21 percent oxygen, the partial pressure of oxygen (P_{O_2}) is 760 mm Hg times 21 percent, or 159.6 mm Hg. Both the relative amounts of gases and their partial pressures in air are quite critical to the survival of mammals. An abnormal increase in the relative amount of any of air's constituent gases presents problems to the animal. The functional adaptations to changes in atmospheric pressures imposed by diving and

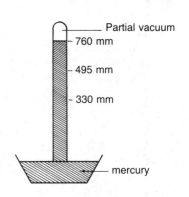

FIGURE 15–1
Diagram of mercury manometer at sea level. Atmospheric pressure at sea level is capable of maintaining a column of mercury 760 millimeters in height (in a vacuum).

high altitude will be discussed in detail in chapter 19, The Physiology of Some Specialized Mammalian Adaptations.

PULMONARY VENTILATION AND ITS REGULATION

The Respiratory Apparatus

The respiratory system of mammals culminates in blind-ended *sacs* in the lungs, into which air is drawn and expelled in a manner very similar to the action of a bellows. The *trachea*, the tube which connects the *pharynx* with the lungs, is elongated and straight except in cetaceans and sireneans. In most mammals the trachea forms two *bronchi*, each of which leads to a lung, where it divides to form *secondary* and *tertiary bronchi*. In pigs, whales, and some ruminants, a third bronchus, termed the *apical bronchus*, is formed on the right side. The division of bronchi into smaller tubes continues until the *terminal bronchioles* are formed. The final tubes through which air passes in the lungs are frequently called the *respiratory bronchioles* because of their thin walls, which occasionally have air sacs enabling oxygen to pass through them and into the blood (see Figure 15–2). Structurally, the difference between bronchi and bronchioles is that bronchi have rings or plates of elastic cartilage, elastic fibers, or both that maintain their shape. These cartilagenous rings are lacking in the bronchioles. Each respiratory bronchiole empties into an *alveolar sac*, which comprises a number of small, well-vascularized compartments called *alveoli*. It is in the alveoli that most gaseous exchange between air and blood occurs.

The lung volume usually bears a uniform relationship among mammalian species. When lung volume to body weight ratios of different species of mammals are compared, a fairly constant positive correlation is found (see Figure 15–3). The equation for the regression line in Figure 15–3 is as follows:

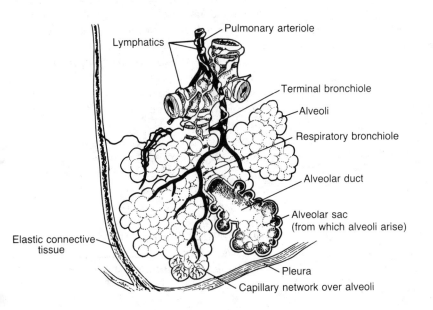

FIGURE 15–2
Microstructure of the lung showing respiratory bronchioles and alveoli

Pulmonary arteriole

Lymphatics

Terminal bronchiole

Alveoli

Respiratory bronchiole

Alveolar duct

Alveolar sac
(from which alveoli arise)

Elastic connective tissue

Pleura

Capillary network over alveoli

$$V = 0.0567 \, m_b^{1.02} \qquad (15.1)$$

where,

$$V = \text{lung volume (liters)}$$
$$m_b = \text{body mass (kilograms)}$$

From this equation, one can approximate the lung volume of a mammal in liters simply by knowing its weight. In a medium-sized dog which weighs 36 kg, lung volume should be 2 liters. In a man who weighs 75 kg, lung volume is approximately 4.5 liters. From these data it is obvious that lung volume is a direct function of body size and does not correlate well with metabolic rate. In other words, smaller mammals do not compensate for their rapid metabolism by having larger lungs

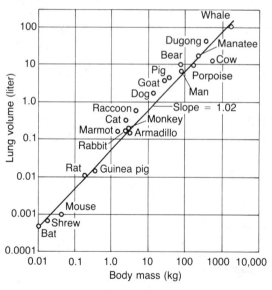

FIGURE 15–3

Lung volume to body size ratio in mammals. From S. M. Tenny and J. E. Remmers, Comparative Quantitative Morphology of the Mammalian Lung: Diffusion Area, *Nature*(London)197(1963):54–56. Reprinted by permission of Macmillan Journals, Ltd., London, U.K.

in proportion to their body volume. If metabolic rate and respiratory volumes showed strong correlation, small mammals would have disproportionately large lungs, and this is not the case. Increased magnitude of the Bohr effect and high P_{50} values (to be discussed later), in addition to increased capillary densities, high cardiac ouput, increased basal ventilatory rate, and increased carrying capacity of the blood are primarily responsible for maintaining oxygen supplies to the tissues of mammals with elevated metabolism.

Respiratory Volumes

During the breathing cycle air is inhaled and exhaled in proportion to the oxygen demand of the tissues. During rest, a volume of oxygen just necessary to maintain minimum metabolism is required. This quantity of air inhaled with one breath when the animal is at rest is referred to as *tidal volume* and varies considerably among species (see Table 15–1). Tidal volume, however, does not correlate well with metabolic rate. Breathing rate is quite similar and compensates for the differences in tidal volume among mammals having different metabolic rates (see Table 15–1). Thus, animals with high metabolic rates usually exhibit high rates of air exchange when compared to mammals whose metabolic rates are low.

When tidal volume is exhaled, a volume of air in excess of this can be forced out of the lungs called the *expiratory reserve volume* (see Figure 15–4). After the tidal volume has been inhaled, another volume can be drawn into the lungs called the *inspiratory reserve volume*. The total amount of air that can be exchanged is called the *vital capacity* and includes all of the lung volumes except a small

TABLE 15–1
Tidal volume and breathing rate (at rest) for several species of adult mammals

Species	Tidal Volume (milliliters)	Breathing Rate (breaths/min)
Horse *(Equus caballas)*	9,060	11.9
Cattle *(Bos taurus)*	2,700–3,400	30.0
Human *(Homo sapiens)*	750	11.7
Dog *(Canis familiaris)*	320	18.0
European rabbit *(Oryctolagus cuniculus)*	21	51.0
Norway rat *(Rattus norvegicus)*	0.86	85.5
House mouse *(Mus musculus)*	0.15	163.0

Source: From P. L. Altman and D. S. Dittmer, *Biology Data Book* (Bethesda, Maryland: Federation of American Societies for Experimental Biology, 1964)

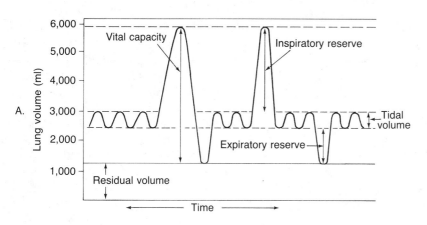

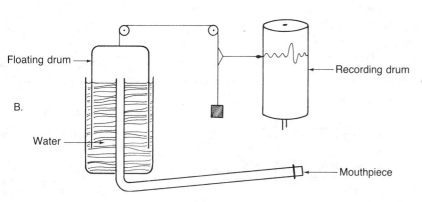

FIGURE 15–4
Measurement of lung capacities in a mammal: (A) chart showing recorded volumes and (B) spirometer for measuring lung volumes

amount of residual air, termed the *residual volume*, which cannot be exhaled. Parts of the respiratory "tree" which lack respiratory surfaces through which gases can be exchanged are referred to as *dead air spaces* or *dead space*. For instance, air in the trachea cannot be exchanged with gases in the blood and is therefore not directly involved with respiration. The volume of dead air space in mammals is quite variable. For instance, the human tidal volume is approximately 500 ml, but 150 ml of dead air space reduces the effective exchangeable quantity of air to about 350 ml. Some mammals with long trachea, such as the giraffe, have a tremendous amount of dead air space and must make up for it with either a rapid rate of breathing or a disproportionately large tidal volume. Some of the diving mammals have very short trachea and bronchi, presumeably as a means of reducing dead air space. The role of dead air space is reduced during exercise simply because it occupies a smaller percent of the total air exchanged. For instance, in humans during heavy exercise the amount of air exchanged with each breath can be as high as 5.0 liters. The dead air space in this case is only about 3.0 percent of the total as opposed to the nearly 30 percent that it occupies of the tidal volume at rest.

The volume of air breathed each minute is usually referred to as *respiratory minute volume*. This rate is closely correlated with oxygen consumption up to about 80 percent of maximum. Respiratory minute volume in the human reaches 150 liters per minute, with a tidal volume of 2.5 liters per inspiration during vigorous work (see Table 15–2). The breathing rate under these conditions is approximately 60 breaths per minute. In the horse, when running at a speed of almost 40 kilometers per hour, respiratory minute volume has been reported to reach 1,372 liters per minute. The repiratory minute volume and breathing rate should not be confused with the *respiratory rate*, which is the rate of oxygen utilization per unit tissue weight per unit time.

Mechanism of Breathing

In order for the mammalian bellows-type lung to function, the volume of the thorax must be changed to force air out of the lungs and draw it back in. This is done by means of the *muscular diaphragm* (which is unique to mammals), the intercostal muscles, and the abdominal muscles. These muscles make it possible to increase both the girth and length of the *thorax*. During inhalation the diaphragm contracts to lengthen the thorax while the external intercostals raise the rib cage and increase the diameter of the thorax (see Figure 15–5). When mammals are relaxed, exhalation is purely passive in nature and involves relaxation of the diaphragm and external intercostal muscles. But during forced exhalation the diaphragm relaxes and

TABLE 15–2
Respiration rate, tidal volume, and minute volume in the human at rest and during vigorous exercise

Calculation	At Rest	During Vigorous Exercise
Respiration rate/min	7–12	40–60
Tidal volume (liters)	0.4–0.6	2.5
Minute volume (liters/min)	2.8–7.2	100–150

Source: From B. Ricci, *Physiological Basis of Human Performance* (Philadelphia: Lea & Febiger, 1967)

EXPIRATION

INSPIRATION

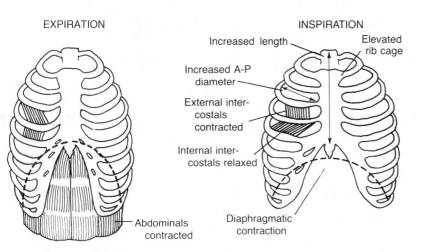

Increased length

Elevated rib cage

Increased A-P diameter

External inter-costals contracted

Internal inter-costals relaxed

Abdominals contracted

Diaphragmatic contraction

FIGURE 15–5

Changes in thorax during expiration and inspiration. Note that during inspiration, both the length and the width of the thorax are increased.

the abdominals contract, forcing the viscera cranially and hence reducing the length of the thoracic cavity. The internal intercostals also contract at this time, reducing the thoracic diameter and thus force air out.

To enable gas exchange in the mammal, the lungs must adhere closely to the shape of the pleural cavity. The outer lining of the lung, the *visceral peritoneum*, must adhere to the inner lining of the thorax, the *parietal peritoneum*, for the lungs to expand with the thorax during inhalation. When air is exhaled, the lungs are compressed by the thorax, causing them to become partially collapsed. As the internal cavities of the lung become expanded during inhalation, lower internal pressure is created which draws air into the lungs. Any adhesion of the epithelial lining within the lungs would prevent this. A phospholipid, *surfactant*, is produced inside the normal lung that acts as an emulsifier to reduce internal surface tension and allows the alveolar membranes to separate during inhalation. This substance thus prevents the adhesion of the internal lung surfaces. In the normal lung the amount of surfactant exceeds the theoretical minimum quantity

needed to cover the pulmonary surface area (see Figure 15–6). The absence of surfactant

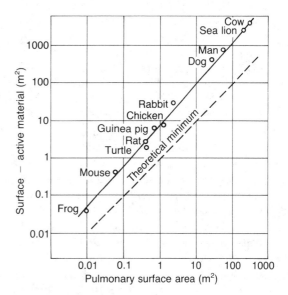

FIGURE 15–6

The amount of surfactant that can be extracted from the lungs of various mammals, compared as a function of the lung surface area in each species. From J. A. Clements et al, Pulmonary Surfactant and Evolution of the Lungs, *Science* 169(1970):603–604, fig. 1. Reprinted with permission. Copyright 1970 by the American Association for the Advancement of Science.

at birth in humans is known as *hyaline membrane disease*. In this condition the lungs of the newborn are unable to expand during inhalation, and suffocation occurs. The name hyaline membrane disease comes from the glossy appearance of adhering membranes inside the lungs when viewed in microscopic sections.

Regulation of Breathing

Breathing rate is regulated in mammals by means of an internal neural cycle, which can be modified by input from stretch receptors, chemoreceptors, and higher nerve centers. Specific neurons in the medulla oblongata and pons have been found to be primarily responsible for *breathing rhythmicity* (see Figure 15–7). The *medullary respiratory center* contains two types of neurons, some of which are associated with inspiration and some of which are associated with expiration. The neurons function as if they were separate oscillators integrated by means of inhibitory neurons. It would appear that oscillation begins in the *inspiratory neurons* (or the *inspiratory center*), which also inhibit the *expiratory neurons* (or the *expiratory center*). Inhibition continues until excitation stops, apparently from refractoriness or fatigue of the neurons, and action then begins in the expiratory neurons. In the resting state, exhalation is passive. But when the mammal is active, the expiratory center inhibits the inspiratory neurons and activates muscles of expiration.

The *pneumotaxic center* is located in the pons, where it affects the oscillatory regularity of the *medullary rhythmicity center*. In the intact animal stimulation of the pneumotaxic center increases breathing rate, thus the name for the center. It is apparently through this center that emotions such as fear and

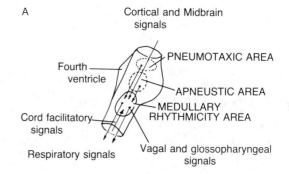

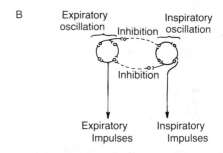

FIGURE 15–7
The respiratory centers of the human located in the medulla and pons (A). Also included is the theoretical mechanism of oscillation between the expiratory and inspiratory neuron (B). From A. C. Guyton, *Textbook of Medical Physiology*, 6th edition (Philadelphia, Pa., 1981), 516, fig 42–1. Reprinted by permission of W. B. Saunders Publishing Co.

excitement from the higher nerve centers stimulate breathing rate. If the centers in the pons are separated from the medulla, the rhythm of breathing is retained, though it lacks the usual regularity seen in the intact animal. The *apneustic center*, also located in the pons, is not necessary for the basic rhythm of respiration. It functions in the intact animal to prolong inspiration and reduce the time of expiration.

Chemoreceptors and control of breathing *Chemoreceptors* which affect respiration are located in various parts of the body. But the locations most generally sensitive to dissolved substances are located near the *carotid sinus*, the *aortic arch* (see Figure 15–8), and the *anterior region of the medulla* (see Figure 15–9). The chemoreceptors appear to respond predominantly to changes in carbon dioxide and hydrogen ion levels of the blood and only secondarily are affected by changes in oxygen concentration. An increase in plasma carbon dioxide or hydrogen ion concentration increases activity of both the aortic and carotid receptors and thus stimulates respiration. A drop in oxygen concentration likewise seems to induce activity in these receptors but does not normally do so because *reduced* or *deoxygenated hemoglobin (HHb)* is a much stronger hydrogen acceptor than is *oxyhemoglobin*. Therefore, *hypoxia* (i.e.,

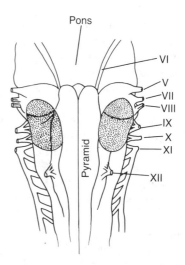

FIGURE 15–9
Ventral view of the brain stem showing respiratory chemosensitive areas on the medulla which respond to changes in pH of the cerebrospinal fluid. From R. A. Mitchell and J. W. Severinghaus, Cerebrospinal Fluid and Regulation of Respiration, *Physiol. Physicians* 3, no.3(1965):3, fig 1. Reprinted by permission of the American Physiological Society, Bethesda, Md.

lack of adequate oxygen) occurs simultaneously with a decrease in plasma hydrogen ion content, which initially negates the effect of oxygen depletion. If the nerve innervating the carotid body is severed, a decrease in oxygen no longer stimulates respiration but instead depresses activity of the respiratory neurons of the pons and medulla. This is apparently because the carotid body has no direct effect upon these centers of the brain and hypoxia is only reflected in their decreased metabolic activity.

The chemoreceptors of the brain stem are stimulated almost exclusively by hydrogen ions within the cerebrospinal fluid. Hydrogen and bicarbonate ions are prevented from entering the cerebrospinal fluid by the blood-brain barrier. But carbon dioxide readily enters the fluid, and with water it is converted to *carbonic acid* in the presence of *carbonic*

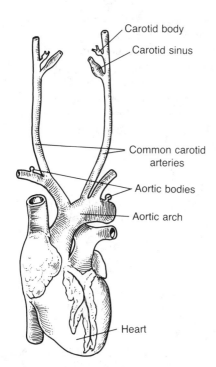

FIGURE 15–8
Location of the carotid and aortic bodies (chemoreceptors) in the human

anhydrase. The increase in carbonic acid lowers the pH of the cerebrospinal fluid, stimulating the chemoreceptors of the pons in a fashion parallel to its action in the carotid sinus and the aortic arch.

Stretch receptors and breathing rate
Stretch receptors that stimulate expiratory neurons of the medulla through the vagus nerve are located in the bronchi and bronchioles. When the stretch receptors are stimulated, the inspiratory center of the medulla is inhibited and the muscles of expiration are activated, causing the animal to force air out of its lungs. This reflex prevents overexpansion of the lungs and is called the *Hering-Breur reflex*. Other receptors located in the muscles and joints of the body also seem to affect respiration when stretched, but such effects are not easily demonstrated in the inactive animal. Yet, during exercise, plasma carbon dioxide, hydrogen ion, and oxygen concentrations usually remain constant in the healthy animal. Inactivity of chemoreceptors during exercise would mean that their influence is negligible and that other factors are involved with increasing breathing rate. It is thought that respiration is stimulated during exercise by activity in the cerebral cortex and by receptors located in the periphery of the body, such as stretch receptors and proprioceptors.

GASEOUS EXCHANGE IN THE LUNGS AND TISSUES

It should be emphasized that the exchange of gases between air and blood and between tissues and blood is primarily dependent upon existing diffusion gradients. In order for diffusion to occur, concentration gradients must be produced and maintained.

The partial pressure of oxygen in the lungs of mammals at sea level is approximately 110 mm Hg, whereas in the tissues it is near 30 mm Hg. The carbon dioxide concentration in the tissues is about 45 mm Hg and about 40 mm Hg in the lungs (see Figure 15–10). Oxygen and carbon dioxide must flow down their respective concentration gradients in order for oxygen to reach the tissues and carbon dioxide to reach the external air. The diffusion of oxygen from higher to lower concentrations between lung and blood and between blood and tissue is the primary mechanism for the exchange of oxygen at these points. This is true for carbon dioxide diffusion at each of these positions also.

It has been known for some time that when carbon dioxide is bubbled through whole blood *chloride ions* disappear from the plasma. In fact, chloride ions shift or move into the red blood cells in the presence of carbon dioxide, hence the name *chloride shift*. Carbon dioxide is produced in the tissues as a result of catabolism of body fuels. The amount of carbon dioxide which can be dissolved in the tissues is not great, and as a

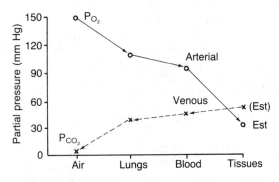

FIGURE 15–10
P_{O_2} and P_{CO_2} values showing concentration differences in various areas of their diffusion paths. From J. M. Kinney, Transport of Carbon Dioxide in Blood, *Anesthesiology* 21(1960):615. Reprinted by permission of J. B. Lippincott, Philadelphia, Pa.

$$CO_2 + H_2O \xrightleftharpoons[\text{Carbonic Anhydrase}]{} H_2CO_3$$

$$\updownarrows$$

$$H^+ + HCO_3^-$$

FIGURE 15–11
Role of carbonic anhydrase in the formation of carbonic acid

result most of it diffuses into the red blood cells, where it reacts with water in the presence of carbonic anhydrase (see Figure 15–11). The carbonic acid formed from carbon dioxide and water ionizes to produce the more soluble *bicarbonate ion* and *hydrogen ion*. As the negatively charged bicarbonate ion accumulates in the erythrocytes, it diffuses from the red blood cells into the plasma. Electrical neutrality is maintained by diffusion of negatively charged chloride ions into the red blood cells. Hydrogen ions produced from the formation of bicarbonate ion

react with oxyhemoglobin to release oxygen and form reduced hemoglobin. The oxygen thus released is free to diffuse into the tissues.

In addition to its reaction with water to form carbonic acid, carbon dioxide reacts with hemoglobin to produce *carbaminohemoglobin* (see Figure 15–12A). The formation of carbaminohemoglobin also reduces the affinity of hemoglobin for oxygen and increases the dumping effect of oxygen in the tissues. This mechanism insures that the tissues undergoing the most rapid metabolism receive maximum amounts of oxygen.

Thus, carbon dioxide is transported in the erythrocyte as dissolved carbon dioxide, as carbaminohemoglobin, and as bicarbonate ion. In the plasma fraction of blood it is transported as dissolved carbon dioxide, bicarbonate ion, and as carbamino compounds formed with plasma proteins. Of these, the bicarbonate ion is by far the most significant

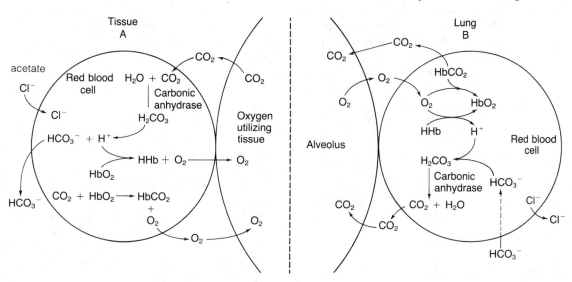

FIGURE 15–12
Reactions associated with oxygen and carbon dioxide transport in the blood: (A) erythrocyte in tissues where oxygen is being utilized and (B) erythrocyte in the lungs

mode of transportation because of its increased solubility in both red blood cells and the plasma.

When venous blood reaches the lungs, carbon dioxide is lost from the plasma into the alveoli in a manner consistent with its diffusion gradient. In addition, diffusion of oxygen into the erythrocytes is enhanced due to the relatively high concentration of oxygen in the alveoli. The reaction of hemoglobin with oxygen is dependent, in part, on the oxygen level (i.e., *mass-action effect*). In the lungs, hemoglobin reacts with oxygen and hydrogen ion is released (see Figure 15–12B). The hydrogen ion formed is free to react with bicarbonate to form carbonic acid. When the erythrocyte is in the lung capillaries, carbonic anhydrase promotes the formation of carbon dioxide and water. The direction of this reaction is controlled by the relative concentrations of the constituents; and, since carbon dioxide diffuses into the alveoli from the blood, more carbon dioxide is formed in the blood from the existing carbonic acid. Since the production of carbon dioxide and water reduces the carbonic acid concentration, more carbonic acid is formed as bicarbonate ion diffuses into the cell and is able to react with hydrogen ion released from the reduced hemoglobin. Chloride shifts from the red blood cells into the plasma and thus stabilizes the electrical charges across the membrane. Note that the reactions of hemoglobin with respiratory gases in the lungs are almost opposite those occurring in the tissues.

HEMOGLOBIN AND GAS TRANSPORT

Hemoglobin functions primarily as an oxygen-binding substance and in humans allows blood to transport about 20 ml of oxygen per 100 ml of blood. The amount of oxygen that can be absorbed per unit volume of blood is its *oxygen-carrying capacity*. The oxygen-carrying capacity of blood varies among species as a function of hemoglobin concentration and of the specific characteristics of hemoglobin within the blood. In some species, such as the horse and the cat, the carrying capacity varies considerably depending upon demand of the tissues for oxygen. These mammals store red blood cells in their spleen and release them into the bloodstream during exercise. In this way they immediately increase the volume of oxygen which can be transported by a particular volume of blood. The carrying capacity of the blood of most mammals increases in situations where there is an increased metabolic demand, such as cold exposure and exercise. Synthesis of erythrocytes and hemoglobin is stimulated as part of the process of becoming cold acclimated or physically fit. Thus, hematocrit increases over a period of a few days to a few weeks, and the carrying capacity of the blood is correspondingly increased.

The hemoglobin content of human blood is approximately 15g to 100 ml blood, or 15g percent, and is a fairly uniform value for other terrestrial species of mammals. For example, average hemoglobin concentration in the mouse is 14.8g percent; in cattle the value is about 11.5g percent; in dogs 14.8g percent; in rhesus monkeys 12.6g percent. It is noticeably low in those animals which can alter their red blood cell volume through spleen storage. For instance, in the resting horse hemoglobin content is only about 11.1g percent; in the domesticated cat, only 11.2g percent.

Mammalian hemoglobin contains four subunits, each consisting of a protein and a

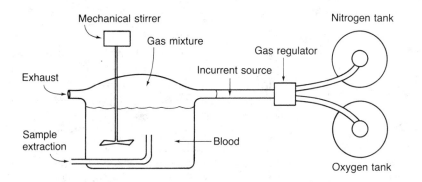

FIGURE 15–13
Apparatus for exposing blood
to gas mixtures in order to
determine saturation curve

porphyrin portion. When each of the sub-units becomes attached to an oxygen molecule, the hemoglobin is said to be *saturated*. When a volume of blood is experimentally equilibrated with a gas containing a partial pressure of oxygen of 110 mmHg, 100-percent saturation of the hemoglobin is achieved (see Figure 15–13). The gas used is usually a mixture of oxygen and nitrogen with a total pressure of 760 mm Hg. As the partial pressure of oxygen is decreased, the percent saturation of hemoglobin also decreases. But the change in saturation does not bear an arithmetic (one-to-one) relationship to the change in partial pressure of oxygen (see Figure 15–14). In fact, the curve is said to be *sigmoid* because of its S-shaped configuration. The basis for the sigmoid hemoglobin saturation curve (or *dissociation curve*) is the changes in the binding states of the individual subunits of the hemoglobin molecule. Oxygen binding alters the positions of the protein strands which form the globin portion of the hemoglobin subunit. The corresponding positions of the heme moieties are said to be in the *relaxed* or *R state*, which favors oxygen binding, and in the *tense* or *T state*, in which oxygen binding becomes difficult. When the first subunit is attached to an oxygen molecule, the hemoglobin assumes the R state. Thus, the second and the third subunits are

easily oxygenated. After the third subunit has been oxygenated the hemoglobin molecule assumes the T state again, and the fourth subunit is relatively difficult to oxygenate. In essence, as each hemoglobin subunit is oxygenated, the quaternary structure of the hemoglobin molecule is altered so that the oxygen affinity of the remaining hemoglobin subunits is changed. Muscle hemoglobin

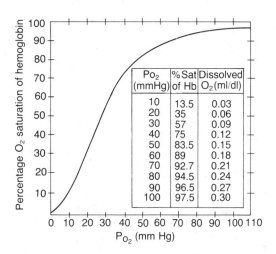

P_{O_2} (mmHg)	%Sat of Hb	Dissolved O_2 (ml/dl)
10	13.5	0.03
20	35	0.06
30	57	0.09
40	75	0.12
50	83.5	0.15
60	89	0.18
70	92.7	0.21
80	94.5	0.24
90	96.5	0.27
100	97.5	0.30

FIGURE 15–14
Oxygen hemaglobin dissociation curve at pH 7.4 and temperature 38° C. Reproduced with permission from Comroe, J. H., Jr., et al.: THE LUNG: Clinical Physiology and Pulmonary Function Tests, 2nd edition. Copyright © 1962 by Year Book Medical Publishers, Inc., Chicago.

(myoglobin) exists as a single molecular entity and therefore does not show a sigmoid saturation curve (see Figure 15–15).

The Affinity of Hemoglobin for Oxygen

The affinity of hemoglobin for oxygen in the organism is altered in several ways, all of which enhance the release of oxygen to the tissues. These factors are pH, temperature, concentration of *2,3-diphosphoglyceric acid (DPG)*, and concentration of carbon dioxide. When an animal exercises there is a local increase in carbon dioxide, hydrogen ion concentration, and temperature in the muscles performing the work. Since metabolism is greatest in those muscles which have performed the most exercise, one might say that there is *specific unloading of oxygen* at the site of maximum utilization. This phenomenon is possible because of the effects of metabolic by-products (i.e., temperature, carbon dioxide concentration, and hydrogen ion concentration) on the arrangements of the molecular subunits of the hemoglobin molecule.

When hemoglobin combines with hydrogen ions or with carbon dioxide, the oxyhemoglobin dissociation curve is shifted to the right (see Figure 15–16). This shift, known as the *Bohr effect*, signifies a decrease in the affinity of hemoglobin for oxygen. The change in affinity of hemoglobin for oxygen is the result of a position change in the beta chains of the hemoglobin molecule. When carbon dioxide or hydrogen ions become attached to hemoglobin or when hemoglobin is warmed as it passes through the capillaries of muscles during exercise, the *beta peptide chains* assume the *T configuration*. When the hemoglobin molecule assumes the T state its affinity for oxygen decreases, which enables more oxygen to be released at the tissue level.

In the lungs, where carbon dioxide is lost into the alveoli, hemoglobin more readily accepts oxygen. As carbon dioxide is lost more carbonic acid is formed, reducing the hydro-

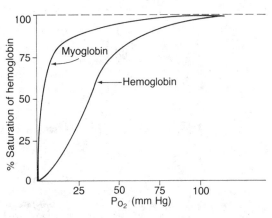

FIGURE 15–15
The saturation curves of myoglobin and hemoglobin

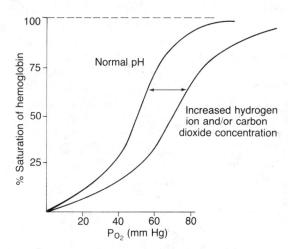

FIGURE 15–16
Effect of hydrogen ion and/or carbon dioxide concentrations and pH on the oxyhemoglobin dissociation curve (the Bohr effect)

gen ion concentration of the blood. Some of the hydrogen ions involved in the reaction of bicarbonate ion with hydrogen ion to form carbonic acid are reabsorbed from hemoglobin. The removal of carbon dioxide as well as hydrogen ion from hemoglobin increases its affinity for oxygen.

The acid 2,3-diphosphoglyceric is found in the red blood cells, where it is formed in the presence of *2,3-diphosphoglycerate acid mutase* (see Figure 15–17). It functions to reduce the affinity of hemoglobin for oxygen. DPG has been reported to increase in concentration after periods of exercise as short as one hour in unconditioned human subjects. Hypoxia is apparently the stimulus for its production; its formation is actually inhibited in well-conditioned atheletes during exercise due to increased concentrations of hydrogen ions in the blood. As pH decreases, glycolysis is inhibited by the increase in hydrogen ion concentration, thus reducing DPG production. In addition to the increase during exercise, the plasma concentration of DPG also increases when an animal ascends to higher altitudes. When ambient oxygen levels fall,

there is a rise in DPG, which reduces the oxygen affinity for hemoglobin and therefore makes more oxygen available to the tissues. Erythrocyte levels of DPG return to normal when the animal returns to sea level. Thus, DPG production is probably an adaptation which allows an individual to function in conditions of reduced oxygen concentration. It is apparently not important as an adaptation to exercise at low altitudes.

There seems to be no readily discernible pattern among mammalian species concerning the presence and effect of DPG. In humans, horses, dogs, rabbits, and guinea pigs the erythrocytes contain significant levels of DPG. On the other hand, several species, including cattle, sheep, goats, and domesticated cats, have low erthrocyte levels of DPG, and their hemoglobin reacts only slightly when exposed to DPG. It should be pointed out that high P_{50} values are found in this latter group (i.e., the partial pressure of oxygen at which 50-percent saturation of the blood is reached), and a general shift of the saturation curve to the right in these animals might not be desirable. The P_{50} value is the best

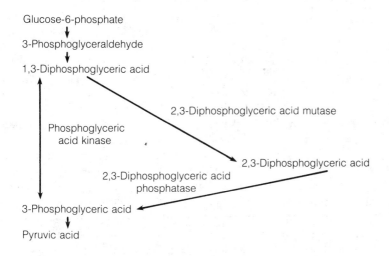

Glucose-6-phosphate

3-Phosphoglyceraldehyde

1,3-Diphosphoglyceric acid

Phosphoglyceric acid kinase

2,3-Diphosphoglyceric acid mutase

2,3-Diphosphoglyceric acid phosphatase

2,3-Diphosphoglyceric acid

3-Phosphoglyceric acid

Pyruvic acid

FIGURE 15–17
Synthesis and degradation of 2,3-diphosphoglyceric acid (2,3-DPG or DPG)

representation of oxygen affinity in mammals. It is a very accurate measure of oxygen affinity because it lies in the center of the sigmoid curve, which forms a point of inflection near 50-percent saturation. Also, it is very difficult to determine maximum absorption because the sigmoid curve forms a horizontal asymptote near 100-percent saturation (refer back to Figure 15–14). In the human, horse, dog, and guinea pig, the P_{50} values are low, and thus their blood can be saturated when alveolar oxygen content is fairly low. There is no phylogenetic relationship which will explain the similarities in oxygen affinities in these groups of animals. But the animals with the low P_{50} values might have evolved at higher altitudes than the species whose blood normally has a low affinity for oxygen. It would also seem possible that animals whose hemoglobin responds readily to DPG have a greater ability to acclimatize to different altitudes than those animals whose hemoglobin has a fixed response to oxygen regardless of the presence of DPG. Note that a number of factors can be associated with an animal's ability to survive and dwell at high altitudes. One should not conclude that one particular factor like blood oxygen affinity or DPG concentration is solely responsible in determining altitude fitness.

Comparative Oxygen Affinities in Mammals

For some time it has been known that oxygen affinity of hemoglobin bears a direct relationship to body size in most mammals. That is to say, the hemoglobin of larger mammals has a greater affinity for oxygen and therefore becomes saturated at a lower partial pressure of oxygen than does the hemoglobin of smaller mammals (see Figure 15–18). Such a condition would tend to support

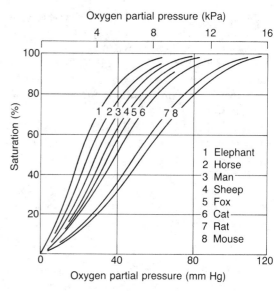

FIGURE 15–18
Oxyhemoglobin dissociation curves in mammals of different body size. From K. Schmidt-Nielsen, *How Animals Work* (London, U.K., 1972). Reprinted by permission of Cambridge University Press.

the greater metabolic demands of smaller animals since more oxygen would be dumped at the tissues where P_{50} values are higher. Since hemoglobin is completely saturated in the lungs regardless of the species, a higher P_{50} value allows more oxygen to be dumped in the tissues. Note that the higher P_{50} value does not mean lower carrying capacity for blood. It only means that the hemoglobin has a reduced affinity for oxygen. Since the affinity of hemoglobin for oxygen is reduced, it can more easily release oxygen in the tissues. This might be more clear if one considers the two curves of Figure 15–19. At 40 mm Hg (the partial pressure of oxygen in venous blood), hemoglobin in the horse is still 70-percent saturated. The hemoglobin of the mouse is only 30-percent saturated at the same partial pressure of oxygen. This means that the hemoglobin of the mouse can deliver 40 per-

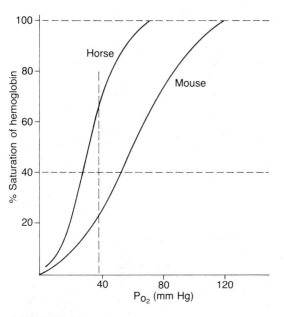

FIGURE 15–19
Oxyhemoglobin dissociation curves of a horse and a mouse

(see Figure 15–20). Even though the P_{50} value for the hemoglobin of the mouse is high, it can still be saturated (or nearly so) in the presence of the partial pressure of oxygen found in the lungs. But when blood reaches the tissues, the presence of hydrogen ions from metabolism causes hemoglobin to change its affinity for oxygen drastically (the Bohr effect). The mouse is therefore able to deliver a greater percentage of oxygen to the tissues per unit volume of blood than can larger animals, because of the greater sensitivity of its hemoglobin for hydrogen ions. An animal with a low metabolic rate, such as the horse or elephant, cannot deliver as much oxygen per unit volume of blood as can smaller mammals, such as the mouse or guinea pig, because of its much lower Bohr effect.

The problem of delivering more oxygen to the tissues can be solved in significantly dif-

cent more oxygen to its tissues under the same environmental conditions.

The generalization that oxygen affinity increases directly with increased body weight should not be carried too far, because there are the numerous exceptions. For instance, the P_{50} value for the guinea pig (*Cavia porcellus*) is 27 mm Hg, which is exactly equal to that of most humans. The camel (*Camelus bactrianies*), which is much larger than a human, has a P_{50} value of only 24 mm Hg.

The ideal situation for sustaining a high metabolic rate would be to have a hemoglobin whose oxygen affinity would be high enough to be easily saturated in alveolar air but could be changed when the tissues are reached, so that oxygen could be easily unloaded. When the magnitude of the Bohr effect is compared among species, it seems that this phenomenon has indeed evolved

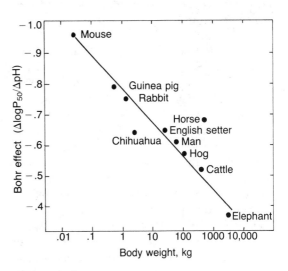

FIGURE 15–20
Bohr effect in mammals having different body size. From A. Riggs, The Nature and Significance of the Bohr Effect in Mammalian Hemoglobin. Reproduced from the *Journal of General Physiology*, 1960, 43:737–752, by copyright permission of the Rockefeller University Press.

ferent ways. During winter when metabolic rate goes up, hemoglobin concentration nearly doubles in the snowshoe rabbit. This is true of many mammals during cold acclimation as well as winter acclimatization. An increase in the concentration of the oxygen-transporting substance is an obvious means of increasing the carrying capacity of blood. As noted earlier, during exercise some animals increase the amount of circulating erythrocytes by releasing additional red blood cells from the spleen. This is, in comparison to the processes of acclimation and acclimatization, a very rapid means of increasing the oxygen-transport capacity of the blood.

The rate at which carbon dioxide is lost from the body also affects the rate that oxygen can be picked up and supplied to the tissues. This loss, known as the *Haldane effect*, is facilitated in the blood primarily by carbonic anhydrase. If the blood lacked carbonic anhydrase, the reaction between carbon dioxide and water to form carbonic acid would be quite slow and the release of carbon dioxide in the lungs would also be slow. The presence of carbonic anhydrase in the erythrocytes greatly accelerates this reaction.

Indirectly, carbonic anhydrase is essential for both oxygen uptake and release by the blood. Animals with high metabolic rates benefit appreciably by having higher carbonic anhydrase activity compared to those animals with low metabolic rates. The activity of carbonic anhydrase in erythrocytes, as expected, is inversely correlated with body weight (see Figure 15–21). Larger species have a much lower activity of carbonic anhydrase in their blood than do smaller species. These data correspond well to the metabolic rates determined for each species.

Blood is in the capillaries of the lungs and other tissues for only a fraction of a second. Therefore, it is essential that oxyhemoglobin

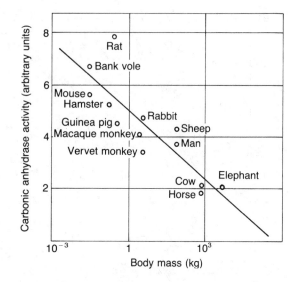

FIGURE 15–21
Carbonic anhydrase activity in different mammalian species as a function of body weight. Reprinted with permission from the *Journal of Comparative Biochemistry and Physiology*, 21:357–360, E. Magid, Activity of Carbonic Anhydrase in Mammalian Blood in Relation to Body Size. Copyright 1967 by Pergamon Press, Ltd.

be formed rapidly, and it is also essential that it be broken down rapidly. Carbonic anhydrase facilitates both of these reactions. In the tissues it enhances the formation of carbonic acid, which immediately ionizes to produce hydrogen ions and bicarbonate ions. The hydrogen ions produced are taken up by hemoglobin. When hemoglobin binds hydrogen ions its affinity for oxygen is reduced. The oxygen release is rapid, and oxygen passes through the capillary wall into the tissues as blood passes through the capillary.

In the lungs, carbon dioxide and water are formed rapidly from carbonic acid in the presence of carbonic anhydrase. This reaction results in the diffusion of carbon dioxide into the alveoli and the diffusion of more bicarbonate ion into the erythrocytes. The presence of additional bicarbonate ion in the red blood cells enhances the removal of hydrogen ions from hemoglobin. When hemoglobin loses hydrogen ions, its affinity for oxygen is increased. The oxygen present in the alveoli is rapidly absorbed by the blood and bound to hemoglobin, ready to be transported to the tissues. These reactions are diametrically opposite from those occurring at the tissue level, where oxygen is released and carbon dioxide is picked up.

CLINICAL DISORDERS OF THE RESPIRATORY SYSTEM

The most common diseases of the respiratory system include *pneumonia, the common cold, influenza, bronchitis,* and *tuberculosis.* These various maladies are caused by microorganisms, and discussion of their etiology is beyond the scope of this text. For a thorough discussion of these diseases the reader is referred to any of a host of textbooks specifically emphasizing pathogenic microbiology. Other disorders of the respiratory system include *bronchial asthma, emphysema, hyaline membrane disease,* and *sudden infant death syndrome.* Bronchial asthma, often caused by an allergic reaction, is characterized by wheezing and dyspnea (difficult breathing) due to the spasmodic contraction of the muscles of the bronchi and bronchioles. Because the air passageways are restricted, the individual has difficulty exhaling and the alveoli may remain partially inflated during expiration. Individuals with this infirmity usually have excessive quantities of mucous from the membranes that line the respiratory tree.

Emphysema is a disease in which the quantity of air that can be exhaled is diminished. This is due to a loss of elasticity of the alveolar walls, which is generally caused by some long-term irritation. As the disease progresses, the chest becomes larger to adjust to the increased lung size due to the permanent inflation of many of the alveoli. Eventually the alveolar tissue is replaced with dense fibrous connective tissue, thus reducing the surface area available for gaseous exchange.

Hyaline membrane disease (HMD) and sudden infant death syndrome (SIDS) are two respiratory disorders affecting the newborn and infant. As already noted, hyaline membrane disease is caused by a deficiency in the amount of surfactant in the lungs of the newborn. Without sufficient surfactant the walls of the alveoli adhere to one another when the lungs are deflated during expiration. Reinflation upon inspiration is often impossible, and the result is the death of the infant.

Sudden infant death syndrome, also called *crib death,* is the leading death-causing disease in children between one week and twelve months of age. It is a very traumatic disorder, because the parents of the child are often left with guilt feelings for something they did or did not do. Crib death occurs suddenly and without warning, though it has been determined that many of the victims suffer upper respiratory tract infections within two weeks prior to death. Some researchers believe the etiological agent to be some type of virus, but no definite causative agent has been isolated.

SUMMARY

Respiration in mammals can be divided into external respiration, which consists of breathing and the delivery of oxygen to the tissues by the circulatory system, and internal respiration, which is restricted to oxidative reactions within the cell.

The physical system of air exchange is based upon compliance of the lungs with the shape of the thorax and the action of the diaphragm, intercostal muscles, and the abdominal muscles. All of these muscles are controlled by the respiratory centers, located in the medulla and pons, during forced ventilation. In some situations exhalation is passive, though inhalation always requires stimulation of the appropriate muscles by the respiratory center.

The volume of air taken in is dependent upon the size and physiological condition of the mammal. In general, the volume of air breathed and the surface area of the lungs correspond to the size of the animal. Quiet breathing without exertion requires the exchange of a minimal amount of air, called the tidal volume. Dead air space, air within the respiratory tree not exposed to the respiratory surface, occupies a significant volume of the tidal air and is relatively negligible in mammals during vigorous exercise.

Breathing rate is controlled by centers located in the medulla and pons. The medullary center is self-regulating, and its rhythm is affected by input from the pneumotaxic and apneustic centers located in the pons. Higher nerve centers associated with the cortex affect the breathing rate through the pneumotaxic center. Breathing rate is also affected by receptors located outside the central nervous system which respond to physical or chemical stimuli. Chemoreceptors located at various points in the body respond to changes in pH, carbon dioxide concentration, and oxygen concentration. When the plasma carbon dioxide and hydrogen ion concentrations increase, breathing rate is stimulated. Proprioceptors and stretch receptors are also important in controlling breathing rate and appear to be primarily effective during exercise.

The transport of oxygen to the tissues depends upon the specific nature of the oxygen-binding substance hemoglobin. The transport of oxygen requires that a hemoglobin molecule change its affinity for oxygen at different positions in the body of the animal. That is to say, it must accept oxygen readily in the lungs and release it at the tissue level. The local metabolic factors which arise from exercise alter the ability of hemoglobin to bind oxygen and insure that maximum oxygen is provided to those tissues carrying out maximum work. The ability of hemoglobin to bind oxygen is directly correlated with the characteristic size of the individuals of a particular species. The smaller mammals have higher metabolic rates than do the larger mammals. This relates well to the higher P_{50} values found in the blood of these smaller mammals. Small mammals also show greater Bohr and Haldane effects, which enable them to deliver more oxygen to the tissues per unit time than is possible in larger individuals.

16

THERMOREGULATION

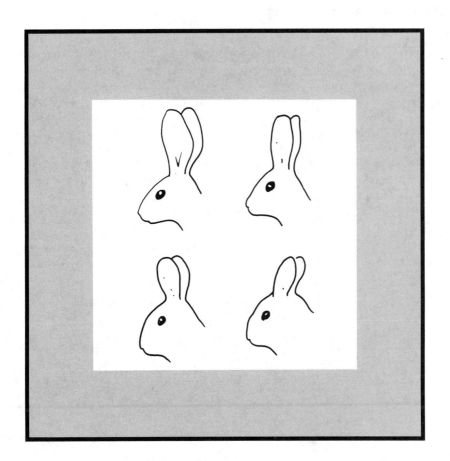

*T*he air temperature on earth is known to vary from a low of −125.3° F
(−87.2° C), recorded in the Soviet Antarctic, to +130° F (54° C) or
more in the desert regions of Africa. Even in the temperate regions
of the United States, animals may be exposed to temperatures between −60° F (−51° C) and +110° F (43° C). In order to survive, most
mammals must control body temperature to within a few degrees so
that normal integrity of biochemical reactions is maintained. Even
when ambient temperatures are ideal, thermoregulation is necessary
to prevent excessive body temperature from building up during exercise. Differences in the ambient temperatures of various altitudes and
latitudes are reflected in many very specific mammalian adaptations.
But in any particular terrestrial environment, a wide variety of temperatures must be met and tolerated if a species is to survive.

EVOLUTION AND ECOLOGICAL THERMOREGULATORY ADAPTATIONS

The great variation in the size of mammals and the wide variety of habitats which they occupy might encourage the novice to suspect that body temperatures vary as much as other physiological characteristics. In fact, body temperatures in most mammals vary only slightly in a *circadian* (daily) cycle, though different portions of a mammal's body might have different temperatures at any point in time. In general, however, the central portion or *core* of a mammal's body is maintained at approximately 37° C (see Table 16–1). This is particularly true of eutherian mammals. It is because of this relatively constant core temperature that the term *warm-blooded* or *homeothermic* (even temperature) is applied. The term *endotherm* is used to describe the condition seen in mammals and birds (as well as certain other animals) which are able to regulate body temperature through the use of heat generated in metabolism. By contrast, other vertebrates are called *ectotherms* as the result of their

TABLE 16–1
Body temperatures charac-
teristic of some mammals
(at rest)

Animal	Normal Core Temperature (°C)
Echidna	30–31
Opossum (*Marmosa*)	33.2–35.7
Armadillo (*Dasypus* sp.)	34–36
Mouse (*Mus musculus*)	37.5–38.5
Ground squirrel (*Ammospermophilus leucurus*)	36
Hedgehog	34–36
Human	37
Camel	38.1
Humpback whale	36

necessity to derive from external sources the body heat needed for activity.

One of the principal driving forces in the evolution of mammals has been their ability to regulate body temperature from within and thus adapt to a wide range of ambient temperatures, from the tropical regions to the poles. The development of homeothermy enabled primitive mammals to search for food in conditions which would have meant certain death from heat or cold to their reptilian ancestors. Homeothermy also meant that food digestion could take place at an even rate and at a wide variety of ambient temperatures. One of the principal characteristics of mammalian reproduction is *viviparity*, the production of live young. Although viviparity is present in other animal forms, it reached its maximum value in mammals, since embryonic development could take place during the winter and young could be born in the spring when chances of survival were greatest. With viviparity, developing embryos can be carried within the mother, leaving the adults free to search for food and still protect the embryos from predation by other species. This is a sizable advantage over birds, which must guard the nest against predators, or such reptiles as the sea turtle, which leave their eggs on sandy beaches to fall prey to humans and other animals.

After the development of homeothermy, mammalian evolution continued along the lines which would lead to better *thermoregulation* (i.e., stable core temperature) under more adverse conditions. One of the first manifestations of the effects of temperatures upon natural selection was observed by Bergmann in 1847. His now classic analysis, which indicated that mammals in the colder climates had larger body sizes than found in more warm-adapted members of the species, is referred to as *Bergmann's rule*. This im-

plies that warm-blooded animals from colder climates are larger in size and therefore have less surface area in relation to body weight than do their relatives found in warmer climates.

The explanation of Bergmann's rule lies in the relationship of surface area to volume (or mass) of an animal's body. Ideally, if mammals were spherical, their body surface area would be described by the following equation:

$$SA = 4\pi r^2 \tag{16.1}$$

where,

$$SA = \text{surface area}$$
$$r = \text{radius}$$

And their volume by the following equation:

$$V = \frac{4}{3}\pi r^3 \tag{16.2}$$

where,

$$V = \text{volume}$$
$$r = \text{radius}$$

Thus, as size increases within these ideal spherical species, the volume increases in proportion to the cube of the radius and the surface area increases in proportion to the square of the radius. The larger of these hypothetical animals would then have a lower surface-to-volume ratio. This would mean that heat-producing tissues (i.e., tissues having rapid metabolism) would occupy greater mass in proportion to the surface area in larger mammals. As a result of these physical relationships, larger animals would be better adapted to survival in cold climates than their smaller counterparts.

For example, assume that an individual of a subspecies found in the southern end of its range had a total mass of 8.45 grams. In that case, the volume would be approximately 8.45 ml. By using equation 16.2, r is found to be equal to 1.26. Then by using equation 16.1, surface area is found to be equal to 20. Surface-to-volume ratio in this case would be $^{20}/_{8.45}$, or 2.36. In a mammal twice this size, it can be shown that the radius is 1.59 and the surface area is 32, giving a surface-to-volume ratio of $^{32}/_{16.9}$, or 1.9. This is considerably less than the ratio expected for the smaller members of the species and, even though hypothetical, has some validity in nature. For example, among humans, Europeans have been found to have a body weight to surface area ratio of 37–39 kg/m^2, whereas people adapted to the tropics (such as the African bushman) have a ratio of only 30.2 kg/m^2. In a number of mammalian species studied by Rensch, 81 percent follow Bergmann's rule in principle. On the other hand, there are numerous exceptions to the rule. Yet the obvious selective advantage of a lower surface-to-volume ratio of warm-blooded animals in cold climates cannot be overlooked.

Obviously, mammals are not spherical and the analogy of surface-to-volume ratio is not a hard and fast rule. But there are many environmental studies of pandemic species which show that subspecies found in colder regions (such as the poles) or at high altitudes are larger than other subspecies living in warmer climates.

Another ecological correlation of significant physiological importance is found in the relationship between body mass and length of the extremities in mammals from different thermal environments. This relationship, known as *Allen's rule*, holds that size of appendages such as ears and limbs of animals found in the northern regions of the range of a species are reduced when compared to warmer-adapted counterparts. Increased surface area means increased area for heat loss, which would be desirable for tropical animals or animals found in the southern deserts of the United States but very undesirable for mammals found in the Arctic.

Allen's rule can be applied to related organisms of different species as well as to the differences in lengths of extremities found among different subspecies (see Figure 16–1). In addition to subspecific genetic differences, size of extremities can vary as a function of the temperature at which mammals are raised. For example, mice raised at 5° C showed a reduction in tail length of 43 percent when compared to the controls raised at 22° C. Also, pigs raised in the cold have shorter legs compared to those raised in warmer environments.

Both Allen's and Bergmann's rules fit the concept of reduced surface area for heat loss with an increase in body size for generation and storage of heat. To conserve energy, mammals found in cold climates must employ every possible mechanism of reducing

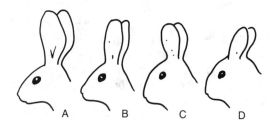

FIGURE 16–1

Example of Allen's rule in the same genus of rabbit: the decreasing size of ears of *Lepus* from south to north. (A) Arizona jack rabbit *(L. alleni)*; (B) Oregon jack rabbit *(L. californicus)*; (C) varying hare from Northern Minnesota *(L. americanus)*; (D) Arctic hare from the barren grounds *(L. arcticus)*. From *Principles of Animal Ecology*, by Warder C. Allee, © 1949 by W. B. Saunders Co. Reprinted by permission of W. B. Saunders, CBS College Publishing.

heat loss to the environment. When metabolic rates are compared among species, they accurately correspond to the surface area of the body and vary widely on a body weight basis (see Table 16–2). This would indicate that surface exposure is a strong force in thermoregulation and is a primary mechanism for regulation of heat production.

METHODS OF HEAT EXCHANGE

During thermoregulation, heat exchange between mammals and their environment follows the principles set down in the laws of physics. Heat is lost or gained from the body surface by *conduction, convection, radiation,* and *evaporation* (see Figure 16–2). Conduction implies that heat is exchanged from regions of high temperature to regions of low temperature between solid or liquid objects by diffusion, without movement of the mass through which the exchange is taking place. Radiation is the exchange of heat by electromagnetic energy flow between objects separated in space. In this way, an animal may be cooled by the radiation of heat from the animal's body to a cooler object in its surroundings. Convection is a type of exchange which implies mass transfer of heat to a current of air or water that the animal may be in con-

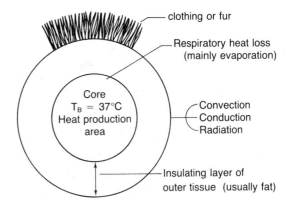

FIGURE 16–2
Schematic cross section of mammalian heat-producing area and insulation showing usual methods of heat loss and heat gain. The layer of insulating tissues which surrounds the core can vary in thickness depending upon peripheral blood flow.

TABLE 16–2
Typical values of basal heat production by humans and various domesticated animals. Values are given as a function of body weight and surface area.

Animal	Body Weight (kg)	Heat Production (Kcal day)			
		Per Animal	Per kg of Body Weight	Per Square Meter of Surface Area	Per kg Weight$^{0.73}$
Rat	0.29	28	97	840	69
Hen	2.1	115	55	701	67
Dog	14.0	485	35	745	71
Sheep	50	1060	21	890	61
Man	70	1700	24	950	77
Pig	122	2400	20	974	72
Cow	500	7470	15	1530	80

Source: From E. S. E. Hafez and I. A. Dyer, *Animal Growth* and *Nutrition* (Philadelphia: Lea & Febiger, 1969). Reprinted with permission.

tact with. In terrestrial mammals water can be lost to the environment, which allows additional cooling by evaporation. But this is a more costly means of body cooling in that energy must be expended by the animal in order to replace water lost by evaporation.

For mammals to maintain a relatively constant core temperature *thermal balance* must be achieved. In other words, heat loss must equal heat gain. In order to maintain thermal balance a wide variety of structural and functional mechanisms are employed by mammals. All of the methods employed must conform with the limits set up by the physical environment in which the animal lives. In some situations heat loss by conduction, convection, and radiation is impossible, and evaporation must be employed to prevent excessive heat gain. In cold climates the opposite situation exists: mammals must reduce the rate of heat loss through insulation and replace lost body heat with metabolic heat.

Aquatic mammals must also regulate thermal exchange, but they have a unique situation in that evaporation, except through respiration, is impossible as a means of cooling the body when excessive heat is present. As a consequence, mammals do not live in water of temperatures exceeding limits of survival. In the polar regions, water may provide

protection from excessive heat loss by mammals which are adequately insulated, because it is never more than a few degrees below zero (Celsius) even in seawater. The thermal environment of the ocean is relatively stable compared to the air temperature. By contrast, arctic air temperature may be as low as $-40°$ C and provide an extremely hostile environment to an unadapted animal.

RESPONSES TO AMBIENT TEMPERATURES

When mammals are exposed to different ambient temperatures, a characteristic metabolic response ensues (see Figure 16–3). In the *thermal neutral zone (TNZ)*, where body temperature can be maintained with little change in metabolism, thermoregulation is performed by changing the physical characteristics of the animal, such as: (1) reducing the surface area by curling up, (2) controlling blood flow to the skin, and (3) increasing the density of the stable air mass around the body by fluffing of the fur *(piloerection)*. Such action to control temperature is referred to as *physical thermoregulation* and usually is only effective over a narrow range of ambient temperatures. When ambient temperatures

FIGURE 16–3
Hypothetical curve of metabolic response to ambient temperature. In the thermal neutral zone, extra metabolic heat is not required, and body temperature is maintained by physically retarding heat flow by means of fur, body position, etc.

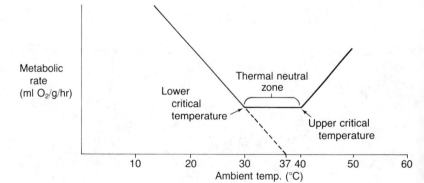

decrease to a point at which physical heat retention is no longer sufficient to maintain body temperature, it becomes necessary to increase metabolism (i.e., increase heat production). Temperature at the lower end of the TNZ, when metabolism increases, is called the *lower critical temperature (LCT)*. At the upper end of the TNZ, increased metabolism is necessary to support such physiological heat-dissipating mechanisms as increased circulation to peripheral areas and increased ventilatory frequency. In addition, increased tissue temperature raises oxygen consumption by the Q_{10} effect. This ambient temperature, when there is an increase in metabolism above the TNZ, is called the *upper critical temperature (UCT)*.

Below the zone of thermal neutrality, the body temperature is largely dependent upon the animal's ability to generate energy from chemical stores in the body. This type of body temperature maintenance is called *chemical thermoregulation*. At temperatures above the thermal neutral zone, metabolic heat-dissipating processes are employed which require that an animal expend chemical energy stored in the body. In other words, metabolism is one of the final mechanisms in maintaining body temperature. When the metabolic processes are insufficient, death from high or low temperatures quickly ensues.

THERMOREGULATION BELOW THE LOWER CRITICAL TEMPERATURE

Excess heat produced during metabolism is lost to the environment, and in so doing the animal functions as a *heat source* while the environment functions as a *heat sink*. This relationship fits nicely into the formula de-

scribed for heat exchange known as *Newton's law of cooling*: When a warm body is placed in a cooler temperature, the rate of heat loss is directly proportional to the difference between the temperature of the heat source (core) and the heat sink (surroundings). The formula can be written in the following form:

$$\Delta H = C(T_B - T_A) \qquad (16.3)$$

where,

ΔH = rate of heat loss (cals/unit time)

T_B = core temperature (°C)

T_A = ambient temperature (°C)

C = a function of proportionality, which is also affected by surface area, conduction, convection, and radiation

Since T_B and C are approximately constant, ΔH varies directly with the difference between T_B and T_A. Thus, the lower T_A becomes, the faster will be the loss of heat from the core. So ΔH is an inverse function of T_A; and since T_B is a constant, ΔH can be represented by metabolic rate *(MR)* (see Figure 16–3). The equation then becomes:

$$MR = C(T_B - T_A) \qquad (16.4)$$

Equation 16.4 fits the line in Figure 16–3 below the lower critical temperature, where metabolic rate is equal to oxygen consumed per gram per hour and C is the slope.

In Newton's equation (16.3), then, C represents the slope of the line below the lower critical temperature. This value is a constant for any mammal under a given set of circumstances but is quite variable among species (see Figure 16–4). By definition C is a constant which affects the rate of heat loss from an animal and is a function of the nature of

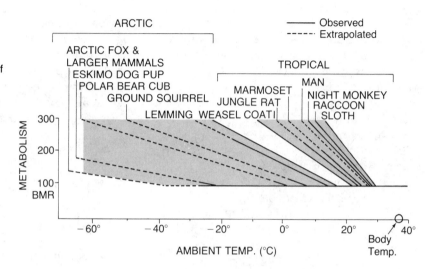

FIGURE 16–4
Metabolic response of arctic and tropical animals to temperatures below their lower critical temperatures. Slope of the lines represents the constant, *C*, from the equation representing Newton's law of cooling. From P. F. Scholander et al, Heat Regulation in Some Arctic and Tropical Mammals and Birds, *Biol. Bull* 99(1950):237–258. Reprinted by permission of Marine Biological Laboratory, Woods Hole, Mass.

the body surface. The larger *C* becomes, the greater the rate of heat loss; it is therefore an inverse function of *insulation,* the resistance to heat loss. In most mammals insulation is related to the amount of fatty tissues and fur or hair surrounding the core.

Insulation can be measured in a variety of ways, the most typical being by a descriptive unit called the *clo.* Insulation was quantified by Burton and Edholm as the amount of heat lost per square meter per hour by a human sitting quietly in an atmosphere of 21° C and less than 50 percent relative humidity. This is equivalent to about 50 cals/m²/hour. If the *insensible evaporative heat loss* (respiratory and nonsweating water loss) of a human, which amounts to about 13 cals/m²/hour, or 25 percent of the total heat loss, is subtracted from 50 cals/m²/hour, one is left with approximately *38 cals/m²/hour,* which has been defined as the clo. A clo is equivalent to the insulation provided by a light business suit.

Insulation is frequently measured in terms of *heat flow,* or in *watts/cm²/hr.* This is a useful term in investigating the comparative in-

sulative values of different types of *integumental covering,* such as hair, fur and wool. It has been shown that animals such as the tundra wolf, which is well adapted to the Arctic, can exist comfortably at −40° C, whereas small mammals such as the lemming cannot be insulated sufficiently to exist in the extreme temperatures of the Arctic because of their size. Instead, lemmings utilize the snow as insulation and exist in a nival habitat for most of the winter.

The integument of most mammals contains a uniform coat of hair. Many of these mammals have a coarse outer covering composed of *guard hairs,* which usually prevents snow from reaching lower layers. In addition, they have a dense inner coat that is capable of holding a large volume of air for insulation. Due to the problems of weight when wet, and resultant lessened mobility, arctic marine mammals have lost most of this external covering and rely upon a heavy layer of fat for insulation.

An interesting aspect for the physiologist is in the utilization of insulation by mammals to survive at low temperatures. Arctic mammals show the greatest increase in insulation during the winter, up to 52 percent in some cases. Insulation can be in the form of fur in some animals, whereas others reduce heat loss with a thick layer of subdermal fat. For example, the domesticated pig, which has a relatively bare skin but thick layer of subdermal fat, exhibits a lower critical temperature of 0° C during winter. Freezing of dermal layers in such bare-skinned animals as the pig is prevented by alternately shunting blood to the periphery.

In the case of marine arctic mammals, which spend most of their lives in the water, fur is of little value. First, winter extremes are never as exaggerated in water as they are on land, and the temperature of marine water reaches only about −2° C as compared to −40 to −60° C experienced on land. Second, these animals, such as whales and porpoises, are usually of such great size that the surface-to-volume ratio is extremely small, thus presenting a reduced area for heat loss. Even in whales, the insulating layer of adipose tissue may be a foot thick. But areas of the body where insulation is thin, such as the flukes and tissues located in the facial areas, are well protected by circulatory mechanisms.

Most arctic mammals can withstand drastic peripheral temperature changes without the usual dire consequences of frostbite and cellular damage seen in mammals adapted to warmer climates. Mammals as a group show an adaptation to cold by ~~allowing the periph~~eral temperature to fall to levels much lower than core temperature. This is sometimes referred to as *regional heterothermy* and is found to occur in tropical as well as arctic mammals. Many studies have indicated that lipid deposits in these peripheral tissues contain more unsaturated fats than do more centrally located sites of lipid storage. It is believed that lower melting points of unsat-

urated fats enable the peripheral tissues to maintain cellular integrity and therefore normal function at low temperatures.

Investigations conducted by R. Henshaw revealed that foot pad temperatures in several species of arctic mammals fall to near freezing and are warmed reflexively by shunting blood into the cooled limb (see Figure 16–5). This allows the limb temperature to approach environmental temperature; heat loss is kept at a minimum and frostbite and subsequent damage to exposed tissues are prevented.

Many organisms reduce the flow of heat to the periphery by means of countercurrent heat exchange between closely aligned blood vessels. Where blood is transported in opposite directions, heat may be exchanged efficiently across a very slight thermal gradient.

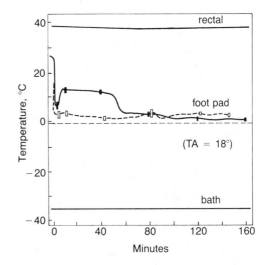

FIGURE 16–5
Temperature in the paw of the wolf approaches the ambient but never reaches freezing due to regular infusion of blood. From R. Henshaw et al, Peripheral Thermoregulation: Foot Temperature in Two Arctic Canines, *Science* 175(1972):988–990. Reprinted with permission. Copyright 1972 by the American Association for the Advancement of Science.

Countercurrent mechanisms are most frequently found in animals which live in cold climates or aquatic environments where efficient heat conservation is mandatory for survival (see Figure 16–6). But in many cases, countercurrent heat exchangers are important mechanisms of thermoregulation in mammals adapted to warm climates. Where countercurrent mechanisms are employed, vessels must closely approximate each other, and in many cases the vessels are broken up into a number of smaller vessels called *rete.* Where rete, or *vascular nets*, are present vascular surface area is maximized, and heat exchange can take place over a very short length of the extremity because of increased exposure between the blood vessels. Very efficient heat exchangers occur in animals such as the muskrat and river otter which spend a great deal of time in the water and must have exposed or uninsulated feet for locomotion. In these animals the countercurrent exchange must be remarkably efficient because of the shortness of the thermal gradient which exists between bare feet and a small but well-insulated body. These mammals have countercurrent heat exchangers in limbs and tail which prevent excessive heat loss from the core while allowing the exposed parts to function at a minimal temperature.

THERMOGENESIS

In order to maintain a constant body temperature, no matter how well insulated, a mammal must produce heat by metabolic processes collectively known as *thermogenesis.* Additional heat can be produced by *shivering*, which provides heat above the normal level of basal metabolism. But shivering is a costly manner of heat production in that it employs muscle contraction without producing useful work. Under some circumstances, a mammal forced to shiver may become exhausted and unable to produce sufficient heat to maintain body temperature. Under these conditions the animal loses body heat faster than it can be produced and subsequently becomes hypothermic.

A more efficient method of heat production and one that does not result in muscle fatigue is produced in animals which have become physiologically accustomed to low ambient temperatures through a process

FIGURE 16–6
Countercurrent heat exchange in the bottlenose porpoise. From P. F. Scholander and W. F. Scheville, Counter Current Vascular Heat Exchange, *J. Appl. Physiol.* 8(1955):279–282. Reprinted by permission of the American Physiological Society, Bethesda, Md.

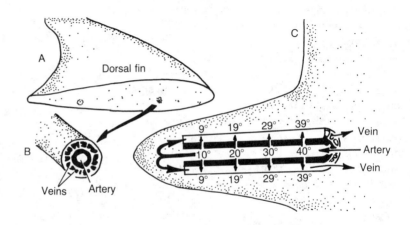

called *acclimation*. This method of heat production, called *nonshivering thermogenesis*, results in the generation of heat in the absence of shivering and does not lead to the obvious sensations of fatigue. Nonshivering thermogenesis is manifest particularly well in animals genetically adapted to cold climates, though it can be produced to varying degrees in practically all mammals tested under laboratory conditions. Animals which exhibit nonshivering thermogenesis have abundant mitochondrial enzymes for the utilization of lipids and produce sufficient heat to maintain body temperatures below the lower critical temperature without shivering.

The ability to regulate heat production through nonshivering thermogenesis can be induced through manipulation of several environmental variables. In particular, long-term exposure to low ambient temperature over a period of time produces a physiological state of cold resistance known as *cold acclimation* (see Table 16–3). Temperature acclimation is accompanied by a number of metabolic changes resulting in an increased production of heat by nonshivering thermogenesis. For instance, there is an increase in the quantity of catabolic enzymes capable of breaking down stored carbohydrates and lipids, particularly in the muscles, along with elevated production of hormones essential to metabolism (thyroxine, norepinephrine, corticosteroids). *Norepinephrine* is a primary hormone in heat generation, since it is essential to the release of fatty acids for energy metabolism, whereas *corticosteroids* enhance metabolism through gluconeogenesis. In addition, the *catecholamines* induce an elevation in oxygen-consumption rate and thus increase metabolic heat production through a variety of calorigenic reactions in the metabolic mill. When animals have been acclimated to cold ambient temperatures, their response to increased circulating levels of norepinephrine is enhanced (see Figure 16–7).

An interesting mechanism for enhancing the cold-acclimated state can be induced through manipulation of the *light cycle* to which mammals are exposed. A reduction in the light cycle simulates the change in *photoperiod* characteristic of the approach of winter. Under natural conditions, this photoperiod change is much more regular and predictable than the changes in ambient temperature. Therefore, change in the light

	Mean Survival Times (min)	
Species	Summer (21 ± 2°C)	Cold-Acclimated (5 ± 1°C)
White rats (n = 9)	50	135
House mouse (n = 2)	36	43
Deer mouse (n = 7)	44	270
Collared lemming (n = 4)	131	2355

TABLE 16–3
Effect of cold acclimation upon survival time (time of exposure to loss of righting response) in several species of rodents exposed to −40° C. Cold-acclimated animals were acclimated at 5° C for twenty-one days.

Source: Data from J. H. Ferguson and G. E. Folk, Jr., Effect of Photoperiod and Cold Acclimation on Survival of Mice in Cold, *Cryobiology* 16(1979):468–472. Reprinted by permission of Academic Press.

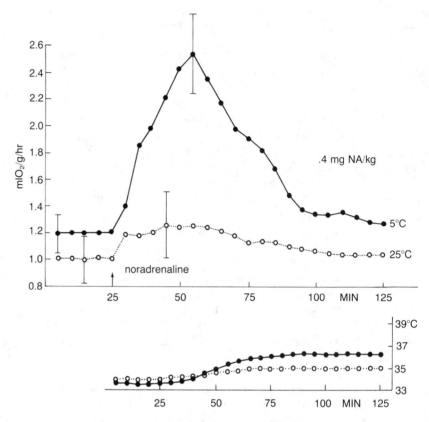

FIGURE 16–7
Response of cold (●) and warm (○) acclimatized rats to infusions of norepinephrine. Lower graph depicts changes in rectal temperature. From L. Jansky et al, Acclimation of the White Rat to Cold: Noradrenalin Thermogenesis, *Physiol. Bohemoslav.* 16(1967):366–372. Reprinted by permission of Ceskoslovenska Akademie Ved, Prague, Czechoslovakia.

cycle is a much more accurate index of approaching winter than is cold ambient temperature. It has been shown experimentally that animals exposed to short photoperiods have higher rates of metabolism than animals maintained on long photoperiods. Likewise, this ability to withstand cold temperatures is enhanced by artifically reducing the daily light cycle (see Figure 16–8).

Diet is also an important factor in resistance to cold. Animals must receive an adequate supply of nutrients to maintain hormonal and energetic functions important to nonshivering thermogenesis. In addition, the nature of specific elements in the diet is important. Animals allowed to consume unsaturated fats increase their lipid stores and are better able to achieve the cold acclimated state than those fed a diet high in saturated fats (see Figure 16–9). Unsaturated fats are utilized as body fuel sources for thermogenesis. They also play an important role in the insulation and maintenance of the fluid nature of the plasma membranes in tissues such as limbs and skin that may drop below normal temperature.

THERMOREGULATION OF ANIMALS IN WARM AMBIENT TEMPERATURES

When mammals are exposed to ambient temperatures above their upper critical temper-

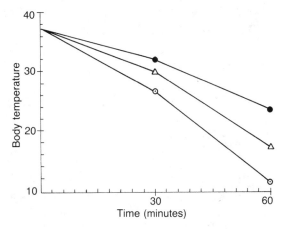

FIGURE 16–8

Effect of acute cold exposure ($-20°$ C) upon cooling of mice maintained in: constant dark (●); constant light (○); and 4 hours light, 20 hours dark (△) while being acclimated to $5°$ C for 21 days. Data from J. H. Ferguson and G. E. Folk, Jr., Effect of Photoperiod and Cold Acclimation on Survival of Mice in Cold, *Cryobiology* 16(1979): 468–472.

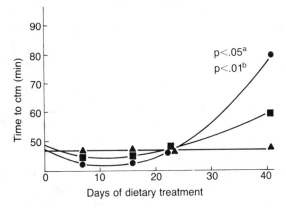

FIGURE 16–9

Effect of dietary lipids on cold survival of mice acclimated to room temperature exposed to $-18°$ C. ctm, critical thermal minimum, or body temperature at which loss of righting response occurs. Unsaturated fat diet (●); saturated fat diet (▲); control diet (■). [a]Probability vs. control group. [b]Probability vs. saturated fat group. Reprinted with permission from the *Journal of Thermal Biology* 5(1980):29–35, fig. 3., C. J. Gordon and J. H. Ferguson, Role of Dietary Lipids in Cold Survival and Changes in Body Composition in White Mice. Copyright 1980 by Pergamon Press, Ltd.

atures, the rate of heat loss to the environment must be increased in order to prevent excessive body temperatures, which might ultimately result in death. Such mechanisms of heat loss involve conduction, radiation, convection, and evaporative cooling, which can be manifested in a variety of ways. Evaporative cooling usually occurs through cooling of the skin through sweat evaporation or evaporation of water from the lungs and respiratory passages.

Sweating is a primary involuntary response generated by the autonomic nervous system in primates and a few other species. Under severe heat stress humans and horses can lose four or more liters of body water per hour through sweat. Other species, such as the rat, are able to lose body water through the skin without the aid of sweat glands by a process called *insensible water loss*. This process is not as effective as sweating because it is apparently not under active physiological control. When exposed to high ambient temperatures such mammals as the opossum, red squirrel, rat, and mouse maintain a steady cooling of the peripheral shell through the evaporation of saliva transferred to the fur by licking.

Evaporative cooling through loss of water from the respiratory membranes also is an important heat-dissipating autonomic response found in panting mammals. This usually involves a rapid exchange of air, which cools the membrane linings of the mouth, nose, and lungs. These animals prevent respiratory alkalosis by means of rapid shallow breathing, which does not affect the concentration of gases in the lungs.

Some mammals survive by relinquishing their ability to thermoregulate and accepting the temperature, within limits, thrust upon them by the environment. A typical example of this is seen in some larger herbivores.

When heat and water stressed, the camel will allow its body temperature to rise several degrees rather than using "precious" water to dissipate heat. For example, to prevent a 1.0° C rise in temperature, the camel requires the evaporative heat loss of 500 kilocalories, which is equivalent to about 862 ml of water. It has been calculated by K. Schmidt-Nielsen that by allowing the body temperature to rise during the hottest part of the day, the camel saves a total of five liters of water per day. Very active animals, such as the antelope, that generate body heat through muscular activity also allow the body temperature to rise, especially under heat stress. Apparently, however, the nervous system cannot tolerate the same increase in temperature absorbed by the rest of the body, and a rete system carries cooled blood from the respiratory membranes of the nose and pharynx to the brain, and thus a critical portion of the nervous system is maintained near *normothermic temperature*. In the hamster, a mammal which lacks a carotid rete, C. Gordon determined that brain temperature is reduced during exercise by arterial blood that is cooled as it passes closely by the cavernous and opthalmic sinuses. At rest, the brain temperature of the hamster was maintained approximately 1° C below body temperature, between ambient temperatures of 18° and 37° C (see Figure 16–10).

HETEROTHERMY

For some small mammals neither heat dissipation in hot environments nor thermogenesis in cold environments is practical because of small body size and hence large surface-to-volume ratio. If challenged with extreme environmental stress, some mammals will forego homeothermy during part of the year or day and assume a condition very

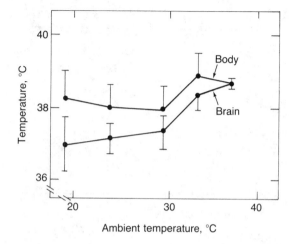

FIGURE 16–10
Mean brain and body temperatures of free-moving hamsters at ambient temperatures of 18–37° C. Vertical bars represent one standard deviation of the mean. From C. J. Gordon et al, Rapid Brain Cooling in the Free-running Hamster, *Mesocricitus auratus, J. Appl. Physiol.* 51(1981):1349–1354, fig. 3. Reprinted by permission of the American Physiological Society, Bethesda, Md.

similar to *poikilothermy* found in cold-blooded vertebrates. These animals are said to be *heterothermic* because they maintain constant body temperature by means of internal metabolism (homeothermy) for part of the time and cease to regulate body temperature for the remainder of the time and take on the temperature of the environment (poikilothermy). In other words, where the maintenance of a constant body temperature is not practical, some mammals shed their homeothermic condition and assume the poikilothermic state. A prime example of this is seen in many bats, in which diurnal dormancy occurs. Many chiropteran species cease to regulate body temperature during dormant periods and allow the core temperature to approach that of the surroundings. This type of heterothermy occurs in a variety of other mammals, usually belonging to such lower evolutionary groups as the marsupials and monotremes.

NEURAL CONTROL OF BODY TEMPERATURE

Any measurable factor, such as core temperature of mammals, that is closely regulated must have a refined mechanism of control. As in many basic regulatory mechanisms, the center for temperature control in mammals resides in the *hypothalamus.* It is here that comparisons are made between temperature sensations from the blood and skin and the hypothetical *set point* for internal temperature regulation, hence the name *set point theory of thermoregulation* (see Figure 16–11). A decrease in core temperature causes the blood flowing into the hypothalamus to become cooler. The temperature of incoming blood is then compared to the *reference temperature* (set point) in the hypothalamic integration center, which signals the effectors of body heat production (shivering, nonshivering thermogenesis) to increase their output, and body temperature is brought back to its normal state of approximately 37° C. An opposite response occurs when core temperature rises and incoming blood temperature exceeds the reference temperature. A similar feedback mechanism occurs when surface temperature changes are picked up by the receptors of the skin. A decrease in skin temperature will result in shivering; an increase in skin temperature causes the reflexive activation of sweating or other mechanisms of heat loss depending upon the species.

TEMPERATURE REGULATION IN DOMESTICATED MAMMALS

In the domesticated mammals which have a carotid rete, panting is usually the predominant method of maintaining body temperature when excessive environmental heat is present or when excessive metabolic heat is generated. In others, such as the cow, camel, horse, and donkey, sweating may predominate as the cooling mechanism, and the release of sweat from the skin may be continuous. In sheep and goats intermittent sweating has been observed, perhaps controlled through an alpha-adrenergic mechanism rather than cholinergic. In the horse, sweat glands are activated by adrenaline in the blood, and evidence indicates that sweating in the donkey is promoted by means of beta-adrenergic receptors in the skin. In the pig, which has a minimum amount of vascularization in the skin, heat loss through sweating is difficult. It must rely upon vaporization of water from its wallow and panting for evaporative heat loss.

In many domesticated species, control of peripheral circulation has become essential

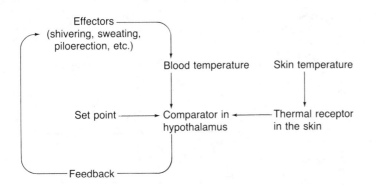

FIGURE 16–11
Schematic of feedback regulation of body temperature showing comparator relationship to set point or reference temperature, blood temperature, and temperature receptors of the skin

to thermoregulation. Increased heat results in increased vascular flow to the ears in the rabbit and to the nose in the cat. Similarly, increased heat results in elevated blood flow to the horns in the domesticated goat and the tail in rodents. Wherever heat loss is conferred through circulatory mechanisms of this type, radiation, conduction, and convection to cooler objects in the environment or to the ambient air are essential.

In ruminants gastric fermentation results in the generation of considerable heat, which is quite variable in amount depending upon the stage of digestion. For this reason, rectal temperature in these animals is not a reliable indicator of core temperature. Because of the increased heat load generated through fermentation in the rumen, a favorable ambient temperature for heat loss is essential. In domesticated cattle, for instance, breeds with compact bodies, such as Angus and Hereford (both of European origin), fare less favorably in warm climates of the southern United States and Mexico than do the less compact types, such as the Brahma, Zebu, and Texas Longhorn, which have greater surface-to-

volume ratios and hence relatively more skin area for heat loss.

CHANGES IN SET POINT: FEVER

The reference temperature or set point of the hypothalamus can be altered by a variety of chemicals called *pyrogens*, the result of which is increased heat production. Also, a number of substances called *antipyrogens* have been found to oppose the action of pyrogens. When a pyrogen is introduced into the mammalian system, the reference temperature is increased. When the reference temperature is altered to a higher position (i.e., from 37° to 39° C) effector mechanisms raise the core temperature to a new level, which is measured as an elevation of body temperature, or *fever* (see Figure 16–12). When the pyrogens are removed from the body the animal feels hot, the reference temperature returns to normal (homeostatic level), and mechanisms such as sweating and panting result in a return of core temperature to its normal level of 37° C. Pyrogens in-

FIGURE 16–12
Alteration of set point by pyrogens in the process of induction and loss of fever

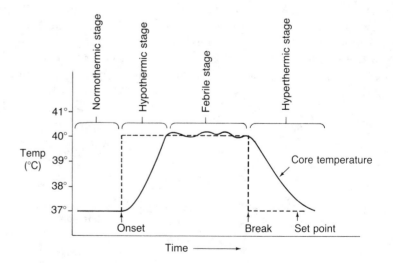

clude bacterial cell walls (bacterial endotoxins) but can be other substances such as antigen-antibody complexes or particles released from neoplastic diseases. Antipyrogens, such as a *salicylic acid* (aspirin) and acetominophen (a nonaspirin analgesic), can be used effectively in many cases to reduce fever by reducing the response of the hypothalamus to pyrogens.

SUMMARY

The thermal environment of mammals varies from the coldest temperatures on earth to some of its warmest. One of the physiological factors which allows mammals to exist and thrive in very harsh environmental temperatures is their ability to regulate body temperature. Through evolution mammals have acquired both physical as well as physiological traits which allow them to exist under seemingly adverse physical conditions. Factors such as viviparity, body surface-to-volume relationships, insulation, and the ability to produce heat internally at a rate which balances the rate of heat loss are essential to mammalian survival. Ways of losing heat through evaporation and other means are also critical elements of their survival repertoire.

A number of very specific mammalian adaptations allow them to readily adapt to drastically different climates. These mechanisms employ basic laws of heat conservation and can be readily analyzed in physical terms. They include countercurrent heat exchangers, insulating layers of tissues, changes in physical dimensions such as curling up and piloerection, differential blood flow to the limbs, and the ability to alter thermogenesis by both shivering and nonshivering means. Many mammals can dissipate heat through evaporative heat loss from sweat and from the respiratory membranes. In addition, specific behavioral mechanisms allow them to seek favorable areas for heat exchange by conduction, convection, and radiation.

Some mammals are able to survive in a seemingly harsh environment by relinquishing their thermoregulatory capacities and allowing body temperature to approach that of the surroundings. For instance, during heat stress the camel can allow its body temperature to rise and thus store body heat, which allows a significant water savings. Other mammals become torpid and allow the body to cool and thus, when inactive, approach the temperature of the surroundings. This reduces the temperature differential between the body and the environment and provides economy of heat conservation.

Body temperature is regulated by means of the central integrative control of the nervous system. A hypothetical temperature called the set point or reference temperature is maintained in the hypothalamus. This temperature is compared to the temperature of the blood and sensations derived from the exteroceptors of the skin. By comparing these temperatures to the set point, the heat-generating mechanisms are accelerated or reduced depending upon the specific temperature involved.

The set point can be modified so that body temperature is regulated at a higher or lower level than normal. Elevated body temperature, called fever, can be induced by means of chemicals released into the blood by invading organisms or other foreign substances (pyrogens). Antipyrogens can be used to reduce the effect of pyrogens and thus lower the hypothalamic set point to its normal level.

17

THE ENDOCRINE SYSTEM

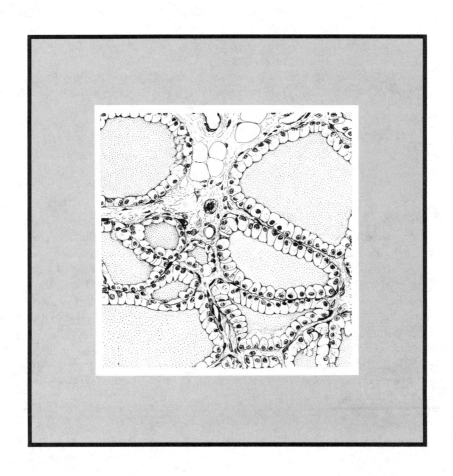

*O*bservations about endocrine glands and their functions were made by Greek philosophers over 2,000 years ago, but the existence of blood-borne substances capable of evoking physiological action in another part of the body was not realized until the early part of the twentieth century. It is probable that most endocrine concepts could not be adequately understood until William Harvey discovered the circulation of blood in the early seventeenth century. Even so, it was still nearly three hundred years after Harvey's work had been published that the first concepts of modern endocrinology became known.

In 1902 the English physiologists Bayliss and Starling discovered that a substance was produced by the intestinal mucosa when the acidic contents of the stomach passed into the duodenum. This substance, which they named secretin because of its physiological action, induced the secretion of pancreatic juices into the intestine and carried out its effects through the bloodstream rather than by means of reflexes involving nerves. Later, Starling accepted a suggestion by W. B. Hardy that this substance fell into the general category of hormone, from Greek meaning to "arouse to activity," and published this interpretation in 1906.

Although slow in its beginnings, the study of the endocrine, or ductless, glands has received a tremendous amount of interest during the twentieth century. Since the work of Bayliss and Starling, a large number of chemical messengers have been discovered, and we now realize that the circulatory system is as essential as the nervous system in the transmission of information throughout the organism.

HORMONES

As presently understood, hormones are chemical substances produced by the endocrine glands and transmitted through the blood to another portion of the body. The endocrine glands lack the means of directly transferring hormones into the bloodstream through valves or tubes. Therefore, all endocrine hormones must reach the blood by diffusion. Some of the glands in the mammal have both endocrine and *exocrine* functions. The exocrine glands have ducts which transmit their products away from their site of origin. The *pancreas* is an example of a mixed endocrine-exocrine gland. The endocrine portion,

the *islets of Langerhans*, produces the hormones *insulin* and *glucagon*, whereas the exocrine portion produces digestive enzymes which are transmitted through the pancreatic duct into the small intestine.

Several classes of chemicals act as hormones (see Table 17–1). The hormones of the pituitary are fairly large polypeptides, as are the hormones of the pancreas. Hormones of this type have a very definite *steric configuration* and their function is dependent upon a fragile *quaternary structure*. The *steroid hormones* provide a very large portion of the mammalian hormones. These are produced by the adrenal cortex and the reproductive glands of both males and females. The function of the steroid hormones is dependent upon specific modifications of the steroid nucleus (see Figure 17–1). Steroid hormones can be synthesized from *acetate* or directly from *cholesterol* (see Figure 17–2). Modification to form the specific hormones occurs in the *ovaries, testes,* and *adrenal cortex.* The mammals synthesize many more steroid hormones than are believed necessary for the control of major physiological systems. For instance, over thirty different steroid-based hormones can be found in the renal cortex, though only a few of these are believed to have major importance. During synthesis, hormones pass through various intermediate

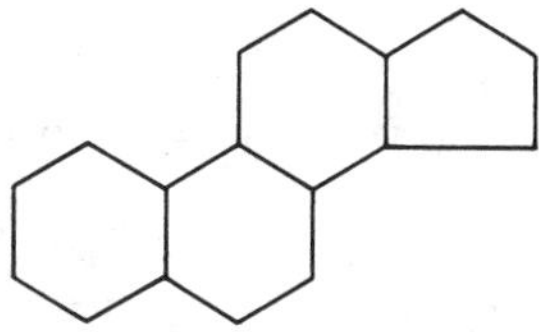

FIGURE 17–1
The cyclopenthanoperhydrophenanthrene nucleus. This forms the basis of the steroid structure.

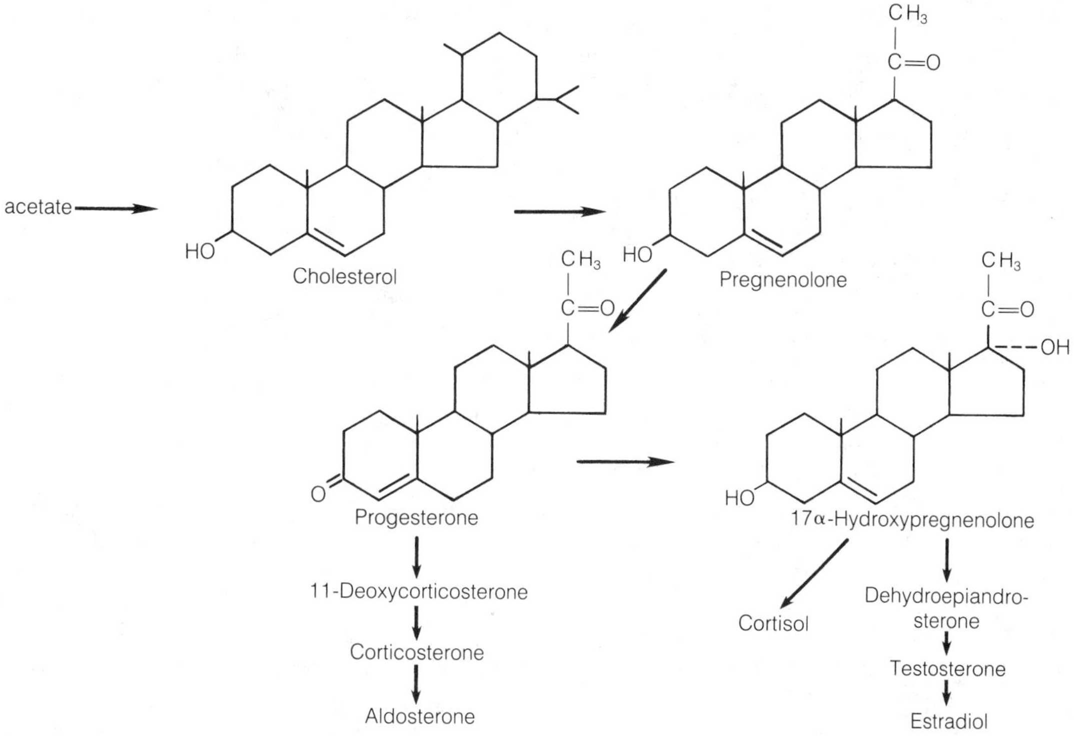

stages. These *intermediates* would induce abnormal activity if allowed to enter the circulation. It is for this reason that accuracy in the synthetic production of these hormones is extremely critical.

FIGURE 17–2
An overview of steroid biosynthesis

TABLE 17–1
Source and chemical class of the various endocrine hormones

Hormone Source	Hormone Name	Chemical Class
Anterior pituitary (adenohypophysis)	Adrenocorticotropic hormone (ACTH)	polypeptide
	Thyroid-stimulating hormone (TSH)	glycoprotein
	Follicle-stimulating hormone (FSH)	glycoprotein
	Luteinizing hormone (LH) or Interstitial cell-stimulating hormone (ICSH)	glycoprotein
	Somatotropic hormone (STH)	polypeptide
	Prolactin	polypeptide
Intermediate pituitary (adenohypophysis)	Melanocyte-stimulating hormone (MSH)	polypeptide
Posterior pituitary (neurohypophysis)	Hormones secreted by the posterior pituitary are produced in the hypothalamus	
Hypothalamus	Vasopressin	octapeptide
	Oxytocin	octapeptide
	Adrenocorticotropic hormone-releasing hormone (ACTH-RH)	polypeptide
	Thyroid-stimulating hormone-releasing hormone (TSH-RH)	polypeptide
	Follicle-stimulating hormone/luteinizing hormone-releasing hormone (FSH/LH-RH)	polypeptide
	Somatotropic hormone-releasing hormone (STH-RH)	polypeptide
	Prolactin-inhibiting hormone (PIH)	polypeptide

Specific structure is very critical in such relatively simple molecules as the *catecholamines* and the *thyroid hormones.* Certain drugs which have structures similar to these hormones are effective in evoking the same or comparable responses. In several cases, the response of an organism to a chemical which resembles the normal hormonal substance is accentuated, and the *mimic* has many times the potency of the natural substance in the body.

Many chemical activators are classified as *local hormones* because they are not carried to target organs at distant locations within the body. The local hormones are usually not produced in specific organs but instead are formed in various locales in the body where they are needed. Good examples of this type of hormone are the *kinins* and *prostaglandins.* The structure of the kinins is poorly understood, but they are known to be polypeptides. They function to dilate blood vessels and perhaps play a role in liberation of secretions from the sweat glands and salivary glands.

The prostaglandins were first discovered in semen but since then have been found in almost all of the body's tissues. They are syn-

TABLE 17–1
(*continued*)

Hormone Source	Hormone Name	Chemical Class
Hypothalamus (continued)	Prolactin-releasing hormone (PRH)	?
	Melanocyte-stimulating hormone-releasing hormone (MSH-RH)	polypeptide
	Melanocyte-stimulating hormone-inhibiting hormone (MSH-IH)	?
	Somatotropic hormone-inhibiting hormone (STH-IH)	polypeptide
Pancreas	Insulin	polypeptide
	Glucagon	polypeptide
Adrenal medulla	Epinephrine	catecholamine
	Norepinephrine	catecholamine
Adrenal cortex	Glucocorticoids	steroids
	Mineralocorticoids	steroids
Ovaries	Estrogens	steroids
	Progestins	steroids
	Relaxin	polypeptide
Testes	Androgens	steroids
Placenta	Chorionic gonadotropin	glycoprotein
	Placental lactogen	polypeptide
	Pregnant mare serum gonadotropin (PMSG)	glycoprotein
Thyroid gland	Thyroxine	iodinated tyrosine derivative
	Triiodothyronine	iodinated tyrosine derivative
	Calcitonin	polypeptide
Parathyroid gland	Parathyroid hormone (PTH)	polypeptide

thesized from the *essential fatty acids (arachidonic, linoleic,* and *linolenic)* and are closely related to these acids in structure. They contain a cyclopentane ring along with the residue of the fatty acids from which they are synthesized (see Figure 17–3). The prostaglandins have a variety of actions. For instance, they are involved with the maintenance of a *patent ductus arteriosus* in the fetus. Some inhibit platelet aggregation, whereas others enhance this reaction. Prostaglandins are thought to be involved in fever; they also lower blood pressure by dilating blood vessels in the splanchnic vascular bed. In actuality, the prostaglandins comprise a whole series of hormones which have a wide range of functions. The exact functions of specific prostaglandins will be under analysis by scientists for some time to come.

Most of the diseases referred to in these sections on endocrinology relate only to humans. This is because in most cases other mammals would be selected against under natural conditions, and these individuals would perish before they could reproduce. It is important for the student to be aware that there are diseases associated with the endocrine organs and their controlling factors.

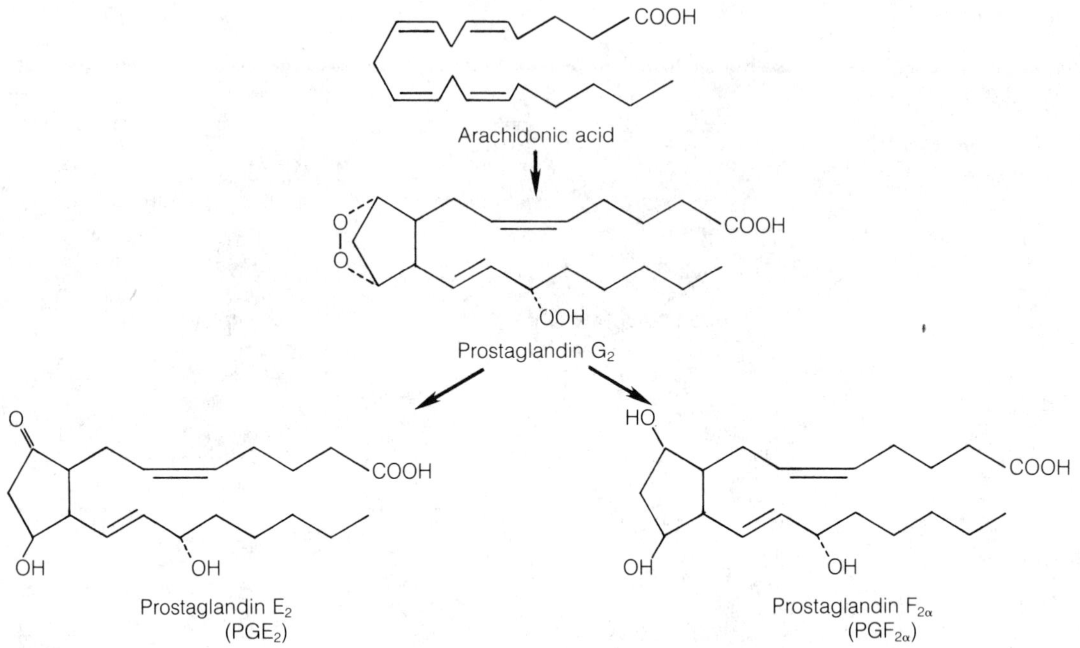

FIGURE 17–3
Three prostaglandins (PG), each with the cyclopentane ring and a fatty acid residue, arachidonic in this case

Therefore, examples of human conditions will be covered in these sections to inform the student of endocrine deficiencies and excesses.

Mechanism of Hormone Action

The function of the hormones varies as widely as their chemical structures. In many cases the mechanisms of specific hormonal actions are well detailed at the cellular level. The mode of action of most, however, is not well understood. Details of the specific nature of hormone action will be taken up at appropriate places in this chapter. In general, their functions in the mammals are directed toward enzyme regulation, membrane permeability, and protein synthesis. Many of these reactions are directly or indirectly related to the production of *cyclic AMP*, also called a *second messenger system*, but this is by no means the universal focus of hormonal action.

The Importance of Feedback Regulation in Hormonal Secretion

The endocrine system provides a means of chemical communication whereby the response following endocrine activity varies with the specific chemical substance (hormone) involved as well as its concentration in the blood. In order to regulate the secretion of chemical messengers over prolonged periods of time, feedback from the target organ or tissue is essential. For example, the *pituitary tropic hormones* increase the production and secretion of other hormones from their target organs. Therefore, *thyroid-stimulating hormone (TSH)* enhances *thyroxine*, and *triiodothyronine* secretion from the thyroid gland, the target organ of this pituitary hormone. These thyroid hormones then feed back to slow the release of TSH through their effect on the hypothalamus and its releasing hormones. Thus, the process is self-regulating. The secretion of all of the hormones is regulated by means of feedback processes of this type. In many such feedback loops, the end product is a blood-borne metabolite, such as glucose in the case of insulin, which retards further production and release of the effector hormone. Details of regulation of each of the hormones will be covered later in this chapter.

THE HYPOTHALAMUS

Although the hypothalamus has already been discussed as a part of the central nervous system, its endocrine function will be mentioned here. It has, in essence, two endocrine functions. First, it produces two hormones, *oxytocin* and *vasopressin*, which ultimately are released from the *posterior lobe of the pituitary*. Second, the hypothalamus produces and secretes *releasing* and *inhibiting hormones* (or *factors*). These hormones are carried through the *hypophyseal portal circulation* to the anterior lobe of the pituitary, which is their target organ. They either stimulate or inhibit the production and release of hormones from the anterior pituitary.

The hypophyseal portal system sequesters blood from capillaries which pass through the *pars tuberalis* of the pituitary and extend to the median eminence of the *tuber cinereum* of the hypothalamus. These capillaries empty into venules, which pass back to the pars tuberalis and then into the *sinusoids* in the anterior lobe of the pituitary. In many mammals, including humans, there is no arterial supply to the anterior pituitary other than a few arterial connections with capillaries from the posterior lobe. In rabbits and some other mammals, arterial blood reaches the anterior pituitary through another set of vessels, but the major portion of the blood supply to this area is transported through the hypophyseal portal system.

Releasing and Inhibiting Hormones of the Hypothalamus

The following is a list of hypothalamic releasing and inhibiting hormones which have either been isolated or for which there is strong evidence to suggest their existence.

Adrenocorticotropic hormone–releasing hormone (ACTH-RH) or corticotropin-releasing hormone (CRH)   There has been a great deal of difficulty in isolating this substance, which is believed to have a disulfide bridge within its structure. In most mammals, ACTH-RH appears to be released from the *median eminence of the hypothalamus*. A number of factors cause the production and release of ACTH-RH and thus stimulate and increase the amount of adrenocorticotropic-hormone (ACTH) secretion by the anterior pituitary. Stress seems to be the most important of these factors. Numerous investigators have demonstrated a positive correlation between environmental factors which upset the general well-being of the mammal and the production of hormones by the adrenal cortex. These studies point to the following sequence. *Stressors*, through some input by either the cerebral cortex or a subconscious effect which could be triggered through the emotional responses associated with the allocortex, initiate release of ACTH-RH. This, in turn, causes more ACTH to be produced and secreted by the anterior pituitary. The increased levels of ACTH result in hypersecretion by the adrenal cortex. This is the basis for the *General Adaptation Syndrome (GAS)*, in which stress stimulates the release of ACTH-RH, which activates the sequence of events mentioned. The adrenal cortex continues to overproduce adrenal corticoids as long as stress persists. These adrenal hormones normally inhibit further production of ACTH-RH and ACTH either through feedback on the hypothalamus or by direct feedback on the pituitary. In many cases, the exact site of feedback inhibition, or *negative feedback*, is not known. Adrenocorticoids possibly inhibit production by action on the higher nerve centers, the hypothalamus or the pituitary. Since one of the functions of the hormones produced by the adrenal cortex is to reduce anxiety and promote a state of wellbeing, an indirect or nonchemical action might be involved with feedback inhibition in this case. At the level of the hypothalamus or pituitary it is probable that feedback inhibition affects an intermediate enzyme in the normal synthetic pathway of ACTH-RH or ACTH.

Other factors which contribute to the control of ACTH-RH release include the presence of both *vasopressin* and *angiotensin II* in the bloodstream. When either of these substances exceeds normal levels in the blood, it stimulates the release of ACTH-RH from the hypothalamus as well as the production of ACTH by the anterior pituitary. In addition to hormones of the adrenal cortex, feedback inhibition of ACTH-RH release by the hypothalamus can also be carried out by ACTH when its concentration reaches high levels in the blood.

Somatotropic hormone–releasing hormone (STH-RH) or growth-stimulating hormone-releasing hormone (GRH) This hormone has an acidic protein structure whose molecular weight is quite variable among species. The major locus for the production of this releasing hormone is thought to be located in the *lateral ventromedial nucleus of the hypothalamus.* Release of STH-RH from the hypothalamus is the result of input from higher centers of the brain and by increased blood levels of arginine, vasopressin, and adrenocorticoids. Its release is slowed or halted again by impulses from higher nerve centers and by high levels of blood glucose, fatty acids, and beta-adrenergic agents. There is also feedback control from the intermediate proteins, which are produced in response to the pituitary growth hormone. These proteins, called *somatomedins*, increase as the growth hormone levels increase. When an optimum level is reached, they inhibit further release of STH-RH from the hypothalamus.

Thyroid-stimulating hormone-releasing hormone (TSH-RH) or thyrotropin-releasing hormone (TRH) The thyroid-stimulating hormone-releasing hormone is a tripeptide that has been isolated from various parts of the hypothalamus and is released into the *hypophyseal portal system* at the *median eminence.* Besides stimulating the release of thyroid-stimulating hormone (TSH), it also stimulates the release of *prolactin* from the anterior pituitary. Thyroid-stimulating hormone-releasing hormone is transmitted by the hypophyseal portal system to the anterior pituitary, where it stimulates the synthesis and release of TSH, which in turn stimulates the thyroid gland to increase its output of *thyroxine* and *triiodothyronine.* Experimental evidence has shown that injection of very small amounts of either of these hormones into the anterior pituitary results in a decrease in TSH release. This reduction is apparently due to a blocking effect of thyroxine and triiodothyronine on the TSH-RH receptor sites in the pituitary. Thus, thyroid hormone production is regulated through a feedback mechanism that affects both the pituitary and the hypothalamus.

Areas for cold and heat reception in the hypothalamus lie very close to the areas of synthesis of TSH-RH. Whether the close approximation of these two areas to the production sites of this releasing hormone is significant remains to be seen. But ambient temperature has a decided effect on the secretion of TSH and thus TSH-RH. Cold exposure enhances the release of TSH-RH and thus TSH. Trauma, restraint, and chronic stress inhibit the release of TSH, presumably through the action of hormones of the adrenal cortex on the secretion of TSH-RH.

Follicle-stimulating hormone/luteinizing hormone-releasing hormone (FSH/LH-RH) There is much controversy over the exact releasing hormone for FSH and LH. Several investigators have indicated that these pituitary hormones have the same hypothalamic-releasing hormone. This hypothesis will be accepted for the sake of discussion throughout the remainder of this text. Since it stimulates the release of both FSH and LH, it may be termed gonadotropin-releasing hormone (GRH). The production and release of this hormone is intimately tied to the levels of the anterior pituitary hormones FSH and LH and the ovarian hormones *progesterone* and *estrogen*. Blood levels of all of these hormones are controlled by means of a feedback-regulation loop. In the human female, levels of these hormones vary greatly during pregnancy. In nonpregnant females, FSH stimulates the *ovarian follicles* to grow. As they increase in size they begin to produce and release higher and higher levels of estrogen into the bloodstream. Ultimately, a precipitous rise in both FSH and LH occurs at the time of ovulation, which is followed by a decrease in blood levels of both of these pituitary hormones. The decrease in release of these hormones apparently occurs through negative feedback.

In the male, LH acts on the *testes*, specifically the *Leydig* or *interstitial cells*, to promote the production of *testosterone*. High levels of testosterone then feed back on the hypothalamus to reduce further secretion of FSH/LH-RH and therefore slow down the release of LH and thus testosterone secretion. Follicle-stimulating hormone secretion could be regulated by a different mechanism, possibly by a protein still to be analyzed called *inhibin*. This protein is believed to be produced by the *seminiferous tubules of the testes*. An increase in plasma levels of inhibin supposedly slows the release of FSH from the pituitary.

Prolactin-releasing hormone (PRH), melanocyte-inhibiting hormone (MIH), and melanocyte-stimulating hormone-releasing hormone (MSH-RH) Releasing hormones for both of these anterior pituitary hormones have been postulated, as has an inhibiting hormone for melanocyte-stimulating hormone. These hormones, however, have not been isolated and little evidence exists for them.

Prolactin-inhibiting hormone (PIH) This inhibiting hormone, produced in the *lateral preoptic area of the hypothalamus*, is believed to be *dopamine*. Its production is stimulated by prolactin; as the level of prolactin increases, it causes the hypothalamus to produce and secrete PIH, which then acts on the pituitary to slow the release of prolactin. If the pituitary stalk is severed, including the hypophyseal portal system, concentrations of all of the anterior pituitary hormones except prolactin are drastically reduced. This hormone, on the other hand, increases its concentration severalfold.

Somatotropic hormone–inhibiting hormone (STH-IH) or somatostatin This is a tetradecapeptide which has been isolated from the hypothalamus and causes inhibition of the release of STH from the anterior pituitary. Its synthesis and secretion are stimulated by high levels of blood glucose, fatty acids, beta adrenergic agents, and somatomedins.

THE PITUITARY GLAND

The pituitary gland, or *hypophysis*, is also called the *master gland* because of the importance of the pituitary hormones in the regulation of activity of other endocrine glands. It is located on the floor of the brain in a depression of the *sphenoid bone* called the *sella turcica* (see Figure 17–4). The hypophysis is attached to the rest of the brain via the infundibular stalk. The pituitary is composed of two parts, the *neurohypophysis* and the *adenohypophysis*, which have separate origins in the embryo. The neurohypophysis is derived from the neural ectoderm, whereas the adenohypophysis arises from a pocket of ectodermal tissue *(Rathke's pocket)* from the embryonic pharynx. Based upon structure in the adult, the pituitary can be divided into three distinct portions: the *anterior, intermediate*, and *posterior lobes*. The anterior pituitary (or *pars distalis*) and the intermediate lobe (or *pars intermedia*) are both part of the adenohypophysis. The posterior pituitary (or *pars nervosa*) represents the entire neurohypophysis. Some authors also include the *supraoptic* and *paraventricular nuclei*, hormone-producing areas of the hypothalamus, as part of the posterior pituitary because the nerve fibers are continuous between the nuclei and the posterior pituitary.

The neurohypophysis is innervated by the *supraoptic-hypophyseal tract*, which enters the posterior pituitary from the hypothalamus through the *infundibular stalk*. The two lobes of the adenohypophysis are not innervated and instead depend upon the hypophyseal portal system for input. It is through this system that releasing and inhibiting hormones from the hypothalamus reach the anterior pituitary and the intermediate lobe of the pituitary and consequently trigger or inhibit release of the hormones from these lobes of the hypophysis.

The Posterior Lobe of the Pituitary

The posterior lobe of the pituitary is composed of the *pars nervosa* and the *hypophyseal stalk*, which connects the median eminence of the hypothalamus with the pituitary gland. The paraventricular and supraoptic nuclei of the hypothalamus are secretory in nature and have axons which terminate in the posterior pituitary. In addition to secretory neurons, there are many *pituicytes*, or modified neuroglial cells, which occur singly and in groups in the pituitary. These cells are supportive in nature and have no secretory function. This region of the pituitary may also contain pigment granules.

In 1895, Oliver and Schafer found that whole pituitary extracts caused vasoconstriction and an increase in blood pressure when administered intravenously to dogs. Later

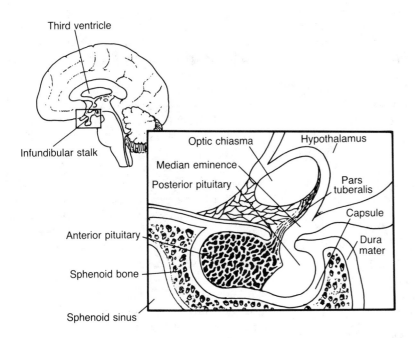

work showed that these effects were attributable to vasopressin from the pars nervosa. Kamm and associates, in 1928, isolated two active fractions from the posterior pituitary, one of which increased blood pressure and the other induced uterine contractions. It was not until the 1950s that Bagmann and the Scharrers discovered that these substances were produced in the hypothalamus. Both of the hormones released from the posterior pituitary (i.e., vasopressin and oxytocin) are polypeptides and are very similar in structure (see Figure 17–5). Both hormones pass down the supraoptic-hypophyseal tract and become associated with carrier proteins called *neurophysins*. Vasopressin and oxytocin are stored in the posterior pituitary in this loose arrangement with the carrier proteins until they are released into the hypophyseal portal system and transferred throughout the body through the bloodstream.

Vasopressin Vasopressin, also called *antidiuretic hormone (ADH)* and *pitiressin*, is well known for its *pressor* (i.e., vasoconstriction) and *diuretic* effects. In addition, vasopressin has a very slight effect on increasing uterine motility. There are two forms of vasopressin

FIGURE 17–5
Chemical structure of oxytocin and vasopressin. It is easy to see that these two peptide hormones overlap in their effects.

in mammals. These chemicals vary only in the placement of *arginine* or *lysine* in position eight of the polypeptide chain. Thus, these hormones are known as *arginine vasopressin* and *lysine vasopressin* depending upon which amino acid is present. Arginine vasopressin, thought to be the more primitive of the two compounds, is present in echidnas and marsupials as well as the higher mammals. Both types of vasopressin are found in the hippopotamus, warthogs, and peccaries. Several strains of domesticated pigs have only lysine vasopressin.

The major physiological effects of vasopressin are in its antidiuretic properties. Vasopressin acts on the epithelial cells of the distal convoluted tubules in the kidney to cause an increase in water permeability (see chapter 14, The Excretory System and Water Balance). This increase in permeability is evidently brought about through increased levels of cyclic AMP. Cyclic AMP is believed to increase tubule cell pore diameter and therefore increase the rate at which water is reabsorbed. The actual release of vasopressin occurs in response to an increase in the osmotic pressure of the blood. This increase in osmotic pressure stimulates the hypothalamic osmoreceptors, which trigger the release of vasopressin. As a result of vasopressin release and consequent water reabsorption by the kidney, plasma osmotic pressure falls. Vasopressin secretion is terminated after the receptors in the hypothalamus respond to the decrease in osmotic pressure of the blood.

A reduction in the blood volume without changing the osmotic concentration of the blood, a situation which might arise during hemorrhage or certain types of shock, also results in release of vasopressin. Volume (pressure) receptors located at strategic points in the circulatory system regulate production of vasopressin by the hypothalamus. This hormone stimulates the production and release of *aldosterone* by the adrenal cortex and also causes an increase in water permeability of the renal tubules. Aldosterone enhances salt retention, which results in increased water retention and hence increased blood volumes.

Kangaroo rats survive on metabolic water derived from oxidation of their food. In these animals the neurohypophysis is relatively large and contains more vasopressin per microgram of tissue than that of similar rodents which must consume water to survive. Laboratory rats, when deprived of water, show an increased secretion of vasopressin and a slowing of food consumption. Decreased food consumption results in reduced feces formation, and therefore less water is lost through the feces.

Release of vasopressin can have many causes besides those mentioned here (i.e., decreased blood volume, increased blood osmotic pressure, and decreased water intake). Other causes for release include: central nervous system stimulation; strong emotions; certain sensory stimuli, such as pain, coitus, and suckling (or milking); changes in environmental temperature; and certain drugs. Among those drugs which decrease the release of vasopressin are caffeine and alcohol; among those which increase vasopressin release are morphine, nicotine, ether, and some barbiturates.

Oxytocin Oxytocin, or *pitocin*, is important in the contraction of smooth muscles in the uterus and for milk ejection in nursing of some mammals (e.g., "letdown" reflex). It may also prevent involution of the lactating mammary gland. Like vasopressin, oxytocin has pressor and antidiuretic effects but these are very minor: 0.5–1.0 percent as effective as vasopressin.

In the female, oxytocin is released during coitus, especially during orgasm, as a result of neurohumoral reflex action involving the hypothalamus. The oxytocin thus released stimulates contraction of uterine smooth muscle, which is important for the movement of sperm from the lower portions of the uterus (cervix) to the upper areas of the uterus, where sperm enter the oviducts. During pregnancy, *progesterone*, which is either produced by the corpus luteum or the placenta or both, inhibits and blocks the effect of oxytocin on the uterus. During parturition, when progesterone and estrogen levels have dropped, the blocking effect of the progesterone is withdrawn and oxytocin enhances uterine contraction and aids in the expulsion of the fetus. Oxytocin is most effective when the uterus has been estrogen primed. When females are hypophysectomized during pregnancy, normal parturition can occur, probably as a result of direct release of oxytocin by the hypothalamus.

When a lactating female is suckled or milked, sensory impulses travel from the mammary glands to the paraventricular and supraoptic nuclei. The stimulation then passes down the axons of these nerves and causes the release of oxytocin and perhaps vasopressin, though vasopressin is five to six times less effective at inducing milk ejection than is oxytocin. These hormones are transmitted through the blood to the mammary glands, where they induce contraction of the *myoepithelial cells*, which surround the alveoli and small ducts. As these cells contract, milk is forced out of the alveoli and small ducts into the larger ducts and subsequently through the nipple or teat.

The Intermediate Lobe of the Pituitary

The pars intermedia, or intermediate lobe of the pituitary, produces a hormone called *melanocyte-stimulating hormone (MSH)* which has an effect on pigmentation in some mammals. In addition to MSH, ACTH may have some function in mammalian pigmentation, though its exact role is still disputed. Both of these pituitary hormones have been found to affect melanocytes in humans, deer mice, and weasels.

Many mammals show an annual color cycle in which a summer pigmented fur is replaced in winter by a fur devoid of pigment. This is usually found in such mammals as the collared lemming, the snowshoe hare, and the weasel, for which the presence of snow during the winter months is an annual event. In these species the lack of pigmentation (i.e., white coloration) is apparently protective in nature, since it allows for better concealment against the white background provided by the snow. It has been shown that the dark coloration in weasels is due to the presence of MSH. Mammals such as the laboratory mouse, whose coat color does not follow a cyclic pattern, become dark when injected with MSH.

The onset of the dark *pelage* (fur) in such animals as the weasel and snowshoe hare appears to be controlled by photoperiod, since color changes in fall and spring in these animals are quite predictable and bear little relationship to other environmental factors (e.g., temperature). This would be an excellent case to show the inhibitory role of *melatonin* on the secretory action of the pituitary, since melatonin production would be expected to increase with the shorter days of fall and decrease with the longer days of spring. But the *pineal gland*, which secretes melatonin, has not been shown to be responsible for the transducer role between day-length and pelage coloration and therefore MSH release in mammals.

The Anterior Lobe of the Pituitary

In most mammals the anterior lobe of the pituitary, or simply anterior pituitary, produces six hormones (see Table 17–1). In animals lacking an intermediate lobe, a seventh hormone, melanocyte-stimulating hormone, is also produced. All of the hormones produced by the anterior pituitary are large polypeptides. Their release seems to be controlled for the most part by humoral rather than neural mechanisms because there are no secretory nerve endings in the anterior pituitary.

The anterior lobe of the pituitary is made up of three types of cells. The *basophils* are cells which secrete both *somatotropic hormone (STH)*, also known as growth-stimulating hormone (GSH), and *prolactin*, which has also been called lactogenic hormone and luteotropic hormone (LtH). The term luteotropic hormone is very common but is somewhat of a misnomer, because its luteotropic effect occurs only in rats and possibly a few other mammals. Many domesticated as well as feral animals have been investigated without additional evidence of this hormone's luteotropic effect. Smaller cells of the adenohypophysis, called *acidophils*, are also secretory in nature. They are responsible for the production of four hormones: *luteinizing hormone* (LH), which is also referred to as *interstitial cell–stimulating hormone (ICSH)* in male mammals; *follicle-stimulating hormone (FSH)*; *thyroid-stimulating hormone* (TSH); and *adrenocorticotropic hormone (ACTH)*. Melanocyte-stimulating hormone (MSH),

whether produced in the intermediate lobe or the anterior lobe, is also secreted by acidophils. A third type of cell found in the anterior pituitary related to hormone production is the *nonsecretory chromophobe.* As the name implies, these cells do not stain readily. Chromophobes are the precursors of the acidophils and basophils and are generally larger than these other cell types. The proportions of these three cell types varies with age, sex, species, reproductive state, various thyroid and other endocrine activities, and pregnancy.

Somatotropic hormone Somatotropic hormone is a polypeptide with a molecular weight of approximately 22,000. There is a similarity in molecular structure among species and in some cases the hormones are interchangeable (see Table 17–2). Human STH is chemically and immunologically related to *human placental lactogen (HPL).* Levels of STH average about 300 micrograms per liter plasma in children and approximately 200 micrograms per liter plasma in adult humans. Somatotropic hormone affects protein, fat, and carbohydrate metabolism and enhances the effects of other hormones.

Effects of STH. Somatotropic hormone decreases protein catabolism and induces a positive nitrogen balance. It also increases the transfer to amino acids across cell membranes. This is especially evident in muscle tissue. This hormone is also *diabetogenic*, in that it causes an increase in blood glucose levels and induces hyperglycemia. It appears to stimulate the *alpha cells* of the islets of Langerhans to secrete glucagon, which causes the release of glucose from glycogen stored in the liver. Somatotropic hormone also enhances *lipid mobilization* and therefore *lipid utilization* by the tissues. An in-

TABLE 17–2
Response of species to interspecific somatotropic hormone types

Test Animal	Source of Somatotropic Hormone or Pituitary Extract*					
	Guinea Pig	Humpback Whale	Pig	Beef	Sheep	Macaque, Human
Mouse				+		+
Rat	+	+	+	+	+	+
Guinea pig	−			−		−
Cat				+		
Dog			+	+		+
Sheep				+		
Goat				+		
Cow				+		
Macaque			−	−		+
Human		−	−	−	−	+

Source: From Molecular Variation and Possible Lines of Evolution of Peptide and Protein Hormones by Irving I. Geschwind. *American Zoologist* 7(1967):89-108.
*Response characteristic of somatotropic hormone was observed in the test animal (+); No such response shown (−).

crease in lipid utilization has a sparing effect on glucose and plasma glucose levels increase. Somatotropic hormone administration also results in an increase in the length of the long bones in young animals. This is accomplished through decreased protein catabolism and increased calcium ion absorption from the gut, with a resultant increase in the width of the epiphyseal cartilages and therefore an increase in the ultimate bone length (see chapter 8, The Skeletal System). Somatotropic hormone also enhances the production of *T cells* by lymphoid tissue. In this action STH augments the production of *cyclic AMP* in lymph tissue, which results in a greater rate of T cell production.

Somatotropic hormone has many synergistic effects when combined with other endocrine hormones. It enhances the effects of ACTH, TSH, FSH, and LH but by itself has little effect on the target organs of these hormones. In these cases it seems to prime the target organs for further hormonal action by their respective pituitary hormones. The combined effect of STH and TSH is especially important, because STH causes an increase in length of the long bones whereas TSH brings about their maturation.

Control of STH release. Control of STH release appears to reside at the hypothalamic level, where both somatotropic hormone–releasing hormone (STH-RH) and somatotropic hormone–inhibiting hormone (STH-IH) are produced and secreted (see Figure 17–6). It has been demonstrated that plasma glucose levels stimulate the production of these control factors. When blood glucose levels are high, STH-IH is released and travels via the hypophyseal portal system to inhibit further release of STH from the anterior pituitary. Low levels of STH result in a decrease in *protein anabolism, fat catabolism,* and *glycogen mobilization.* When the plasma glucose levels drop below normal, the hypothalamus releases STH-RH, which promotes the release

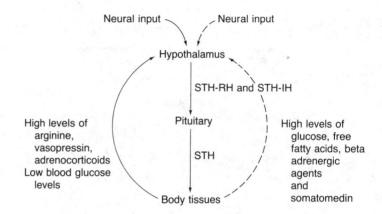

FIGURE 17–6
Feedback regulation of somatotropic hormone (STH). Dashed lines indicate inhibition; solid lines show stimulation.

of STH from the anterior lobe of the pituitary. There is a subsequent rise in protein anabolism, fat catabolism (and therefore free fatty acid levels), and blood glucose levels. Stress, exercise, and amino acid levels also affect the release of STH.

Effects of variation in STH levels. Hypophysectomy in young animals results in immediate cessation of skeletal growth. In rats there is a suppression of their response to carcinogenic agents due to the effect on lymphoid cell production. Administration of STH restores this response. Exogenous administration of STH and testosterone in hypophysectomized animals also restores the male accessory sex glands to their normal function. The administration of STH alone results in a little improvement in the histological appearance of some of the other endocrine glands and other tissues in hypophysectomized mammals.

Prolonged administration of high doses of STH causes a number of pathological problems, one of which is permanent diabetes in dogs. In this case the beta cells in the islets of Langerhans are thought to be destroyed because they are too heavily taxed in the production of insulin to combat the diabeto-

genic effect of STH. In rats there is hypertrophy of the muscles, skin, and connective and lymphoid tissues. There may also be neoplastic growth in the lungs, adrenal medulla, and reproductive organs.

Three diseases specific to the concentration of STH are observed in mammals. *Pituitary* or *ateliotic dwarfism* results from STH insufficiency. Such individuals look like miniature adults with normal body proportions. This condition is due to the slow growth of the bones and epiphyseal closure before adult height is reached. *Giantism* is a result of hypersecretion of STH during early development. This results in a rapid increase in bone length and individuals of unusually large stature. Hypersecretion after epiphyseal closure results in a condition known as *acromegaly*. This disease is characterized by the continued increase in length and thickening of the bones of the hands, feet, jaw, and cheeks. Other soft tissues in the eyelids, lips, nose, and tongue continue to grow, and furrows form on the forehead and soles of the feet.

The effects of hyper- and hyposecretion of endocrine hormones will not be discussed extensively in this text. This subject is well covered in most medical physiology textbooks, and the reader is therefore directed to any of the excellent medically oriented texts.

Thyroid-stimulating hormone Thyroid-stimulating hormone is a glycoprotein with a molecular weight of approximately 33,000. It has two subunits which may be interchangeable with subunits of LH, FSH, *human chorionic gonadotropin (HCG)*, and *pregnant mare serum gonadotropin (PMSG)*. Thyroid-stimulating hormone is the main factor controlling activity of the thyroid gland.

Effects of TSH. Thyroid-stimulating hormone (or *thyrotropin*) acts on the thyroid gland to cause the production and secretion of *thyroxine* and *triiodothyronine*. This increase in synthesis and release of these thyroid hormones is accomplished in many ways. First, TSH increases the cleavage of the *thyroglobulin peptide* in the *thyroid follicles*, resulting in the hydrolysis of thyroxine and triiodothyronine. TSH also enhances iodide uptake by the thyroid gland, with a subsequent increase in iodination of *tyrosine*, the thyroxine and triiodothyronine precursor, in the *follicular colloid*. Thyroid-stimulating hormone also increases the size and number of thyroid cells.

Control of TSH release. Control of TSH release from the anterior pituitary may reside in the pituitary itself as well as within the hypothalamus (see Figure 17–7). There is some evidence that high levels of thyroxine in the blood feed back directly on the pituitary to inhibit further release of TSH. This feedback loop can be observed in rabbits in which the *hypophyseal portal vein* has been destroyed. In these animals an injection of thyroxine causes a decrease in the release of TSH from the pituitary. To further isolate the anterior pituitary from hypothalamic-releasing hor-

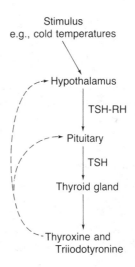

FIGURE 17–7
Feedback regulation of thyroid-stimulating hormone (TSH). Dashed lines indicate inhibition.

mones, it can be transplanted to the anterior eye chamber of hypophysectomized rabbits. In both of these cases there is no intact hypophyseal portal system, but, thyroxine effectively inhibits TSH release from the anterior pituitary. In normal intact animals it is believed that thyroxine feeds back on the hypothalamus to reduce the amount of TSH-RH that is secreted and therefore the amount of TSH released by the pituitary.

Effects of variation in TSH levels. Surgical removal of the thyroid gland, termed *thyroidectomy*, may result in the formation of tumors in the anterior lobe of the pituitary. Tumor formation is apparently due to the lack of feedback inhibition of thyroid hormone on the pituitary. This leads to increased activity and size of the pituitary as it increases production and release of TSH. These tumors produce exceptionally high levels of TSH because there is no feedback from the thyroid to stop the production and secretion of TSH.

The importance of the feedback mechanism between these two glands can also be observed upon ablation of the pituitary. In this case, the thyroid gland atrophies. There is a reduction of iodine uptake, the secretory epithelium becomes flattened, and the production and secretion of thyroxine and triiodothyronine decrease dramatically. Exogenous administration of purified TSH or a fresh pituitary implant will cause the thyroid to regain its normal appearance and function.

In some cases the pituitary produces and secretes sufficient TSH but the thyroid is unable to produce enough thyroxine and triiodothyronine for maintenance of normal function. This failure is due to insufficient iodine concentrations and results in development of an enlarged thyroid, known as an *endemic goiter*. The goiter is the result of the trophic action of TSH on the thyroid gland. Because of the release of insufficient levels of thyroxine and triiodothyronine from the thyroid, the pituitary continually releases TSH. The goiter is then the result of *thyroid cell hyperplasia* and *hypertrophy*. Goiter formation may also be induced by the administration of high levels of *thiouracil* and *thiourea*. These compounds prevent the synthesis of thyroxine and triiodothyronine, which then results in an increase in TSH secretion and a subsequent increase in the size of the thyroid gland. Agents such as thiouracil are termed *goiterogenic agents*.

Adrenocorticotropic hormone Adrenocorticotropic hormone is a rather small, straight-chain polypeptide containing 39 amino acid residues and has a molecular weight of approximately 4,500. The structure of the hormone varies from species to species, but the active site of the molecule remains the same. This hormone has been synthesized *in vitro* and has been found to have sequences of amino acids common to those of melanocyte-stimulating hormone.

Effects of ACTH. The *adrenal cortex* is the main target organ of this hormone. Adrenocorticotropic hormone activates the enzyme *adenyl cyclase*, which converts ATP to cyclic AMP. The increase in cyclic AMP accelerates the conversion of cholesterol to *pregnenolone*. Pregnenolone is the precursor of many of the *adrenocorticoids*. In any case, there is an increased synthesis and subsequent secretion of *glucocorticoids* from the adrenal cortex. This increase in production and secretion of adrenal hormones results in an enlargement of the *adrenal gland.* The administration of ACTH can reverse atrophy in the adrenal cortices of hypophysectomized individuals. There is also some evidence that ACTH may directly affect carbohydrate and fat metabolism throughout the body.

Control of ACTH release. Control of ACTH release from the anterior pituitary resides in the hypothalamus, as does the release of many of the anterior pituitary hormones (see Figure 17–8). The hypothalamus produces a peptide, *adrenocorticotrophic–hormone releasing hormone (ACTH-RH)*, which when released into the hypophyseal portal system stimulates the production and release of ACTH from the pituitary. The ACTH which is thus released acts on the adrenal cortex to promote the production and secretion of *adrenocortical steroids*, which feed back to slow the release of ACTH-RH. This feedback decreases the rate of release of ACTH.

The General Adaptation Syndrome (GAS)
In the 1950s, Hans Selyé demonstrated that mammals under stress exhibited a general alteration in a number of major bodily functions which ultimately become deleterious.

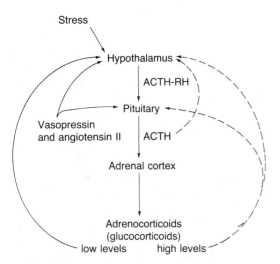

FIGURE 17–8
Feedback regulation of adrenocorticotropic hormone (ACTH). Dashed lines indicate inhibition; solid lines show stimulation.

This set of responses has subsequently become known as the *General Adaptation Syndrome*. Any disturbance or deviation from the normal in functional mechanisms essential to the survival of the mammal can be manifested as *stress*. Stress can be used to describe emotional as well as physical trauma felt by an animal. Examples of factors which have been considered to constitute stress are temperature extremes, pain, overcrowded conditions, and physical injury. Mammals may be stressed by one or several factors but in the final result show a general response involving more than one physiological mechanism. Examples of the functional response to stress are increased ACTH production, increased adrenal activity, and increased plasma fatty acid levels. All of these factors are in one way or another related to adrenal gland activity and could be initiated through an effect on the hypothalamus and its production and release of releasing hormones.

If the stress is not removed from the organism or population, the ultimate result is death of the organism or population decline. Some specific effects which usually precede death of the individual are decreased clotting time, elevated blood pressure, heart hypertrophy, and gastric ulcers. Population decline is sometimes very rapid once a certain density has been reached, referred to as a *population crash*. This type of rapid decline is seen in the much-emphasized lemming population cycle. Analysis by R. Andrews and associates of the physiological changes in lemmings during an apparent population high revealed adrenal hypertrophy, high basal levels of adrenal steroid secretion, high pituitary ACTH levels, cardiac hypertrophy, and an increased incidence of renal disease.

It is probable that stress, whether emotional or physical, activates certain areas of the hypothalamus which control the production of ACTH-RH. This in turn results in increased ACTH production and ultimately in elevated blood levels of adrenocortical hormones, which lead to the debilitating factors characteristic of the General Adaptation Syndrome. The persistence of the stress factor must in some way block or override the feedback regulation of ACTH production and allow the production of adrenal corticoids to increase to an abnormally high level. During this time, though the animal's sense of well-being is increased and inflammatory responses are retarded, white blood cell production is reduced, which reduces the animal's resistance to disease. In most cases, animals under stress are very susceptible to disease. This is one of the reasons for the importance of the GAS theory to medicine. A number of diseases, such as certain types of heart disease and types of cancer which have not been linked to an infectious organism, may be stress related.

Follicle-stimulating hormone Follicle-stimulating hormone (FSH) is one of the *gonadotropic hormones* of the pituitary, and thus certain aspects of this hormone will also be covered in chapter 18, The Reproductive System. Follicle-stimulating hormone, a glycoprotein with a molecular weight of about 30,000, is composed of two subunits. In some cases these subunits can hybridize with subunits from a different hormone and still be biologically active. That is, the alpha subunit of FSH may hybridize with the beta subunit from LH and still have FSH-like activity.

Effects of FSH. Follicle-stimulating hormone binds to the *granulosus cells* of the *ovarian follicles* in the female. In these animals FSH stimulates young ovarian follicles to form antra and many granulosus layers. In female mammals, there is an increase in the cytogenic activity of these follicular cells. Besides increasing the activity and number of granulosus cells in the developing follicles and therefore increasing the size and complexity of the follicle, there is also a stimulatory effect on these cells to produce and secrete *estrogen.* In order for the follicles to attain their full size and be able to secrete estrogen, LH must also be present. The interaction of these two hormones is closely related in many aspects. During the ovarian cycle, there is a preovulatory surge of both FSH and LH in most mammals. This surge contributes to the actual process of the release of the ovum from the follicle. In some experimental animals FSH was shown to be capable of inducing ovulation without the presence of LH.

In male mammals, FSH binds to the epithelial cells of the *seminiferous tubules.* This hormone is important for *gametogenesis* in that it stimulates the formation of *secondary spermatocytes* from *primary spermatocytes.*

It also stimulates the Sertoli cells to form *androgen binding proteins.* These proteins enhance the transfer of testosterone from the Leydig cells to the germinal epithelium. Follicle-stimulating hormone alone, when administered to hypophysectomized male rats, stimulates the seminiferous tubules but not the Leydig cells.

Control of FSH release. Follicle-stimulating hormone production is controlled by means of a releasing hormone (FSH/LH-RH) from the hypothalamus (see Figure 17–9). As FSH is released from the anterior pituitary, it binds to the granulosus cells in the ovary. These cells increase in size and number and eventually begin to produce estrogen. Estrogen then feeds back on the hypothalamus to slow the

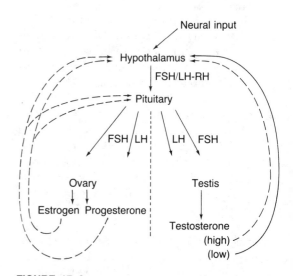

FIGURE 17–9
Feedback regulation of the gonadal steroids and follicle-stimulating hormone and luteinizing hormone from the pituitary. High concentrations of these steroids cause a decrease in FSH/LH-RH release. There may also be some feedback control on the pituitary itself. Dashed lines indicate inhibition; solid lines indicate stimulation.

release of FSH/LH-RH. Lack of this peptide slows the production and secretion of FSH.

Luteinizing hormone Like other pituitary gonadotropins, LH has its primary effect on the reproductive system in mammals. Luteinizing hormone, as its name implies, brings about the luteinization of *granulosus* and *thecal cells* in the ovary. This hormone is composed of two subunits very similar to those found in FSH. It is also chemically similar to human chorionic gonadotropin and is immunologically similar to TSH. There is a loss of biological activity when LH is treated with chymotrypsin, but the immunological activity remains fairly high. This finding suggests that there are two different activity sites on the LH molecule.

Effects of LH. In the female, LH binds to the thecal cells of ovarian follicles and to the *luteal cells* of the corpus luteum. It also works synergistically with FSH to stimulate the secretion of *estrogen* from the granulosus cells. Just prior to ovulation there is a rapid increase in the levels of FSH and LH. This LH surge may be responsible for the preovulatory swelling and rupture of the *Graafian follicle*. Luteinizing hormone is directly or indirectly responsible for the formation of the corpus luteum after ovulation and may indirectly affect the maintenance of the corpus luteum by its effect on ovarian interstitial cells. The ultimate effect of this hormone is to stimulate the production of progesterone by the corpus luteum. In rats LH acts synergistically with prolactin to bring about the production of *progesterone* by the luteal cells. This secretion of progesterone is very important in the maintenance of the ovarian cycle and the preparation of the uterus for the implantation of blastocycts in the pregnant female. Once implantation has occurred, progesterone must be produced either by the corpus luteum or the placenta or both in order for the pregnancy to be maintained.

In the male mammal, LH binds to the Leydig cells of the testes. Here, the LH stimulates the production of *androgens*. When the LH binds to the Leydig cells, it activates the production of *adenyl cyclase*, which in turn causes the conversion of ATP to cyclic AMP. Steroidogenesis increases as the intracellular concentrations of cyclic AMP increase. This may be due to the action of cyclic AMP on cholesterol in steroid production. This same mode of action is hypothesized in the production of progesterone in the female.

Control of LH release. *Testosterone* produced in the testes by males and *progesterone* produced in the corpus luteum and placenta of the female feed back on the hypothalamus to slow production and release of FSH/LH-RH (see Figure 17–9). This peptide stimulates the production and release of LH, as well as FSH, from the anterior pituitary. High levels of estrogen have also been shown to inhibit release of LH. When the levels of progesterone or testosterone decrease, more FSH/LH-RH is released by the hypothalamus, which causes a subsequent release of LH. This increase stimulates the Leydig cells and ovarian tissue to produce more steroids and the feedback loop is once again complete.

There is also a *neuroendocrine mechanism* which is hypothesized for the release of LH. This hormone has been shown to increase the receptivity of some mammalian females during the breeding season. Induced ovulation may be brought about through the nervous stimulation achieved during copulation in the rabbit, ferret, and cat. In bulls there is often an increase in the circulating levels of LH due to sexual excitement. This rise in LH levels may be caused by the mere sight of a cow or solely by the act of coitus, but most often by sniffing the vulva of a cow in heat. In these experiments it was noted that if testosterone levels were concomitantly high, LH did not cause these levels to rise further; but if the testosterone levels were low, LH resulted in a definite increase in testosterone levels.

Prolactin Prolactin, or *luteotrophic hormone*, is composed of approximately 200 amino acids, and its molecular weight varies depending upon the species in question. The molecular weight of human prolactin is about 22,000; that of sheep and oxen about 25,000. Prolactin is produced and secreted by the *acidophil cells* of the anterior pituitary and binds the *interstitial cells of the ovary* and the *cells of the corpus luteum.* It also must bind areas of the *mammary glands*, because of its pronounced effect on lactation and development of the mammary glands. Because it elicites lactation in mammals, it has been termed the *lactogenic hormone.*

Effects of prolactin. This hormone is found in most, if not all, vertebrates. Its effects and modes of action are as varied as the animals in which it is produced. There is some question as to whether all of the following actions are attributable to prolactin alone or whether they are the result of impure preparations of this hormone. Prolactin has been separated from STH in humans. This impurity could be part of the reason that prolactin has been shown to stimulate growth in some mammals. Probably the best-known effects of prolactin in mammals are related to reproduction and care of the offspring. As already

mentioned, prolactin is essential for the maintenance of the corpus luteum in the rat and possibly some other mammals. In mammals in general, prolactin stimulates the development of the mammary gland and subsequently brings about lactation. In male mammals it acts synergistically with testosterone in stimulation of *prostatic growth* and may also stimulate the *seminal vesicles* in some way. In male rabbits there is a decrease in copulatory behavior with an increase in prolactin concentration. In some species of mammals it also reinforces certain aspects of parental care of the young. Maternal behavior is enhanced in laboratory rats that are administered prolactin.

Some of the other effects of prolactin in mammals include its actions related to metabolism. Besides its reported effects on growth, it has been shown to be *diabetogenic* (or *hyperglycemic*) in its action. It may also increase lipid deposition and stimulate the production of red blood cells. How these effects are brought about is presently unknown. Again, some of these may be connected with other hormones; or, at the very least, there may be synergistic effects with other hormones. Prolactin seems to increase the size and activity of sebaceous glands in general and in this way also affects the mammary glands. In addition, there is some evidence that prolactin may affect hair maturation. For more information on the development of the mammary glands as a function of prolactin, see chapter 18, The Reproductive System.

Control of prolactin release. Release of prolactin is under the control of the hypothalamic hormone *prolactin-inhibiting hormone (PIH)* (see Figure 17–10). This inhibitory hormone maintains normal prolactin levels at relatively low concentrations. During preg-

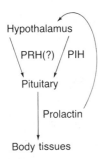

FIGURE 17–10
Feedback regulation of prolactin release by the pituitary. Note that prolactin feeds back directly on the hypothalamus to increase release of prolactin-inhibiting hormone (PIH). Solid lines indicate stimulation of PIH release.

nancy and lactation, however, prolactin levels increase. Once pregnancy is terminated and lactation has continued for a period of time, the prolactin levels again decrease.

THE GONADS

In both male and female mammals the reproductive organs are paired structures of mesodermal origin. The *gonads*, as they are called, have both cytogenic and endocrine functions. The cytogenic aspect is covered in Chapter 18, The Reproductive System. Only the endocrine functions will be discussed here.

The Ovaries

The mammalian *ovaries* are responsible for the production of as many as four or more hormones. Of special importance are the hormones *estrogen* and *progesterone*, or more precisely the classes of *estrogens* and *progestins*. These two hormonal classes maintain the reproductive organs in the female. These classes of hormones are also essential in establishing and maintaining the *female secondary sex characteristics*. These secondary sex characteristics, such as mammary gland development, hair distribution, certain aspects of behavior, a higher-pitched voice, broader pelvic girdle, and a typical distribution of subcutaneous body fat, are obvious in the human female. Two other hormones which are produced and secreted by the ovaries are *androgens*, which occur in relatively minute quantities in most female mammals, and *relaxin*, which is generally only produced during pregnancy. Ovariectomy of the prepuberal female halts further development of the reproductive tract. In the postpuberal female ovariectomy induces atrophy of the uterus, oviducts, and vagina and brings on a premature climacteric.

Estrogens The estrogens are a class of *steroid hormones* which include *estrone, estriol,* and *estradiol* (also *equilin* and *equilenin* in horses). Estradiol is the most potent of the three. All members of this class are composed of a *cyclopenthanoperhydrophenanthrene nucleus*. These steroids are found in all female vertebrates and are produced from cholesterol not only in the ovaries but also in the adrenal cortices and the placenta (see Figure 17–11). In males they are synthesized in the adrenals and the testes. Synthetic chemicals with estrogenic properties include *diethylstilbestrol, dimethylstilbestrol, hexestrol, dienestrol,* and *benzestrol* (see Figure 17–12).

Effects of estrogens. No matter where the estrogens are formed, once in the bloodstream they travel to the liver, where they become bound to protein carrier molecules, which then transport them to their target organs. Estrogens are inactivated in the liver, finally processed through the kidney, and ex-

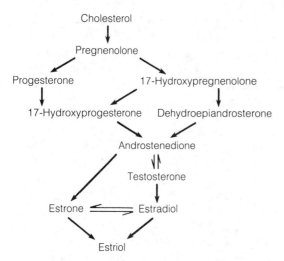

FIGURE 17–11
Pathways for the biosynthesis of the estrogens

creted in the urine, mainly in the form of *glucuronide* and *sulfate conjugates.* Some of the estrogens are reabsorbed into the bloodstream from bile.

The effects of the estrogens are most noted in the *female reproductive tract.* This becomes apparent when H^3-labeled estradiol is injected into experimental animals. This radioactive material binds to uterine, oviduct, and vaginal tissue and to the nuclei of the granulosus and thecal cells of the ovary and the interstitial cells of the testes. It also binds to the tissues concerned with feedback control of estrogen synthesis and secretion: the amygdala, hypothalamus, and anterior pituitary. Such injection shows that the estrogen-binding areas of the brain are identical in the male and female and that these areas do not bind progesterone or testosterone. Cytoplasmic estrogen receptors have been isolated from rat and calf uterine tissue.

The most important effects of estrogens in the female are on the state of the reproductive tract. During maturation of the human

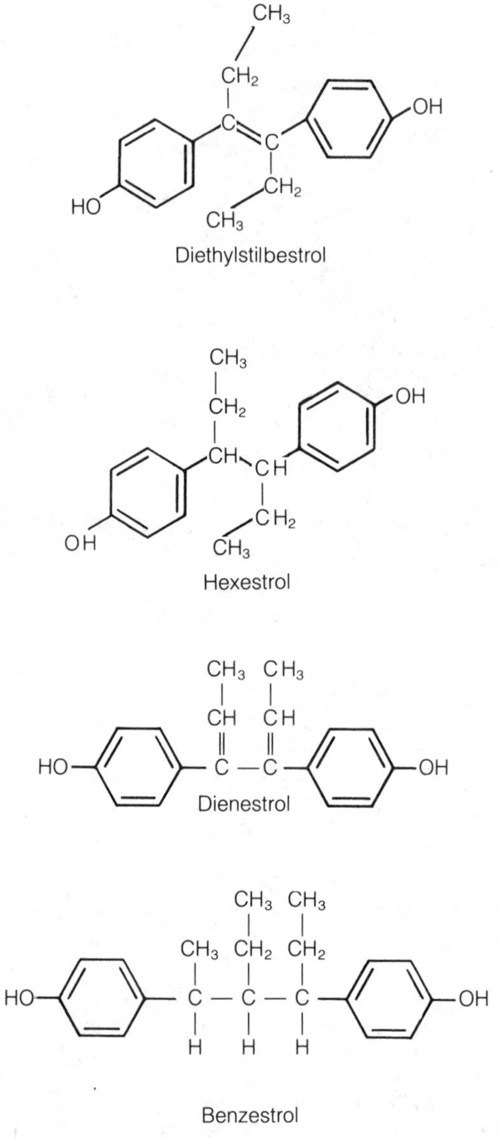

FIGURE 17–12
Four synthetic estrogenic compounds

female, there is a twentyfold or more increase in the amount of estrogen produced and secreted by the ovaries. The large amounts of estrogens produced during puberty greatly increase the size of the *oviducts, uterus,* and *vagina* as well as cause an increase in fat deposition in the external genitalia and the mammary glands. Estrogen secretion by the ovaries increases the motility of the *uterine tubes* and increases the amount of *glandular tissue* present in these structures. Estrogens also cause an increase in the number of ciliated epithelial cells which line the *Fallopian tubes.* Such changes occur not only in the human reproductive tract but also in most other mammalian species as well.

The effects of estrogens on the uterus are, in some cases, very similar to those occurring in the oviducts. The size of the uterus increases two- to threefold, and there are great changes in the endometrium at the time of puberty and during successive ovarian cycles. Upon secretion of estrogen from the ovaries or after exogenous administration of estrogen in ovariectomized animals, there is a dramatic increase in size of the uterine endometrium due to an increase in mitosis of the stromal and epithelial cells and an increase in individual cell size. There is also an increase in the size of the endometrial glands and an increase in vascularization of the endometrium. Estrogen influences hypertrophy and hyperplasia of the myometrium and increases smooth muscle contraction in the uterus and oviducts. In pigs estrogen causes contraction of the sphincter muscle of the cervix as well.

Estrogens also act on the vaginal epithelium to increase the number of cells present. Due to the rapid growth of these cells many of them are pushed further toward the lumen and away from their blood supply. Being isolated from the circulation in this way, these cells become *cornified* (or thickened). The degree of cornification can be used as a diagnostic tool in identifying certain phases of the estrous cycle. During the cornification process there may be a decrease in pH of the vagina, a slight amount of edema, and a slight increase in the vascularity of the vaginal epithelium, but not enough to prevent the cornification process from taking place.

Mammary gland development is under the control of estrogen as well as other hormones which will be discussed later. Estrogens are responsible for the characteristic fat deposition in the human female which occurs during puberty. Besides the more obvious changes in breast size there is a concomitant increase in stromal tissue and growth and development of the *glandular duct system.* In order for the mammary glands to become milk-producing structures it is necessary for other hormones to take over once the duct system has been increased.

Secondary female sex characteristics are more apparent in some mammals than in others. In certain species of monkeys there is a brightly colored *sex skin* in the region of the buttocks. Before puberty and in ovariectomized animals this skin is rather pale. As puberty begins, or as estrogens are given in the case of the ovariectomized animal, the color of the sex skin brightens considerably. In those animals in which the female is sexually dimorphic from the male of the species, she is generally smaller than the male. This is due, in part, to the effects of estrogens on skeletal growth. Due to the high estrogen levels during puberty, there is an increase in osteoblastic activity and an increase in the rate of calcium ion and protein deposition during bone formation. After a period of time, however, estrogen causes epiphyseal closure of the long bones. In the human female, and possibly many other mammals as well, there is a *broadening of the pelvis,* which is also brought about by estrogens. This accommodates the development and birth of the fetus. Estrogens are also responsible for the resorption of the pubic bones and ligaments in sexually mature female pocket gophers.

There are a number of miscellaneous effects that occur due to estrogen activity that would be difficult if not impossible to place in any specific category. There is a slight retention of sodium and chloride ions, which causes a decrease in the volume of urine excreted and an increase in blood volume, which could lead to an increase in blood pressure. These effects are generally negligible except possibly in the pregnant animal, when estrogen levels are maintained for long periods of time. In pigs, horses, and humans there is an increase in physical activity with increased estrogen levels. In lactating rats injection of estrogens triggers implantation of blastocysts. *Erythropoiesis*, the formation of red blood cells, is inhibited by high levels of estrogen. It is unknown whether this is due to the estrogenic effects on bone growth or to the direct action of estrogens on erythropoietin production.

The actual mode of action of estrogens or how they bring about their specific effects is only known in part. It is known that they increase cell hypertrophy and hyperplasia through their effect on *protein synthesis.* Estrogen binds to the nucleus of its target cells. Here, estrogen stimulates the synthesis of specific messenger RNA, which allows for the production of specific proteins. This action can be blocked by the administration of *actinomycin D*, an antibiotic which inhibits DNA-dependent RNA synthesis. Estrogen also stimulates a transfer enzyme involved in the oxidation of *reduced nicotinamide adenine dinucleotide phosphate (NADPH)* to *nicotinamide adenine dinucleotide phosphate (NADP)*. This results in an increase in the amount of

energy available to the cells undergoing increased metabolite synthesis.

Control of estrogen release. Estrogens are produced by the *placenta*, the *corpus luteum*, the *adrenal cortex*, the *testes*, and the *granulosus* and *thecal cells* of the *developing follicle*. Here, attention will be directed to the estrogens produced in the *ovaries* (i.e., developing follicle and corpus luteum). These levels of estrogens are under direct control of the anterior pituitary hormones FSH and LH. Estrogens can in turn affect the levels of these hormones by their feedback control on the hypothalamus and possibly directly on the anterior pituitary itself (see Figure 17–9).

Progestins Progestins are a class of steroid hormones that produce secretory changes in an estrogen-primed uterus. Progesterone is the most common progestin in mammals. It is essential for the preparation of the female reproductive tract for pregnancy, implantation of the blastocyst, and the maintenance of pregnancy. Progesterone and its derivatives are also formed from cholesterol and provide intermediate precursors to the formation of estrogens and androgens as well as the adrenal steroids *11-deoxycorticosterone* and *cortisone* (see Figure 17–13). Progestins are produced primarily by the *corpus luteum* in the nonpregnant female and some pregnant animals and secondarily by the *placenta*, with minute amounts being produced by the *adrenal cortex* and *testes*. In the latter two cases the progestins produced may just be precursors to the corticosteroids and androgens, respectively.

The effects of progestins. The most important target organ of the progestins is the *uterus*. The most important function of this class of steroids is to bring about the secre-

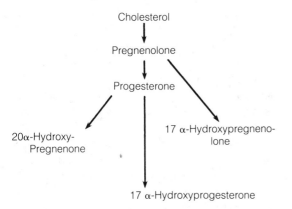

FIGURE 17–13
Pathways for the biosynthesis of the progestins

tory changes of the *endometrium* which prepare the uterus for the implantation of the fertilized ovum. In many cases progesterone acts synergistically, as in the preparation of the uterus, with estrogens. During the luteal or proliferative phase of the ovarian cycle, the progesterone secreted by the corpus luteum causes an increase in the thickness of the uterine endometrium. The blood vessels in this tissue become dilated, and the uterine glands become tightly coiled and highly branched and begin to secrete endometrial fluid actively. There is also an increase in the amount of cytoplasm in the stromal cells along with an increase in glucose and lipid deposits. The endometrium at this stage is called a *lace curtain* because of its appearance. The uterus is now ready to receive a fertilized egg (see Figure 17–14). Note that for progesterone to induce its particular effects on the uterus, the tissue must first be estrogen-primed.

The presence of the ovaries and therefore the presence of progesterone is of an absolute necessity in the early stages of pregnancy in all mammals. Removal of the progesterone source results in immediate termination of the pregnancy in its early stages, either through abortion or through resorption of the embryo. In many mammals, such as humans, horses, and guinea pigs, the

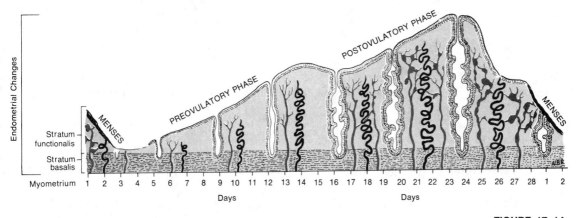

FIGURE 17–14
Estrogen- and progesterone-primed endometrium ready for blastocyst implantation. From G. J. Tortora and N. P. Anagnostakos, *Principles of Anatomy and Physiology*, 3rd edition (New York, N. Y., 1981), 727, fig. 28–17. Reprinted by permission of Harper and Row Publishers.

ovaries may be removed in the last part of the pregnancy, the acceptable time of removal depending upon the species involved. In these animals the placenta takes over most of the progesterone producing duties, so the corpus luteum may be removed without having adverse effects on the pregnancy.

One of the many ways progesterone helps to maintain pregnancy, especially in the later stages, is by its effect on *uterine motility*. Progesterone acts antagonistically to estrogen and oxytocin to reduce smooth muscle contraction of the uterus. This same reduction of motility can be observed in the oviducts.

The estrogen-primed mammary glands are also greatly affected by progesterone. This steroid hormone stimulates the development of the *mammary lobules* and *alveoli*. The alveolar cells increase in number, enlarge, and become secretory in nature, though the actual process of milk secretion into the alveoli is triggered by a different hormone, prolactin.

In humans there is a cyclic change in the awakening basal body temperature which corresponds to the steroids secreted during normal ovarian cycling. During the early part of the cycle, estrogen predominates and the basal body temperature remains constant. Just before ovulation there is a slight decrease in temperature, followed by a rise which corresponds to the increasing levels of progesterone secretion. This higher body temperature remains somewhat constant as long as the progesterone levels also remain high.

Exogenous administration of progesterone prevents further ovarian cycles from occurring and maintains the uterus in a state of readiness for blastocyst implantation. This same reaction occurs during normal pregnancy, when the corpus luteum is maintained due to the presence of gonadotropic hormones from the placenta. Within two or three days after cessation of the progesterone administration, the cyclic pattern returns to normal. Exogenous administration during pregnancy in some species may prolong the gestation period. Once progesterone therapy is discontinued in these animals, parturition occurs rather rapidly.

The cellular mode of action of progesterone is to increase the uterine concentration of RNA and DNA, *glucose-6-phosphate dehydrogenase*, and *isocitric dehydrogenase*, along with a concomitant decrease in *pyruvate kinase* activity. Progesterone also increases carbonic anhydrase activity and may have a slight effect on protein catabolism.

Control of progesterone release. Because progesterone is produced mainly by the corpus luteum in nonpregnant female mammals, any hormone that affects the growth and maintenance of the corpus luteum will also affect progesterone levels. Two anterior pituitary hormones, FSH and LH, help to maintain the corpus luteum. High levels of progesterone feed back on the hypothalamus to reduce the amount of FSH/LH-RH released and therefore the amounts of FSH and LH released from the anterior pituitary (refer back to Figure 17–9).

Relaxin Relaxin is produced not only in the *ovaries* by the corpus luteum of pregnancy but also in the *placenta* and the *uterus* of some mammals. It is believed that this hormone is produced only during pregnancy, at least in humans, because no detectable levels have been isolated from nonpregnant women or men. Relaxin disappears from the blood within twenty-four hours after parturition. Purified *porcine relaxin* is composed of two protein chains; one has 22 amino acid residues and the other has 30 residues. The molecular weight of this hormone is 6,500.

Effects of relaxin. The major target organs of relaxin are the *uterus* (with its muscular cervix) and the *pelvic girdle*. In most cases, relaxin acts on estrogen-primed tissue. In rats that are ovariectomized, estrogen-primed, and then injected with relaxin, the uterus shows a marked increase in glycogen concentration and water content. There is also inhibition of uterine motility in these animals. Relaxin causes an increase in water imbibition by the rat uterus whether it has been estrogen-primed or not. Relaxin also acts directly on the cervix, softening the tissue and then causing its dilation. All of these actions facilitate the process of parturition.

The second effect of relaxin in a number of mammals is to relax the pelvic girdle during the latter part of gestation. This may occur in conjunction with other hormones. In the cow and sheep there is a mobilization of the *sacroiliac joints*. In other mammals there is a relaxation of the *fibrocartilage* which connects the *pubic symphysis*. This is brought about by an increased vascularization of the pubic symphysis and imbibition of water in this area. There is a subsequent *depolymerization* of the *colloidal components* of the joint and a *disaggregation* of the fibers which make up the fibrocartilage.

There is also evidence that relaxin may act in the development of the mammary gland, along with estrogen and progesterone. It may also inhibit lactation before parturition.

The Testes

The testes are the major source of *androgens* in male mammals; lesser amounts are produced by the adrenal glands. Androgens are a class of steroid hormones which have physiological and masculinizing effects similar to testosterone. The biosynthetic pathways of the androgens are shown in Figure 17–15. The most abundant and most potent of these hormones is *testosterone*. Other androgens include *dihydrotestosterone, androstenedione,* and *dehydroepiandrosterone*. Many male accessory organs convert testosterone to dihydrotestosterone. The development of the *testes, scrotum,* and *penis* in the male fetus is stimulated by this dihydrotestosterone, whereas the development of the *seminal vesicles, vas deferens,* and *epididymis* are all stimulated by testosterone. In the male, some events of puberty are also influenced by dihydrotestosterone. Androstenedione has a weaker action than testosterone and generally undergoes reduction to testosterone. Great quantities of androstenedione are produced in juvenile ungulates as opposed to adult ungulates, which primarily produce testosterone. Dehydroepiandrosterone is a very weak androgen and is produced in greatest quantities by the adrenal glands.

The *Leydig* or *interstitial cells* of the testes are the major source of testosterone pro-

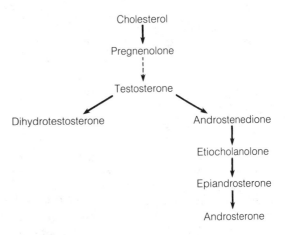

FIGURE 17–15
Pathways for the biosynthesis of androgens

duction in mammals. The Leydig cells contain prominent Golgi apparatuses, extensive smooth endoplasmic reticulum, many liposomes, and fat droplets. These fat droplets are more prominent during periods of relative inactivity of the Leydig cells. These cells usually contain no granules or vacuoles, and there is very little rough endoplasmic reticulum. It is in the interstitial cells that *acetate* and sometimes *preformed cholesterol* from the blood are used in the synthesis of androgens. Different pathways of biosynthesis predominate in different species. Once formed, some of the androgens pass into the bloodstream and testicular lymph. In the bloodstream, testosterone is bound to protein carrier molecules which aid in the transport of testosterone to its target organs. Testosterone that is not taken up by the cells of the target tissues is metabolized rather quickly by the liver into inactive products which are then excreted in the urine.

Effects of androgens Testosterone and its derivatives are responsible for the masculine characteristics observed in adult male mammals. During fetal development the *genital ridge* in the male produces testosterone, which promotes the formation of the male reproductive system. As the testes develop, they take over the synthesis of the androgens. Testosterone is also responsible for the descent of the testes in at least some, if not all, mammals. During puberty in the human male, testosterone stimulates an increase in muscle mass, causes a deepening of the voice, and stimulates growth of the penis and scrotum. At this time dihydrotestosterone influences prostatic growth, development of facial hair, a temporary recession of the hairline, and the development of acne. In adult and subadult mammals in general, testoster-

one affects various systems of the body, but most importantly it is responsible for the development and maintenance of the *male secondary sex characteristics*, the function of the male *accessory sex organs*, and *gamete formation*. Other systems affected by testosterone include the integument, skeleton, and musculature. Testosterone also affects mammary gland development, certain aspects of behavior, and certain metabolic factors.

The maintenance of the accessory sex organs is totally dependent upon the presence of androgens. There is a good correlation among testicular weight, rate of testosterone production, and the weight of androgen-dependent organs. Castration results in atrophy and cessation of function of the prostate, seminal vesicles, and Cowper's glands, and there is a decrease in height of the epithelial lining of these organs. Because of the necessity of LH in testosterone formation, hypophysectomized male mammals are affected in this same manner. The effects on these accessory sex organs can be observed by close scrutiny of the composition of the seminal fluid, which is closely correlated with androgen concentrations. Testosterone also appears to prolong the life span of *epididymal spermatazoa* and to stimulate *gametogenesis*.

One of the best-known effects of testosterone is the increase in *protein synthesis*. As protein synthesis increases there is a direct effect on the skeletal and muscle systems of the body. There is an increase in the thickness of muscle fibers as well as an increase in tensile strength of the muscles and their working ability. Certain skeletal muscles are particularly susceptible to androgen stimulation. In mice the *levator ani muscle* and in guinea pigs the *masticator muscles* are especially affected by androgens. Because of this increase in protein anabolism, and possibly a decrease in protein catabolism as well, there is an increase in the protein matrix in bone. In animals possessing antlers there is also a marked effect on antler growth. If these animals are castrated early in life no antlers are formed. If they are castrated while still in velvet, after the antlers have formed, the remaining velvet is not shed, as normally occurs. But if they are castrated after the velvet has been shed, the antlers themselves will be shed immediately. The next set of antlers that grows remains in velvet permanently. If ovariectomized females of these species are given testosterone, they too will produce antlers.

The exact effect of testosterone on the integument is not known. It has been shown that the *sebaceous glands* in the skin of human males may be regulated by testosterone. Androgens, especially testosterone, induce growth and development of the ducts and alveoli of the mammary glands. It has also been shown that men with the *baldness hereditary factor* usually do not show this trait if castrated before the phenomenon becomes apparent.

As far as the effects of testosterone on metabolism are concerned, the most marked effect is that of the increase in protein synthesis. Besides increasing the muscle mass and increasing the protein matrix of bone, there is also an increase in *nitrogen retention* by the kidneys. This decrease in nitrogen loss in the urine adds to the availability of nitrogen for amino acid synthesis, which is necessary for increased protein synthesis.

In some species erythrocyte counts and hemoglobin concentrations are greater in males than in females. In castrated males levels of hemoglobin and erythrocytes are lower than those found in normal males. Exoge-nous administration of testosterone returns these levels to normal.

The effect of testosterone on behavior in general and sexual behavior in particular has been well documented. The human male sex drive is dependent to a great extent on the levels of testosterone present. In bulls, boars, and rabbits, if males are used as teasers, that is if they are exposed to females in heat but are not allowed to mate with them, sex drive is lost. Some of these animals will even refuse to mate even if they are finally given the chance. Testosterone has also been shown to affect butting order in cows as well as libido in bulls.

Most evidence for the mode of action of testosterone shows that it promotes synthesis of RNA. The testosterone becomes bound to receptor proteins in the cytoplasm of the target organ cells. Here, testosterone is transported to the nucleus, where it binds to a nuclear protein. In the nucleus the DNA-dependent RNA transcription of certain genes takes place, and there is an increase in cellular protein content. After a few days there is also an increase in DNA content of the organ due to the increase in cell number as well as cell size. These effects have been noted particularly in the seminal vesicles and prostate, two organs drastically affected by testosterone levels in the blood. Some of the effects attributed to testosterone can be blocked by the administration of RNA-synthesis inhibiting drugs.

Control of testosterone release from the testes As with many other hormones, there is a feedback control mechanism of testosterone secretion. This hormone feeds back on the hypothalamus to decrease the amount of FSH/LH-RH released into the hypophyseal portal system (refer back to Figure 17–9). This decrease in FSH/LH-RH causes a subsequent decrease in LH release but has little effect on the release of FSH unless the testosterone levels are extremely high. In those animals with distinct *breeding seasons* (i.e., sexual activity takes place only at specific times of the year), external and internal mechanisms stimulate the release of LH from the anterior pituitary, resulting in a surge of testicular activity, which includes both testosterone production and spermatogenesis. The exact mechanism for this phenomenon is not known, but some hypotheses have been made. For more information on breeding seasons see chapter 18, The Reproductive System.

THE PLACENTA

The placenta is the bond between the mother and the developing embryo in all of the mammalian species except the monotremes. This structure is formed from both maternal and embryonic tissues and serves as a passageway for nutrients, gases, and waste products. It also acts as a selective filter in that it restricts the passage of certain substances from the mother to the embryo. In addition to these functions, the placenta also serves as an endocrine organ, though a rather short-lived one compared to others in the body. As an endocrine organ it produces and secretes many hormones, such as *estrogens*, *progesterone*, *chorionic gonadotropin*, *relaxin*, and possibly *intermedin*. The various levels of some of these hormones in human females is shown in Figure 17–16. In some mammals the placenta also produces *placental lactogen*. During gestation in the mare, the placenta also produces *equine gonadotropin*, or *pregnant mare serum gonadotropin (PMSG)*.

Hormones of the Placenta

Chorionic gonadotropin This hormone is characteristic of primates and may be produced by lower mammals as well. A glycoprotein which contains *galactose* and *hexosamine*, it comprises two subunits like those of the glycoproteins of the anterior pituitary. The *alpha subunit* is quite similar to the alpha subunits of LH, FSH, and TSH, with only five amino acids being different. The molecular weight of this subunit is 18,000. The *beta subunit* has a molecular weight of 28,000. Chorionic gonadotropin has a luteotropic effect on the corpus luteum, prolonging its life span, increasing its size, and enhancing its secretion of estrogen and progesterone. This luteotropic effect has been observed in humans by *human chorionic gonadotropin (HCG)*, as well as in rabbits, pigs, and rats. By maintaining the corpus luteum and its endocrine functions, the uterine endometrium is also maintained and therefore so is the pregnancy.

Chorionic gonadotropin is produced and secreted by cells of embryonic origin which later give rise to the cells of the *chorionic villi*. In the human, it can be detected as early as eight days after ovulation and subsequent fertilization and reaches a peak around the sixth week of pregnancy, at which time it drops to a low maintenance level until shortly after parturition. In monkeys and chimpanzees it is only produced for a short time and then disappears. It is present in the maternal blood and urine during pregnancy and is the basis for most of the pregnancy tests.

Estrogens and progesterone Estrogens and progesterone are produced and secreted by the *syncytial cells* of the *trophoblast*, as is chorionic gonadotropin. These hormones are

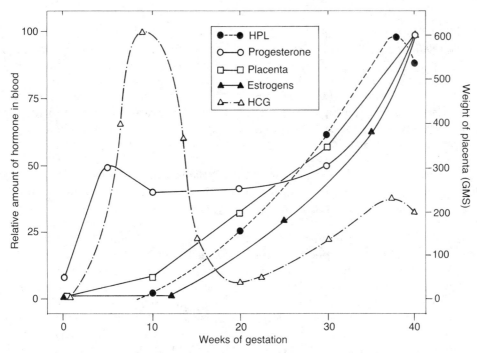

FIGURE 17–16

Changes in blood levels of HCG, HPL, progesterone, and estrogens during pregnancy in the human. Also note increase in placental weight. From E. E. Selkurt, *Physiology*, 4th edition (Boston, Mass, 1976), 813. Reprinted by permission of Little, Brown and Co.

not, however, produced from acetate as they are in the ovary. Instead, *dehydroepiandrosterone,* a steroid compound produced by the fetal adrenal glands, is transported to the placenta where it becomes the precursor of the steroids. This is the reason that very little of these hormones is produced during the early stages of pregnancy. In the pregnant human female, estriol is produced in very high quantities. By comparison, the nonpregnant female produces only very small amounts of this particular estrogen. Thus, although the pregnant female produces as much as 300 times as much estrogen as a nonpregnant female, the actual estrogenic activity is only increased 30 times due to the types of estrogen produced. Since a large

portion of estrogen and progesterone in the blood is filtered but not reabsorbed by the kidneys, all of these hormones can be monitored through the urine of the pregnant female. *Pregnanediol* and *pregnanetriol* are also excreted in large amounts in the urine.

Just like the estrogens and progesterone produced by the ovary, these hormones produced by the placenta help maintain the *endometrium* and therefore are essential to pregnancy. Estrogens also cause an enlargement of the mammary glands through growth of the glandular tissue, in preparation for lactation, enlargement of the uterus, and enlargement of the external genitalia. In some animals the estrogens also relax the pelvic ligaments and help loosen the pelvic joints for an easier passage of the fetus during parturition. Progesterone helps to maintain the *decidual cells* of the endometrium, which aid in nutrition of the developing embryo. This hormone also helps to prevent uterine contraction by its quieting effect on the smooth muscles of the uterus. Like the estrogens, progesterone also helps to prepare the mammary glands for lactation.

Placental lactogen Placental lactogens have been found in humans and rats. In the rat this hormone has effects on the mammary glands as well as a luteotropic effect. This hormone is very similar in many ways to the growth-stimulating hormone and prolactin, which are produced by the anterior pituitary. Because of this similarity there is also in humans a growth-stimulating effect from this hormone. This attribute has not been recorded for the rat. *Human placental lactogen (HPL)* is very similar to STH in its chemical make up. Both of these hormones have 191 amino acid residues, of which 161 are identical, and two disulfide bridges, which are located in analogous positions. Production and secretion of placental lactogen from the syncytial cells of the trophoblast in humans begins at about the fifth week of pregnancy and continues until parturition.

Relaxin Relaxin is produced by the placenta in some mammalian species. It is a nonsteroid polypeptide which causes relaxation of the estrogen-primed pubic ligaments. More information on this hormone is contained in the section on the ovary.

Pregnant mare serum gonadotropin Evidence brought forth in the early 1970s established the site of synthesis of this hormone (also known as equine gonadotropin) as the *fetal allantochorionic cells* and not the uterus, as was supposed earlier. These fetal cells become attached to the *uterine mucosa*, where they develop into specialized areas called *endometrial cups.* It is now evident that these endometrial cups are fetal in origin rather than maternal, as was previously hypothesized. Pregnant mare serum gonadotropin (PMSG) first appears in the blood on about the fortieth day of gestation with a peak concentration occurring about day 120 and disappearance of the hormone about day 180.

This hormone is a glycoprotein with FSH-like and LH-like activity depending upon the dose. It has a molecular weight of approximately 68,000 and is most probably a tetramer. It is different from FSH and LH in that it is retained by the kidneys and very little is excreted in the urine. For this reason, and because it is not readily broken down by the liver, its half-life in the circulation is much longer than that for FSH or LH.

There is some evidence that this hormone stimulates the growth of small follicles during the early stages of pregnancy of the mare. These follicles grow and some may ovulate. Whether or not ovulation occurs, these follicles soon undergo luteinization due to the presence of pregnant mare serum gonadotrophin. These *accessory corpora lutea*, as they are called, are essential for the production of sufficient quantities of progesterone to maintain the pregnancy. The levels of pregnant mare serum gonadotrophin correspond well to the appearance and then disappearance of these accessory corpora lutea. One hundred eighty days after fertilization, the placenta produces enough progesterone to maintain the pregnancy and the accessory corpora lutea are no longer necessary.

In addition to its effects on the ovarian tissue, PMSG also affects the fetal ovaries and testes. The fetal ovaries increase greatly in size until they are larger than the mare's. The fetal testes also increase in size and are larger at this time than at birth.

THE ADRENAL GLANDS

The adrenals are *paired glands* which lie in the *retroperitoneal region.* They have been called the *suprarenals* because of their position with respect to the kidneys. These glands were first described by Eustachius in 1563, and it was not until 1805 that Cuvier described the two separate regions that compose each of the glands. Later, Addison described the condition, which bears his name, that results from the degeneration of these glands.

Adrenal tissue exists in all vertebrates, and in mammals these organs are divided into two separate and distinct areas: the *inner adrenal medulla* and the *outer adrenal cortex* (see Figure 17–17). In prototherians, medullary cords penetrate the cortex, and these two areas are not nearly as distinct as they are in the higher mammals. The adrenal medulla is derived from the ectoderm; the adrenal cortex from the mesoderm. The difference in embryonic origin will become apparent when the different functions of these two regions are discussed. The size of these two areas differs among species as well as within a species. In some mammals, such as rats, there is sexual dimorphism, in which the adrenals of the female are larger than those of the male. The reverse is true in hamsters. There may also be a difference in size within the same animal, as is the case with nutria, a small rodent, in which the left adrenal gland is 50 percent larger than the right adrenal. One region (i.e., the medulla or cortex) may predominate in size. In the guinea

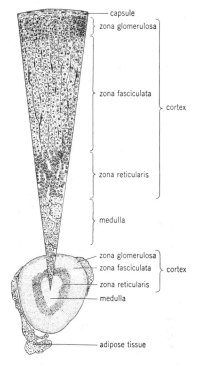

FIGURE 17–17
Cross section of the adrenal gland showing the medulla and cortex. Note composition of the adrenal cortex: zona glomerulosa, zona fasciculata, and zona reticularis.
From C. K. Weichert, *Anatomy of the Chordates,* 4th edition (New York, N.Y., 1970). Reprinted by permission of McGraw-Hill Book Co.

pig and porcupine the cortex is larger than the medulla, and in chimpanzees and porpoises the reverse is true. The size of the adrenal cortex is variable among different populations of wild and domesticated Norway rats. The adrenal glands of animals from wild populations are larger than the adrenal glands from domesticated individuals. Once tamed, the adrenals of the once wild rats decrease in size. A somewhat analogous study has shown that an increase in population density in mice causes an increase in aggressive behavior and an increase in plasma concentrations of hormones of the adrenal cortex (adrenocorticoids). Thus, the ecology of these animals is reflected in their behavior, whether wild, domesticated, or in crowded conditions, and has a definite effect on the size and function of the adrenal cortex.

The Adrenal Medulla

The adrenal medulla is responsible for the synthesis and secretion of a group of hormones called *catecholamines*. The two principal catecholamines secreted are *epinephrine* and *norepinephrine*. The cells responsible for the production of these hormones are called *chromaffin cells*, which are so named because they contain cytoplasmic granules that stain yellowish brown with salts of chromic acid. The color, in this case, indicates the presence of epinephrine. There are also scattered groups of cells located elsewhere in the body that resemble cells of the adrenal medulla. Some of these cells are located in the *carotid glands*, the *organs of Zuckerkandl* (which are near the origin of the inferior mesenteric artery), near the capsules of the *sympathetic nerve ganglia*, and scattered throughout the *heart, liver, kidney*, and *gonadal areas*. Besides producing epinephrine, the chromaffin cells also produce *serotonin*.

The chromaffin cells of the adrenal medulla are surrounded by a series of blood sinuses. The basal ends of the medullary cells abut against the capillaries, and the other ends are in close proximity to a vein. Cells of the adrenal medulla are *modified postganglionic cells* of the sympathetic nervous system and therefore, like most nerve cells, do not regenerate if damaged. These cells are innervated directly by preganglionic fibers of the sympathetic nervous system. They are unlike most target organs, in which the preganglionic fibers of the sympathetic nervous

system first synapse with a postganglionic nerve before innervating the effector organ. The chromaffin cells are therefore postganglionic sympathetic nerve cells which are secretory in function.

Hormones of the adrenal medulla Both epinephrine and norepinephrine are produced by the adrenal medulla. The ratios of these hormones produced by the adrenals vary from species to species. In humans and dogs the adrenal medulla produces approximately 80 percent epinephrine, with lesser amounts of norepinephrine and dopamine being produced. Naturally aggressive mammals, such as lions, tigers, and domesticated cats, have a tendency to produce higher levels of norepinephrine than do less aggressive species, such as rabbits and hamsters. Psychological factors also cause the concentration of each of these hormones in the adrenal medulla to vary. Stimulation of the sciatic nerve, painful stimuli, reduction in blood glucose levels due to exogenous administration of insulin, and stimulation of specific areas of the hypothalamus result in secretion of epinephrine from the adrenal medulla but not norepinephrine. Norepinephrine secretion can be increased by clamping the carotid artery and by stimulation of specific areas of the hypothalamus. Because these various types of stimuli result in the release of specific catecholamines, it has been postulated that each of the chromaffin cells can produce only one of the catecholamines, but insufficient evidence has been accumulated for this to be substantiated.

Biosynthesis of catecholamines in the adrenal medulla. The biosynthesis of these amines has already been discussed in chapter 5, The Autonomic Nervous System. As stated there, the amino acids *phenylalanine* and *tyrosine* are precursors which are converted to *dihydroxyphenylalanine (Dopa)*. Dopa is decarboxylated to form *dihydroxyphenylethylamine (dopamine)*, which is hydroxylated to form norepinephrine. Here the similarity with other tissues ceases. The adrenal medulla and brain are the only tissues of the body which have the enzyme *phenylethanolamine-N-methyltransferase (PNMT)*, which converts norepinephrine to epinephrine (see Figure 17–18). This conversion is stimulated in the presence of *adrenocorticotropic hormone (ACTH)* from the anterior pituitary and by *glucocorticoids*, which are secreted by the adrenal cortex in response to ACTH stimulation. Removal of the pituitary results in a decrease in epinephrine synthesis.

Once formed these amines are stored in the *medullary cells* in granules in which they are bound to ATP and in binding proteins called *chromogranin*. High concentrations are accumulated in these cells as the result of active transport, which tends to concentrate the substances after they are produced. Secretion of the catecholamines is initiated by *acetylcholine* release from the sympathetic preganglionic fibers in the adrenal medulla. Acetylcholine causes an increase in the permeability of the cells to catecholamines as well as to their binding proteins and ATP. All three of these substances are released from the cells by the process of exocytosis. From the cells of the adrenal medulla the catecholamines are released into the nearby blood sinuses. Once in the bloodstream epinephrine is usually bound to blood proteins, but norepinephrine is usually not protein-bound once in the blood. Due to their rapid metabolism, these amines are not retained in the blood for very long periods of time. The major metabolites of catecholamines which appear in the blood and urine are: *3-methoxy-4-hydroxymandelic acid*, or *vallinylmandelic acid* (VMA); *3-0-methylepinephrine*, or *metanephrine*; and *3-0-methylnorepinephrine*, or *normetanephrine* (see Figure 17–19). These substances are found in free and conjugated forms and are inactive.

Effects of catecholamines. In general, both epinephrine and norepinephrine contribute to the *fight or flight response* described by Walter Cannon (see chapter 5, The Autonomic Nervous System). This is accomplished through an increase in heart rate and systolic blood pressure, vasoconstriction of some areas of the body, free fatty acid mobilization, and stimulation of metabolic rate. Each of these effects is brought about by differences in the levels of circulating catecholamines as well as differences in the actual types of catecholamines present. A review of the effects of epinephrine and norepinephrine is given in Table 17–3. There is a conspicuous paucity of information regarding dopamine and its actions in various physiological functions. This catecholamine is a precursor to norepinephrine and thus epi-

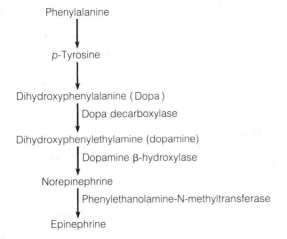

FIGURE 17–18
Formation of the catecholamines in the adrenal medulla

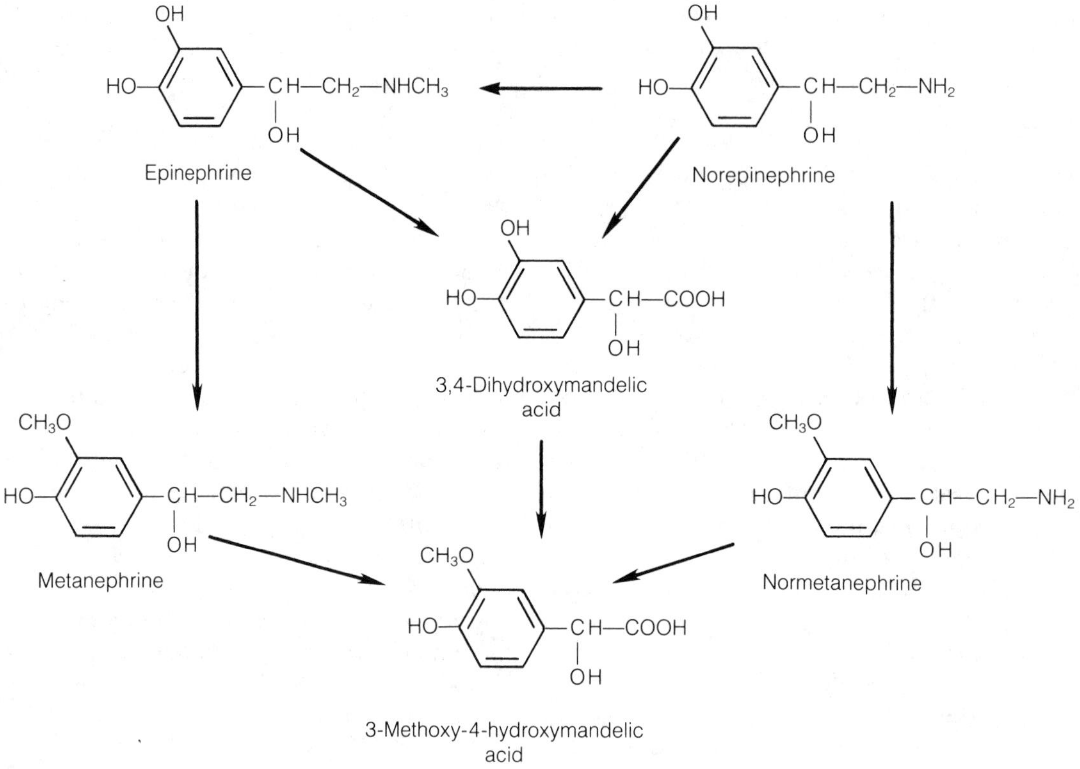

FIGURE 17–19
The formation of blood and urine metabolites of the catecholamines

nephrine in the adrenal medulla, and it is estimated that 50 percent of the dopamine found in the plasma is of adrenal medullary origin.

The effects of catecholamines on the cardiovascular system are varied. Epinephrine has a greater effect on the heart than does norepinephrine, though both cause an increase in the force of contraction and an increase in the rate at which the heart beats. Norepinephrine causes an increase in both systolic and diastolic blood pressures, whereas epinephrine causes an increase in systolic pressure but has little or no effect on the diastolic pressure. Some of these effects are due to a reduction in peripheral resistance brought about by the *vasodilation* of blood vessels in the skeletal muscles, heart, brain, and liver. Overall, however, there is a net vasodilator effect of epinephrine and a net vasoconstrictor effect of norepinephrine.

Both norepinephrine and epinephrine cause an increase in carbohydrate metabolism, with epinephrine having a much greater effect. This is accomplished through an increase in glycogenolysis in the skeletal muscles and liver. By this process glycogen is converted to glucose phosphate and there is a subsequent rise in blood sugar levels due to the action of phosphorylase in the liver.

TABLE 17–3
Some effects noted with epinephrine and norepinephrine secretion from the adrenal medulla

	Epinephrine	Norepinephrine
Heart rate	increase	increase
Force of contraction of heart	increase	increase
Systolic blood pressure	increase	increase
Diastolic pressure	no effect	increase
Peripheral resistance	decrease (net vasodilation)	increase (net vasoconstriction)
Blood flow to skeletal muscle, liver, and brain	increase	no effect or slight decrease
Renal blood flow	decrease	decrease
Vasoconstriction of capillaries in the skin	increase	increase
Respiration	increase	increase
Oxygen consumption	increase	no effect
Blood sugar	increase	slight increase

Low plasma concentrations of epinephrine also cause the pituitary to release ACTH, either by direct feedback or by the production of hypothalamic releasing hormone. In any case, the results are the same. The adrenal cortex is stimulated to produce and release more glucocorticoids, which then also cause a rise in blood glucose levels. There is some evidence that epinephrine may also cause a decrease in cellular uptake of glucose as well as a decrease in glucose catabolism on the cellular level. These catecholamines also stimulate free fatty acid mobilization and a subsequent increase in metabolic rate. This is believed to be brought about through the action of the catecholamines on cyclic AMP production.

Secondarily, the catecholamines result in a reduction of circulating *eosinophils*. This is accomplished by augmentation of production of ACTH-RH by the hypothalamus, which in turn sets up a sequence of reactions including formation and release of ACTH followed by production of adrenal corticosteroids. Exogenous administration of epinephrine causes a decrease in blood clotting time. Administration of this hormone also causes nervous system changes in some mammals by causing general restlessness, and in humans causes anxiety and fatigue. The effects of epinephrine and norepinephrine on the respiratory system and other functions are outlined in chapter 5, The Autonomic Nervous System.

Control of catecholamine release from the adrenal medulla. Since the chromaffin cells of the adrenal medulla are innervated by the sympathetic nervous system, any stimulation of this part of the nervous system will also increase the production and secretion of catecholamines. Catecholamine synthesis is also promoted by ACTH and the glucocorticoids by virtue of their effect on the enzyme phenylethanolamine-N-methyltransferase, which converts norepinephrine to epinephrine. Therefore, anything that causes an increase in the amount of circulating ACTH and therefore glucocorticoids will also increase the amount of epinephrine formed, if not secreted.

The Adrenal Cortex

The adrenal cortex or outer region of the adrenal glands comprises three distinct areas or regions (see Figure 17–17). The outermost layer, or *zona glomerulosa*, is responsible for the production of a group of steroid hormones called the *mineralocorticoids*. The zona glomerulosa is a group of deep-staining cells which are arranged in alveolarlike units. The next two layers are called the *zona fasciculata* and the *zona reticularis*. Both of these regions produce steroid hormones classified as *glucocorticoids*. Some of the sex steroids can also be found in these layers of the cortex, but they are not released into the general circulation in large quantities under normal circumstances. All of these steroid hormones together are termed the *adrenocorticoids*. There are nearly fifty different steroids produced by the adrenal cortex, though only a very few are known to have any real importance in normal mammalian function. Those most important are *aldosterone* (a mineralocorticoid), *cortisol* and *corticosterone* (both of which are glucocorticoids), and, to a much lesser extent, the *gonadal* or *sex steroids*.

Hormones of the adrenal cortex All of the hormones produced and secreted by the adrenal cortex are lipids having the basic cyclopenthanoperhydrophenanthrene nucleus characteristic of all steroid hormones (refer back to Figure 17–1). The adrenocorticoids fall into two basic classes (i.e., mineralocorticoids and glucocorticoids) based upon

structure and biological activity. In many cases the intermediates involved in the synthesis of the corticoids have functions which resemble the functions of the gonadal steroids. This has led some authors to include a third class of adrenocorticoids called *gonadocorticoids*. But in most cases these compounds play an insignificant role in reproduction and maintenance of the secondary sex characteristics.

Biosynthesis of the adrenocorticoids. All of these hormones are formed from cholesterol (refer back to Figure 17–2). In the biosynthetic pathway the first important intermediate and the first 21 carbon (C-21) compound that is produced is *pregnenolone.* Pregnenolone is converted to progesterone, which can then be altered to form either *1-α-hydroxyprogesterone* and finally *cortisol* or *11-deoxycorticosterone*, which is later converted to aldosterone. The biosynthetic pathways for the sex steroids are covered in the section in this chapter dealing with gonadal hormones. In the glucocorticoids and mineralocorticoids, a hydroxyl group at the *C-21 position* is important for sodium ion retention and related activities and is also necessary for carbohydrate metabolic activity. This effect on carbohydrate metabolism is further enhanced by a second hydroxylation at the *C-17 position*. Oxygenation at the *C-11 position* has little effect on electrolyte metabolism, but it does enhance carbohydrate and protein metabolic activity. It should be noted that all of the *C-21 steroids* that are secreted by the adrenal cortex have both mineralocorticoid and glucocorticoid effects. Those hormones in which the effects on sodium and potassium ion concentrations predominate are called mineralocorticoids, and those in which the effects on carbohydrate and protein metabolism predominate are termed glucocorticoids. For instance, aldosterone is 10,000 times more effective as a mineralocorticoid than as a glucocorticoid, so it retains the mineralocorticoid designation.

The life span of the adrenocorticoids in the circulation is rather short. These steroids are generally inactivated by the liver and to a lesser extent by the kidneys. Most of the steroids are excreted in the urine as glucuronic or sulfuric acid conjugates.

Glucocorticoids: introduction and functions. These adrenocorticosteroids are known as the *11-oxygenated adrenocorticoids* and are very important in protein and carbohydrate metabolism. Generally, the most abundant of the glucocorticoids is *cortisol* (or *hydrocortisone*), with corticosterone and cortisone being found in lesser quantities. The actual ratios of these compounds is species dependent. For instance, cats, sheep, monkeys, and humans secrete predominantly cortisol; rats and mice secrete predominantly corticosterone; and dogs secrete almost equal amounts of these two hormones. There are also a number of synthetic glucocorticoids available.

Once in the bloodstream the glucocorticoids are bound to plasma proteins, specifically an alpha globulin named *transcortin*. Binding of the glucocorticoids to these proteins reduces the rate at which they are destroyed by the metabolism. This particular protein, also called *corticosteroid-binding globulin (CBG)*, is produced in the liver. Various physiological conditions affect the synthesis of transcortin. The high levels of estrogen produced during pregnancy are known to result in elevated levels of CBG, whereas cirrhosis of the liver decreases their production. As cortisol becomes bound to plasma protein, a new balance must be reached between the free and bound concentrations of these glucocorticoids. As it becomes bound to the carrier protein, there is a temporary decrease in the amount of free cortisol. This triggers release of more ACTH from the anterior pituitary, which causes a rise in glucocorticoid levels, and a new balance is obtained. Free cortisol is metabolized in the liver to *tetrahydrocortisol*, which is conjugated to *glucuronic acid.* This is dissolved in the blood and taken to the kidneys, where it is excreted in the urine.

Glucocorticoids decrease carbohydrate metabolism by the tissues, promote deposition of liver glycogen, and promote gluconeogenesis from proteins and fats. Some of these effects lead to an increase in blood glucose levels. The positive effect on gluconeogenesis is brought about through the ability of cortisol and related substances to increase the rate of transport of amino acids from the extracellular fluid and muscle cells into the liver, where gluconeogenesis takes place. In the liver some of these amino acids are used to synthesize new proteins necessary as enzymes for the process of gluconeogenesis, whereas others are deaminated to form *alpha keto acids*, which are used as carbohydrate intermediates. Glucocorticoids may inhibit the phosphorylation of glucose to *glucose-6-phosphate* and they may decrease the oxidation rate of NADH, thereby slowing down the process of glycolysis by the cells. In the liver cortisol causes an increase in *glucose-6-phosphatase* which catalyzes the removal of phosphate from glucose. All of the above reactions contribute to the net effect of glucocorticoids on carbohydrate metabolism and result in elevated blood glucose levels.

Overall there is a reduction in cellular protein in the presence of glucocorticoids. This is due in part to the increased catabolism of proteins already present in the cells and to a decrease in protein anabolism in the tissues, with the exception of the liver. This difference is probably the result of the increased mobilization of amino acids from extrahepatic tissues (especially the muscles) to the liver, where gluconeogenesis and increased protein synthesis of liver and plasma proteins takes place, and also because of the depressing effect that glucocorticoids have on RNA synthesis and therefore protein synthesis. Because of the increase in gluconeogenesis and therefore elimination of urinary nitrogen from amino acid catabolism, there is a negative nitrogen balance and a lowered *respiratory quotient (RQ)* (see chapter 13, Metabolism).

In addition to the change effected on protein and carbohydrate metabolism, the glucocorticoids increase the mobilization of fatty acids from adipose tissue. There is also a decrease in the rate of conversion of carbohydrates to fats in the presence of these hormones. These two factors, along with the decrease in glucose availability, allow the body cells under stimulation by cortisol to increase cellular oxidation of free fatty acids in the plasma. The increased use of fatty acids as an energy source also results in a lower RQ.

One of the most important effects of cortisol is in the body's response to stress. Nearly any type of physical or emotional trauma is followed by an increase in ACTH levels and subsequently by an increase in cortisol levels. It is fairly easy to see how physical trauma might be resisted by cortisol. Some of these mechanisms probably include increased gluconeogenesis and therefore an increase in the amount of glucose present for an energy source in times of stress. Cortisol also has an anti-inflammatory effect, which may be accomplished in a number of different ways. First, cortisol stabilizes lysosome membranes to keep them intact and thereby

reduce the destruction of tissue by the hydrolytic enzymes contained in these organelles. Second, cortisol decreases the rate of formation of *bradykinin* and thereby reduces vasodilation, which would otherwise ensue. Increasing blood flow to a tissue increases capillary leakage and, hence, swelling of the traumatized area. Third, cortisol decreases the effects of *histamines* (i.e., vasodilation and increased capillary permeability). And fourth, cortisol augments the effects of epinephrine and norepinephrine on the blood vessels.

While enhancing resistance to physical and emotional trauma, glucocorticoids also reduce the number of circulating white blood cells. This reduction tends to decrease the body's ability to resist diseases through a decrease in the amount of circulating antibodies and lymphocytes that participate in cell-mediated immunity. Glucocorticoids are given as therapy for certain diseases, such as rheumatoid arthritis, in which inflammation is a problem. Indeed, the glucocorticoids reduce the amount of inflammation, but they also make the animal more susceptible to infection.

Mineralocorticoids: introduction and functions. The mineralocorticoids are essential to life, unless some type of therapy is given to counteract the effects of their absence. These hormones are produced by the zona glomerulosa, which in mammals does not depend on ACTH for the production of these mineralocorticoids, though ACTH can enhance their production. It is because of this lack of dependence on pituitary hormones that hypophysectomy does not appreciably affect synthesis or secretion of aldosterone and related hormones. This group of adrenocorticoids comprises two different types of mineralocorticoids, those which are oxygenated in the *C-11 position* and those which are not. Those which lack the oxygenation at this carbon are less potent and include *11-deoxy-corticosterone* and *17α-hydroxy-11-deoxycor-ticosterone*. These mineralocorticoids have an effect on the sodium and potassium ion concentrations in the blood and control electrolyte and fluid changes in the body but to a much lesser extent than does aldosterone. Aldosterone is a member of the first group of mineralocorticoids, those which are oxygenated at the C-11 position. Aldosterone is the most potent of the mineralocorticoids and is responsible for as much as 95 percent of the mineralocorticoid activity in the body.

In general, the mineralocorticoids increase the reabsorption of sodium ion from the body fluids, such as sweat, urine, saliva, and gastric juices. These hormones also increase the release of potassium ion by the kidneys and the reabsorption of anions in the distal tubules and collecting ducts of the kidney. The reabsorption of sodium ions from the kidney tubules, especially the ascending loop of Henle, the distal tubules, and the collecting ducts, is brought about by the action of aldosterone and other hormones with mineralocorticoid activity. Although the specific mechanism responsible for this action is unknown, it is known that aldosterone increases messenger RNA synthesis and subsequently increases protein synthesis. There is a possibility that the proteins formed act as permeases to actively transport the sodium against the concentration gradient from the tubular lumen into the epithelial cells. It is also possible that the proteins are used in oxidation processes to increase energy available for the active transport of the sodium. Aldosterone may also be directly involved with the sodium pump in the kidney. Any or all of these hypotheses may be correct, and there may be still other undiscovered mechanisms.

As sodium ions are pulled out of the glomerular filtrate, there is an exchange of positive ions, with potassium and hydrogen being passed into the distal tubules and collecting ducts. This exchange is assumed to take place because of the noticeable negative charge left in the lumen of the tubule as the positively charged sodium ions are being pulled out. This action is essential because it is the major method by which the body rids itself of extracellular potassium ion. As the hydrogen ions are transmitted into the lumen of the tubule, bicarbonate ions are left behind as a result of the ionization of carbonic acid to bicarbonate and hydrogen ions. This results in a slight alkalosis, but due to the excellent buffer systems found within the body the change is usually compensated elsewhere.

Because many of the electrolytes are being pulled out of the tubules and into the extracellular fluid, there is an osmotic gradient set up which also draws water out of the kidney tubules and into the extracellular fluid.

Mineralocorticoids: control of release. Adrenocorticotropic hormone from the anterior pituitary has little effect on the production and release of the mineralocorticoids, though it greatly increases the concentration of glucocorticoids. Secretion of mineralocorticoids is controlled by plasma levels of sodium and potassium. A high concentration of potassium ions or a low level of sodium ions stimulates the production and release of the mineralocorticoids. These hormones then act on the kidney tubules to increase sodium ion reabsorption and potassium ion secretion.

Aldosterone secretion is also controlled by the *renin-angiotensin pathway*. Here, decrease in blood volume, whether caused by hemorrhage or other factors, results in a release of renin from the juxtaglomerular cells which surround the afferent renal arterioles. As was described in previous sections of this text, renin causes the conversion of *angiotensinogen* to *angiotensin I*. Angiotensin I is converted to *angiotensin II* by a plasma enzyme. Angiotensin II then enhances the release of aldosterone from the adrenal cortex. Elevated blood volume and consequently blood pressure results in a decrease in renin secretion from the juxtaglomerular cells. It has also been observed that pregnancy and emotional stress increase the secretion of aldosterone. The increase during pregnancy may be due to the increased circulating levels of *progesterone*. When progesterone is added to the zona glomerulosa of beef adrenal slices in tissue culture, it is converted to aldosterone. It has not been established if this is the case *in vivo*.

The Fetal Adrenals

The fetal adrenal glands are very large and contain an extra layer of cells not present in the adult mammal. This layer, called the *boundary zone* (or *fetal zone*, or *X zone*, or *androgen zone*) lies between the adrenal medulla and the zona reticularis of the adrenal cortex. This is the first part of the fetal cortex to become differentiated. It stains differently from the adult adrenal cortex and involutes after birth in the normal animal. This zone has been described for the human, mouse, and hamster fetuses and the fetuses of a few other mammals. Persistence of this zone after birth or the oversecretion of androgens from other adrenal cortical zones results in a more masculine appearance in females (i.e., the clitoris enlarges to the size of the penis, the voice deepens, menstruation fails or ceases to begin, and there is an increase in body hair and a thickening of the musculature). In males when this zone fails to disappear it re-

sults in precocious puberty, but the testes remain infantile.

Adrenal Abnormalities

If the adrenal glands are removed (adrenalectomy) death occurs within one or two weeks. Symptoms which occur in these adrenalectomized animals include the following: severe depletion of liver glycogen, low blood glucose levels, decrease of glucose absorption from the gut, and an eventual loss of glycogen from the muscles. These symptoms are all caused by the increased use of carbohydrates due to the lack of glucocorticoids. In these animals there is a decrease in gluconeogenesis and an increase in the utilization of available carbohydrates. This results in a higher RQ. These animals also show drastic signs of mineralocorticoid insufficiency with hemoconcentration, reduced blood pressure, and kidney failure. There is also extreme muscle fatigue because of hypoglycemia; a reduction in body temperature, probably due to the lack of glucose and fats available for thermoregulation, and an inability to tolerate stress of any kind. There is also an excessive loss of sodium, chloride, and bicarbonate ions and a decrease in potassium ion loss in the urine. The lymph nodes and thymus gland become enlarged and there is an increase in the number of lymphocytes. Death can be prevented if substantial amounts of the depleted salts are replaced, either in the diet or in the drinking water.

Addison's disease   This syndrome is attributed to the destruction of the adrenal cortices in a rather slow manner, as is found in adrenal tumors and complications of tuberculosis. In these cases there is atrophy of the cortical tissue and a slow decline in the levels of circulating adrenocorticoids. This slow adrenal insufficiency results in many of those symptoms already mentioned, but there is a slower onset of symptoms than those manifested due to bilateral adrenalectomy. In humans there is an increase in melanin pigmentation in the mucous membranes of the lips and in the nipples, elbows, and torso. This action is presumed to be due to the lack of cortisol available to inhibit release of ACTH and MSH by the pituitary. Both of these anterior pituitary hormones result in increased pigmentation. Individuals with this disease generally die of secondary infections due to the loss of resistance to some disease or due to shock related to the decrease in blood volume and consequent increase in hemoconcentration.

Cushing's disease Unlike Addison's disease, Cushing's disease is due to an oversecretion of adrenocorticoids, especially cortisol. This results in a redistribution of body fat, which results in a large fatty deposition on the back ("buffalo hump"), a moon-shaped face, an enlarged abdomen, and small extremities. There is also a marked increase in protein catabolism, which adds to the smallness of the extremeties. The skin of the face becomes flushed, and there is a significant increase in the bruisability of the skin and a marked decrease in wound healing.

Adrenogenital syndrome This disease may be due to the presence of an adrenal tumor or to the hypertrophy of the adrenal cortices. In this ailment the adrenal glands secrete extremely high levels of androgens. In human females with this disease, there is marked masculinization of the body, with increased facial and body hair, increased muscle development, and development of the cli-

toris. In the adult male there may be no overt signs of the disease, and diagnosis can only be made through analysis of the urine. Prepuberal males show precocious puberty.

THE THYROID GLAND

The thyroid gland originates in the mammalian embryo as an *outpocketing* or *evagination of the pharyngeal floor*. The size of the gland fluctuates with age, diet, season, and reproductive state. It produces and secretes many hormones, the most important of which are *thyroxine* (T_4), *triiodothyronine* (T_3), and *calcitonin* (or *thyrocalcitonin*). Both thyroxine and triiodothyronine have the same effect, but triiodothyronine is more potent than thyroxine. Thyroxine is produced in greater quantities than is triiodothyronine and therefore has a greater net effect. Both of these hormones affect metabolism and development, whereas calcitonin affects calcium balance. The thyroid gland is richly supplied with blood and is innervated by postganglionic sympathetic fibers of the cervical ganglia and by the vagus nerve. The thyroid gland continues to function even when denervated, probably owing to its dependence on the anterior pituitary hormone, thyroid-stimulating hormone.

The thyroid gland contains many cystlike *follicles* which function in the storage of thyroid hormones (see Figure 17–20). On the surface, each follicle is surrounded by a *basement membrane* and is lined with a layer of *secretory epithelial cells*. The center of the follicle is filled with a *globulin* (or *thyroglobulin*) called the *colloid*. This substance accumulates when the thyroid gland is inactive and decreases as thyroid activity increases. The thyroglobulin is taken up during increased thyroid activity by the epithelial cells

FIGURE 17–20
Histology of the rat thyroid gland. Note large, colloid-containing follicles. From *General Endocrinology*, 5th edition, by Clarence D. Turner and J. T. Bagnara. Copyright © 1971 by W. B. Saunders Co. Reprinted by permission of W. B. Saunders, CBS College Publishing.

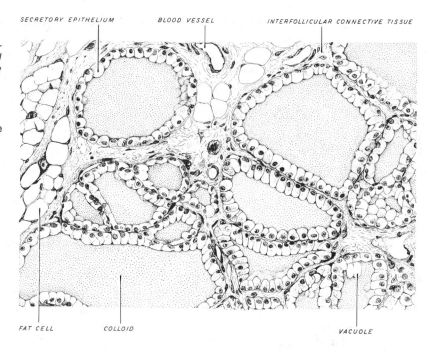

SECRETORY EPITHELIUM   BLOOD VESSEL   INTERFOLLICULAR CONNECTIVE TISSUE

FAT CELL   COLLOID   VACUOLE

surrounding the follicle. Once inside the epithelial cells, the thyroglobulin undergoes proteolysis and is converted to thyroxine and triiodothyronine, which are then released into the circulation. The innermost part of the epithelial cells, which is adjacent to the follicle space containing the colloid, is lined with numerous *microvilli* which protrude into the colloid. The increased surface area provided by the microvilli allows the thyroid cells to rapidly absorb the colloid by pinocytosis.

Calcitonin is produced by the *ultimobranchial glands* of fish, amphibians, reptiles, and birds. In mammals this tissue is not present as a specific gland but rather is incorporated into either the thyroid or parathyroid glands. In humans a part of the thyroid gland is made up of *parafollicular* or *C cells*, which occur throughout the gland and surround the follicles. These are the cells of ultimo-branchial origin which produce and secrete calcitonin in the human.

Hormones of the Thyroid Gland

Thyroxine and triiodothyronine Thyroxine (or *tetraiodothyronine*) and triiodothyronine are synthesized in the colloid from *tyrosine* and *iodine* as they are attached to the thyroglobulin molecule. Thyroglobulin is a large polypeptide with a molecular weight of approximately 670,000. It is usually not found in the blood and is easily hydrolyzed to a number of iodinated amino acids. The molecule itself contains 25 tyrosine residues which become iodinated to form *monoiodotyrosine* which is iodinated again to form *diiodotyrosine.* Two diiodotyrosine molecules combine to form tetraiodothyronine (thyroxine). Triiodothyronine synthesis involves the combination of monoiodotyrosine and a diiodotyrosine molecule (see Figure 17–21). There is a ratio of about nine thyroxine to one triiodothyronine molecules. These hormones remain attached to the thyroglobin and are stored in the follicles, or they are cleaved from the thyroglobin moiety and released into the bloodstream. The thyroglobin molecules remain in the colloid where they are reused.

Iodide accumulation by the thyroid gland
The thyroid gland, which sequesters iodide from the circulation, contains more than 90 percent of the body's iodide. There is at least twenty times as much iodide in the thyroid gland as there is in the blood plasma. This difference may become more exaggerated during periods of active hormone formation. The thyroid cells accumulate iodide by

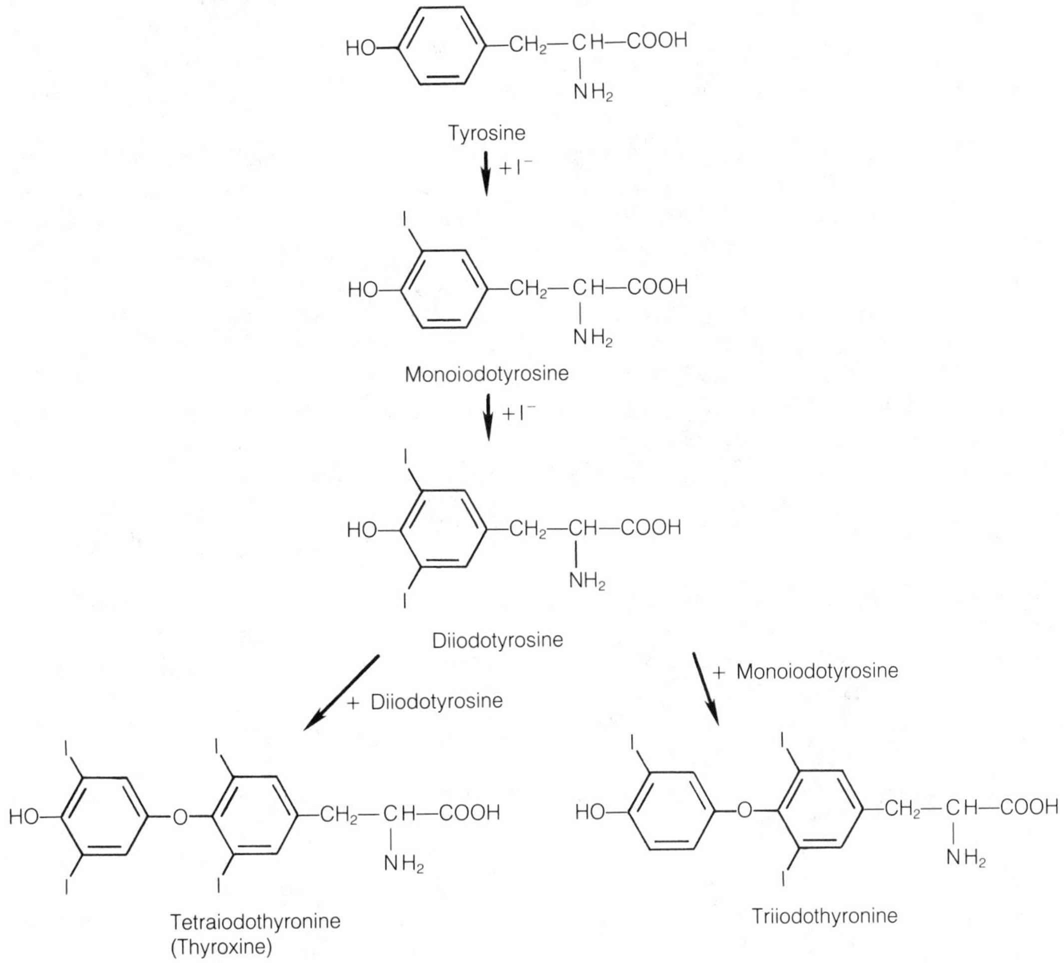

FIGURE 17–21
Biosynthesis of thyroxine and triiodothyronine

means of an active transport mechanism which is referred to by some authors as an *iodide trapping system*. Once inside the follicle the iodide passes into the colloid and is oxidized. It is in this oxidized form that iodide is bound to tyrosine.

Secretion of thyroxine and triiodothyronine. Thyroglobulin with its attached thyroxine and triiodothyronine is brought back into the epithelial cells lining the follicular space, where the colloid globules merge with lysosomes inside. Proteases in the lysosomes fragment the thyroglobin and cleave the thyroxine, triiodothyronine, diiodotyrosine, and monoiodotyrosine molecules from their "carrier." The last two classes of compounds are readily deiodinated by *iodotyrosine dehalogenase*, and the iodide is recycled and used again in the colloid to iodinate more tyrosine. This enzyme attacks the iodinated tyrosines but not the iodinated thyronine; therefore, the thyroxine and triiodothyronine are not deiodinated. These two hormones are instead released, and they pass into the blood. Once in the blood they readily combine with plasma carrier proteins such as *thyroxine-binding globulin (TBG)*, *thyroxine-binding prealbumin (TBPA)*, and *albumin*. These last two carriers bind significantly less thyroxine than does TBG. Very little free hormone is present in the plasma, but it is the free thyroid hormone that feeds back on the pituitary to regulate production of TSH. There is a very slow release of these thyroid hormones to the tissues because of the high affinity of thyroxine and triiodothyronine for their protein carriers. This is more noticeable with thyroxine than with triiodothyronine. Therefore, triiodothyronine, which has less affinity for its carrier, is released more quickly to the tissues.

Catabolism of thyroxine and triiodothyronine. The *liver* and *kidney* are the two major organs of catabolism of the thyroid hormones in this group. These hormones are deiodinated in the liver and salivary glands, and the iodide is recycled back to the thyroid gland for reuse in the formation of more thyroid hormones. In the liver, thyroxine and triiodothyronine are conjugated to *glucuronides* and *sulfates*. These substances are passed through the bile into the small intestine, where they pass out of the body with the feces. Some of the compounds may also be reabsorbed once they are hydrolyzed.

Effects of thyroxine and triiodothyronine. The major effect of these hormones is to increase the rate of metabolism. This is true in all tissues except the brain, spleen, lungs, uterus, lymph nodes, testes, and retina (see Figure 17–22). Most of the action is brought about by thyroxine, since it is the most prevalent of these two hormones; but once inside the tissues, it is converted to triiodothyronine. Thus the contribution of one hormone type over another is moot. Nevertheless, with equal availability, triiodothyronine is as much as seven times more potent than thyroxine, even though thyroxine is produced in much greater quantities.

Increase in metabolic rate is brought about by an increased uptake of glucose by the cells, increased gluconeogenesis, glycolysis, liver glycogenolysis, increased insulin secretion due to increased blood glucose levels, and increased monosaccharide absorption from the gut. These actions promote a marked increase in oxygen consumption by the tissues. This is therefore called a *calorigenic effect*. To add to this effect there is also a net increase in fat catabolism. This is accomplished through increased mobilization

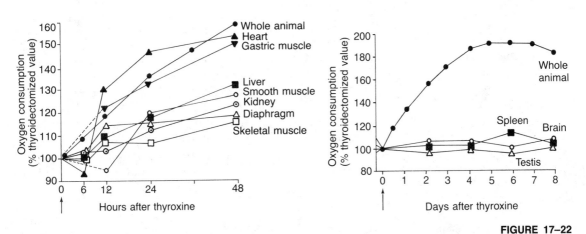

FIGURE 17–22

Comparative metabolic rates of different tissues of thyroidectomized rats after a single injection of thyroxine. From S. B. Barker and H. M. Klitgaard, Metabolism of Tissues Excised From Thyroxine–injected Rats, *Am. J. Physiol.* 170 (1952):81. Reprinted by permission of the American Physiological Society, Bethesda, Md.

of free fatty acids, with a subsequent increase in fatty acid oxidation by the cells. Along with these changes there is also an increase in the ATP-forming enzymes such as *cytochrome oxidase, cytochrome c,* and *succinoxidase.* These allow many of these increases in energy utilization. Because of the increase in energy utilization there may be an increase in body temperature.

In addition to the increase in carbohydrate and fat utilization, there is also a considerable effect on protein metabolism. Both protein catabolism and protein anabolism are increased. The *catabolic effect* adds to the process of gluconeogenesis and also frees amino acids for energy releasing reactions. The *anabolic effect* is most dramatic in younger mammals, in which thyroxine and triiodothyronine are important for normal development of the musculature and bones. Eventually these hormones will contribute to the epiphyseal closure and therefore a cessation of growth in the long bones. In the meantime, however, bone growth is stimu-

lated through the effect of these hormones on the laying down of the protein matrix necessary for bone formation. It should be noted that the thyroid hormones, along with STH from the anterior pituitary, have a synergistic effect on the rate of growth of the individual. These thyroid hormones and STH are necessary to promote normal growth and development.

Thyroxine and triiodothyronine affect the cytogenic and endocrine functioning of the ovaries and testes, possibly because these hormones tend to lower the circulating levels of cholesterol, which is a precursor for the formation of the sex steroids. It is the sex steroids, or lack thereof, that would affect the reproductive system. It has also been shown that these thyroid hormones affect the release of hypothalamic releasing hormones, which in turn affect the amounts of gonadotropic hormones secreted by the anterior pituitary. The evidence suggesting that thyroid hormones cause alteration in reproductive cycles includes their effects on the ovaries, on subnormal fecundity in mammals follow-ing thyroidectomy, and on increased suscep-tibility to ovarian cysts. It has been established that the gonads of young animals are more affected by thyroid deficiencies than those of older individuals.

Thyroxine and triiodothyronine increase certain activities in the brain. There is an in-crease in synaptic activity, which may ex-plain an increase in tension, restlessness, and irritability. There is also an increase in mentation. There appears to be a shortening of reaction time for certain stretch reflexes. In hypothyroidism, there is an increased sen-sitivity to light, sound, narcotics, and dimin-ished alpha waves.

The cardiovascular system is influenced by the release of thyroxine and triiodothyro-nine. The most noted effect is the increase in heart rate. Due to the increased metabolic rate there is a need for more rapid exchange of gases in the respiratory system, and a buildup of carbon dioxide occurs which stimulates the rate and depth of breathing. This buildup of metabolic waste products in the blood stimulates vasodilation, as does the increase in blood temperature due to the higher metabolic rate. To compensate for in-creased blood flow to the tissues the cardiac output also increases. Besides increasing car-diac output, these hormones cause a slight increase in the strength or force of the heart-beat.

Mode of action of thyroxine and triiodothyro-nine. At present there are so many actions of these hormones that there is no known ex-planation for how all of these effects are brought about. There is an increase in cyclic AMP and so the *second messenger idea* may be very important as a basis for many of the reactions that follow increased levels of these thyroid hormones. It has been established that these hormones enter the cytoplasm and are carried to the nucleus, where they increase protein synthesis, especially in mus-cle tissue. This has been confirmed because the protein synthesis inhibitor *actinomycin D* will also inhibit the actions of thyroxine in some if not all tissues. There is some evi-dence that thyroxine and triiodothyronine may also increase the permeability of cellular membranes.

Calcitonin   Calcitonin, also called *thyrocal-citonin* is produced by the *parafollicular cells* of the thyroid gland in humans and by one or both of the thyroid and parathyroid glands in other mammals. Calcitonin is a polypeptide composed of 32 amino acid res-idues and has a molecular weight of approx-imately 3,000. This hormone decreases the plasma calcium levels by causing an increase in the calcification of bone. Its effects are much more noticeable in younger animals than in adult animals owing to the reduction of calcium turnover in the adult. Calcitonin also prevents the reabsorption of bone. Thus, it may be seen that calcitonin acts antago-nistically to parathyroid hormone, which in-creases blood calcium levels. For further dis-cussion of the role of calcitonin in calcium metabolism, see chapter 8, The Skeletal System.

Thyroid Abnormalities

Hyposecretion of the thyroid gland in adult humans is associated with the disease *myx-edema*. Myxedema is usually the result of degeneration of the thyroid gland. It is manifested by an accumulation of *mucopoly-saccharides* in the interstitial spaces. This re-action is apparent in facial puffiness and bagginess under the eyes. There is also an increase in plasma cholesterol levels, which often leads to severe arteriosclerosis. There is also a dulling of the mental capabilities, and affected individuals retain fluid and show an increase in weight.

Children who are *hypothyroid* from birth are said to have *cretinism*. These children are characterized by a slow rate of growth and development. Along with the retarded growth, which often results in dwarfism, there is also retardation of the mental capabilities. These children show slower tooth formation and eruption, a lower body temperature, protrusion of the abdomen, and thickness of the tongue. These symptoms are mostly the result of a lack of proper balance between growth of the skeletal system and that of the soft tissues.

Endemic goiter may affect individuals of any age and will result in the symptoms already described for cretinism and myxedema. In this case the cause of the lack of thyroid hormones can be directly traced to an *iodine deficiency*. In this disease there is a decrease in the levels of thyroxine and triiodothyronine resulting from insufficient amounts of iodine in the diet. Because of the low concentrations of these hormones in afflicted individuals, the anterior pituitary continues to release TSH, which results in increased stimulation of the thyroid gland. As TSH production proceeds unchecked, there is follicular cell hyperlasia, which results in hypertrophy of the entire gland. Once the iodine levels return to normal and the thyroid hormones are produced in normal concentrations, TSH production is reduced by means of the normal feedback mechanism. Another type of goiter, called a *simple colloid goiter*, can result when more thyroid hormone is stored in the colloid than can be re-

leased. This is due to a lack of sufficient TSH secretion and stimulation.

Hyperthyroidism, or the hypersecretion of thyroxine and triiodothyronine, results in marked hyperplastic growth of the thyroid gland. This type of goiter formation is called *toxic goiter* or *exopthalmic goiter*. The latter term came into use when it was found that this type of thyroid malfunction resulted in *edema* behind the eye, which causes the eye to bulge noticeably. This type of malady is also characterized by a very high metabolic rate, muscle tremors, loss of weight, sweating, increased nervousness, and increased body temperature. In these individuals there are more than sufficient supplies of the thyroid hormones. The anterior pituitary continues to release TSH even though external evidence of feedback regulation is present.

THE PARATHYROID GLANDS

The parathyroid glands are usually located in the neck region near the thyroid gland. In sheep, rabbits, and oxen, the parathyroids are completely separate from the thyroid gland. There may be one or more pairs of these glands. A single pair of parathyroids is found in the rat, mouse, shrew, seal, and pig. There are two pairs in the human, dog, cat, horse, guinea pig, rabbit, and opossum. These glands originate from the *dorsal part of the third and fourth pharyngeal pouches*. Each gland is surrounded by a capsule of connective tissue which extends into the interior of the gland and separates it into *lobes*. There is little innervation of these glands, but there is a rich blood supply from the *inferior* and *superior thyroid arteries*.

The parathyroid glands are composed of densely packed epithelial cells of two different types. The most prevalent type by far in mammals is the *chief* or *principal cells;*, only a few *oxyphil cells* are present in most mammals. The function of the oxyphil cells is unknown, but that of the chief cells is production and secretion of *parathyroid hormone (PTH)*, or *parathormone*. The oxyphil cells are rich in mitochondria, contain little or no glycogen, and have a rather granular cytoplasm. It is possible that these are older chief cells and that they may produce small reserve quantities of PTH. The chief cells contain a great deal of glycogen. These cells are small and have a large nucleus and agranular cytoplasm.

Hormones of the Parathyroid Glands

Parathyroid hormone Parathyroid hormone is the only known hormone produced and secreted by the parathyroid glands. In humans this hormone is composed of 84 amino acids in a straight-chain formation and is derived from a larger protein called *pre-pro-parathyroid hormone*. This larger protein contains 115 amino acids. During synthesis of parathyroid hormone, 25 of these amino acids are cleaved to leave *pro-PTH*, which then contains 90 amino acids. Just prior to release into the bloodstream, the 84 amino acids which constitute the active PTH are cleaved from pro-PTH.

Effects of parathyroid hormone. There are two target organs directly affected by circulating PTH. These are the *kidneys* and *bones*. In the kidneys PTH causes an increase in release of phosphate ions from the blood into the urine. It also increases removal of calcium and magnesium ions from the glomerular filtrate by increasing their reabsorption. The increased rate of renal excretion of phos-

phates is due to a decrease in tubular reabsorption of the phosphate. Parathyroid hormone's action on the bones is brought about through an increase in osteoclast activity. These bone cells increase the demineralization and reabsorption (breakdown) of bone. In doing this there is destruction of bone collagen and apatite crystals, which then causes release of calcium and phosphate into the blood plasma. This increase in calcium release from bone and increased calcium reabsorption in the kidney both contribute to the increase in plasma calcium levels observed with release of PTH. In addition to these effects already noted, PTH also increases formation of *1,25-dihydroxycholecalciferol* (i.e., the active form of vitamin D). For more information on the effects and mode of action of PTH, see chapter 8, The Skeletal System.

Control of PTH release. The circulating level of calcium ion is the major controlling factor in the control of PTH release from the parathyroid glands. As plasma calcium levels drop, the parathyroid glands are stimulated to produce and secrete more PTH. As the PTH levels rise, there is an increase in plasma calcium ion concentration, which then retards further PTH release. There is some evidence that increased blood phosphate levels may also increase the release of PTH (see Figure 17–23).

Abnormalities of the Parathyroid Glands

Hyperparathyroidism As might be expected, there are many adverse effects that can be attributed to hyperparathyroidism. One of the first symptoms is *hypercalcemia* due to the close correlation of blood calcium levels with the PTH levels. These high levels of calcium ions cause anorexia, nausea, and

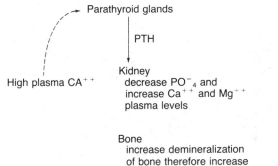

FIGURE 17-23
Parathyroid hormone (PTH) and calcitonin act as antagonists. As blood calcium ion levels rise, PTH secretion slows and calcitonin secretion increases. The reverse is true when plasma calcium ion levels drop. The dashed line indicates inhibition.

a softening of the bones due to demineralization. There may also be calcium deposits in soft tissues and organs due to the excess calcium concentrations. *Hyperphosphatemia* can occur in conjunction with the increased calcium levels. Other symptoms include decreased sensitivity of the neuromuscular system due to increased excitability of the nerves. Again, this is probably due to the calcium overload. In humans the hypersecretion of the parathyroid gland is known by the name *von Recklinghausen's disease* or *osteitis fibrosa.*

Hypoparathyroidism Studies on the effects of parathyroidectomy using dogs have shown the following results: subnormal body temperature, vomiting, anorexia, salivation, diarrhea, and tetany. The tetany leads to an increase in body temperature, and at the same time the respiratory rate increases and becomes deeper. The blood becomes more alkaline because of the decrease in carbonic acid concentration. This alkaline blood condition leads to an inhibition of calcium ioni-

zation, which then results in greater tetany. Goats show a definite muscular tremor but no tetany. For some reason herbivores are more tolerant to parathyroidectomy than are carnivores. In humans the problems of hypoparathyroidism are more pronounced in children and in pregnant or lactating women because of their increased calcium demands.

Other symptoms of parathyroidectomy include reduced plasma citrate levels, increased plasma inorganic phosphate concentrations, and decreased urinary excretion of phosphate and calcium. The decreased plasma levels of calcium, besides leading to the obvious tetany, also contribute to the actual cause of death, which is asphyxiation resulting from spasms of the laryngeal muscles. Another interesting result of parathyroidectomy is the development of cataracts in the lenses of the eyes of dogs, rats, and humans.

THE PANCREAS

The pancreas is the second largest digestive gland in the mammalian body. It arises from the *ectoderm of the primitive gut* and usually lies in a loop between the intestine and the stomach. The pancreas is both exocrine and endocrine in function. The exocrine function is as a gland of digestion. The endocrine activity is carried out by the *islets of Langerhans*, small areas of endocrine tissue that are scattered among the exocrine cells, or the *alveoli* (see Figure 17-24). These islet cells comprise only about 1.0 to 2.0 percent of the pancreatic tissue, with the most numerous groups lying closest to the spleen. Innervation is by the right vagus nerve of the autonomic nervous system, though both alveolar and islet cells continue to function after denervation.

FIGURE 17–24
Histology of the pancreas showing many pancreatic alveoli (acini) and islets of Langerhans. From *General Endocrinology*, 5th edition, by C. D. Turner and J. T. Bagnara. Copyright © 1971 by W. B. Saunders Co. Reprinted by permission of W. B. Saunders, CBS College Publishing.

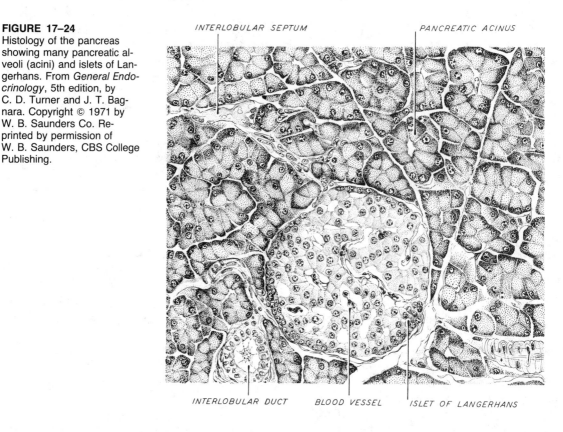

INTERLOBULAR SEPTUM   PANCREATIC ACINUS

INTERLOBULAR DUCT   BLOOD VESSEL   ISLET OF LANGERHANS

Each group of islet cells contains at least three types of cells. The *alpha* or *A cells* are usually located around the periphery of the islet. These cells, which make up approximately 20 to 25 percent of the total islet, contain large water-soluble granules and stain red with modified Mallory aniline blue stain. The alpha cells produce and secrete glucagon. The *beta* or *B cells* are the source of insulin in the pancreas and make up the bulk of the cells composing the islets. These cells contain smaller alcohol-soluble granules and stain a blue purple with Mallory's stain. Other cells which make up the islets of Langerhans include the *delta* or *D cells*, the *C cells*, and other as yet unnamed cells. All of these cells of the islets are derived from cells lining the pancreatic ducts and are in close apposition to the many capillaries that perfuse the pancreas. Pancreatic endocrine hormones are secreted into these capillaries and are carried by the *hepatic portal vein* to the liver, where a great many of their effects are observed.

Hormones of the Pancreas

Insulin   Insulin is a protein molecule with a molecular weight of approximately 6,000. The actual weight and amino acid sequence varies from species to species, though there are two subunits with two disulfide bridges common to all types of insulin thus far studied. Rats produce two types of insulin which differ somewhat in their amino acid sequence, but both carry out principally the same function, that of carbohydrate, fat, and protein anabolism. Insulin is synthesized from a single-chain protein precursor called *proinsulin*. After cleavage of proinsulin, the insulin molecule is stored in the granules of the beta cells, where it is released by means of exocytosis. Once in the bloodstream it is generally bound to protein carriers. Approximately half of the secreted insulin is trapped in the liver and degraded by a series of proteolytic enzymes. Insulin not trapped and destroyed by the liver becomes tightly bound to the cells of its target organs.

Effects of insulin. Nearly all of the tissues of the body respond to insulin. In the tissues insulin has a tendency to increase anabolism of carbohydrates, fats, and proteins, These actions are in opposition to those of glucagon, which is also secreted by the pancreas.

The effect of insulin on carbohydrate metabolism occurs at several different levels. Insulin first promotes the uptake or transport of glucose from the blood into other tissues. This decreases blood glucose levels but increases the level of glucose in the tissues. Glucose uptake by the cells may be increased as much as twentyfold in animals previously deprived of insulin. The tissues in which glucose transport is most noticeable include skeletal muscle and adipose tissue. There is also an increase in glucose uptake by cells of the heart, the smooth muscles, the mammary glands, and pancreatic islets. Tissues not affected in their uptake of glucose include most parts of the brain, the kidney tubules, and the intestinal mucosa.

Glucose enters the cells by means of *facilitated transport*. That is, energy is expended and carriers are necessary but glucose does not move against its concentration gradient.

The exact mechanism by which insulin stimulates this process is unknown. It is known, however, that insulin attaches to a receptor protein on the membrane surface of these cells. In the liver, glucose enters the cells by passive diffusion rather than facilitated transport. Once inside the liver cells, the glucose is phosphorylated by means of the enzyme *glucokinase*, whose production is stimulated by insulin. Once the glucose is phosphorylated, it is trapped within the cell and cannot diffuse back out.

When there is an excess amount of both glucose and insulin, certain tissues are stimulated to increase the formation of glycogen. This is brought about by the buildup of glucose and its metabolites in these cells. Some of the metabolites resulting from excess carbohydrate utilization, indicative of high levels of available glucose sources, are ATP and citrate ion. These two compounds inhibit the activity of *phosphfructokinase*, an enzyme important in the glycolytic pathway. This slowdown in glycolysis results in further buildup of glucose concentrations in the cells. At this point there is activation of a glycogen-forming enzyme, *glycogen synthetase*, which then increases the conversion of glucose to glycogen. There is a concomitant inactivation of *phosphorylase*, which normally leads to the destruction of glycogen.

Protein metabolism is also greatly affected by insulin. There is a marked increase in protein anabolism in the liver, skeletal muscle, and adipose tissue, which increases the movement of amino acids into these tissues. Once inside these cells there is an increase in RNA translation into proteins. There may also be some increase in RNA transcription, though some studies have shown that the effects of insulin on protein anabolism are generally not blocked by the administration of RNA-inhibiting antibiotics.

Control of insulin release. Many actions regulate the secretion of insulin from the islet cells of the pancreas (see Figure 17–25). The foremost regulator is blood glucose levels. When blood glucose levels rise there is a subsequent rise in insulin release. This acts on various target organs to decrease the amount of glucose liberated by the tissues and increases the amount of glucose taken up by the tissues. High concentrations of amino acids and fatty acids also stimulate the release of insulin. Other factors contributing to insulin production and secretion include: increased cyclic AMP levels; the drug theophyllin; other hormones such as STH and ACTH from the anterior pituitary; glucocorticoids from the adrenal glands; glucagon from the pancreas; thyroxine from the thyroid gland; and intestinal hormones such as secretin and gastrin. Both epinephrine and norepinephrine inhibit the secretion of insulin. These effects are brought about by the beta adrenergic receptors which are located near the islet cells.

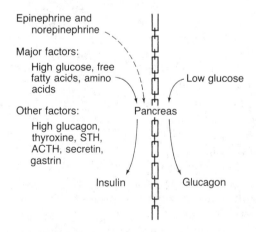

FIGURE 17–25
Feedback regulation of the major pancreatic hormones, insulin, and glucagon. The dashed line indicates inhibition; solid lines indicate stimulation.

Hyposecretion of insulin. The hyposecretion of insulin results in a disease in mammals known as *diabetes mellitus*. In this situation there is a dramatic increase in blood glucose levels *(hyperglycemia)*. This condition may be caused by pancreatectomy, by the administration of alloxan, a drug which selectively destroys the beta cells of the pancreas when given in proper concentrations, or by some other means. The resulting hyperglycemia is in part due to the rapid depletion of liver and muscle glycogen stores, a halting of further formation and storage of glycogen by the liver and other tissues, and the impairment of the catabolism of glucose in the tissues. Because of these high concentrations of blood glucose, there is an increase in excretion of glucose by the kidneys, a process called *glucosuria*. Because of the high levels of solutes in the urine during glucosuria, there is also an osmotic gradient into the kidney tubules and, therefore, and increase in water lost in the urine with a subsequent increase in urine output *(polydipsia)*. Along with these direct effects on carbohydrate metabolism, the metabolism of fats and proteins is also altered with detrimental effects. There is an increase in protein and fat catabolism to make up for the lack of carbohydrate that can be used by the tissues as an energy source. This results in weight loss and an increase in *ketone bodies* as a result of lipid oxidation. These ketone bodies (*acetoacetic acid, beta-hydroxybutyric acid,* and acetone) accumulate in the blood. The acetone can be smelled on the breath and is also excreted in the urine. In addition to this *ketosis* that results from fat oxidation, the acetoacetic and beta-hydroxybutyric acids also decrease the pH of the blood. The resulting *acidosis* stimulates the respiratory center in the brain, which causes a rapid, deep respiratory rate. Because of the low pH of the urine, sodium and potassium ions are also eventually lost in the urine, with a dramatic effect on the individual. There is dehydration, loss of perception, hypotension, and *hypovolemia* (decreased blood volume), the last of which contributes to the hypotension. The eventual result of these physiological consequences is a diabetic coma and death.

The basis for this disease is that the islets of Langerhans no longer secrete insulin or the normal amounts are not able to enter the bloodstream. This may be brought about by a growth-onset type of diabetes in young animals. This type of diabetes mellitus responds to treatment by insulin injection because there is an actual deficiency of the hormone. In maturity-onset type of diabetes mellitus, which occurs in middle-aged animals, there is usually no positive response to insulin injections. This is because the problem is not one of deficiency of the hormone, since it is present in normal concentrations in the blood but for some reason cannot reach the target tissues. Individuals with this type of diabetes can usually be treated by altering the diet and lowering the intake of glucose.

Hypersecretion of insulin. An excess secretion of insulin is most often due to a tumor of the islet cells or an insulin overdose. Individuals with this problem show a dramatic decrease in blood glucose levels. These low glucose levels have their most marked effect on the brain, which preferentially uses glucose as an energy source. Therefore, symptoms of hypersecretion of insulin result in hypoglycemia, which in turn causes weakness, dizziness, and confusion in the individual. There is also an increase in the activity of the sympathetic nervous system, which causes an increase in the release of epinephrine. High levels of epinephrine induce increased heart rate, sweating, tremors, and anxiety. If blood glucose levels are not returned to normal, the individual lapses into a coma, and death results from asphyxia caused by depression of the respiratory center.

Glucagon Glucagon is a straight-chain polypeptide composed of 29 amino acids and has a molecular weight of approximately 3,500. This hormone is sometimes called the *hyperglycemic-glycogenolytic factor (HGF)* and has a rapid hyperglycemic effect. Most of its effects on the body are exactly opposite to those observed for insulin, and there is mutual regulation of secretion of insulin and glucagon.

Effects of glucagon. The major actions of glucagon are exhibited preferentially on the liver. These actions are increased glycogenolysis and increased gluconeogenesis, both of which increase blood glucose levels. The glycogenolysis in the liver is the result of direct action of glucagon on the activation of *adenyl cyclase*, which promotes the formation of cyclic AMP. The increased level of cyclic AMP results in the activation of *protein kinase regulator protein*, which in turn activates *protein kinase*. Next there is an activation of *phosphorylase b kinase* and a conversion of *phosphorylase b* to *phosphorylase a*. It is the phosphorylase a which stimulates the degradation of glycogen to *glucose-1-phosphate*. The glucose is then dephosphorylated and is released from the liver cells (see Figure 17–26). This is one of the cases in which cyclic AMP acts as a second messenger in hormone action, and in this case the entire sequence of events is known.

The rate of gluconeogenesis in the liver is also increased, even after all of the stored glycogen is released. In this action there is an

FIGURE 17–26
Mode of action of adenyl cyclase in the breakdown of glycogen

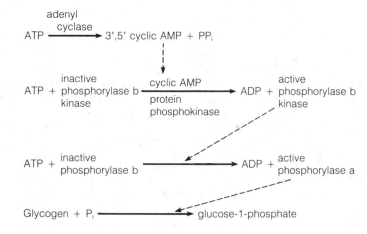

increase in the transport of amino acids into the cells of the liver. These amino acids are then converted to glucose precursors. Increased amino acid transport to the liver is a result of an increase in protein catabolism in tissues other than the liver. This increased transport, along with an increase in the oxidation of fats to fatty acids and glycerol (which supplies glycerol for gluconeogenesis), causes an increase in the precursors necessary for gluconeogenesis to occur.

Control of glucagon release. The level of glucagon is primarily controlled by the concentration of blood glucose (see Figure 17–25). When the level of plasma glucose drops for any reason, there is a stimulatory effect of the alpha cells of the pancreas to increase glucagon production and secretion. Other factors which contribute to the secretion of glucagon include: high amino acid concentrations in the blood, as would occur following a high protein mean; exercise, due to the subsequent decreases in blood glucose levels; starvation, for the same reason; cortisol; infection; gastrin; theophyllin; and stimulation of the beta adrenergic nerve endings. Factors known to inhibit the release of glu-

cagon include: high glucose levels; a lack of insulin, since glucose cannot enter the alpha cells to slow release of glucagon; the presence of free fatty acids and ketones; and high levels of somatostatin from the hypothalamus, which then slows release of somatotropic hormone from the anterior pituitary.

Other hormones secreted by the pancreas By far the major hormones of the pancreas have already been discussed, but there are two more hormones which are secreted by this organ. *Somatostatin* is also produced in the pancreas and tends to decrease the levels of both insulin and glucagon. It also is produced by the gastrointestinal tract and may have some hormonal effect on it. Its major role, however, is that of inhibition of secretion of somatotropic hormone. Another substance, *pancreatic polypeptide*, has also been desribed as being produced in the pancreas, but its function is not known.

THE PINEAL GLAND

The pineal gland develops from the *diencephalon*, almost opposite to the site of formation of the pituitary. No neural connections from the diencephalon are retained in the adult, though it does receive innervation from sympathetic neurons. The pineal has received the interest of physiologists the world over who have described several substances which might possibly be produced by it as well as a number of its possible functions. The pineal was discovered by early Greek anatomists, who in the absence of any definitive data proposed various and sometimes unrealistic functions of this gland. Probably the most famous reference to the function of the pineal was made during the seventeenth century by Descartes, who thought the structure was the seat of the soul.

Recent data would indicate a variety of pineal functions. Most of the definitive data on pineal function have involved the use of nonmammalian species as experimental animals. Experiments to reveal the function of the pineal in mammals cover a wide range of possibilities, but no well-established function or mechanism of function has been thoroughly demonstrated which would allow generalization for the mammals as a group. One of the first modern experiments of the endocrine function of the pineal, reported by Bagnara, revealed that some secretions from the amphibian pineal caused blanching of the skin. It was demonstrated that pineal function regulates circadian (daily) rhythms in birds. Evidence drawn from human cases of pineal tumors has indicated that the pineal might function in maturation. In these cases it appears that hyposecretion of *melatonin*, the major pineal secretory product, results in early maturation, apparently through removal of its inhibitory action on pituitary gonadotropin synthesis and release. A possible function which has eluded investigators working with mammals is the pineal's role in circadian rhythms. It is quite probable that it functions in some circadian capacity in mammals since some of the enzymes as well as products follow a diurnal periodicity in their synthesis and accumulation.

In the rat the pineal has been shown to produce melatonin as the final product of an anabolic pathway beginning with *5-hydroxytryptophan* (see Figure 17–27). It has been shown that injections of melatonin into rats retard the estrous cycles and cause a general decrease in ovarian weight. When rats were maintained in various light cycles, melatonin production reached a maximum in reduced light. This is correlated with an elevated level of the enzyme *hydroxyindole-o-methyltransferase (HIOMT)*, which promotes the forma-

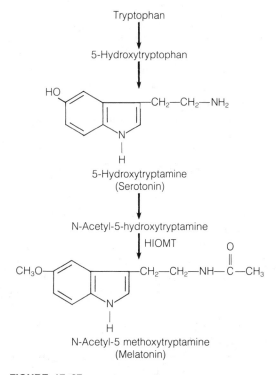

FIGURE 17–27
Melatonin synthesis in the pineal gland

tion of melatonin from serotonin. It has been reported that when the transmission of light information was interrupted in rodents by blinding the animal or by cutting the sympathetic nerves to the pineal, the gonadal response to photoperiod was also abolished. But a working hypothesis for the role of the pineal in mammalian physiology still eludes investigators in this field.

SUMMARY

Hormones produced and secreted by the endocrine glands are chemical messengers which alter the action of their target organs. There are several classes of hormones (i.e., steroid, glycoprotein, etc.) but regardless of their specific chemical configuration all hormones evoke some sort of response from the target tissues. The mode of action of hormones on their target organs is generally directed toward protein synthesis, membrane permeability, or enzyme regulation.

The hypothalamus is responsible for the production of two hormones released by the posterior pituitary (vasopressin and oxytocin) and for the production of releasing and inhibiting hormones, which have the anterior pituitary as their target organ. This latter group of hormones is released into the hypophyseal portal system, which carries them to the anterior lobe of the pituitary.

Adrenocorticotropic hormone-releasing hormone (ACTH-RH) controls the release of ACTH from the pituitary, which in turn increases the synthesis and secretion of adrenocorticoids from the adrenal cortex. Factors which enhance the release of ACTH-RH include stress, vasopressin, and angiotensin II. Adrenocorticoids and ACTH act to slow the release of ACTH-RH.

Somatotropic hormone-releasing hormone (STH-RH) is an acidic protein which enhances the release of STH from the anterior pituitary. Secretion of STH-RH is stimulated by nervous action, increased blood levels of arginine, vasopressin, and adrenocorticoids. Release of STH-RH is slowed by increased plasma levels of glucose, free fatty acids, and beta adrenergic agents as well as by stimuli from the higher nerve centers.

Thyroid-stimulating hormone-releasing hormone (TSH-RH) controls, to a great extent, the release of TSH from the pituitary. Levels of TSH-RH are increased by low levels of thyroxine and triiodothyronine and by low ambient temperatures. There is a decrease in TSH-RH secretion when the animal is under stress, restrained, and traumatized or when there are high levels of thyroxine and triiodothyronine.

A single releasing hormone has been postulated for control of the secretion of FSH and LH. Secretion of this releasing hormone, FSH/LH-RH, is regulated by circulating estrogen and progesterone levels. When the plasma concentration of either of these hormones is high there is an inhibition of FSH/LH-RH release.

Prolactin-releasing hormone, somatrophic-inhibiting hormone, melanocyte-inhibiting hormone and melanocyte-stimulating hormone-releasing hormone have all been postulated, but not much data have been accumulated on these hypothalamic factors. Prolactin-inhibiting hormone reduces the secretion of prolactin and maintains normal prolactin levels at a low concentration, except during pregnancy and lactation in mammals.

The pituitary, or "master gland," is composed of three lobes: the anterior and intermediate lobes make up the adenohypophysis and the posterior lobe makes up the neurohypophysis. The latter of these two parts is innervated by the supraoptic-hypophyseal tract. The adenohypophysis is not innervated and depends on the hypophyseal portal system for a major part of its control.

The posterior pituitary secretes two hormones, vasopressin and oxytocin, which are produced in the supraoptic and paraventricular nuclei of the hypothalamus. Vasopressin, or antidiuretic hormone, increases the permeability of the convoluted tubules of the kidney, which results in an increase in water reabsorption and a decrease in osmotic pressure in the blood. An increase in osmotic pressure stimulates release of vasopressin, as does decreased blood volume, nervous stimulation, certain emotions, pain, suckling, and changes in ambient temperature.

Oxytocin, which is released by the posterior pituitary, is important in milk ejection during nursing and for contraction of smooth muscles of the uterus and oviducts. Release of oxytocin is brought about through nervous stimulation due to coitus, parturition, and tactile stimulation of the nipples or teats.

The intermediate lobe of the pituitary produces melanocyte-stimulating hormone, which effects pigmentation in mammals.

The anterior pituitary produces six and sometimes seven hormones. Somatotropic hormone causes an increase in blood glucose levels, lipid mobilization and utilization, and bone length and decreases protein catabolism. High blood glucose levels decrease STH secretion through feedback on the hypothalamus.

Thyroid-stimulating hormone is a glycoprotein and consists of two subunits. The main target organ of TSH is the thyroid gland, where it causes an increase in iodine uptake by this gland and an increase in the synthesis and release of thyroxine and triiodothyronine. The feedback control of TSH is maintained through plasma levels of thyroxine and triiodothyronine. These hormones may affect either the hypothalamus or the pituitary in their feedback regulation.

Adrenocorticotropic hormone is a small, straight-chained polypeptide whose main target organ is the adrenal cortex. As adrenocorticoid production increases, these hormones feed back to decrease ACTH release. In animals under stress, the normal feedback relationships are somehow blocked or overridden, and there is a greater than usual release of adrenocortical steroids. This set of conditions leads to the General Adaptation Syndrome first described by Hans Selyé.

Follicle-stimulating hormone and luteinizing hormone are two of the pituitary gonadotropic hormones. In the female FSH causes the growth and development of the ovarian follicle and then the production of estrogen. Luteinizing hormone triggers ovulation and then luteinizes the follicular cells, which remain in the follicle after the egg has been released. The resulting structure, the corpus luteum, produces progesterone. In the male, FSH is important for gametogenesis and LH is necessary for testosterone production.

Prolactin is a lactogenic hormone produced and secreted by the anterior pituitary. Difficulty in purification of this hormone has presented many problems in identifying actions on target organs which are attributable to pure preparations of this hormone. The major effects of prolactin are in the development of the mammary glands and in its role in lactation.

The gonads (the ovaries and testes) are the paired primary reproductive organs in mammals. The major hormones produced by the ovaries (estrogens and progestins) are responsible for the maintenance of the reproductive organs, the female secondary sex characteristics, and the normal reproductive cycle observed in the female. Estrogens are responsible, in part, for the development of the female reproductive tract and the mammary glands. They stimulate the development of the endometrium and vaginal cornification during successive ovarian cycles. Progestins are necessary for the preparation of the female reproductive tract for implantation and maintenance of pregnancy. These effects predominate in the uterine endometrium. Progestins also act on the mammary tissue to stimulate the development of the mammary lobules and alveoli.

Relaxin, thought to be a hormone of pregnancy, is produced by the ovaries, placenta, and uterus. The major target organs of this polypeptide are the uterus and pelvic girdle. During parturition, relaxin softens and dilates the cervix and, in the later stages of pregnancy, also mobilizes the sacroiliac joints and relaxes the fibrocartilage in the pubic symphysis.

Androgens, another class of steroid hormones, are produced and secreted by the testes. Estrogen and progesterone in the female are responsible for the development and maintenance of the reproductive tract and maintenance of the secondary sex characteristics; testosterone takes over these responsibilities in the male. The effect of testosterone on increased protein anabolism and libido have been well documented and are two of the most noticeable effects of this hormone.

The placenta produces and secretes many hormones. Among these are estrogens, progestins, and relaxin. Chorionic gonadotropin is a luteotropic hormone secreted by the placenta which helps to maintain the corpus luteum, especially during the early stages of pregnancy. Placental lactogen affects the mammary glands and in humans also has growth-stimulating effects. Pregnant mare serum gonadotropin is produced by the endometrial cups in the uterus, which are of fetal origin. This hormone is luteotropic and may stimulate the formation of accessory corpora lutea in the horse.

The adrenal glands comprise an inner medulla and an outer cortex. The adrenal medulla produces and secretes a group of hormones called catecholamines. This area of the adrenal gland is innervated directly by preganglionic fibers of the sympathetic nervous system. The catecholamines (specifically, epinephrine and norepinephrine) generally tend to increase heart rate and its force of contraction, increase systolic pressure, increase carbohydrate metabolism, and therefore increase blood glucose levels.

The adrenal cortex is responsible for the synthesis and release of the mineralocorticoids and glucocorticoids, all of which are steroid hormones. A third group, the gonadal or sex steroids, is also produced by the adrenal cortex, but the effect of these hormones of the adrenal glands is small in comparison to those produced by the gonads. The glucocorticoids increase gluconeogenesis from fats and proteins and increase the deposition of liver glycogen. There may also be a decrease in glycolysis in the target cells. The anti-inflammatory action of cortisol, one of the glucocorticoids, is well known.

The mineralocorticoids, of which aldosterone is the most potent, increase reabsorption of sodium ion from the body fluids and by doing so also leads to an increase in water retention by the kidneys. There is also an increase in potassium and hydrogen ion release and an increase in anion reabsorption by the kidneys. Secretion of the mineralocorticoids is controlled by plasma concentrations of sodium and potassium and by a decrease in blood pressure, which activates the renin-angiotensin pathway.

Thyroxine and triiodothyronine are produced in the thyroid follicles from thyroglobulin. Iodide, necessary for the formation of thyroxine and triiodothyronine, is accumulated against a concentration gradient in this organ. These two hormones tend to increase the metabolic rate by increasing the rate of glucose uptake by the cells and by increasing gluconeogenesis, glycolysis, liver glycogenolysis, glucose absorption from the gut, and insulin secretion. There is also an increase in free fatty acid mobilization and utilization.

Calcitonin is produced and secreted by cells of ultimobranchial origin. In the human these cells are located in the thyroid gland. This polypeptide hormone causes a decrease in plasma calcium ion levels and acts antagonistically to parathormone produced by the parathyroid glands.

Parathyroid hormone, or parathormone, is the only hormone known to be produced and secreted by the parathyroid glands. In the kidneys PTH causes an increase in release of phosphate ions and an increase in reabsorption of calcium and magnesium ions. Parathyroid hormone acts on the bones to cause demineralization and thereby increases plasma calcium levels in this way, too.

The two hormones of major concern produced by the pancreas are insulin and glucagon. Insulin stimulates an increase in uptake of glucose by the cells of the target organs and sometimes an increase in glycogen synthesis. Insulin also causes an increase in protein anabolism. Most of the effects brought about by glucagon are in opposition to those brought about by insulin. Glucagon tends to increase blood glucose levels through an increase in glycogenolysis and gluconeogenesis by the liver.

The pineal gland is considered to be an endocrine gland by most investigators, though its major effects in mammals are not well documented. It is apparently important in the production of melatonin, which controls blanching in amphibians and affects circadian rhythms in birds. This hormone is thought to be important in controlling circadian activity in mammals, but definitive data in this regard have not been obtained.

18

THE REPRODUCTIVE SYSTEM

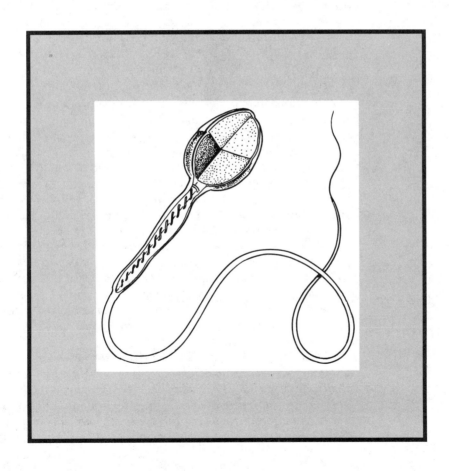

*T*he reproductive system of mammals comprises the primary reproductive organs, the ovaries and testes, and a number of accessory organs. The majority of these are paired structures. The primary organs give rise to the reproductive cells, which are eggs (or ova) in the case of the female and the sperm in the case of males. Both male and female primary organs are also endocrine in function, since they produce and secrete most of the sex steroids found in mammals. The accessory sex organs store, protect, and nurture the gametes and allow their union. In addition, female accessory sex organs provide a suitable environment for the embryo after fertilization of the egg. Once produced by the primary reproductive organs, the ova and sperm pass through their respective duct systems and, when successful, unite to form a zygote or fertilized egg. All male mammals possess a copulatory organ, the penis, for the transfer of sperm into the reproductive tract of the female, and all mammals except the monotremes are viviparous (i.e., give birth to live young). Although there are many variations in the basic mechanism, all mammalian reproduction involves the formation of the zygote, development of the embryo, and some type of maternal care. In all mammals other than monotremes, reproduction also involves zygote implantation in the inner lining of the uterus and subsequent parturition.

All mammals nourish their young by means of the mammary glands, but in many cases this is where the similarity ends. In the class Mammalia there are several different and unique methods of gestation and birth of the young (see Table 18–1). The class Mammalia is divided into two subclasses, Prototheria and Theria. The latter group contains the infraclasses Metatheria and Eutheria. The subclass Prototheria contains three living species, all of which are in the order Monotremata. These include the duckbill platypus and two genera of echidnas (or spiny anteaters). In this subclass the Müllerian ducts, which give rise to the female reproductive tract, do not fuse, as is the case in most mammals. These mammals incubate the developing embryo outside of the body in eggs covered by a leathery shell. Once the neonates are hatched, they are nourished by means of the mammary glands, which in these animals do not have nipples or teats. After secretion, the milk flows into a small depression in the skin and the young lap it up.

In the platypus, the female possesses two ovaries but only one is functional. As the fertilized eggs pass down the oviduct a thin layer of albumin is added. Once inside the uterus a horny shell is added, and the egg continues to increase in size, from about 4.0 mm to nearly 10 mm in diameter. At this time, calcium salts are added and the egg again continues to increase in size until the time of hatching, *when it may reach 17 mm. These eggs are incubated outside of the body for about two weeks before they hatch. In the echidnas the mother lays the eggs and then places them in her temporary* brood *pouch, which is located on her abdomen. Mammary glands are located on either side of this pouch and serve to nourish the young after they have hatched.*

In the infraclass Metatheria (such marsupials as the kangaroo and the opossum), the young are born in an extremely undeveloped condition. After birth, they migrate to the mother's pouch, attach to one of the nipples, and then undergo further development. At this undeveloped stage they cannot suckle, so the mother ejects milk into their mouths. This is accomplished by the contraction of the mother's abdominal muscles. Because the trachea opening is in the back part of the nasal passages at this stage of development, the milk does not pass into the lungs through the trachea, as one might expect from a knowledge of adult anatomy. As is true of the prototherians, the Müllerian ducts remain separate in the metatherians so that there are two separate vaginae, two cervixes, *and two* uterine horns. *The male mammals of these species have a forked* glans penis *which is capable of penetrating each of the vaginae simultaneously. In the metatherians, unlike the eutherians, there is no true placental attachment of the embryo. The embryos derive their norishment while* in utero *from the* uterine glands, *which secrete uterine "milk."*

The infraclass Eutheria, as its name implies, is the only group of mammals which form a true placenta. A detailed discussion of the placenta is included later in this chapter. Additional information on the endocrine function of the placenta is covered in chapter 17, The Endocrine System.

THE FEMALE REPRODUCTIVE TRACT

The Ovaries

In all mammals the ovaries are paired structures and remain near the kidneys in the lumbar or pelvic region. The outer portion of the ovary, the *cortex*, is made up of connective and interstitial tissue, whereas the inner portion, the *medulla*, is richly supplied with blood and lymph vessels, connective tissue, and nerves (see Figure 18–1). The cytogenic and endocrine functions take place in the cortex. The ovaries receive blood from the ovarian artery, which branches directly from the dorsal aorta. Circulation and nerve supplies are received through a distinct region of the ovary called the *hilum*. The shape of the ovaries is quite variable among species. *Polytocous animals* (i.e., those animals which are habitually litter-bearing) have ovaries which are berrylike in appearance because of multiple mature follicles. This is in contrast to *monotocous mammals*, which are single-

TABLE 18–1
Summary of the major reproductive characteristics of various mammalian groups

Class Mammalia
  Subclass Prototheria
    Order Monotremata
      Müllerian ducts not fused
      Oviparous (lay eggs)
      Mammary glands do not possess nipples or teats
  Subclass Theria
    Infraclass Metatheria
      Müllerian ducts not fused
      No true placental attachment of the embryo
      Viviparous
      Young born in extremely undeveloped (altricial) condition
      Mammary glands with nipples
    Infraclass Eutheria
      Some fusion of the Müllerian ducts
      True placenta formed
      Viviparous
      Young born at various stages of development (altricial to precocial)
      Mammary glands with nipples or teats

FIGURE 18–1
Cross-sectional view of the ovary showing ovarian cortex and medulla

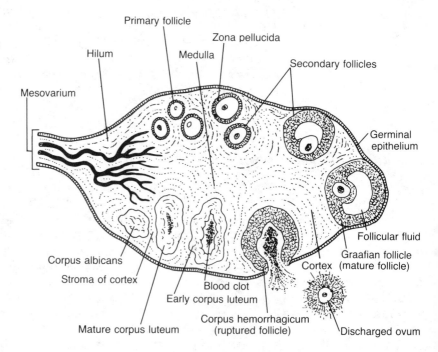

Primary follicle

Zona pellucida

Hilum

Medulla

Secondary follicles

Mesovarium

Germinal epithelium

Follicular fluid

Graafian follicle (mature follicle)

Cortex

Corpus albicans

Stroma of cortex

Blood clot

Early corpus luteum

Mature corpus luteum

Corpus hemorrhagicum (ruptured follicle)

Discharged ovum

bearing and have ovaries that are more oval-shaped and smooth. The mare, which usually produces single offspring, has somewhat kidney-shaped ovaries.

Ovarian histology An in-depth study of the histology of the ovaries is not appropriate here, but a generalized overview will be given to acquaint the reader with the basic aspects necessary to understand ovarian function. The *follicles*, the site of egg production, are separated by connective tissue. There are three stages of follicular development within the ovary: the *primary stage*, the *growing stage*, and the *mature stage* (see Figure 18–2).

During the primary stage, the *primary* or *primordial follicle* contains the *primary oocyte* and is composed of spindle-shaped cells.

During the growing stage of follicular development, the primary follicle begins to increase in size, and the oocyte becomes surrounded by *granulosus cells*. A membrane called the *zona pellucida* forms around the oocyte, and a small space begins to form inside of the follicle, which is now called a *secondary follicle*. During growth the follicle migrates toward the medulla of the ovary and growth continues. The space (or *antrum*) inside of the follicle grows as the volume of fluid filling it increases. The antrum is bound by the granulosus (or follicular) cells and is filled with *liquor folliculi*, or *follicular fluid*. A small mass of granulosus cells forms around the ovum and later protrudes into the antrum. This mass, known as the *cumulus oophorus*, comprises the zona pellucida and the *corona radiata*, as well as the ovum (see Figure 18–3). The corona radiata is made up of granulosus cells more columnar in shape than the remainder of the follicular cells. At this point in development the follicle is called a *tertiary follicle*. During growth the *theca folliculi* forms and surrounds the follicle. It is composed of two distinct layers, the *theca interna* and the *theca externa*. The cells of the theca interna are rounded; those of the theca externa are more spindle-shaped. Both of these cell types are essential to the formation of the *corpus luteum* and take part in the secretion of estrogens.

The *Graafian follicle* is the last or mature phase of follicular development. It is at this point that there occurs the release of the egg from the ovary, or *ovulation*. During this stage the *first polar body* and *secondary oocyte* are formed. Size is the major factor which separates this phase from the tertiary follicle.

At any time during the development of a follicle it may begin to degenerate, though this occurs most often during the tertiary stage. At this time there is an accumulation of fat droplets and the formation of coarse granules inside of the egg itself. This process seems to be triggered by degeneration of the ovum.

When the Graafian follicle is mature, a sequence of hormonal events promotes its rupture. When the follicle breaks, the liquor folliculi, along with the ovum, is expelled into the space between the ovary and the *infundibulum* of the oviduct. The surface of the ovary immediately reveals a *reddish spot* or *blood spot*, which lasts for an hour or so in most species. The cells of the follicle which remain in the ovary continue to provide vital endocrine functions for the physiological events to follow.

The formation of the corpus luteum
Shortly after ovulation occurs the antrum may become filled with blood and lymph, resulting in a structure called the *corpus hemorrhagicum*. The corpus hemorrhagicum is

FIGURE 18–2
Various stages of follicular
development and subsequent
corpus luteum formation

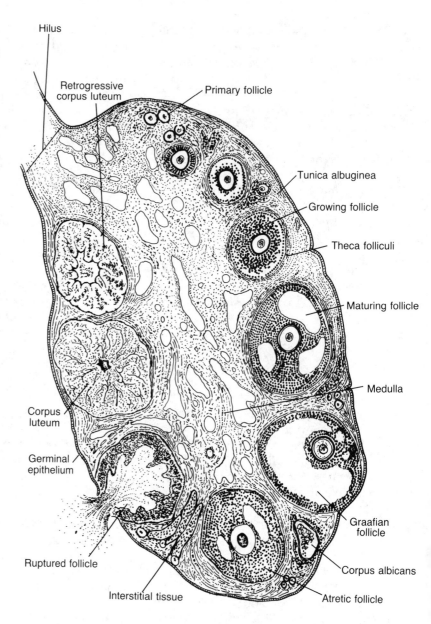

Hilus

Retrogressive
corpus luteum

Primary follicle

Tunica albuginea

Growing follicle

Theca folliculi

Maturing follicle

Medulla

Corpus
luteum

Germinal
epithelium

Graafian
follicle

Ruptured follicle

Corpus albicans

Interstitial tissue

Atretic follicle

absent in some species. In pigs there is a
large accumulation of fluid in the follicle after ovulation, and the area becomes distended. In cattle and sheep there is very little
fluid accumulation. Gradually the blood clot

is reabsorbed, and the resulting structure
takes on a yellowish appearance in humans,
cattle, and a variety of other mammals. This
yellowish color has given rise to the name
corpus luteum, or yellow body. The yellow

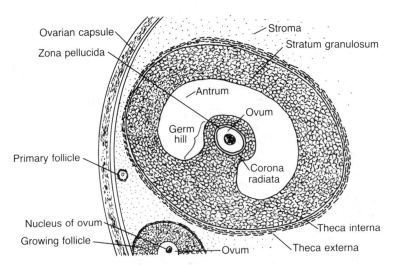

FIGURE 18–3
Close-up of a mature follicle

color is attributed to lipids which accumulate among the granulosus cells. This is followed by a proliferation of the granulosus cells, which, under the influence of *luteinizing hormone (LH)* from the anterior pituitary, begin to produce and secrete progesterone. This hormone prepares the uterus for the possibility of an ensuing pregnancy by enhancing the proliferation of the endometrium. These cells are now called *luteal cells*, and the entire area which was previously known as the follicle develops into a corpus luteum. The corpus luteum is quite variable in size among species. In the blue whale it measures 9.0 inches in diameter, but in most species it is less than an inch in diameter. It is interesting to note that in the African elephant shrew there is a proliferation of the luteal cells prior to ovulation. In this species the proliferation of luteal cells actually triggers the follicle to rupture and expel the ovum. Preovulatory luteinizing also occurs in some perissodactyls and some rodents.

When there is no fertilization, the corpus luteum persists for only a short period of time and is called the *corpus luteum of ovulation.* As LH secretion slows, the luteal tissue is invaded by connective tissue and begins to decrease in size and degenerate. The color of the structure changes to a white or light brown and is called a *corpus albicans.* If pregnancy does occur, the corpus luteum enlarges and may be called the *corpus luteum of pregnancy* or *corpus luteum verum.* The corpus luteum may continue to function as an endocrine gland throughout pregnancy, or it may degenerate at any time during gestation, depending upon the species. In mice, goats, and rabbits it remains functional over the entire pregnancy but finally begins to degenerate near the time of parturition. In dogs, cats, ewes, and guinea pigs the corpus luteum is functional only during the first part of the pregnancy. Where the corpus luteum becomes nonfunctional during pregnancy, progesterone secretion is assumed by the placental tissue.

In horses, elephants, and the blue antelope of India, a number of follicles begin to grow simultaneously. When they reach the Graafian follicle stage, many of them do not ovulate, but they nevertheless undergo luteinization and take on an accessory endocrine function. In this stage they are known as *accessory corpora lutea*.

The Oviducts

The oviducts or Fallopian tubes are paired structures which arise from the embryonic Müllerian ducts. In addition to the oviducts, the Müllerian ducts also give rise to the uterus, cervix, and vagina. These ducts are present in all mammals regardless of sex; that is, they form a part of the male reproductive system also. Near the ovary the oviduct flares out and enlarges to form the infundibulum, which sometimes possesses

fingerlike projections called *fimbria* (see Figure 18–4). The actual opening of the oviduct near the ovary is called the *ostium*. The fimbria usually envelopes the ovaries at least partially, though in some species these structures only lie near the ovary. When the oviduct completely encloses the ovary the resulting structure is called the *bursa ovarii*. In the dog, fox, and mink the bursa has a slit through which the ova pass into the oviduct, and in the rat and mouse there is a small hole through which the ova pass.

Histology of the oviducts   The oviducts are composed of three layers of tissue. The outermost layer is the *serous membrane*. The middle layer is made up of an inner layer of

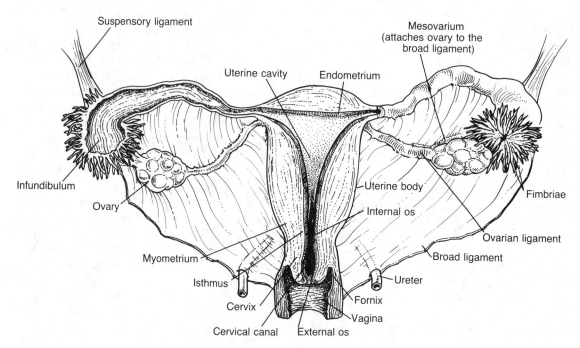

FIGURE 18–4
Close-up of the human female reproductive tract. Note simplex uterus. Most of the other structures are common to all mammalian species.

thick circular muscle and an outer layer of thin longitudinal muscle which runs the entire length of the oviduct. The third and innermost layer of the oviduct is a mucosal layer which is composed of ciliated columnar epithelium and secretory cells. The secretory cells are thought to be important to the nutrition of the ovum as it passes down the oviduct toward the uterus.

The Uterus

The uterus varies in structure among species and is extremely interesting and important from a comparative point of view. In the subclass Prototheria the Müllerian ducts retain the primitive, completely separated structure (see Figure 18–5). In these animals each of the uteri end in the *urogenital sinus*. Note that only the left side of the female reproduc-

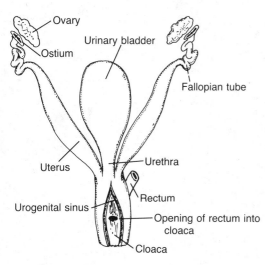

FIGURE 18–5
Female reproductive tract characteristic of monotremes. From C. K. Weichert, *Anatomy of the Chordates*, 4th edition (New York, N.Y., 1970). Reprinted by permission of McGraw-Hill Book Co.

tive tract is functional in monotremes. The metatherians also retain the complete separation of the Müllerian ducts, with two vaginae which terminate in the urogenital sinus. There are four uterine types, based upon gross morphology, found in the eutherians (see Figure 18–6).

The *duplex uterus* is composed of two completely separate uterine horns, each with its own cervix, no uterine body, and one vagina. This type of uterus is found in rabbits, many rodents, elephants, some bats, pikas, and the aardvark.

The *bicornuate uterus* has two uterine horns, a very small uterine body, one cervix, and one vagina. This uterine type is characteristic of pigs, insectivores, whales, most bats, some carnivores, and many hoofed mammals.

The *bipartite uterus* has two uterine horns, a prominent uterine body, one cervix, and one vagina. Frequently, depending upon the species, a septum separates the two uterine horns. The bipartite uterus is found in some rodents, a few bats, some carnivores, cattle, and horses.

The *simplex uterus* is characterized by a complete fusion of the Müllerian ducts, except for the presence of two Fallopian tubes. There are no horns present, and the uterine body is very prominent. This type of uterus is found in primates and the armadillo.

Histology of the uterus   The uterine wall is composed of three general layers: the *serous membrane* on the exterior, the *myometrium* in the middle, and the *endometrium* bordering the lumen. The myometrium is in turn made up of three distinct layers: an external longitudinal muscle layer, an intermediate vascular layer, and an internal circular muscle layer. The two muscle layers contract in

FIGURE 18–6
Eutherian uterine types: (A & B) duplex uterus, (C) bicornuate uterus, (D & E) bipartite uteri, and (F) simplex uterus. From *Reproductive Physiology of Mammals and Birds*, 3rd edition, A. V. Nalbandov. Copyright © 1976, W.H. Freeman and Co. All rights reserved.

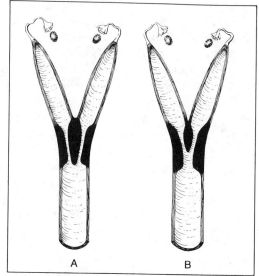
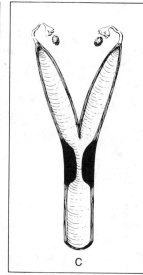
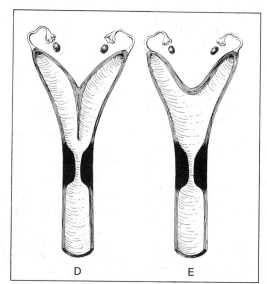
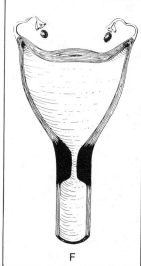

response to hormonal as well as autonomic stimulation. There are three layers in the endometrium: an outer layer of connective tissue, a glandular intermediate layer, and an inner epithelium. Endometrial development is regulated in sequence with the ovarian cycle and undergoes dramatic changes from one period of the ovarian cycle to the next. For more information, see chapter 17, The Endocrine System.

The Cervix

The cervix is the opening between the uterus and vagina. It forms a muscular sphincter lined on the inside by a mucous membrane. The amount and viscosity of the mucous secreted is dependent upon the phase of the ovarian cycle. In some instances the mucous completely isolates the uterus from the vagina. This mucous lining of the lumen has many interdigitating ridges called *annular rings*, which are very prominent in the cow, a little less obvious in the pig, and least apparent in the horse. During pregnancy the cervical secretions harden to form a *cervical plug* which is resistant to invasion by microorganisms. Disruption of the plug in cattle usually leads to abortion or mummification of the fetus. Such termination of pregnancy is probably due to bacterial or viral infection and can be prevented in some cases by the use of antibiotics.

The Vagina and External Genitalia

The vagina serves as a receptacle for the penis during copulation and as part of the birth canal during parturition. It is a muscular, tube-shaped organ lined by a mucous membrane. The muscular wall of the vagina is much less developed than that of the uterus. Epithelial cells line the lumen and undergo periodic changes during normal reproductive cycling. These changes are prompted by the hormonal changes associated with the ovarian cycle. Since there are no glands in the vagina, the mucous found there is formed, for the most part, by the mucous lining of the cervix.

The external genitalia (or *vulva*) are composed of the *labia majora*, the *labia minora*, the *clitoris*, and the *glands of Bartholin* (or *greater vestibular glands*). These glands correspond to *Cowper's glands* (or *bulbourethral glands*) in males. The labia majora are comprised of thin muscle layers intermixed with fatty tissue. These structures are homologous to the *scrotum* in males. The labia minora are composed of spongy connective tissue with an external epithelium which also contains many sebaceous glands. The clitoris is the embryological homologue of the penis and contains erectile tissue. In some species a bone is also present in the clitoris. This bone is the homologue of the ossified penis found in certain carnivores.

THE MALE REPRODUCTIVE TRACT

The Testes

The testes are paired structures which are cytogenic and endocrine in function. They develop near the kidneys and then descend into the pelvic region, except in the monotremes, where they remain near the site of development. Depending upon the species, the testes may remain in the pelvic region or descend further and pass into the scrotum (see Table 18–2). In some groups, the testes descend into the scrotum during the breeding season, after which they are brought back into the abdominal cavity; during the time they are located in the abdomen they decrease in size and become inactive (called *testicular regression*).

Histology of the testes Internal membranes divide the testes into lobules which contain continuous *seminiferous tubules*. The seminiferous tubules make up about 90 percent of the testicular mass (see Figure 18–7). Their walls are formed by a basement membrane, which supports an inner layer of *Ser-*

TABLE 18–2
Position of the testes of various mammalian groups

Group	Intra-abdominal Testes	Periodic Descent into Scrotum	Permanently in Scrotum
Monotremata	all		
Metatheria			all
Insectivora	some	some	some
Chiroptera		all	
Edentata	most		some
Pinnipedia	family Phocidae family Odobenidae		family Otariidae
Cetacea	all		
Proboscidea	all		
Hyracoidea	all		
Sirenia	all		
Perissodactyla	some		most
Rodentia		most	
Carnivora		some	most
Tubulidentata		all	
Artiodactyla		some	most
Primates			all

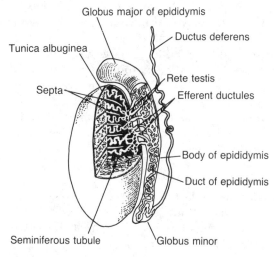

Globus major of epididymis

Tunica albuginea

Ductus deferens

Rete testis

Efferent ductules

Septa

Body of epididymis

Duct of epididymis

Seminiferous tubule

Globus minor

FIGURE 18–7
The duct system of the mammalian testis

toli cells and *spermatagonia* (see Figure 18–8). The diploid spermatagonia located near the basement membrane give rise to the haploid *spermatids* in several steps. First, they form diploid *primary spermatocytes* and then divide by meiosis to form haploid *secondary spermatocytes*, which then become spermatids. The spermatids give rise to *spermatozoa*, the male sex cells (or gametes), by the process of *spermiogenesis.*

The Sertoli cells, or *sperm mother cells*, produce a specific androgen-binding protein which aids in the transfer of male hormone from its origin to the germinal epithelium. They are also believed to be important as "nurse" cells since the spermatids undergo spermiogenesis, a differentiation process, to become spermatazoa while attached to the Sertoli cells. Sperm differentiation requires the presence of follicle-stimulating hormone

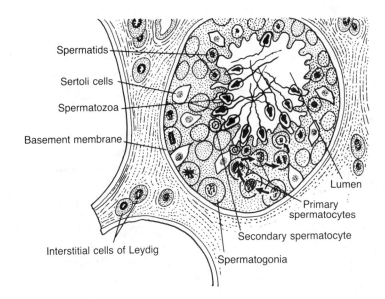

FIGURE 18–8
Cross-sectional view of the seminiferous tubule. Note Sertoli cells and various stages of spermatogenesis.

(FSH) from the anterior pituitary and vitamin E. Once spermiogenesis has occurred, the spermatozoa are released from the Sertoli cells by a process known as *spermiation*.

Many interstitial cells, or *Leydig cells*, are interspersed among the seminiferous tubules. These cells are present in all males during the breeding season. Most evidence indicates that these are the only cells in the testes which produce the androgens. Androgens are important in the production of sperm and in the maintenance of the accessory sex glands and the male secondary sex characteristics.

Spermatozoa The male gametes in mammals are called spermatozoa. They have three parts: the *head*, the *neck* (or *middle piece*), and the *tail* (see Figure 18–9). The head contains the nucleus and a small amount of cytoplasm and varies in shape depending upon the species. The *acrosome*, which is derived from the Golgi apparatus of the spermatogonia, lies at the anterior end of the head. Alteration in the shape of the acrosome modifies the shape of the head and provides much of the variability in sperm appearance seen among species (see Figure

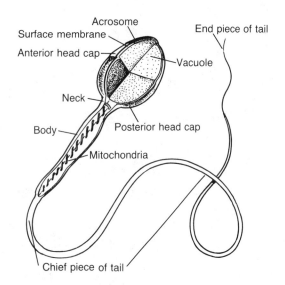

FIGURE 18–9
Human sperm

18–10). The acrosome usually produces an enzyme which breaks down the material composing the egg membrane, thus allowing entry of the sperm into the egg. Both the neck and the tail contain several strands, forming an *axial filament* enclosed in a sheath. The tail, long and whiplike, is used for locomotion. Energy used in the swimming action and enzyme synthesis by the sperm is derived from the ATP produced in the mitochondria of the neck region. The sperm are nonmotile as long as they remain in the testes and the epididymis, but they become motile after being exposed to the fluid from the male accessory glands. This fluid secretion of the male accessory glands when combined with the sperm is called *semen,* or *seminal fluid.* The ensuing movement of the sperm may be influenced by the pH of the fluid and other environmental factors provided by the surrounding medium.

Survival of sperm Sperm usually do not live for more than a few hours once they leave the male reproductive tract and become motile. The environment found in the female reproductive tract is somewhat hostile to sperm and is one of the primary factors which reduces longevity. In humans the sperm usually live 20 to 30 hours in the vagina and up to 72 hours in the cervix. The short life span of mature sperm does not hold true as long as they remain in the male reproductive tract, especially if they remain in the epididymis, where the sperm have not yet come into contact with the seminal fluid. In bulls the sperm may survive for as long as 60 days in the epididymis but are motile for

FIGURE 18–10
Some variations in mammalian sperm

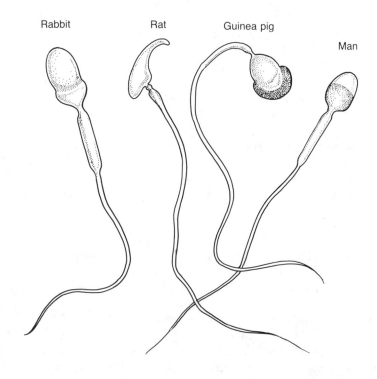

Rabbit Rat Guinea pig Man

only 72 hours in the ampulla of the vas deferens. Note that sperm usually remain motile for longer periods of time than they remain virile (see Table 18–3).

The Scrotum

The scrotum is a two-lobed pouch into which the testes drop either permanently or seasonally, depending upon the species. It is composed of a thin integument which is often folded many times and has slightly more pigment than the surrounding tissue. The dermis contains a smooth muscle layer, the *dartos tunic,* which also extends into the *septum,* which divides the internal aspect of the scrotum into lobes. This muscle responds to changes in temperature by contracting when cold and relaxing when warm. As it contracts it brings the testes closer to the abdomen, where the temperature is higher. The *cremaster muscle* lies between the dartos tunic and the parietal layer of the *tunica vaginalis,* which envelopes each of the testes. This muscle also controls the position of the testes in response to temperature changes. The *gubernaculum,* which provides a path for the descent of the testes into the scrotum, is composed of the *ligamentum testis* and the *scrotal ligament.* It forms during development of the male fetus and attaches the testes to the base of the scrotum in the adult.

Cryptorchidism is a condition characterized by the retention of normally scrotal testes in the abdominal cavity. The condition may be due to a hormonal deficiency, in which case hormone therapy may result in descent of the testes into the scrotum. Cryptorchidism may also be due to an anatomical obstruction which can be surgically corrected to allow the testes to descend into the scrotum. Cryptorchid animals are invariably sterile because sperm development is inhibited by the high temperatures of the body core, where the testes are kept. Although the testes of cryptorchid mammals remain smaller than normal, there seems to be no decline in normal androgen production, and they usually show the same physical and be-

TABLE 18–3

Survival time and retention of fertility of sperm in the epididymis and in the female reproductive tract

Species	Retention of Sperm Motility		Retention of Sperm Fertility	
	Epididymis	Female Repro. Tract	Epididymis	Female Repro. Tract
Guinea pigs	60 days	41 hours	20–35 days	21–22 hours
Rats	42 days	17 hours	21 days	14 hours
Mice		13 hours		6–12 hours
Cattle	60 days	15–56 hours		28–50 hours
Sheep		48 hours		30–48 hours
Humans		60–96 hours		28–48 hours
Rabbits		43–50 hours		30–36 hours
Horses		12 days		12 days

havioral adaptations seen in other males of the same species.

Temperature regulation of the testes

The major function of the scrotum is to maintain the testes at an optimum temperature, which is usually 1.0° to 8.0° F below that of the body core. This lower temperature is necessary for the production and subsequent survival of sperm. In addition to the temperature regulation by movement of the testes with respect to the body, testicular temperature is also maintained by the *pampiniform plexus* (which is described in detail in chapter 8). This plexus is composed of tightly coiled blood vessels located on the surface of the epididymis and follows the *spermatic cord* as it passes through the *inguinal canal*.

In a few species the testes do not become scrotal and usually lie within a shallow pocket of skin in the abdominal region. In kangaroos the "scrotum" is homologous to the pouch of the female. If male young are castrated and administered injections of estrogen, the pouch will develop like that of the female. The testes of elephants and whales normally remain within the abdomen.

The spermatic cord

The spermatic cord comprises: the *testicular artery*, which supplies the testes with blood; some nerves; the cremaster muscle, which elevates the testes; and the testicular veins and lymphatics that drain the testes. The spermatic cord passes through the inguinal canal and enters the abdomen.

The Duct System of the Male Reproductive Tract

The function of the duct system is to provide passage of the sperm from their point of origin in the testes to the outside of the body during copulation. It is largely derived from the *Wolffian ducts* in the embryo. Androgens are essential to the development and maintenance of all such derivatives. The Müllerian ducts give rise to a part of the male reproductive tract which is not affected by the male sex hormones. That part does, however, continue to respond to the female sex steroids.

The seminiferous tubules empty a compact series of ducts, the *rete testes*, which then give rise to the *vasa efferentia*, or *efferent ducts* (see Figure 18–7). The vasa efferentia eventually fuse to form the *epididymis*, which is made up of three parts: the *head*, or *caput epididymis*; the *body*, or *corpus epididymis*; and the *tail*, or *globus minor* or *cauda epididymis*. The epididymis is greatly convoluted, and it is here that the spermatazoa undergo maturation, which may be aided by glandular secretions from the epididymal epithelium.

The lumen enlarges, and the epididymis increases in thickness and finally joins the *vas deferens*, or *ductus deferens*. The vas deferens is less convoluted than the epididymis and is surrounded by three muscle layers. The inner muscle layer is longitudinal and is surrounded by an intermediate circular layer and an outer longitudinal layer. In mammals with scrotal testes, the vas deferens enters the pelvic area and eventually loops over the ureter and finally enters the urethra.

Accessory Glands

The *ampulla*, a chamber formed from the vasa deferentia, may function as a temporary storage place for spermatazoa, in ruminants, shrews, carnivores, primates, and some rodents (see Figure 18–11). In some mammals the seminal vesicles may also be derived from the vasa deferentia. These accessory

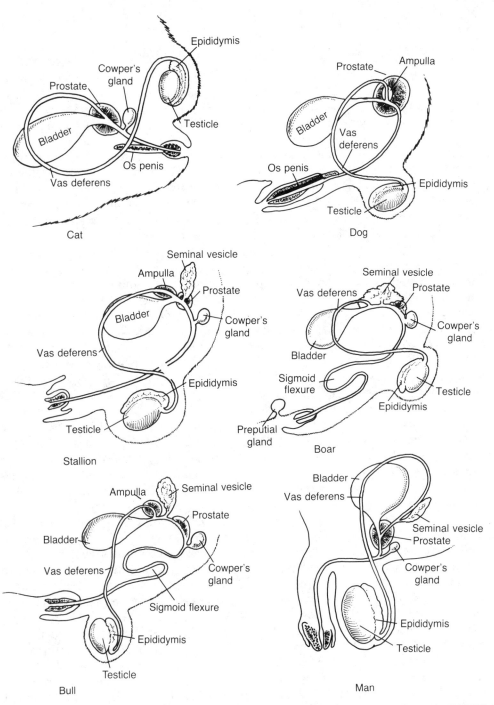

FIGURE 18–11

Comparative anatomy of the mammalian male reproductive organs. From *Reproductive Physiology of Mammals and Birds,* 3rd. edition, by A. V. Nalbandov. Copyright © 1976, W. H. Freeman and Co. All rights reserved.

glands are missing in the wolf, fox, dog, cetaceans, marsupials, and monotremes. The common duct between the ampulla and the seminal vesicles forms the *ejaculatory duct*, which aids in the ejection of sperm from the male copulatory organ, the penis. Near the ampulla the ducts of the seminal vesicles, the urethra, and the many prostatic ducts empty into a common tube which is joined by the duct leading to the bulbourethral glands (Cowper's glands). At this point the duct is called the *prostatic urethra*.

The seminal vesicles, prostate, and Cowper's glands function as accessory glands in the male. The seminal vesicles and Cowper's glands are both paired structures. The seminal vesicles are secretory in nature and do not store sperm. The secretory epithelium lining the seminal vesicles secretes a mucoid substance which is high in fructose and other compounds. These materials supply nutrients and a fluid environment for the sperm. The Cowper's glands secrete a clear, mucoid, alkaline fluid which helps to neutralize the acidity of the urethra. The *prostate gland* is a single structure in most mammals, though in rats it is composed of three lobes. This organ produces a milky fluid containing a clotting enzyme. Semen coagulates after ejaculation; and in some mammals, particularly rodents, it forms a vaginal plug which prevents further copulation. The pH of the prostatic fluid is also alkaline and aids in the neutralization of both the male and female reproductive tracts. Seminal fluid formed in these glands is added to sperm during ejaculation and contains electrolytes (specifically sodium and potassium chloride), prostaglandins, nitrogen, citric acid, fructose, ascorbic acid, inositol, vitamins, ergothionine, and phosphatase. The amount of fluid contributed by the different glands and its exact composition varies from species to species.

In the human, the prostate contributes 15 to 30 percent of the total ejaculate, with the seminal vesicles adding 40 to 80 percent. In the boar, 2.0 to 5.0 percent of the seminal fluid is derived from the testes and epididymis, 10 to 25 percent from Cowper's glands, and the remainder from the urethral glands. Even though the seminal fluid is rich in electrolytes and acts in suspending and activating the previously nonmotile sperm, it is not essential to virility.

The *preputial glands* found in some mammals are not accessory glands *per se* but are still of some importance to the reproductive process. These are sebaceous glands which secrete *smegma* at the base of the glans penis. In several species they secrete a sexual attractant. The preputial glands are the only accessory glands present in marsupials.

The Penis

The penis is the copulatory organ of the male mammals. In monotremes the penis lies on the floor of the cloaca, but in other mammals it is completely separate from the gastrointestinal tract. In the penis, the urethra is surrounded by erectile tissue called the *corpus spongiosum* and the *corpora cavernosa* (see Figure 18–12). The penis of monotremes differs from all other mammals by having a separate opening for the urethra, which empties into the cloaca. In humans the *glans penis*, or enlarged anterior end, contains erectile tissue and is covered by a fold of skin called the *prepuce*. In echidnas and the platypus the glans is forked to accommodate the two vaginae present in the female reproductive tract of these mammals. The tip of the penis in some marsupials is also bifurcated (see Figure 18–13).

In most mammals the penis is covered by a *sheath* from which it can protrude during

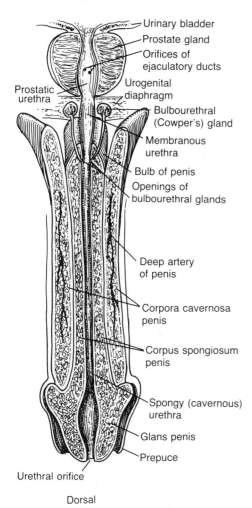

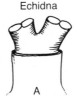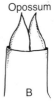

FIGURE 18-13
Bifurcated glans penis of the echidna and marsupial.
From C. K. Weichert, *Anatomy of the Chordates*, 4th
edition (New York, N.Y., 1970). Reprinted by permission
of McGraw-Hill Book Co.

FIGURE 18-12
Longitudinal and cross-sectional views of the human
penis

copulation. In primates the *foreskin* is the
only visible remaining part of the sheath. In
many species there is an ossified portion of
the corpus cavernosa which is usually a
spongy layer of tissue. This structure is
known as the *os penis,* or *baculum,* and helps
increase the rigidity of the erect penis.

THE OVARIAN CYCLE

The ovarian cycle in female mammals includes the development of the follicle, ovulation, and subsequent corpus luteum formation. Changes in the reproductive tract and
accessory sex organs are representative of
the hormonal changes associated with the
cycle. In general, the reproductive cycle is
under hormonal control of the pituitary as a
result of the trophic action of its hormones
upon the endocrine glands essential to reproduction. The segments of the cycle are
regulated by the interaction between the pituitary and its target organs through feedback regulation (see Figure 18-14).

As has been discussed previously, there
are at least two and sometimes three anterior
pituitary hormones that directly regulate the
ovarian cycle. *Follicle-stimulating hormone
(FSH)* has the primary responsibility in female mammals of stimulating growth of the

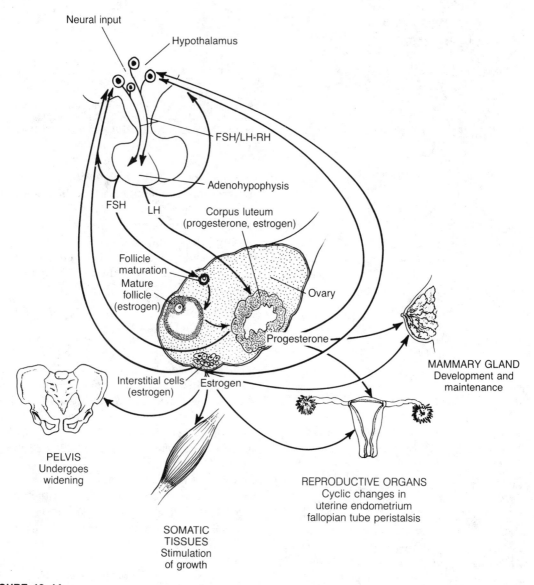

FIGURE 18–14
Hormonal regulation of the ovarian cycle. Note ovarian hormone feedback regulation on the hypothalamus. From *Animal Physiology,* by R. Eckert and D. Randall. Copyright © 1978 by W. H. Freeman and Company. All rights reserved.

ovarian follicles. This hormone seems to act particularly on the granulosus cells, which increase in number and produce greater quantities of estrogen. The estrogen which is produced inhibits further release of FSH and stimulates release of *luteinizing hormone (LH)*. There is a surge of both FSH and LH prior to ovulation. After the ovum has left the ovary the corpus luteum begins to form under the stimulation of LH. In the rat, *prolactin* is also luteotropic in nature. After ovulation the production of progesterone increases due to the effect of the luteinizing hormone on the luteal cells. As the concentration of progesterone increases it inhibits further release of LH by the anterior pituitary. As the amount of LH in the plasma decreases, the production of progesterone declines. At this time the *menses* occurs in primates. In mammals which have successive breeding periods, the next cycle begins with the release of FSH once again.

One of the functions of the steroids that are produced by the ovaries is preparation of the uterus for possible pregnancy. The estrogen secreted by the developing follicle primes the uterus and initiates the hypertrophy and hyperplasia that occurs in the uterine endometrium. Later in the cycle it also prolongs the life of the corpus luteum. The progesterone is of primary importance in priming and then maintaining the uterus in a state of readiness for the implantation of the blastocyst.

Ovulation

The steps in the development of the follicle have already been discussed in a previous section of this chapter. Rupture of the Graafian follicle occurs due to the influence of LH. The *cumulus oophorus*, which contains the

egg, separates from the rest of the follicle as the follicle ruptures. This cumulus mass is extruded into the coelom and may stick to the ovary until it is removed by the cilia of the fimbria, which push the mass through the ostium and into the Fallopian tube. Flagellar action by the cilia and peristaltic movements of smooth muscles in the oviducts are responsible for the passage of the cumulus mass down the oviduct and into the uterus. The peristaltic movements may be higher at this time due to the fairly high levels of estrogen, which promote smooth muscle contraction. Note that not all ova shed into the Fallopian tubes are destined to be fertilized and implant. In the elephant shrew, the female of the species ovulates over 100 eggs at a time, but only one or two implant. In many mammals the ovulation rate rises to a peak with increasing age and then begins to drop off.

Mammals can be divided into two basic categories based upon patterns of ovulation: those animals which have regular, repeating cycles in which ovulation is part of the cycle; and those animals which have a reproductive cycle represented by hormonal as well as uterine changes but do not ovulate unless the female is allowed to breed. The first type of ovulation is termed *spontaneous ovulation;* the second type is called *induced* or *reflex ovulation*. The hormonal events in both spontaneous and induced ovulation are shown in Figure 18–15.

Spontaneous ovulation usually occurs shortly before or shortly after the end of a heat period, or in the middle of the menstrual cycle in the case of primates. This type of ovulation is found in most mammals and occurs at regular intervals when the female is not pregnant. Mammals in which spontaneous ovulation occurs include the Primates,

FIGURE 18–15
Ovarian cycles of (A) spontaneous and (B) induced ovulators. From *Reproductive Physiology of Mammals and Birds*, 3rd edition, A. V. Nalbandov. Copyright © 1976, W. H. Freeman and Co. All rights reserved.

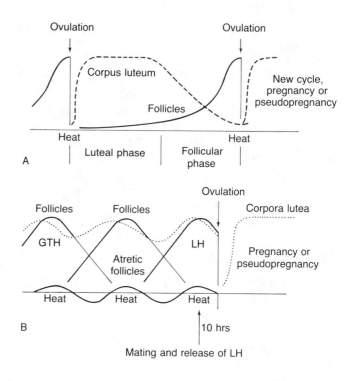

Marsupalia, Cetacea, Proboscidea, Perissodactyla, Artiodactyla, and some Carnivora.

In the most prevalent example of induced ovulation, the ovum is shed within a few hours after copulation takes place. The manipulation and stimulation of the cervix causes reflex release of LH from the pituitary, which activates rupture of the Graafian follicle. But note that other stimulating factors for induced ovulation are sometimes involved. These usually include sight or smell of the male of the same species. The neural portion of the reflex can be blocked by severing the sensory nerves which innervate the cervix. The impulse is transmitted to the hypothalamus, where FSH/LH-RH is released. In animals which show induced ovulation there is no true *estrous cycle*, as seen in other mammals. During much of their reproductive cycle they are in a state of constant receptivity. There is usually a short heat period followed by an equally short *anestrus phase*, which corresponds to the growth and *atresia* of the ovarian follicle. During estrus the follicles are stimulated, and estrogen production increases until further pituitary hormone release is inhibited. This decrease in pituitary gonadotropins causes a subsequent decrease in follicular growth and results in follicular atresia. The atresia leads to a decrease in steroid production by the ovaries and a consequent increase in pituitary hormones, which starts the cycle all over again. During this type of cycling there is no large LH surge unless copulation occurs. Almost all insectivores, some carnivores, lagomorphs, and several rodents all have this type of reflex ovulation. In rabbits it has also been observed that about 1.0 to 5.0 percent of the females will spontaneously ovulate without copulation.

The factors which stimulate ovulation, such as contact with other animals of the same species, sight of a male, smell, and so on, as well as factors which might inhibit ovulation, are covered later in this chapter.

Fertilization *Internal fertilization* occurs in all mammalian species. The penis is inserted into the vagina and sperm are placed at or near the cervix of the female. In some species, such as the horse, the penis may actually enter the uterus. Fertilization usually takes place in the upper one-third of the oviduct, except in some insectivores in which intrafollicular fertilization occurs. Muscular contractions of the uterus and oviducts transport sperm toward the ovaries, a process which only takes a few minutes. Thus, sperm movement is not caused solely by flagellar action of the sperm, as was suspected at one time. This has been confirmed by placing dead sperm and inanimate objects inside the uterus and showing that they move equally as swiftly as the motile sperm. This neuro-endocrine reflex begins when nerve endings in the cervix are stimulated during coitus and transmit impulses to the brain. The stimulation of the neurohypophysis results in the release of *oxytocin*, which is carried through the bloodstream to the smooth muscle of the uterus and oviducts. The oxytocin enhances the uterine and oviducal motility. Uterine muscle tone is also affected by secretions of the sympathetic nervous system.

Only a few sperm ever reach the ovum, though more than one may penetrate the zona pellucida. *Hyaluronidase*, an enzyme which hydrolyzes glycoproteins, is contained within the acrosome of the sperm and helps to disperse the follicular cells that may still be clustered around the ovum. Even though more than one sperm may penetrate the zona pellucida, there is only one sperm that actually enters the ovum. This results in fertilization of the egg. The two nuclei fuse and the zygote begins to develop.

Sperm capacitation, or *adaptation*, to the uterine environment is required in some mammals. This process necessitates that the sperm be exposed to the female reproductive tract for a certain period of time before they are able to fertilize the ovum. The exact mechanism of sperm capacitation has not been delineated.

Transport of the ovum through the oviduct is accomplished by means of ciliary action. About 75 percent of the time spent by the egg in the oviduct is in the upper part of the Fallopian tube near the ovary. This is true regardless of whether the egg is fertilized or not. Note that the general fertilizable life span of the ovum is approximately 12 to 24 hours. Sperm which survive for longer periods may be present at the time of ovulation. If fertilization does not occur, the egg passes out of the oviduct and a new ovarian cycle ensues.

Delayed fertilization There is some evidence that sperm may be stored in the female reproductive tract for long periods before fertilization occurs. The evidence for this is still somewhat in doubt. The only group of mammals for which this phenomenon has been suggested is the order Chiroptera (bats).

Implantation

Implantation is the first step in the attachment of the developing *blastocyst* to the uterine endometrium. The presence of the blastocyst apparently signals the pituitary to continue to release LH, which maintains the corpus luteum in order for production of progesterone to continue. Foreign particles stimulate the uterus in the same manner as the true blastocyst. It has been shown that the presence of beads in the uterine lumen of sheep and guinea pigs can cause an increase in the length of the luteal phase of the estrous cycle.

There are three types of implantation that may occur in mammals. In one of these, which is specific to carnivores and ungulates, the blastocyst enlarges and fills the uterine cavity, which then triggers implantation. This reaction is termed *central implantation*. In rodents a type of implantation called *eccentric implantation* involves the embedding of the small blastocyst in a fold of the uterine lumen. In the third method of implantation, called *interstitial implantation*, the embryo buries itself among cells of the uterine epithelium and loses contact with the uterine lumen completely. Implantation of this type is observed in guinea pigs, insectivores, and humans.

The actual time of implantation of the blastocyst is quite variable. It depends upon the species and the physiological condition of the female at the time of ovulation. A previous litter which may still be suckling or the season of the year may modify the physiological condition of the female. Under normal conditions the blastocyst will usually implant within a short period after ovulation (see Table 18–4).

Delayed implantation Some mammals exhibit a delay in the implantation of the blastocyst, which may be either *obligate* or *facultative*. In those animals which have an obligate type of delayed implantation, the delay is a consistent part of the reproductive

TABLE 18–4
Time of implantation relative to time of ovulation

Species	Number of Days From Ovulation to Implantation
Humans	6–8
Mice	5
Guinea pigs	6
Cattle	40
Horses	96*
Sheep	18
Cats	13
Pigs	11–20

*Days to complete attachment

cycle. The delay may last anywhere from 12 days to 11 months depending upon the species. During this time there is little if any growth of the blastocyst. The Jamaican fruit bat is somewhat of an exception to this rule in that the embryo continues to undergo cell division but only at a very slow rate. When implantation is delayed, growth of the blastocyst is usually arrested at the 100–400 cell stage of development. During this time the blastocyst becomes covered by a thick acellular layer and continues to float free in the uterine lumen prior to implantation. This type of delayed implantation is a part of the normal cycle in bears, badgers, roe deer, seals, mink, armadillos, and some marsupials.

Facultative delayed implantation has been observed in some marsupials, some insectivores, and some rodents, such as mice and rats. In this manifestation of delayed implantation the actual trigger for the implantation process to begin is dependent upon certain conditions to which the female is subjected. In rats and mice, as long as there is another litter that continues to suckle, the blastocysts become spaced in the uterine horns and then settle onto the uterine epithelium. They adhere to the epithelial tissue of the uterus until suckling by the other litter is terminated. Suckling apparently provides a signal which prevents implantation. After suckling is terminated, the decidua begins to form, probably under the influence of estrogen, and the implantation process ensues. At this time, it has been postulated, some sort of uterine proteins (such as blastokinin) are responsible for the growth and differentiation of the blastocysts.

In some marsupials a rather unique type of delayed implantation occurs. It will be remembered that marsupials have two distinct uteri. In one group of marsupials the macropodids, only one uterus becomes pregnant with the first copulation. During development of the embryo there is a prepartum copulation, which results in the previously nonpregnant uterus receiving a blastocyst. In the nonmacropodid marsupials, the females mate in a postpartum heat period. In either the prepartum pregnancy or the postpartum pregnancy, the newly formed blastocyst does not implant until the previous offspring has been removed from the mother's pouch. It is the continual suckling of the newborn that prevents the implantation of the blastocyst, which remains in the 70–100 cell stage of development. During this time the blastocyst is covered by a layer of albumin and a shell membrane. Once the blastocyst becomes implanted, it develops at a normal rate. After leaving the pouch, the offspring of the previous litter continue to return to suckle the mother. The suckling period after leaving the pouch is longer than the gestation period of the newly implanted embryo, and it is born while the first offspring are still periodically returning to suckle. After the neonate finds its way to the mother's pouch, it attaches itself to one of the mother's nipples and re-

mains attached there for some time while development continues. During this time both litters continue to suckle, though the older offspring only return to suckle periodically. It is fascinating that the milk secreted early in the suckling period is very low in fat, whereas that produced farther along in the development of the young has as much as 20 percent fat. When two young of different ages are suckling, the nipple that is only suckled periodically by the older of the two offspring releases milk which is higher in fat content than the nipple which is continuously suckled by the neonate.

Factors influencing delayed implantation There are many factors which are capable of inducing implantation. In rabbits, the exogenous administration of progesterone will induce implantation, though less progesterone is needed if a small amount of estrogen is administered simultaneously. In rats, implantation can be induced experimentally as the result of estrogen administration. In the European badger, implantation cannot be induced by exogenous administration of any of the sex steroids. In armadillos, which normally have a four month delay period, if the pregnant female is ovariectomized after two months the blastocysts will implant normally after a subsequent 30 days. This would suggest that in these animals the delay is maintained by some type of nonovarian tissue or some tissue in addition to the ovaries. In wallabies, delayed implantation can still occur after hypophysectomy.

Environmental factors can also affect the length of delay encountered in some facultatively delayed implanters. In martens, implantation can be delayed up to six months or can be shortened from the regular delay length by exposure to longer photoperiods. This decrease in delay using increased day length can also be accomplished in mink. In mink the gestation period ranges anywhere from 39 days, the normal gestation period with no delay, to 74 days, which includes a delay period. The length of gestation in these animals is dependent upon environmental temperature and frequency of mating.

Migration of Blastocysts

Polytocous mammals have the added element of the spacing of the blastocysts. This spacing may be due to the muscular contraction of the uterus when it is stimulated by the presence of the blastocysts away from the one which triggers the contractions. In some mammals, such as the pig, which has a *bicornuate uterus*, some of the blastocysts may migrate from one horn to the next until the number on each side is evenly balanced. In the mouse the ovarian end of the uterine horns is not as favorable for implantation. Blastocysts which implant near the ovaries develop into smaller fetuses and are more prone to having cleft palates and cleft lips than those which develop nearer to the cervix.

Stages of Uterine Adjustment to Pregnancy

There are three basic stages in the adaptation of the uterus to the pregnant condition. The first stage is one of uterine preparation, which occurs during the regular ovarian cycle. Estrogen produced by the developing follicle primes the uterine tissue and causes an increase in the supply of blood to the endometrium. Progesterone is then secreted in high concentrations by the corpus luteum. This hormone causes an increase in cell division, especially in the smooth muscle layers. The second stage of adjustment begins immediately after implantation. The embryo

increases in size and stimulates hypertrophy of the myometrium. This accounts for the increase in uterine size during middle and late pregnancy. The final stage is characterized by the stretching of those cells which were enlarged during the previous period of accommodation. It is during this phase that growth begins to diminish.

These stages do not occur to the same extent in the *nongravid uterus* of a pregnant female. That is, in those mammals which have duplex uteri it is possible to have one-half of the uterus with implanted blastocysts (*gravid*) while the other side remains barren (*nongravid*). Even with all of the extra circulating hormones, the nongravid side still does not get as big as the gravid uterus. This is probably due to the fact that a great deal of the increase in size of the gravid uterus is in response to the physical tension generated by the developing embryo.

The Placenta

The placenta, literally "flatcake," provides for the passage of nutrients and oxygen to the developing fetus and the removal of waste products from the embryo. It develops in the early stages of pregnancy, and at least part of it is expelled during the birthing process. The placenta also serves as an endocrine organ, which helps to maintain the state of pregnancy. It acts as an "accessory" pituitary gland in that it produces gonadotropins and as an "accessory" gonad in that it produces sex steroids which are normally produced by the ovaries. Another very important function of the placenta is to serve as a barrier against chemicals and bacteria.

Development of the placenta There are two basic parts to the placenta, the maternally derived tissues and those derived from the embryo. The maternal tissues result from proliferation of the uterine endometrium and an increased vascularization of this tissue. The amount of maternally derived placental tissue lost after parturition depends upon the type of placenta formed. The *extraembryonic tissues*, which compose the fetal part of the placenta, include the *amnion, chorion, yolk sac*, and *allantois* (see Figure 18–16). These fetal membranes are always expelled as part of the afterbirth regardless of the type of placentation.

Classification of placentae There are two types of mammalian placentae, the *choriovitelline placenta* and the *chorio-allantoic placenta*. The chorio-vitelline placenta, or *yolk sac placenta*, is found in all marsupials except the Peramelidae. In this type of placenta the yolk sac enlarges and serves as one of the organs of nutrition and for the removal of wastes. Here, the blastocyst sinks into a shallow depression in the uterine mucosa during placentation. This somewhat tenuous attachment is strengthened by the wrinkling of the blastocyst wall next to the uterine surface, which also increases the amount of surface area for nutrient transfer. Most nourishment is obtained from the uterine glands, which

secrete uterine "milk," and there is a limited diffusion of nutrients and waste products. Poor efficiency of nutrient and waste transfer in this type of placentation limits the duration of gestation in these animals.

The chorio-allantoic placenta is found in the Peramelidae and all eutherians. In the placenta of the peramelids, which is slightly different from that of the eutherians, the allantois enlarges and becomes highly vascularized. The allantois makes contact with the chorion at the point of contact between the embryo and the endometrium. The chorion soon disappears, and the uterus becomes well-vascularized at the point of contact. Uterine milk continues to supply nourishment to the embryo throughout gestation. Again, due to the rather limited capacity for exchange through this kind of placenta, the gestation period of the peramelids, like that of other marsupials, is fairly short.

In the eutherian chorio-allantoic placenta, the blastocyst first adheres to the uterine endometrium and then sinks into it. As the chorionic villi are formed they protrude still further into the endometrium. At the same time there is a local breakdown of the endometrium which allows the villi to push still further inward. The tissue derived from the

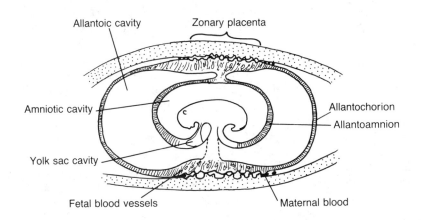

Allantoic cavity   Zonary placenta

Amniotic cavity

Allantochorion
Allantoamnion

Yolk sac cavity

Fetal blood vessels   Maternal blood

FIGURE 18–16
Fetal membranes in the dog. From H. H. Cole and P. T. Cupps (eds.), *Reproduction in Domestic Animals*, 3rd edition (New York, N.Y., 1977). Reprinted by permission of Academic Press, Inc.

local destruction of the uterine wall is utilized by the developing blastocyst as a temporary nutrient source until the placenta is completed. The numerous, highly vascularized villi provide a large surface area for the diffusion of nutrients and waste products to occur. The large surface area also contributes a great deal to the efficiency of this type of placentation.

The degree of separation of the maternal and fetal bloodstreams is another method used in the classification of variations of the chorio-allantoic placenta. The *epitheliochorial placenta* is found in the pig, horse, donkey, and lemurs. This placental type is very diffuse in shape and, most importantly, there is no intimate fusion between the fetal and maternal tissues. Not only is there little contact between the two parts, but the distance over which the materials must pass to get to and from the fetus also results in poor efficiency. The materials must pass through the uterine blood vessels, then through layers of connective tissue and epithelium, and finally through the endothelium of the fetal capillaries before they reach the circulation of the embryo. At parturition the fetal placenta is easily separated from the uterine endometrium, which remains intact. Because of the easy separation of the two membranes, there is no uterine bleeding during parturition. Since neither the endometrium nor its related tissues are lost, this type of placenta is also referred to as being *apposed* or *nondeciduate*.

The *syndesmo-chorial placenta* is also apposed or nondeciduate, because there is no loss of maternal tissues during parturition. This is again the result of the lack of intimate contact between fetal and maternal parts of the placenta, though unlike the epitheliochorial type of placentation there is some local erosion of the uterine epithelium. At parturition the fetal placenta separates easily from the uterine endometrium, and this does not result in major damage or bleeding. The syndesmo-chorial placenta is found in sheep, goats, cows, and other ruminant artiodactyls.

The final three categories of placentae, based upon separation of the maternal and fetal circulations, are all *conjoined* or *decidual* placenta types. In all three there is intimate connection between the two circulatory systems. During parturition there is a difficult separation of the tissues with bleeding and a tearing of the maternal tissues. This is due to the close apposition of the circulations and the high degree of endometrial erosion.

The *endothelial-chorial placenta* is found in cats, ferrets, dogs, and other carnivores. Here, erosion is greater than that seen in the syndesmo-chorial type. Because the uterine epithelium is so eroded, the chorion is in close contact with the uterine circulation. The *hemo-chorial placenta* is found in bats, some rodents, some insectivores, and all primates except lemurs. In this category there is extensive erosion of the uterine wall during development, including the vascular endothelium. This creates blood sinuses in the endometrium, which allows the chorionic villi to come into direct contact with the maternal blood. There is of course no exchange of blood between the mother and the fetus because the fetal blood is still physically isolated from the maternal blood supply by the walls of the vessels in the chorionic villi. The *hemoendothelio-chorial placenta* shows the greatest degree of erosion and the closest contact of the two circulatory systems. The only separation between maternal and fetal circulations is the endothelial lining of the blood vessels of the chorionic villi. This type of placentation is found in the rat, guinea pig, and rabbit.

The arrangement and positioning of the villi over the chorion greatly influences the shape of the placenta and thus lends itself to another form of classification. There are four kinds of arrangement: the *diffuse*, the *cotyledonary*, the *zonary*, and the *discoidal*. The diffuse pattern is found in perissodactyls, some artiodactyls, and lemurs. It is characterized by having villi covering the entire surface of the chorion. This allows for a large surface area over which diffusion can occur. The diffuse arrangement is important because it is found in those animals which have an epithelio-chorial type of placenta formation. Here, there is little intimate contact between the fetal and maternal circulations, which places more importance on having a large surface area for diffusion.

The cotyledonary arrangement of villi is only found in ruminant artiodactyls. It will be remembered that these animals also have the syndesmo-chorial placenta. In this type of zonation there are a number of somewhat evenly spaced masses of villi which occur over the surface of the chorion. The zonary pattern is characteristic of carnivores and other mammals which have either endothelio-chorial or hemoendothelio-chorial placental formation. This kind of arrangement of villi forms a band which circles the equator of the chorion, hence the name zonary. The discoidal scheme, as its name implies, is formed by the presence of one or two disc-shaped areas of villi which are located on the chorion. The villi of insectivores, bats, rabbits, rodents, and some primates are arranged in this pattern.

Hormones produced by the placenta Because these hormones were covered in chapter 17, only a brief mention of them will be made here. Major hormones produced and secreted by the placenta are the sex steroids (estrogen and progesterone), chorionic gonadotropin, human placental lactogen, and relaxin. All of these are in some way important for the maintenance of pregnancy, either through their effect on the gonads or through their effect on the pituitary through the hypothalamus. Relaxin is the only exception to this, since this hormone is important during parturition.

Hormonal Control of Pregnancy

Whether its source is the ovary or the placenta or both, progesterone seems to be the most important hormone for the maintenance of pregnancy. It is this hormone that maintains the quiescent nature of the uterus. Exogenous administration of progesterone to ovariectomized females can prevent the death of the blastocyst. It should be noted that smaller amounts of progesterone are necessary if estrogen is also administered. In monotocous species the placenta is the major source of progesterone, especially during the last half of pregnancy. On the other hand, the corpus luteum is the principal source of progesterone throughout the entire pregnancy in polytocous mammals.

The ovaries are required for the implantation of the blastocysts and the maintenance of the pregnancy unless there is another source of progesterone, such as the placenta. The length of time that the ovaries alone are required for the maintenance of pregnancy is species dependent. It has been shown that ovariectomy in some species during the blastocyst stage prevents implantation and placentation, which results in death of the blastocyst. The presence of the ovaries is required during the entire gestation period in the opossum, mouse, rat, rabbit, golden hamster, 13-lined ground squirrel, and goat. In the horse, sheep, cat, dog, guinea pig, and pig, the ovaries are necessary at least during the first half of the gestation period while the placenta is forming and just beginning to secrete progesterone. In humans and monkeys, the presence of the ovaries is only necessary for a short period of time for maintenance of pregnancies.

The production and secretion of luteotropic hormone by the placenta has been documented in the primates, horses, and possibly other animals. This hormone is called *chorionic gonadotropin,* and in humans it is termed *human chorionic gonadotropin (HCG).* The chorio-allantoic cells of the embryo in pregnant mares serves this same purpose as it produces and secretes copious amounts of *pregnant mare serum gonadotropin (PMSG).*

The importance of the pituitary during pregnancy depends upon the time of gestation and the species involved. Removal of the pituitary during any part of the gestation period results in abortion or resorption of the fetuses in cats, dogs, and rabbits. In the mouse, rat, guinea pig, and monkey when hypophysectomy is done after the first half of gestation, there is usually no effect on the maintenance of the pregnancy. The pituitary is essential in the mouse during the first half of pregnancy because it releases prolactin, which helps to maintain the corpus luteum in these animals. This release of prolactin is triggered by stimulation of the female reproductive tract during coitus.

Hormonal Levels During Pregnancy

The levels of the steroid hormones in particular vary from species to species during pregnancy (see Figure 18–17). The number of developing embryos may influence these levels. It has been observed that there is a higher level of progesterone present in ewes bearing twins than in those bearing single offspring. In some species, such as the pig, there is no correlation between the number of embryos and the progesterone levels. It has been noted that there is generally a sharp decrease in the amount of progesterone secreted just before parturition.

The urinary levels of hormones during pregnancy give an idea of the plasma concentrations. During pregnancy the human kidney excretes tremendous amounts of estrogen metabolites, especially *estriol glucuronide,* which is fairly inactive. The levels of these metabolites in the urine fall shortly before parturition. In nonpregnant women the amount of estriol glucuronide excreted is 300 units per day as opposed to 20,000 units per day in pregnant women. The same increase is observed in the mare, where levels increase from 2,000 units per day to 1,000,000 units. It is also interesting to note that the estrogenic steroids produced by the mare during pregnancy are not of ovarian origin. The progestin metabolite that is primarily excreted by the human female during pregnancy is *pregnanediol glucuronide.* These levels rise after the second or third month of pregnancy and then fall abruptly after parturition. Pregnant cows excrete very high levels of androgens in their feces. These high levels are not observed in bulls and nonpregnant cows.

Gestation Periods

The *gestation period,* the time from fertilization to parturition, varies tremendously among species. The time required for gestation is genetically determined and usually remains fairly constant under normal conditions of pregnancy. If the fetus is surgically removed from the rhesus monkey, rat, or rab-

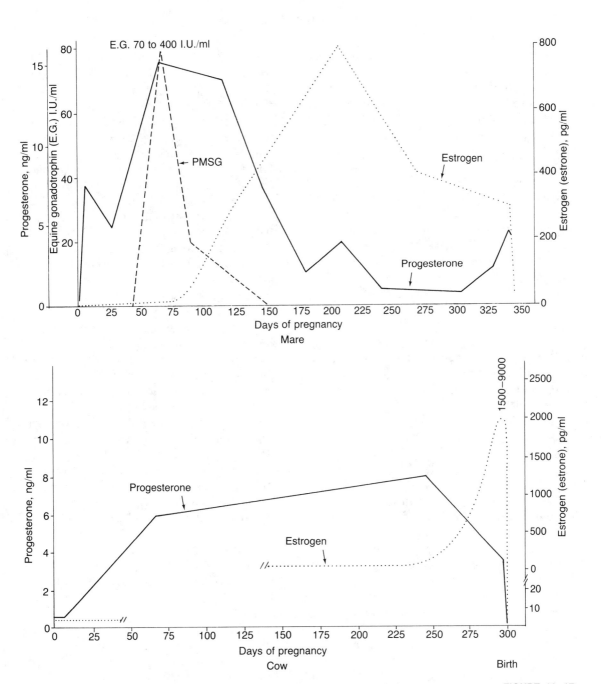

FIGURE 18–17

Levels of various hormones during pregnancy in different mammals. From H. H. Cole and P. T. Cupps (eds.), *Reproduction in Domestic Animals,* 3rd edition (New York, N.Y., 1977). Reprinted by permission of Academic Press, Inc.

437

bit, leaving only the placenta and extraembryonic membranes in place, a normal gestation period results, with the embryonic membranes and placenta being delivered at their normal time. This also demonstrates that for these animals the fetus does not determine the time of parturition. It is interesting to note that in monotocous mammals the female fetuses are usually carried for a shorter period of time than are the male fetuses.

In certain breeds of dairy cattle the normal gestation period of 278 to 290 days is lengthened to 330 days. The calves continue to grow *in utero* and may weigh as much as 200 pounds at birth. Many require surgical delivery because the calves have grown too large for regular vaginal delivery. In these cattle there is no drop in progesterone levels just prior to delivery. Attempts at prolonging gestation past the normal delivery time by exogenous administration of progesterone have failed.

Parturition

Parturition is the result of many synchronized events. During gestation the uterus is relatively quiet, but as parturition nears, the myometrium becomes more susceptible to hormones, and there is an increase in motility and contraction. The endocrine organs which usually provide most of the hormonal control for this event are the ovaries, placenta, and pituitary. The pituitary is generally thought to be expendable because its major (and possibly only) contribution to parturition is the release of oxytocin, which is not necessary for a normal delivery.

The ovaries and placenta maintain the pregnancy through the production of estrogen and progesterone. As the time of parturition nears the concentration of progesterone generally begins to drop, sometimes precipitously. It is progesterone that helps maintain the uterus in its quiet state. In many mammals there is a concomitant rapid rise in estrogen levels. Estrogen has a tendency to promote smooth muscle contraction. At this time there is a release of relaxin from the placenta and ovaries which acts on connective tissue such as the *pubic symphysis* (relaxes the fibrocartilagenous ligament) and the *sacroiliac joints* (mobilizes them). Oxytocin also takes part in the process of parturition. In some animals there is no demonstrable release of oxytocin at the onset of labor. But others show an appreciable increase in plasma oxytocin levels during the second stage of labor, when the head of the fetus appears. Exogenous oxytocin has also been used to induce labor in a number of species. In humans, at least, this method does not work unless the natural time for parturition is close at hand. It has been observed in several species that as parturition nears there is an increase in the maternal plasma concentration of *prostaglandin* $F_{2\alpha}$ *(PGF$_{2\alpha}$)*, which stimulates smooth muscle contraction. It has been used to induce abortion in humans but requires intravenous injection of very high doses above normal physiological levels. These high doses lead to a number of gastrointestinal side effects and therefore are of questionable value. Prostaglandins have also been found to shorten the normal gestation period in pigs by a few days.

As stated earlier, it is possible to remove the fetus and still have continuation of the pregnancy and a normal delivery of the placenta. In those animals tested which responded in this way, it may be assumed that the presence of the fetus has nothing to do with the maintenance of pregnancy or the onset of parturition. But in some species this is not the case. For instance, it has been shown that the fetal adrenal glucocorticoids may induce labor in sheep. If the fetal adrenal glands are removed or the fetal pituitary is removed or destroyed, the pregnancy will continue past the normal time of parturition. Administration of exogenous ACTH triggers labor in hypophysectomized sheep fetuses which have their adrenal glands left intact. Labor also commences if the adrenalectomized lamb fetuses are given injections of glucocorticoids.

DEVELOPMENT OF THE YOUNG

The stage of development of the young at birth is perhaps as varied as the number of mammalian species. Except for the marsupials, mammalian young are relatively well developed at birth, but there are still a number of differences and gradations of development. At birth the young of marsupials, after just two weeks of gestation, still resemble the embryo stage of most other mammals.

Three criteria are often used to judge the level of maturation of the neonate. The first of these criteria is the ability of the animal to get around by itself. The differences in this category range from herd ungulates that must be able to move and keep up with their mothers within hours after they are born, to the helpless young of cats, dogs, mice, and so on. The ability of the neonate to thermoregulate is also an important guideline for the assessment of development of the newborn. Some animals, such as the jack rabbit, are fully furred at birth and can maintain their own body temperature; others, such as mice, are naked. But the ability to thermoregulate is dependent upon development of internal mechanisms of thermogenesis and has little to do with the presence or absence of hair. These animals, which lack the thermoregulatory ability, must be kept warm by the parents during the cold weather or they quickly perish. The third standard for establishing the degree of maturation of the young is whether the eyes are open or shut at birth, and, if they are shut, how long it takes for them to open. Carnivores and most rodents are totally blind at birth and remain so for some time, whereas deer, domesticated livestock, and the jack rabbit are all born with their eyes open. Of course there are gradations for each of these criteria, and an animal may be fairly well developed in one criterion and not another. Those animals which are born generally alert, able to thermoregulate, and able to get around on their own are termed *precocial*. Those that are blind, unable to thermoregulate, and generally not ambulatory at birth are said to be *altricial*.

PSEUDOPREGNANCY

Pseudopregnancy is a neurohumoral phenomenon. Stimulation of sensory receptors in the cervix induces the hypothalamus to release FSH/LH-RH, which acts on the pituitary to release LH. In the presence of LH the corpus luteum persists, and the endometrium is maintained in its receptive state. During normal copulation this action prepares the uterus for the implantation of blastocysts. A state of pseudopregnancy results when there is no fertilization because of the sterile condition of the male, the female, or both or because of a noncopulatory stimulation of the cervix. This condition can also be induced by adrenalectomy or, in some species, by the stimulation of the nipples of the female. Pseudopregnancy may also result spontaneously with no apparent stimulation in dogs, foxes, rabbits, and cats. It is important to note that all of these animals are induced ovulators.

In the pseudopregnant animal, the ovaries and uterus resemble those of normally pregnant animals. That is, there is an increase in the size of the uterus and an increase in the size of the mammary glands. Lactation occurs in some dogs during pseudopregnancy, and specific pregnantlike behavior has been observed, such as retrieval of foster young and nest building.

HEATS AND OVULATION DURING PREGNANCY

In general, *heat periods* do not occur during pregnancy. But in some species there is a *psychological heat* in the absence of *true* or *physiological heat* at this time. Such heats are frequently observed in laboratory rodents, ewes (nearly 30 percent), and cows (approximately 10 percent). Psychological heat periods occur at random and without a predictable rhythm. In some mammals there are true physiological heats during pregnancy with subsequent ovulation, and *superfetation* may result if these mammals were allowed to mate. Superfetation is the implantation of a fertilized egg in an already gravid uterus. This phenomenon has been observed in horses, mice, rabbits, cattle, and sheep. Heats during pregnancy are common in marsupials, which may have delayed implantation of a blastocyst, a neonate suckling on one nipple in the mother's pouch, and an older offspring returning to the pouch periodically to suckle a different nipple.

THE MAMMARY GLANDS AND LACTATION

These glands are peculiar to mammals and may be located anywhere along the abdomen or thorax, with their exact location being a particular characteristic of the species. Primates, sirenians, and elephants have mammary glands located in the thoracic region. Ungulates and cetaceans have mammary glands located in the inguinal region. Litter-bearing mammals usually have two rows of glands which extend from the thoracic to the inguinal region. Note that most mammals possess more glands than the usual number of young born at one time.

The prototherians have the least complex and most primitive type of mammary glands. The glands themselves are of the *compound-tubular type* and open directly onto a depression in the skin. Milk is secreted into the depression, and the young grab onto hair tufts and lap the milk from the depression. The metatherians and eutherians have either *nipples* or *teats*. The nipple is a raised area on the breast, with the mammary ducts opening directly to the outside (see Figure 18–18). Some rodents, marsupials, and insectivores possess a single duct, whereas some carnivores and humans have numerous ducts. The teat, or *false nipple*, is formed when the skin of the mammary grows outward to form a protrusion. The mammary ducts open into a *cistern* at the base of the teat. The cistern then has a single duct which allows passage of milk to the outside of the body.

Anatomy of the Mammary Gland

Mammary glands are highly modified sebaceous glands which are usually only func-

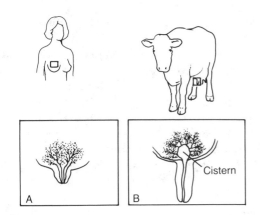

FIGURE 18–18
Cross-sectional view through (A) nipple and (B) teat

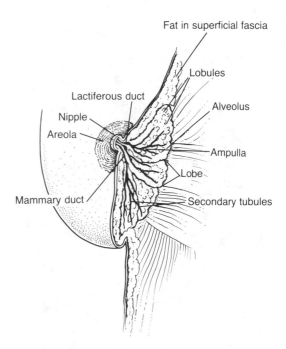

FIGURE 18–19
View of the human female mammary gland showing
duct system typical of most mammals

tional in the recently pregnant female. In the human female each mammary is composed of from 16 to 25 *lobes* (see Figure 18–19). These lobes are made up of *alveoli* lined by a layer of milk-secreting epithelial cells (see Figure 18–20). This layer of cells is in turn covered by a basement membrane, a number of fine capillary networks, and the *myoepithelial cells.* The myoepithelial cells are affected by histamine, oxytocin, vasopressin, and acetylcholine, all of which cause contraction of smooth muscle. The myoepithelial cells cause the alveoli to contract, which releases milk into the duct system. This system starts at the alveoli which enter the *capillary milk duct.* The capillary milk duct empties into an *intralobular duct,* which then empties into the *lactiferous duct.* Each of the lobes is drained by a much branched lactiferous duct which dilates to form a sinus called the *ampulla.* Here, milk collects and then passes through a narrow constriction to the nipple or cistern. In mammals other than monotremes, each breast or mammary has its own excurrent duct which leads to the nipple or to the teat. The number of ducts varies con-

siderably among species. The simplest duct system is found in domesticated cattle, which possess a single excurrent duct per teat. As has already been pointed out, the human mammary gland has a number of excurrent ducts which drain the gland through the nipple.

At birth the mammary glands are rather small in size but may be somewhat enlarged due to the effect of maternal hormones present during gestation and parturition. The mammary glands of the offspring may even expell a small amount of milk at birth. This is sometimes called *witches' milk.* The maternal hormones have a fairly short half-life, and the fetal mammary glands soon become nonfunctional and reduced in size. In females

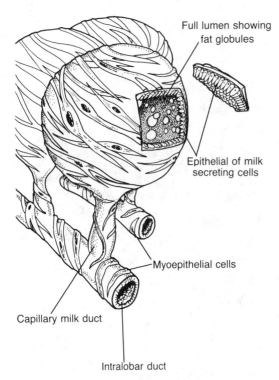

Full lumen showing fat globules

Epithelial of milk secreting cells

Myoepithelial cells

Capillary milk duct

Intralobar duct

FIGURE 18–20
View of a mammary alveolus showing the duct system and myoepithelial cells

the glands increase in size and complexity from birth until maturity, with a maximum amount of development occurring during pregnancy and pseudopregnancy.

Mammogenesis

The mammary glands of males and immature females are very simple, unbranched structures. Puberty in females results in an increase in the growth and branching of the duct system and a rapid deposition of fat in the breasts. Estrogen is usually considered to be important for the growth of the duct system, with progesterone being primarily responsible for alveolar and lobular develop-

ment (see Table 18–5). Follicle-stimulating hormone and LH affect the ovary and stimulate it to produce and secrete the estrogen and progesterone necessary for the growth and development of the mammary glands. It has also been found that ACTH and the subsequent release of glucocorticoids from the adrenal glands, TSH and the subsequent release of thyroxine, and STH all have a positive effect on the development of the mammary glands. In the rat, prolactin is also necessary for their development. Prolactin and STH evidently act directly on the mammary tissue, whereas ACTH and TSH influence mammary development through the hormones produced by the target organs.

Postpuberal virginal females may have slight fluctuations in their mammary glands during normal ovarian cycles. An increase in the branching of the duct system and formation of secretory alveoli in the mammary glands of pregnant females are also due to hormonal influences. After parturition, milk secretion increases due to the release of prolactin from the pituitary gland. During pregnancy prolactin secretion is inhibited by the high concentrations of estrogen and progesterone. Eventually, the mammary glands involute, and lactation stops until the next pregnancy occurs. It is interesting that in marsupials gestation does not affect the mammary glands. It has been shown that young can suckle mature virginal females which are in proestrus.

Lactogenesis

The anterior pituitary has been shown to be indispensible in the production of milk (*lactation*), and corticosteroids are necessary for at least the initiation of lactation. It appears that recently divided cells in the mammary glands are primed by corticosteroids. Once

Hormone	Physiological State		
	Puberty	Pregnancy	Lactation
Estrogen	X	X	
Progesterone	X	X	
Glucocorticoids	X	X	X
Insulin	X	X	
Prolactin	X	X	X
Placental lactogen		X	
Somatotropic hormone	X	X	
Oxytocin			X

TABLE 18–5
Hormonal control of mammary gland development in the rat during puberty, pregnancy, and lactation. Levels of these hormones will vary with the physiological state of the animal.

these cells have been primed, prolactin or placental lactogen or both can cause them to become secretory and begin milk synthesis. Female mice which have undergone adrenalectomy during pregnancy deliver normal litters but do not produce enough milk to sustain the neonates. Lactation can be induced in pseudopregnant rats by the injection of adrenocorticoids and prolactin. In these cases, exogenous administration of prolactin alone does not bring about lactation. In hypophysectomized rats and guinea pigs the administration of either prolactin and ACTH or prolactin and corticosteroids induce lactation. Somatotropic hormone from the anterior pituitary also plays some part in lactation, since STH, along with ACTH and prolactin, increases the amount of milk secreted. This could be due to its ability to elevate plasma glucose levels. It has also been shown in dairy cattle that specific levels of TSH and therefore thyroxine will also increase milk production.

The actual initiation of milk secretion (lactogenesis) is dependent upon the time of decrease in estrogen. This normally occurs immediately before or within a short time after parturition. The decrease in the amount of estrogen is necessary because it blocks the release of prolactin. Once the estrogen levels drop, prolactin levels increase, and the mammary glands begin to secrete milk. There is also evidence that a concomitant rise in corticosteroids may stimulate the onset of postpartum lactation.

Composition of milk Mammals are born with the necessity to obtain nourishment by suckling (nursing) the mother. The composition of milk varies widely among species (see Table 18–6), and no exact rationale for the differences is readily available. This is not the case, however, for energy-yielding compounds. Precocial mammals, like the herbivores, which are able to keep up with adults within a few hours after birth require a great deal of energy for locomotion as well as growth. One would expect the milk of these species to be high in energy-rich compounds such as fats and carbohydrates. Aquatic mammals such as the whale and seal not only require high levels of energy for locomotion and growth, but are also born under conditions which require a high percentage of energy intake to be used in thermoregulation.

The problem of thermoregulation of the young is obvious in the reindeer, which pro-

THE REPRODUCTIVE SYSTEM

TABLE 18–6
Composition of milk in several mammalian species*

Species	Fat	Lactose	Protein			Ash
			Total	Casein	Whey	
Rodents						
Rat	11.9	2.9	8.9	7.2	1.7	1.4
Guinea pig	6.6	3.0	8.1	6.6	1.5	0.8
Carnivores						
Cat	10.9	3.4	11.1	—	—	0.8
Dog	8.4	3.8	7.4	3.9	3.5	1.2
Herbivores						
(non-ruminants)						
Rabbit	14.1	1.9	12.0	9.2	2.8	2.2
Horse	1.5	6.2	2.4	1.3	1.1	0.4
Elephant	15.2	3.5	4.9	—	—	0.8
Rhinoceros	0.3	7.2	—	—	—	0.4
Hippopotamus	4.5	4.4	0	—	—	0.1
Ruminants						
Reindeer	22.5	2.5	10.3			
Sheep	6.6	4.5	5.6	4.3	1.3	0.9
Goat	4.1	4.5	3.5	2.7	0.8	0.8
Buffalo (Indian)	7.6	4.9	3.8	3.2	0.6	0.8
Bovine	3.8	4.8	3.6	2.9	0.7	0.7
Omnivores						
Pig	7.9	4.7	5.7	3.9	1.8	0.9
Primates						
Human	4.2	7.0	1.6	0.9	0.7	0.2
Marsupials and						
monotremes						
Kangaroo	2.1–16.2	2.4†	6.2–16.8	—	—	1.2–2.0
Echidna	19.6	3.8	11.3	8.4	2.9	0.8
Aquatic mammals						
Whale	38.0	2.0	13.6	7.0	6.6	1.1
Seal	53.2	2.6	11.2	—	—	0.7

Source: From *Veterinary Physiology* by J. W. Phillis. Copyright © 1976 by W. B. Saunders Co. Reprinted by permission of the author.
*Figures (where available) are grams of whole milk
†Carbohydrate other than lactose

duces 22.5 percent fat (by weight) in its milk, as opposed to the Indian buffalo, a warm-climate mammal, which only produces 7.6 percent fat in its milk for the nourishment of its young. Many mammals, particularly ro-

dents, cannot thermoregulate in colder climates by means of internal heat production until they are several days or weeks of age. These young are maintained in the nest and conserve heat through close contact with littermates or the mother. The marsupials, which are maintained in the mother's pouch, also have a reduced demand for fat because of their protected condition.

Colostrum *Colostrum* is the first milk of gestation and pregnancy. It contains virtually no fat and has less lactose than milk produced and secreted later. In some mammals the colostrum is essential for conferring passive immunity on the newborn. This is true in horses, pigs, ruminants, humans, and to some extent dogs.

Milk Ejection

Milk ejection is very different from milk secretion, though both processes are the result of neural reflexes. As previously discussed, milk secretion involves the production and release of milk from the mammary alveolar cells. This process requires the presence of prolactin primarily and other hormones secondarily. Milk ejection, on the other hand, involves the reflex release of oxytocin from the posterior pituitary. This reflex can also be brought about by the electrical stimulation of the paraventricular nucleus of the hypothalamus.

The actual neural arc begins with the stimulation of the mammary glands as a result of suckling. Nerve impulses travel up the sensory neurons of the mammaries and eventually reach the nuclei of the hypothalamus. This action potential travels down the supraoptic-hypophyseal tract to the posterior pituitary, where oxytocin is released into the blood. Once the oxytocin reaches the mammary gland it causes contraction of the myoepithelial cells, or *basket cells*, that surround the mammary alveoli and some of the short ducts. As they contract they force milk out of the alveoli and into the duct system.

The actual release of milk from the secretory cells has already occurred due to the stimulation provided by prolactin. Vasopressin (ADH), which is also released by the posterior pituitary, will cause milk ejection but to a lesser extent than does oxytocin. The actual milk-ejection reflex is an interesting one since it may become conditioned in some animals. Most diary farmers are aware that it is best to milk their cows at about the same time every day and that the sounds and environment of the milking barn facilitate milk ejection.

Because milk ejection is dependent upon a neurohormonal reflex there are many factors which can inhibit this process, not the least of which is the severence of the pituitary stalk. Other ways this reflex can be blocked include the ablation of specific parts of the hypothalamus which are involved with lactation, the absence of suckling, exogenous administration of epinephrine, and strong emotions such as fear, worry, and embarrassment. If the sensory neurons to all of the nipples are severed, milk ejection will cease. But, if the sensory neurons to some of the nipples are left intact, milk ejection will occur from all of the nipples as long as suckling occurs on the innervated nipples. There is also a radical drop in milk release from anesthetized nipples.

The formation of milk continues and is under the same hormonal control as milk initiation until shortly after the young are weaned. As the young get older they tend to suckle less and less. This decrease in suckling stimulus consequently decreases the amount of milk produced and secreted by the mammary glands. When the young are weaned, the mammary glands involute and no longer produce or secrete milk. Glandular involution has been experimentally retarded in rats and mice by the exogenous administration of prolactin. Hypophysectomy at any time during lactation causes an abrupt cessation of that process.

REPRODUCTIVE CYCLES

There is an important relationship between the gonads and the hypothalamic-pituitary axis. The condition of the accessory sex organs and glands, the secondary sex characteristics, and the feedback regulation of the pituitary hormones all depend on the production of steroid hormones by the gonads. The gonads, on the other hand, require almost continuous stimulation by hormones from the pituitary (gonadotropins). When the pituitary hormones are absent the animal is in a nonreproductive state. This occurs regularly in seasonal breeders.

Several different cycles will be referred to here. Each of these has a somewhat different emphasis, but each has a definite relationship to the state of the reproductive readiness of the breeding members of a population. The reproductive cycle is reflected in the physiological changes which regularly occur between two successive reproductive periods. The changes occurring in the ovaries between two ovulatory periods is called the *ovarian cycle*, and the hormones contributed by the ovary regulate the condition of the uterus. The estrous cycle seen in most mammals is primarily observed as a behavioral change which denotes the state of copulatory receptivity of the female. When this type of behavior occurs in males, it is referred to as the *rut period*. In most cases the estrous cycle is also reflected in the physiological state of the uterus, and the behavioral state of sexual readiness is usually described in terms of the physiological condition of the uterus. The uterus cycles between states of

preparedness for reception of the zygote during the ovulatory periods. The menstrual cycle is a very specific type of ovarian cycle, occurring only in primates, in which the outer layer of endometrial cells of the uterus are shed in a periodic fashion that reflects the hormonal changes undergone by the female.

The ovarian cycle includes the development of the ovum, its release from the ovary (ovulation), and transport of the ovum to the uterus. As pointed out earlier, the ovarian cycle, which is reflected in the reproductive cycle, can be divided into two major phases, the follicular phase and the luteal phase. The hormonal control of the reproductive cycle begins with the release of FSH/LH-RH from the hypothalamus. This stimulates the anterior pituitary to produce and secrete FSH, which promotes the growth and development of the ovarian follicle. As the follicle develops, estrogen production is elevated. Increased plasma levels of estrogen reduce the release of FSH/LH-RH and somehow stimulate the release of LH from the pituitary. The LH, which is subsequently released by the anterior pituitary, stimulates further pre-ovulatory development of the FSH-primed follicle, which continues to produce estrogen. Both FSH and LH are required for maximum secretion of estrogen. At this time there is a surge of both FSH and LH, and ovulation occurs soon afterward. The LH continues to act on the "empty" follicle, which collapses after the egg is released. Luteinizing hormone causes the luteinization of the follicular cells, which then begin to produce progesterone. Eventually, the progesterone levels increase to the point where they cause a decrease in the amount of LH released from the pituitary. The declining levels of LH result in a decrease in progesterone secretion by the corpus luteum. In the primates, menses begins with the decline in progesterone levels.

In mammals which have estrous cycles, the cycle goes into a quiescent stage (anestrus) or begins another estrous cycle initiated by the release of FSH. Both progesterone and estrogen inhibit the release of FSH. As long as there is sufficient progesterone present, new follicles will not develop except in very rare cases. In rats, prolactin is also required for the maintenance of the corpus luteum and therefore high progesterone levels.

Differences Between Estrous and Menstrual Cycles

The menstrual cycle occurs only in primates and differs from the estrous cycle in several ways. One of the major differences is the presence of a bleeding phase, which is referred to as *menstruation*. Menstruation is characterized by the regular sloughing of the superficial layers of the endometrium, which is accompanied by bleeding from the spiral arteries. The menstrual cycle is quite pronounced in most primates except the New World monkey, which shows only a very slight amount of bleeding. The bleeding phase lasts for four to seven days and is counted as the beginning of the cycle. For example, day one of the menstrual cycle is the first day of bleeding, whereas day one of the estrous cycle is counted as the day of ovulation. The menstrual cycle is also characterized by a constant state of sexual receptivity, whereas the estrous cycle is punctuated by specific heat periods in which the female is receptive to the male.

The Estrous Cycle

The estrous cycle is characteristic of most mammalian species. It can be divided into four stages: *proestrus, estrus, metestrus,* and *diestrus.* These four stages can be catego-rized in terms of their relationship to the ovarian cycle. Proestrus and estrus occur during the follicular phase of the ovarian cycle and are characterized by a predominance of estrogen secretion. Metestrus and diestrus are both marked by a predominance of progesterone secretion as opposed to high levels of estrogen. The increased levels of progesterone are secreted by the corpus luteum during the luteal phase.

The actual length of the estrous cycle is dependent upon the life span of the corpus luteum and varies from species to species. The estrous cycle is lengthened when the life span of the corpus luteum can be extended. In cattle, and less commonly in horses, ovarian cysts sometimes occur which secrete high levels of estrogen and progesterone. Not only does this alter the estrous cycle, but it is also frequently associated with nymphomania in these animals. Other factors such as age may also alter the length of the estrous cycle. In pigs the cycle length increases with age. Virginal cows have a tendency toward shorter and less intense heats than do parous cows. Anything that affects thyroid function also affects the length of the ovarian cycle because of the stimulatory effects of thyroxine on ovarian function. In horses the estrous cycle is influenced by the breed and by the time of year, with the shortest cycles occurring in August and September. Also, mares in temperate regions do not have estrous cycles from about September through February. Photoperiod seems to affect the estrous cycle in mares, and it has been found that estrus can be induced in January and February by the use of artificial lighting. Also, the last estrous cycle or heat period occurring in September frequently is reflected in behavioral receptivity of the mare to the stallion but is not accompanied by ovulation. Estrus sometimes occurs in mares without causing a behavioral display. This is referred to as a *quiet heat* and is fairly difficult to detect.

Although there is no uterine bleeding or regular sloughing of the superficial layers of the endometrium during the estrous cycle, there is a periodic sloughing of the *uterine epithelium*, a part of the endometrium. In sheep, parts of the uterine epithelium are shed which resemble casts of the uterine horns. This happens midway between two ovulations during the early follicular phase. Cows and sows produce uterine casts in the late luteal phase. Female rats experience an almost constant sloughing of the uterine epithelium.

Many mammals exhibit a *postpartum heat* within a few days after parturition, even though they are nursing young. Rats exhibit such a heat, usually within 48 hours of the birth of the young. Sows show a heat three

to seven days after parturition, but there is no ovulation unless the litter dies or is removed from the mother soon after birth. Mares go through a heat five to ten days after foaling, and it lasts from one to ten days. Ovulation may or may not occur at this time. Cows exhibit no postpartum heat.

The rat estrous cycle Rats are spontaneous ovulators and go through a complete ovarian cycle in four to five days (see Figure 18–21). Proestrus lasts about 12 hours and is the beginning of the follicular phase. The small follicles in the ovary begin to increase in size under the influence of FSH from the pituitary. These follicles become swollen, continue to grow and produce increasing amounts of estrogen. When the estrogen level rises to a peak, the hypothalamus is prevented from releasing additional FSH/LH-RH. Usually there is a short surge of FSH and LH,

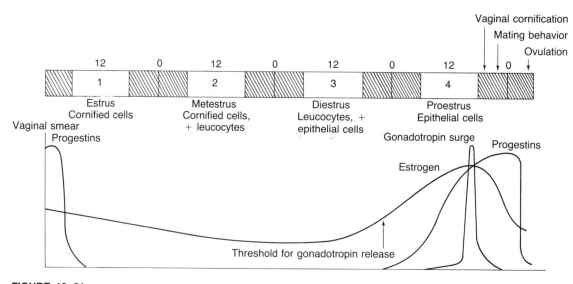

FIGURE 18–21
Diagram of the rat estrous cycle showing plasma hormone levels. From M. S. Gordon, *Animal Physiology: Principles and Adaptations*, 2nd edition (New York, N.Y., 1972). Reprinted with permission from Macmillan Co.

with LH reaching a peak about one hour after the estrogen peak. There is also a preovulatory progesterone peak due to the release of LH and prolactin. During this phase, water retention causes the cervix to harden, and retention of water in the uterine walls results in a ballooning effect. Vaginal smears taken during this time reflect an increase in mitosis of the vaginal epithelium.

The estrus phase, or *heat period*, lasts about 9 to 15 hours. It is only during this time that copulation is permitted. The heat is characterized by increased activity. This increase in activity is also observed in other domesticated species. Other behavioral aspects of heat, including *lordosis* (arching of the back in preparation for acceptance of the male) are also noted. These behavior patterns are due to the high levels of circulating estrogens. Ovulation finally occurs near the end of estrus or, according to some investigators, at the beginning of metestrus. Nevertheless, it does occur within approximately 10 hours of the LH surge. By this time, levels of estrogen, LH, FSH, and progesterone in the blood are all decreasing. The uterine ballooning effect reaches a maximum, and there may be a loss of luminal fluid before ovulation occurs. The endometrium contains simple unbranched uterine glands at this time which are typical during estrogen stimulation. The cervix secretes increasing amounts of mucous, and the pH approaches neutrality. The vagina, however, becomes more acid, and the epithelium undergoes a great deal of mitosis and some cornification. These changes are also due to the high levels of estrogen. At the end of estrus, the cornified vaginal epithelium begins to slough off into the vaginal lumen and form a cheeselike mass.

There are two interesting deviations in estrus which occur in cattle and horses. Quiet heats are especially predominant in March and April. This type of heat is characterized by the absence of psychological heat (behavioral heat) but is physiologically the same as the regular heat. A *split heat* is frequently observed in some animals. In this type of heat the female is sexually receptive, then suddenly is nonreceptive, and then after a few hours in cows and one or two days in horses the female becomes receptive again.

Metestrus is the beginning of the luteal phase. It begins immediately following ovulation and lasts for 10 to 14 hours in the rat. The corpus luteum is formed and then maintained as a result of the trophic action of LH and prolactin. There is an increase in progesterone, which causes an increase in uterine gland activity and a decrease in uterine vascularity and contractility. The vaginal epithelium begins sloughing as cornification breaks down due to the decrease in estrogen levels. At this time copious amounts of leukocytes invade the vaginal lumen.

Diestrus is the final stage of the luteal phase. It lasts nearly one-half of the entire reproductive cycle, or about 60 to 70 hours. The corpus luteum begins to degenerate, resulting in lower progesterone levels. This triggers the release of FSH/LH-RH, which stimulates growth of the follicles and secretion of small amounts of estrogen. The follicles remain small until the end of this stage. The uteri become small and anemic and show little contractility. The vaginal mucosa is thin, and vaginal smears contain primarily leukocytes with only a few nucleated epithelial cells. The vagina also becomes more alkaline at this time.

In animals which do not undergo continuous breeding cycles, anestrus provides a fifth stage of the reproductive cycle. This phase is characterized by a complete degeneration of the corpus luteum, and low cuboidal-type cells with no cornification predominate in the vaginal epithelium. Plasma steroid levels are characteristically low at this time. This stage may also be described as a modified diestrus by some investigators.

The Menstrual Cycle

The menstrual cycle only occurs in primates and is characterized by a menstrual phase in which the superficial layers of the endometrium are sloughed. The length of the cycle varies according to species, with the rhesus monkey and humans having a 28-day cycle and chimpanzees having a 35-day cycle. In all primates the cycle is said to begin on the first day of bleeding. The hormonal levels and subsequent uterine and ovarian changes are depicted in Figure 18–22.

The menstrual cycle is also composed of four stages or phases. The *menstrual phase* begins on day one with bleeding from the *spiral arteries* (except in the New World monkey) and the shedding of the upper two-thirds of the endometrium. Only the basal part of the uterine glands remains. The onset of this phase is due to the decrease in progesterone levels and is therefore termed *withdrawal bleeding*.

The *follicular* or *proliferative phase* runs from the end of menstruation up to ovula-tion. During this phase there is an increase in FSH levels, the development of the follicle, a thickening of the endometrium, and a heightening of the uterine epithelium. There is also a return of vascular and glandular patterns to the endometrium. This is known as a *midcycle type* of endometrium. Within a particular species this phase is somewhat variable in length.

During the short *ovulatory phase*, there is no conspicuous change in the uterine endometrium. Basal body temperature increases at the time of ovulation and remains high until the next cycle begins. The rise in basal body temperature as well as the actual ovulation is controlled by hormonal levels.

The final phase, the *luteal* or *progestational phase*, is marked by the development and then finally the degeneration of the corpus luteum. During the first part of this phase the *secretory stage* occurs. There is an increase in estrogen and progesterone secretion by the corpus luteum due to the action of LH. These two steroids promote changes in the uterine endometrium, including the dilation of the spiral arteries. The stroma becomes edematous and highly vascularized, and the uterine glands begin to secrete after becoming tightly coiled and convoluted. This is termed a progestational type of uterus and

FIGURE 18–22
Diagram of the human menstrual cycle showing plasma hormone levels and changes in the endometrium. From *General Endocrinology*, 5th edition, by C. D. Turner and J. T. Bagnara. Copyright © 1971 by W. B. Saunders Co. Reprinted by permission of W. B. Saunders, CBS College Publishing.

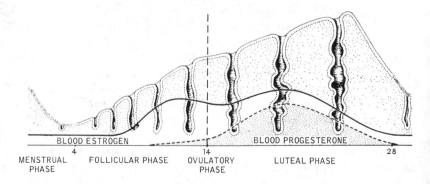

BLOOD ESTROGEN   BLOOD PROGESTERONE

| 4 | 14 | 28 |

MENSTRUAL PHASE   FOLLICULAR PHASE   OVULATORY PHASE   LUTEAL PHASE

is ready for the blastocyst to implant. If pregnancy and implantation do not occur, the corpus luteum begins to degenerate about 8 to 10 days after ovulation, and less and less progesterone is secreted. Leukocytes invade the endometrial tissue, the uterine glands involute, and necrotic changes occur in the stroma. The endometrium continues to decrease in thickness while the spiral arteries become constricted and more coiled. This is known as the *ischemic stage* of the luteal phase. Because plasma progesterone concentrations fall, FSH production by the pituitary decreases and withdrawal bleeding is triggered. Within a species the length of this phase is not variable under normal circumstances.

Menopause When female mammals reach middle age they undergo a regressive change in their reproductive cycles. In primates this is called *menopause*. At this time the ovaries cease to undergo their normal cyclic changes, and the menses no longer occurs. In mammals with an estrous cycle there is no longer a heat period. Because the normal ovarian cycle ceases and there are fewer steroids being produced, there may be a change in the secondary sex characteristics at this time.

FACTORS CONTROLLING THE REPRODUCTIVE CYCLES

The triggers which initiate the reproductive cycles in both males and females may be environmental *(exogenous rhythms)* or genetic *(endogenous rhythms)*. Those mammals that are *seasonal breeders* have evolved with reproductive cycles which allow the young to be born at the most favorable time of the year. This insures a better survival rate for the neonates. Generally a seasonal breeder has one and perhaps two breeding periods per year. Between these cycles the gonads become inactive. In the females the ovaries involute completely, and in the males the testes regress. In some cases, the testes are withdrawn from the scrotum into the abdominal cavity, a process termed *testicular regression*. When the next breeding season begins, the testes descend back into the scrotum, and gametogenesis and testosterone production start once again. This process is called *testicular recrudescence*. Note that domestication usually has its effects on the reproductive cycles in mammals. Many mammals which are seasonal breeders in the wild become continuous breeders after domestication, or at least breed more often than they did in the wild. Even though the seasonal cycles are lost, domesticated animals may show peak periods of fecundity which correspond to the breeding seasons of feral individuals.

Endogenous rhythms in the female *(cycling)* are governed by the hypothalamus through the anterior pituitary gland and depend upon feedback regulation by the gonadal steroids. This type of cycling is genetically controlled. Exogenous rhythms, on the other hand, can be modified by cues from the environment. Environmental cues which trigger physiological rhythms are termed *zeitgebers*. Zeitgebers allow all of the mammals in a particular population to be in the same reproductive state at any given time. This is an excellent mode of increasing mating efficiency and insures the optimum time for birth of the young. One would expect to find this type of breeding sequence especially important in environments where conditions are extreme (i.e., arctic and desert biomes), since the need for an optimal time of birth of the young is magnified in such environments.

Breeding cycles are generally placed in one of two categories, the *continuous breeders* and the *seasonal breeders.* Continuous breeders have constantly repeating reproductive cycles with no reproductive quiescent period. Seasonal breeders do exhibit at least one anestrous period during the year. The frequency of heats during a breeding season can be further delineated. *Monoestrus mammals* are those animals which have only one reproductive cycle per breeding season. *Polyestrus animals* may be seasonally polyestrus, as are pigs, sheep, and cattle, or they may be continually polyestrus, as are many laboratory animals. Some animals which are continually polyestrus show greater fecundity at certain times of the year. An interesting point is that seasonal breeders may be changed to continuous breeders by anterior hypothalamic lesions and, in some species, by the administration of a single dose of steroids in the prepuberal animal.

The importance of zeitgebers in seasonal breeders cannot be overemphasized. It is the zeitgeber which sets off the release of pituitary hormones, which begin the ovarian cycles and prepare the testes for gametogenesis and hormone production. Most mammals that live in temperate zones bear their young during the spring or summer months. This is synchronized by receptivity to appropriate cues. The most important zeitgebers include photoperiod, temperature, social factors, moisture, and nutrition.

Photoperiod, because of its regularity and therefore dependability, is probably the most important single zeitgeber in mammals. Light is received by the animal, and impulses are sent to the hypothalamus, which then releases certain releasing hormones which trigger the production of gonadotropic hormones by the pituitary. The reproductive cycle of the *short-day* or *fall breeders*, such as domesticated sheep and goats, is triggered by decreasing day length. *Long-day* or *spring breeders* respond to an increasing day length. Horses, cattle, wolves, coyotes, and ferrets are all long-day breeders. Whether for short-day or long-day breeders, the photoperiod causes the gonads to enlarge or recrudesce and become fully functional.

An increase in temperature usually results in gonadal recrudescence and a decrease in temperature usually brings on gonadal regression. There are, however, some notable exceptions to this rule, especially in such short-day breeders as the ram. Here, there seems to be an interaction between the shorter photoperiod and the cooler temperatures of fall.

It is very difficult to differentiate between the direct effect of rainfall or moisture on the reproductive cycles and the indirect effect of food availability. *Microtus californicus* is a continuous breeder when it lives in irrigated habitats. In drier habitats it has fewer breeding cycles. The actual cycle may be determined by the quantity and quality of the food being consumed. Experiments using this animal showed that groups fed sprouted wheat had larger litters, more litters, quicker onset of puberty, increased number of maturing follicles (tertiary follicles), and increased uterine weight as opposed to control groups.

Other examples of the interrelationship of moisture and nutrition are observed in the small desert mammals. Pocket mice and kangaroo rats bear most of their young just after the winter rainfall when the spring vegetation is present. The Jamaican fruit bat bears two litters when the main fruit crops are present. Parturition of the insectivorous bats in Mexico corresponds to the increased insect populations after the rainy season.

It has been shown that the reproductive cycles may be altered by visual, olfactory, auditory, and possibly tactile stimulation. In sheep, visual contact is required for the female to come into estrus. Visual contact between the sexes in mink will increase the number of developing follicles. It has also been found that female mice become anestrus when kept in crowded conditions with other females or when kept singly in small cages.

Of the social factors which affect reproductive cycles, olfactory stimulation seems to be the most outstanding. Some of the observed effects of olfactory stimulation include hastened vaginal opening and an earlier first estrous cycle in infantile female mice exposed to male mouse odor. In *Microtus*, the female remains in proestrus until the male is brought near. Removal of the olfactory bulbs in sexually mature female pigs resulted in either cessation or at least an irregularity of subsequent ovarian cycles. At necropsy the ovaries contained no corpora lutea, presumeably because not enough LH was secreted by the anterior pituitary to induce ovulation. The Bruce and Whitten effects observed in mice are both related to olfactory events. The *Bruce effect* occurs in mice when recently pregnant females abort after being put in a cage previously occuped by a male mouse of a different strain. This effect could be reversed by the exogenous administration of prolactin or progesterone. Prolactin release is evidently inhibited by the ''strange'' odor, the corpora lutea are no longer maintained, and implantation fails to result. In the *Whitten effect*, the pheromones produced by the male affect the time of ovulation in the female and seem to synchronize the female reproductive cycles. Synchronization of female ovarian cycles has also been reported in human females.

CLINICAL DISORDERS OF THE REPRODUCTIVE TRACT AND MAMMARY GLANDS

Probably the most widely recognized diseases of the reproductive system are the *venereal* or *sexually transmitted diseases*. This group includes *genital herpes (herpes simplex II*, a virus), *gonorrhea (Neisseria gonorrhoeae*, a bacterium), and *syphilis (Treponema pallidum*, also a bacterium). Further information on these diseases may be obtained from any of the excellent texts on pathogenic or medical microbiology.

Many of the maladies involving the male reproductive system are attributed to disorders of the prostate gland. *Prostatitis*, both acute and chronic, and *enlargement of the prostate gland* are two of the most common diseases of middle-aged and older males. In both cases the prostate gland becomes enlarged and tender. If the enlargement is great, the urethra may become blocked, leading to obstruction of urine flow. Blockage may subsequently lead to damage of the bladder, ureters, and kidneys. Tumors of the prostate are also common, with prostate cancer being the second leading cause of cancer-related deaths in American males.

Disorders of the female reproductive system revolve around the uterus, ovaries, and pituitary gland. Anything that adversely affects the endocrine function of these organs may subsequently be reflected by changes in the menstrual cycle. Ovarian cysts, fluid-filled tumors, are a common ailment concerning the female reproductive tract. *Endometriosis*, a pervasive disorder in middle-aged women, is caused by the growth of endometrial tissue anywhere in the pelvic cavity, including the abdominal wall, cervix, and bladder. Symptoms of endometriosis, which include unusual premenstrual and menstrual pain, are due to the sloughing of this extrauterine tissue at the same time as the tissues within the uterus.

The mammary glands of both males and females are subject to cysts and tumors, though some breast cancers are much more common in women than in men. *Fibroadenoma*, a benign tumor of the breast, frequently occurs in young women. Breast cancer, involving malignant tumors, is much more prevalent in women than in men and generally occurs in older women.

SUMMARY

Reproduction in mammals is a cyclic process involving development of the ovum and sperm, copulation, fertilization of the ovum, development of the embryo, and parturition. In all mammals there is some type of maternal care of the young. In the monotremes, the only mammals which are not viviparous, the young receive milk from the mother which is secreted from the mammary glands into depressions on her abdomen. The marsupials give birth to very altricial young, which become attached to nipples in the maternal pouch. They receive milk which is injected into their mouths as a result of contraction of the maternal abdominal muscles. Members of the infraclass Eutheria are born in various stages of development depending upon the species. The neonates are nourished through a lactation period by milk suckled from the mother.

In the mammalian female the ovaries undergo regular cycles which normally end in ovulation or expulsion of the egg or ovum from the ovarian follicle. The changes manifest in the ovary are under the control of the pituitary hormones, whose release is controlled by inhibiting and releasing hormones secreted by the hypothalamus. During the development of a mature Graafian follicle, more estrogen is produced which slows further FSH and LH production by the pituitary, except for a preovulatory surge of both of these hormones.

After ovulation the granulosus cells take on a yellow coloration and begin secreting progesterone. This is the luteal phase of the ovary, which results in the proliferation of endometrial cells of the uterus. As a result, the endometrium becomes thick and well-vascularized in preparation for acceptance of the embryo. If fertilization occurs, the corpus luteum persists and continues to supply progesterone, which is required to sustain additional growth and vascularization of the endometrium. In some species the corpus luteum is retained throughout the pregnancy, whereas in others it degenerates following the development of the progesterone-secreting capacity of the placenta.

Fertilization usually occurs in the Fallopian tubes, and the embryo passes into the uterus where implantation occurs. In some species implantation is delayed until favorable environmental conditions exist for raising the young. In most species, however, copulation is aligned with development in such a way that the young are born at an appropriate time with respect to the environment.

Milk production from specialized glands called mammary glands is an exclusive characteristic of mammals. There is increased development and complexity of the mammary glands and milk secretion with the evolution of more advanced mammalian species. Milk production and ejection is a very complex phenomenon involving several hormones produced by the ovaries, hypothalamus, and pituitary. The development of the mammary glands prior to parturition is also regulated by hormones from the placenta.

In some species, the males undergo cyclic hormonal changes similar to those seen in females. In these species a pattern of hormonal changes occurs which prepares the animal for reproduction. These males respond to environmental zeitgebers, which evoke hormonal responses leading to testicular recrudescence with increased androgen and sperm production. The males of most domesticated species do not show this pattern and retain their reproductive readiness throughout the year.

19

THE PHYSIOLOGY OF SOME SPECIALIZED MAMMALIAN ADAPTATIONS

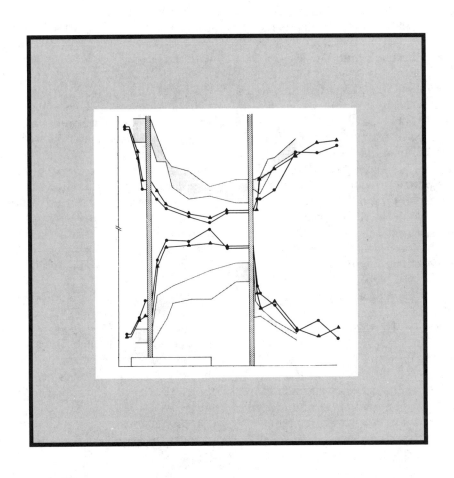

M ammals are found in an array of environmental situations requiring unique specializations. In order to survive in these environments the mammals must draw from several different systems or cope by means of modification of several different physiological processes. For these reasons, survival at high altitudes, in semiaquatic situations (diving), and during severely cold seasons (hibernation) are discussed separately in this chapter. It is obvious that many aspects of these phenomena utilize more than one organ system and represent parts of other adaptive mechanisms. In this chapter, an attempt has been made to isolate diving, hibernation, and survival at high altitude by treating each as an individual phenomenon.

ALTITUDE

Barometric pressure, which changes with altitude, is approximately 760 millimeters of mercury (mm Hg) at sea level. Of this pressure, 21 percent is contributed by oxygen. No matter what altitude is reached in a terrestrial environment, the percent of the total pressure occupied by a particular gas does not change. In other words, at sea level the partial pressure of oxygen is approximately 160 mm Hg. If a mammal resides at a higher altitude where barometric pressure is 400 mm Hg, the partial pressure of oxygen is still 21 percent, but 21 percent of 400 mm Hg equals only 84 mm Hg. Although most mammals are found near sea level, terrestrial environments in North America reach 6,400 meters (21,000 feet) on Mount McKinley. The greatest terrestrial altitude is found on Mount Everest, which reaches 8,839 meters (29,028 feet).

The question of terrestrial residence at high altitude includes a number of limiting factors in addition to the obvious one of oxygen availability. Four specific factors must be considered when analyzing the abilities of animals to exist at a particular altitude: (1) *light intensity*, (2) *food availability*, (3) *temperature*, and (4) *oxygen density*.

With the decrease in atmospheric density as high altitudes are approached, there is an increase in the amount of solar radiation reaching the surface. This is particularly true with such shorter wavelengths as ultraviolet which are normally filtered out at sea level by the great atmospheric density. Vegetational types are altered by decreasing temperatures and changing water conditions, which ultimately restrict the growth of trees altogether. The altitude where trees no longer grow, called the *tree line* or *timber line*, varies considerably depending upon latitude, soil conditions, direction of slope, wind patterns, and available moisture. In many cases, microhabitat selection reduces the effects of temperature as well as food availability. For instance, the pika avoids minimum temperatures at high altitudes by selecting a nival habitat (i.e., beneath the snow) in winter. It also avoids starvation when plant production is reduced by storing food in its den. Many small mammals at high altitudes hibernate. Larger mammals, such as deer and elk, are forced to migrate to lower elevations during the coldest parts of the year in order to obtain food.

With increasing altitudes the faunal changes approach in some ways those encountered in arctic environments. In North America, for instance, one might find the woodland caribou above 1,525 meters in northern Idaho and Montana. With truly high altitudes, above 3,500 meters, there are no faunistic resemblances with the Arctic, though all of the species which reside and reproduce at this altitude exhibit a strong resistance to low ambient temperatures. The abundance of mammalian species decreases as the altitude increases; at the highest elevations only a few species are found, and these are well adapted to resist both low temperatures and low oxygen tensions. In this text, *adaptation* is used to describe functional genetic changes, whereas physiological modification of an existing function when mammals are exposed to alpine terrain is referred to as *acclimatization*. Note that *acclimation* differs from acclimatization in that the former term is used to describe functional modifications induced by a *single variable*. Animals which are taken from sea level to high altitudes must respond to changes in several environmental variables, and thus acclimatization rather than acclimation becomes the term of choice for describing the physiological and morphological changes which occur under varying field conditions.

For mammals living near the equator, high altitude, mountain habitats may be reached if food availability is not one of the primary limiting factors in an animal's survival. At such elevations oxygen availability becomes the limiting factor and the mammal is faced with the problem of delivering sufficient oxygen to the tissues to maintain normal metabolism. When mammals are exposed to low ambient temperatures, metabolic heat production must be elevated to replace heat lost to the environment. Increased oxygen consumption necessary for elevated metabolism during cold stress is not

a difficult or unusual condition to be met by temperate zone or arctic mammals under the conditions found at sea level. But under alpine conditions, where the atmospheric pressure reduces the availability of oxygen, the achievement of this elevated metabolic rate becomes difficult or impossible. Therefore, the critical partial pressure of oxygen (P_{O_2}) may not be obvious under ordinary experimental conditions. For instance, an experimental animal may fare well at reduced barometric pressures in an investigator's laboratory at room temperature; but when these same reduced pressures are coupled with the ambient temperatures normally encountered at high altitudes, survival may be impossible. In other words, the mammal must be able to maintain a fairly constant body temperature at all times in order to survive. If its respiratory and circulatory systems are unable to deliver enough oxygen to the tissues to maintain sufficient metabolism, body temperature decreases and the animal succumbs to hypothermia. Another critical factor here is that hypothermia might result in central nervous system failure, which would be the actual cause of death. But in this case ambient temperature is again only secondary: the true limiting factor is the availability of oxygen. In this way both oxygen availability and ambient temperature play important roles. In other words, if sufficient oxygen is available to support adequate thermogenesis, ambient temperature may not be a limiting factor. Yet this same ambient temperature, which is not a stress factor at sea level, may result in severe hypothermia at high altitudes where ambient oxygen content is not sufficient to maintain adequate metabolic rate.

Thus, sufficient oxygen delivery to the tissues is the primary limiting factor for the survival of mammals in alpine habituation, though other factors are certainly significant.

It follows, then, that the mechanisms of delivery of sufficient oxygen to the tissues under the conditions of rarified air found at high altitudes are extremely important. There are two principal means of oxygen delivery employed by mammals, diffusion and blood circulation, and changes in either (or both) would depend upon adaptations in the lungs and circulatory system. For instance, one might expect that *alpine animals* (i.e., mammalian species capable of survival and perpetuation at high altitude) would have one or more of several possible functional adaptations which would allow increased availability of oxygen to the tissues. In order to enhance diffusion of oxygen from the inspired air into the bloodstream, greater lung volume is essential. An increased lung volume also implies that the surface area for diffusion is increased so that more rapid exchange between the blood and alveolar spaces is possible. An increased lung volume might also be associated with greater tracheal diameter and nostril size in order to get more air into the lungs with a given inspiratory effort.

Oxygen and carbon dioxide diffusion gradients can be maximized by increasing the breathing rate and increasing pulmonary circulation. By flushing the lungs with fresh air more often, the diffusion gradient based upon oxygen and carbon dioxide concentrations in the lungs approaches that of inspired air, which increases the diffusion gradients for both of these cases between the alveoli and blood. Since the gradient depends upon venous blood concentrations of oxygen and carbon dioxide, the diffusion gradient becomes steeper for both gases if the rate of pulmonary circulation of blood is increased. The rate of pulmonary circulation is proportional to cardiac output, which is the product of stroke volume and heart rate. One might expect survival of mammals in alpine conditions to be enhanced by factors which increase cardiac output. In some mammals survival might be reflected in increased heart size and heart rate, whereas in other species either heart size or heart rate alone might be greater than expected when compared to sea level values. Either rate or size would be important as long as an increase in the cardiac output was sustained. When heart hypertrophy is accompanied by increased rate of contraction in lowland species, it usually indicates a pathophysiological condition. But rate as well as size sometimes increases with no ill effects when animals become adapted to high altitudes.

Another adaptation which would be expected of mammals capable of residing at high altitudes would be an elevated diffusion gradient between blood and the tissues. As observed in some species with high metabolic rates, this is accomplished by increasing capillary density, which reduces the area over which oxygen must diffuse. Reduced diffusion distance increases the diffusion gradient and effectively increases the ease with which the cells are supplied with oxygen (see chapter 10, The Circulatory System and Blood Pressure).

Other possible adaptations for the delivery of oxygen to the tissues would be increased numbers of red blood cells (i.e., hematocrit) or increased hemoglobin content of the red blood cells. Some mammals might employ both of these functional mechanisms for matching the rigors of increased oxygen demand, whereas others might employ only one. Note that these changes are quantitative rather than qualitative in nature. Mammals therefore reflect changes in these variables as a matter of *degree*. Some mammals might be better suited than others for life in alpine regions, because acclimatization or change in oxygen carrying capacity occurs more rapidly and with greater magnitude in some species than in others. A limiting factor here is the degree to which the hematocrit can safely increase before blood viscosity reaches a critical level. With increased viscosity, peripheral resistance is elevated, which in turn forces greater energy expenditure by the heart. It is possible, therefore, that increased hematocrit would induce circulatory problems that could result in cardiac failure and death.

Oxygen delivery in highland species could be enhanced by altering the saturation characteristics of hemoglobin. Oxygen could be picked up more readily in the lungs if the affinity of hemoglobin for oxygen was increased. At the tissue level, more oxygen could be released from a given volume of blood if the affinity of hemoglobin for oxygen was reduced. In other words, oxygen release would be enhanced if the P_{50} value of hemoglobin could be increased and its saturation would be enhanced if the P_{50} value was reduced.

More oxygen would also be available for metabolism at the tissue level if myoglobin was in greater abundance. This would allow the mammal to maintain a higher oxygen concentration in the tissues. An increase in tissue myoglobin would enhance the storage capacity for oxygen and make more oxygen available for metabolism when a combination of barometric pressure and temperature effects was present for short periods of time. Also, oxygen storage in this manner might allow a mammal to exhibit short bursts of activity followed by appropriately long rest periods. In many mammalian species of the smaller variety, such as rodents and lago-

morphs, activity related to food gathering and reproduction is thus restricted even at sea level.

Adaptations of Alpine Species

Large mammals   There are few purely alpine mammalian species, since a number of mammals migrate to high altitudes for short periods of time and then return to lower elevations. Species such as the bighorn sheep and mule deer are found at higher altitudes in North America during the warmer parts of the year but at lower elevations during winter temperature extremes. A few species, however, can survive and reproduce under truly alpine conditions, and many of their adaptations have been investigated. The most conspicuous of these are members of the Camelidae family, such as the llama and vicuña of South America. These species have adapted to year-round residence at altitudes which exceed 3,000 meters and have solved the problem of limited atmospheric oxygen supplies in an expected but unusual way. The hemoglobin of species of the family Camelidae is unique in that it has a high affinity for oxygen, which enables their blood to become saturated at low atmospheric pressures (see Figure 19–1). In these species P_{50} values are characteristically low, and hemoglobin saturation occurs at a P_{50} of only half that required for other mammals. In other words, these organisms have adapted to alpine conditions through a genetic change that resulted in a qualitative shift in oxygen affinity. Other species of this family living at low altitudes also show this trait. It is interesting, however, that the family Camelidae is not the only group with hemoglobin having high oxygen affinity (see Figure 19–2). The elephant, for instance, equals or even exceeds

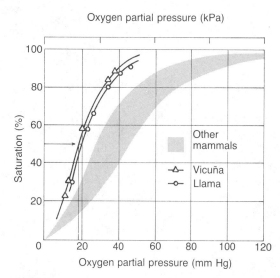

FIGURE 19–1
Oxygen dissociation curves of two well-known high altitude tolerant species, the llama and vicuña, in comparison to other mammals (shaded area). From F. G. Hall et al, Comparative Physiology in High Altitudes, *J. Cell. Comp. Physiol.* 8(1936): 301–313. Reprinted by permission of Alan R. Liss, Inc., New York, N.Y.

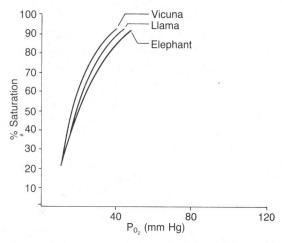

FIGURE 19–2
Oxyhemoglobin dissociation curve for the vicuña, llama, and elephant. Data from F. G. Hall et al, Comparative Physiology in High Altitudes, *J. Cell. Comp. Physiol.* 8(1936): 301–313, and K. Schmidt-Nielsen, *How Animals Work* (London, U.K., 1972). Reprinted by permission of Alan R. Liss, Inc., New York, N.Y. and Cambridge University Press.

the affinity found in the vicuña and llama. Perhaps Hannibal was better informed than anyone realized when he used elephants in 218 B.C. to cross the Alps and invade Italy during the Second Punic War. It should be noted that Hannibal lost half of his men in crossing the Alps, but all the elephants survived.

In addition to hemoglobin changes, members of the family Camelidae also have smaller volumes of red blood cells when compared to lowland mammals. This allows them, by virtue of a relative increase in the surface-area-to-volume ratio of the red blood cells, to load and unload oxygen more rapidly. In fact, a cursory review of the hematocrit of members of this family would lead one to believe that they are anemic. But the erythrocytes of the llama have a higher density of hemoglobin than expected when com-

pared to the hemoglobin concentration of erythrocytes found in typically lowland species. As a result of greater cellular hemoglobin concentrations, hemoglobin levels in the blood of these mammals are quite normal when compared to lowland species. It would be expected that such mammals as the llama and vicuña, which have hemoglobin with high oxygen affinity, would increase the amount of oxygen available to the tissues by means of an increased Bohr effect. But such is not the case. Other dissolved substances (such as DPG) which cause a shift in the P_{50} values of hemoglobin in lowland species are in low concentration in these alpine species.

Note that all of the highland species studied by a number of investigators seem to have a genetically fixed hematocrit. For example, even when a llama is raised at low elevations, its hematocrit is as characteristically low as the hematocrits of llamas raised at high altitudes. When taken to higher altitudes, the llamas raised at lower elevations do not compensate by increasing red blood cell production. In fact, as pointed out in chapter 9 (Blood as a Tissue), hematocrit increase can lead to certain deleterious effects as a result of heightened blood viscosity. It is probable that activity in these animals at high altitudes is possible as a result of the high hemoglobin–low hematocrit relationship.

In addition to elevated blood hemoglobin content and hemoglobin with a greater affinity for oxygen, highland species tend to have greater heart and lung size and increased airway passage capacity. The breathing rate and heart rate in alpine species are more rapid than in lowland animals, even when due consideration is given to acclimatization. It is surprising that little shift occurs in the P_{50} values of these alpine species due to lowered pH or elevated carbon dioxide concentrations.

A striking situation occurs in domesticated sheep, which fare well at a simulated altitude of 6,200 meters. When exposed to low barometric pressures, sheep compensate by increasing the red blood cell content of the plasma from splenic stores and by increasing the heart rate (see Figure 19–3). In addition, sheep have two hemoglobin types, called *hemoglobin A* and *hemoglobin B*. The relative amounts of A and B differ among different strains. When subjected to low barometric pressure, hemoglobin A is replaced by a third type called *hemoglobin C*, which has a greater affinity for oxygen and a greater Bohr effect than the other two types. Hemoglobin C is ideally suited for an animal residing at high altitudes and is a controlling factor in this animal's ability to thrive on alpine terrain.

Small mammals A number of small mammals that reside at high altitudes have been studied. The Andes Mountains of South America provide a suitable habitat (above 3,900 meters) for many species, including vole mice of the genus *Akodon*, several species of the family Chinchillidiae, the guinea pig, feral mice, and the laucha. In addition, the pericote (*Phyllotis*) ranges from sea level up to 4,000 meters. As in most alpine species, the hematocrits of these animals appear to be genetically controlled. Transfer of high altitude species to low altitudes results in no appreciable change in hematocrit after several months of acclimatization. In addition, the offspring of individuals captured at high elevations have hematocrits undistinguishable from their parents. Also, these mammals have greater hemoglobin concentrations in their blood in comparison to lowland species: 295–316 grams per liter versus 256–278 grams per liter, respectively. The only species from this group which shows changes in hematocrit after being maintained at an alien altitude is the feral mouse (*Mus musculus*). All other species have a highly intriguing "genetic architecture" that is suitable for the altitude to which they are adapted.

Acclimatization of Lowland Species to Higher Altitudes

When lowland species are taken to higher elevations, several profound physiological changes occur which render them more suitable to function in an alpine environment. Almost all lowland or subalpine species show some degree of acclimatization. As a general rule, acclimatization of lowland species to alpine environments results in: higher hematocrit as a result of erythropoiesis, increased respiratory rate, increased heart size and heart rate, and decreased affinity of hemoglo-

FIGURE 19-3

The effect of barometric pressure changes in hemoglobin, hematocrit, and cardiac output in sheep and llama. From N. Banchero and R. F. Grover, Effect of Different Levels of Simulated Altitude on Oxygen Transport in Llama and Sheep, *Am. J. Physiol.* 222, no. 5 (1972): 1239, figs. 3 & 5. Reprinted by permission of the American Physiological Society, Bethesda, Md.

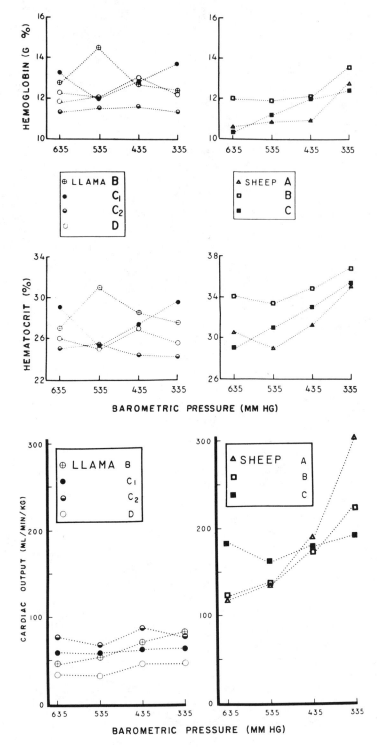

bin for oxygen. On the other hand, the reverse of acclimatization to high altitude rarely occurs when highland species are brought to sea level.

When exposed to high altitude, the horse acclimatizes partly as a result of increased capillary density in its skeletal muscles. This acclimatization technique perhaps occurs in other species as well. The horse does not acclimatize to altitudes greater than about 4,270 meters (14,000 feet). Yet, mules are able to survive at much greater altitudes and have been used to transport heavy equipment at 5,490 meters (18,000 feet).

In humans, acclimatization can occur as the result of either long-term residence beginning at birth or early childhood or as the result of short-term residence of a few days or weeks at high altitudes. The long-term situation involves developmental changes in addition to several circulatory modifications also known to occur during short-term acclimatization. Those native to the Andes Mountains of South America are able to live at 5,000 meters and work at even higher elevations, which would be prohibitive to unacclimatized individuals. These people have relatively large lung capacities and large hearts in comparison to total body mass. These two characteristics are developmental and do not appear to be genetic, because their offspring born and raised at sea level fail to show these traits.

When humans raised at sea level are taken to higher elevations (short-term acclimatization) several changes occur which are similar to some of the modifications found in long-term residents of high altitudes. These changes, which include increased hematocrits and decreased affinities of hemoglobin for oxygen, are found in other lowland species which become acclimatized to high altitudes. The mechanism by which hemo-

poietic tissue is stimulated to increase the production of red blood cells is unknown, but stimulation is believed to be triggered by a hormone called *poietin*, which is formed under situations where sufficient oxygen is unavailable for maximum metabolic rate. How poietin is formed and from what tissue is not clearly understood. Even the chemical nature of the hormone has not been described.

The second change which occurs during short-term acclimatization results in the decrease in the affinity of hemoglobin for oxygen. But the change usually occurs in a matter of 15 to 20 hours in humans and is not the result of change in the hemoglobin molecule, as might be expected. This change in the affinity of hemoglobin for oxygen is not the result of an increase in hydrogen ion concentration of the blood, as might be supposed, but rather occurs as the result of increased concentration of *2,3-diphosphoglyceric acid (DPG)*. At high altitudes, hemoglobin is not completely saturated. In the unsaturated condition hemoglobin molecules become excellent hydrogen ion acceptors, which means that the plasma hydrogen ion concentration decreases when lowland species are taken to high altitudes. As pointed out in chapter 15 (Respiration), reduction in hydrogen ion concentration causes a shift of the hemoglobin saturation curve to the left rather than to the right, as noted during altitude acclimatization. Yet simultaneously with the increase in pH there is an increase in DPG. It appears that the increase in DPG is the primary cause in the decreased affinity of hemoglobin for oxygen. The decrease in oxygen affinity of hemoglobin results in an increase in the amount of oxygen that can be released at the tissue level. This in effect makes more oxygen available to the tissues, though by a totally different mechanism than that found in such alpine species as the llama and vicuña, whose blood becomes completely saturated at very low partial pressures of oxygen.

In addition to changes in the carrying capacity of blood and its ability to deliver more oxygen to the tissues, an increase in heart rate occurs during acclimatization which allows more blood to be carried to the tissues. The exact mechanism for the increased heart rate is not known. Ascent to higher altitudes induces an increased ventilation rate, which subsequently increases venous return. It is possible that the increase seen in the heart rate of individuals results from increased venous return, since it is seen in both highland and lowland animals at high altitudes. Another result of the increased ventilation rate of mammals at high altitude is the depletion of carbon dioxide from the blood (see Figure 19–4). The production of DPG, however, counteracts the effects of carbon dioxide depletion. It is well known that the carbamino compounds decrease the affinity of hemoglobin for oxygen. When carbon dioxide concentration in the blood is reduced, the affinity of hemoglobin for oxygen is increased. Hence, the presence of DPG is thought to maintain a high P_{50} value for hemoglobin even when the blood P_{CO_2} is abnormally low.

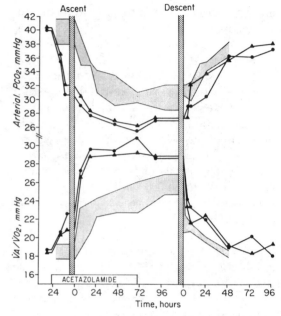

FIGURE 19–4

Changes in arterial P_{CO_2} and ventilation-oxygen consumption ratios in two groups of humans after ascent to 4,509 meters and descent to sea level. Triangles and dots represent subjects whose blood was made acidic through administration of acetazolamide. Normal subjects are indicated by uninterrupted lines. From C. Lenfant et al, Shift of O_2–Hb Dissociation Curve at Altitude: Mechanism and Effect, *J. Appl. Physiol.* 30, no. 5 (1971): 625–631. Reprinted by permission of the American Physiological Society, Bethesda, Md.

DIVING PHYSIOLOGY

Numerous observations have been made of diving organisms. Modern technology has allowed researchers to investigate many of the physiological changes that occur during a dive. Truly aquatic animals have no need for a specialized *diving response* because they are able to obtain oxygen directly from the water and thus sustain themselves indefinitely in the aquatic medium. Here, aquatic animals comprise those which live in either fresh or marine water. Terrestrial or land mammals, on the other hand, have in many cases gone back to the aquatic mode of living (to some extent) and have adapted to the aquatic habitat with varying degrees of success. In animals which have returned to the aquatic mode of life, the problem of obtaining the necessary gas exchange with only the physical attributes of a terrestrial mammal has arisen. Many mammals, however, have adapted so well to the aquatic habitat that they have achieved almost complete freedom in the water.

All classes of truly terrestrial vertebrates (birds, mammals, and reptiles) contain species which either spend part of their lives underwater or seek food or shelter by becoming submerged for a period of time. For example, a freshwater mammalian species, the North American beaver, stores food in the form of green branches beneath the surface of the water. It also employs a subaquatic entrance to its den. Each time a beaver submerges for food or for entry into its den, certain autonomic responses occur (i.e., functional changes resulting from autonomic stimulation) which enable it to remain beneath the surface of the water for a period of time longer than would be possible for a nonadapted terrestrial mammal.

Physiological Characteristics of Diving Mammals

One of the first attempts to explain the ability of diving animals to remain submerged for long periods of time was made in 1870 by Paul Bert, who measured blood volume in birds and mammals and related it to breath-holding ability. Diving mammals, and diving homeotherms in general, have larger blood volumes than nondiving animals and can remain submerged for truly remarkable periods of time (see Table 19–1).

One of the first changes noted in animals that normally dive beneath the surface of the water is a reduction in heart rate, or *brady-cardia*. Almost all terrestrial animals show some degree of bradycardia when diving or when forced to submerge in water. But mammals that traditionally utilize aquatic habitats show a more pronounced reduction in heart

rate in a much shorter time. For instance, the normal resting heart rate of beavers is approximately 140 beats per minute, whereas after two minutes of submergence the heart rate falls to less than 20 beats per minute. Another animal which is well adapted to the aquatic mode of life, the hair seal, shows a decrease in heart rate of 95 beats per minute in less than 30 seconds. Some of the changes in heart rate seen in diving vertebrates are shown in Figure 19–5. Note that warm-blooded animals show a more rapid response to submergence than do reptilian species. Likewise, such animals as seals, which traditionally are found in open ocean environments and are thus forced to depend upon their aquatic skills for feeding and eluding predators, show the most dramatic response of all.

In addition to bradycardia, blood flow to specific muscles and various organs is decreased or stopped altogether during the dive. Autonomic activity results in constriction of vessels carrying blood to skeletal muscle, kidneys, and the periphery of the body. Lactic acid produced as a result of anaerobic glycolysis in muscles isolated in this way is less likely to enter the systemic circulation and affect such vital organs as the brain and heart. This response also reduces the likelihood that hydrogen ions will accumulate in the blood and be available to stimulate the chemoreceptors that control breathing. An important consequence of the alterations in blood flow seen in diving mammals is that the most essential organs (i.e., brain, heart, and lungs) receive uniform blood flow and pressure both before and during the dive. This allows for uniform blood and oxygen delivery to the essential organs at all times.

The hemoglobin of diving mammals is not distinct from nondivers in its ability to be-

TABLE 19–1
Blood volume, oxygen capacity, and duration of dives in several mammalian species

Species	Blood Volume (% of body weight)	Oxygen Capacity Volume (%)	Duration of Dive (min)
Rabbit	6.5	15.6	—
Dog	6.2–10.5	21.8	—
Human	6.2–7.0	20.0	2.5
Horse	7.0–10.7	16.7, 14.0	
Beaver (Castor canadensis)		17.7	15.0
Muskrat (Ondatra zibethica)	10.0	25.0	12.0
Seal (Phoca vitulina)	15.9	29.3	20.0
Sea lion (Eumetopius stelleri)	9.0–11.0	19.8	—
Porpoise (Phocaena communis)	15.0	20.5	—
Blue whale* (Balaenoptera musculus)	—	14.1	60.0
Fin whale* (Balaenoptera plupalis)	—	14.1	
Sperm whale* (Physeter catadon)	—	29.1	90.0

*Blood samples taken from carcasses several hours after death

come saturated with oxygen. This is to be expected, since most divers, except for some of the freshwater species (e.g., beavers, muskrats), reside at sea level, where oxygen availability from the atmosphere is not a major problem. An increase in the Bohr effect in these mammals would allow for greater oxygen delivery to the tissues in the same fashion as it does in animals at high altitudes or animals with high metabolic rates. It is surprising that a pronounced Bohr effect is not found in diving mammals.

Other changes in the bodies of divers are also apparent. For instance, the principal energy sources of muscles in divers (such as glycogen and adenosine triphosphate) are in ample supply and appear to be stored for that time when they are most needed. Diving mammals also have high concentrations of myoglobin in their muscles, which gives them a remarkable ability to store oxygen.

In contrast to the apparent fright reaction to submergence seen in nondivers, diving mammals are accustomed to the physical sensations of diving and usually do not show signs of struggling. The divers relax and thus conserve energy which would otherwise be spent in useless struggling during an experimental dive. This ability to relax under water appears to be a purely behavioral reflex which is just as essential as the other functional changes discussed above.

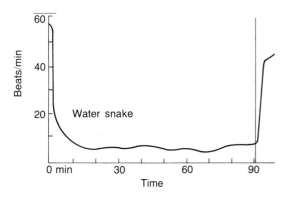

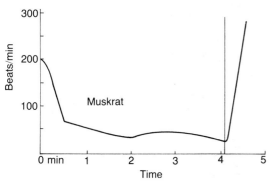

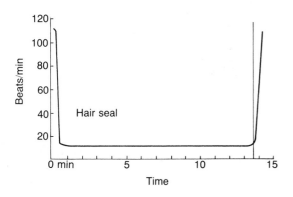

FIGURE 19–5

Effect of diving on heart rate in several vertebrates. From J. H. Ferguson, Diving Physiology, in *Encyclopedia of Science and Technology,* 5th edition, S. Parker, ed. (New York, N.Y., 1982). Reprinted by permission of McGraw-Hill Book Co.

Biochemical Adjustments in Diving Mammals

From a teleological standpoint, diving mammals would be expected to have expanded abilities to derive energy by means of anaerobic glycolysis when compared to nondiving mammals. This has led to a great deal of speculation that diving mammals have enhanced potential for generation of energy by the Embden-Meyerhoff pathway. But from the existing data on the subject it would appear that only a few diving mammals are able to utilize energy derived from anaerobic glycolysis in the skeletal muscles to greater than average advantage. In fact, it appears that the role of anaerobic glycolysis is negligible in explaining the ability of most divers to exert muscular energy for long periods of time while diving. On the other hand, several of the organs of divers can withstand ischemia for protracted periods and probably do have a greater than average facility for utilizing energy obtained from anaerobic glycolysis. This has drawn attention to the fact that metabolism among different organs of the body in certain diving mammals can be decidedly unique and contributes to the understanding of mechanisms which allow for long periods of anoxia in diving species. As pointed out earlier, the less essential organs of divers receive reduced blood flow during the dive. When activities of *lactate dehydrogenase (LDH)* and *phosphokinase (PK)* of diving and nondiving mammals are compared, it appears that the liver and kidney have an abundance of enzymes for developing and releasing oxygen debt (see Table 19–2). The abundance of LDH in these organs would indicate that the reduction in blood circulation to them is compensated by an elevated ability to obtain energy from the Embden-Meyerhoff pathway. These mammals probably

TABLE 19–2
Tissue enzyme activity levels (mean ± SD)*

	Heart	Brain	Liver	Kidney Cortex	Kidney Medulla	Muscle
LDH (pyruvate to lactate)						
Marine	813 ± 323	210 ± 29	538 ± 188	382 ± 133	322 ± 99	1,021 ± 203
Terrestrial	801 ± 102	214 ± 30	310 ± 182	312 ± 149	233 ± 93	1,086 ± 418
Rank	WS,D,B,HS	M,SO,WS,D	HS,M,WS,SL	WS,B,SL,HS	SO,B,WS,SA	WR,HS,WS,SA
LDH (lactate to pyruvate)						
Marine	189 ± 84	53 ± 9	155 ± 45	116 ± 49	84 ± 21	272 ± 60
Terrestrial	177 ± 28	53 ± 8	78 ± 46	69 ± 39	53 ± 19	315 ± 170
Rank	WS,B,HS,M	WS,M,SO,D	HS,M,WS,SO	WS,SL,HS,D	SO,B,SA,WS	WR,WS,HS,B
PK						
Marine	187 ± 98	150 ± 35	23 ± 7	47 ± 23	89 ± 48	697 ± 255
Terrestrial	225 ± 131	198 ± 45	32 ± 17	24 ± 12	66 ± 61	806 ± 374
Rank	WS,SO,M,D	M,D,WR,WS	M,D,SL,HS	HS,SL,WS,B	B,HS,SO,SL	SA,WR,WS,P

Source: From Physiology of Diving Mammals by G. L. Kooyman. Reproduced, with permission, from the *Annual Review of Physiology*, Volume 43, © 1981 by Annual Reviews, Inc.

*Activities are expressed as international units (μmoles of substrate converted to product per minute) per gram wet mass tissue at 37°C, pH 6.8. All tissues are from adult animals. Muscle activities are pooled averages for all sites measured for each animal. Marine mammals: Weddell seal, *L. weddelli* (WS); harbor seal, *P. vitulina* (HS); sea otter, *E. lutris* (SO); sea lion, *Z. californianus* (SL); and porpoise, *Stenella attenuata* (SA). Land mammals: white mouse, *Mus musculus* (M); white rabbit, *Oryctolagus cunniculus* (WR); dog, *Canis familiaris* (D); domestic pig, *Sus scrofa* (P); and Beef, *Bos taurus* (B). Rank shows the highest four activities in decreasing order. Significant difference at 95% level (students t-test), shown by underlined values.

are able to store lactate in the liver and kidneys during a dive, which is, in a definitive way, the ability to maximize oxygen debt. The presence of elevated tissue LDH probably also allows these mammals to eradicate oxygen debt rapidly after surfacing. Several interesting observations on the changes of pH in these organs during a dive could no doubt be made.

It is known that cardiac metabolism of terrestrial mammals is primarily aerobic. This is based upon the respiratory quotient (RQ) of heart muscle tissue, which approaches 0.7. That figure is quite different from the RQ of skeletal muscle tissue, which varies widely, depending upon the state of exercise and other environmental factors, between 0.7 and 1.0. A different picture seems to be emerging based upon the concentrations of PK and LDH in heart muscle tissue of diving mammals. Several investigators have found that PK and LDH are in greater concentrations in the cardiac tissues of divers when compared to nondivers. It appears that the activities of these enzymes, as well as their prevalence, increases in the heart with the ability of the animal to perpetuate a dive. Because of the presence of supranormal concentrations of PK and LDH, the heart, liver, and kidneys of diving mammals have an increased ability to withstand anoxia. This same situation based upon enzyme activities does not hold true for neural tissue. Investigations of brain tissue show the divers as being no more able to tolerate neural ischemia than totally terrestrial species. Some data support the claim that gluconeogenesis in the lungs results in the formation of glucose, which is transported to the brain for metabolism. This presents a rather novel interdependence of organs in the diving mammals and should receive further study. But, as similarly shown in cold-acclimated animals, new and diverse mechanisms of energy metabolism have not been found in divers. Rather, metabolic alterations seen in diving mammals result from emphasis of certain pathways to the exclusion of others through changes in enzyme activities and concentrations.

In addition to the expected dependence upon the development of oxygen debt, it has been found that metabolic rate is reduced when divers are submerged and that body temperature falls two to three degrees below normal. The change in body temperature occurs in both freshwater and marine species. Although direct methods of determining metabolism during the dive have not been used, metabolic rate has been estimated through analysis of turnover rates of labelled metabolites. In fact, because of the Q_{10} phenomenon, a fall of $2.0°$ to $3.0°$ C in body temperature would result in about a 25-percent decrease in total metabolism. This and other data, such as the reduction in body core temperature during the dive, have allowed investigators to assume that metabolic rate during the dive is depressed by 20 to 25 percent below the resting metabolism. Lending further support to such an assumption is that during a dive blood circulation to the periphery is reduced. That reduction in turn enhances insulation. A decrease in metabolism is a possible explanation when body temperature decreases while insulation increases, because under normal circumstances when insulation increases core temperature also rises because of insufficient heat dissipation.

Some Specific Examples of Diving Mammals

Seals Some of the best known of the diving mammals are the seals, which range from the colder waters of the Antarctic and Arctic to the equator. The Weddell seal, found in the

Antarctic, has been studied in its natural habitat by G. Kooyman. This species dives to a depth of 600 meters and remains submerged for as long as 43 minutes. This is indeed remarkable when one considers that pressure in water increases by approximately 14.7 pounds per square inch for every 10 meters (about 33 feet) of submergence. Thus, the pressure withstood by the Weddell seal must vary from atmospheric to 883 pounds per square inch. In order to descend to this depth, the seal must also withstand the effects of water temperatures as low as 2.0° C, which means that this species has adapted to a very demanding and rapidly changing environment.

Whales Of all the divers, the whales are probably the best adapted. But for most whale species comparatively little data have been collected. The sperm whale *(Physeter catodon)* has been observed to remain under water for as long as 75 minutes, sometimes reaching a depth of 900 meters. The bottlenosed whale *(Hyperoodon ampullatum)* can remain submerged for two hours, though the maximum depth to which it dives is not known. Another species, the blue whale *(Sibbaldus musculus)* can dive for 49 minutes and reach a depth of 100 meters. Contributing to the remarkable depth and consequent pressure which these whales attain may be their ability to collapse their lungs during a dive. This would eliminate part of the problem of *nitrogen narcosis* and the development of the *bends* associated with absorption of nitrogen gas. As the whale descends, pressure apparently forces air out of the lungs and into the trachea, which is expanded in these species and impermeable enough to prevent gas exchange with the blood. Whales seem to have an excellent means of storing oxygenated myoglobin in the muscles. They have also de-

veloped thermoregulatory mechanisms which allow them the freedom of both temperate and arctic waters.

Muskrats The muskrat *(Ondatra zibethica)* is a freshwater mammal which has numerous physiological adaptations for diving, such as high oxygen-storage capacity in the blood and pronounced bradycardia. It is also able to survive cold ambient air and water temperatures as a result of insulation provided by its dense, nonwettable fur. Body insulation is also enhanced by peripheral vasoconstriction, which reduces blood flow to the tail and feet when this animal is exposed to cold.

It has also been shown that exposure to cold water in this species affects heart rate and that bradycardia is more pronounced at lower water temperatures (see Figure 19–6). Metabolic rate of the muskrat apparently decreases when exposed to cold ambient water temperatures, since body temperature drops from a normal of about 37° C to 34° C when

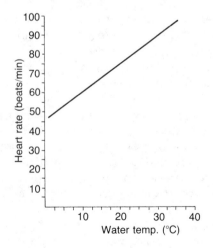

FIGURE 19–6
Effect of water temperature upon heart rate during submergence of the muskrat *(O. zibethica).* Data from C. J. Gordon, personal communication.

the animal is forced to dive in water at 2.0° C. These data were acquired using captive animals during forced dives, but the muskrat experiences similar water temperatures in nature. Investigators have observed the muskrat foraging in ice-covered water. Here, the same observation can be made concerning increased insulation during a dive in cold water as was pointed out for the seal. The deep-body temperature of the muskrat drops even though insulation increases due to vasoconstriction. This would indicate that metabolism has decreased as a part of the response to the stimulus provided by the dive. Diving in warm water presents a completely different situation from diving in cold water in terms of heat dissipation. When diving in warm water, increased peripheral vasodilation necessitates an increase in heart rate in order to maintain adequate blood flow to peripheral tissues.

Humans Humans have a poor diving ability when compared to such excellent divers as seals and whales. But almost all humans experience bradycardia when diving or even when the face is submerged in water. For example, the heart rate will fall from a resting rate of 72 beats per minute to 60 beats per minute after less than a minute of facial submergence. This bradycardia is identical to the bradycardia observed when diving and, like the bradycardia observed in the muskrat when diving, is affected by temperature.

In the Orient, where industries for both food and jewelry have been built up around the ability of divers to obtain shellfish, the principal divers are women, who withstand both cold and anoxia for extraordinary periods of time. The diving women of Japan and Korea frequently dive to depths of 80 feet and remain submerged for up to two minutes in water temperatures of 10° C. Most divers can-

not remain submerged for more than three minutes without the aid of artificial air supplies.

Problems related to artificial apparatuses in diving Very early it was deemed necessary for humans to perform work underwater. Devices were developed which would allow them to survive for extended periods beneath the surface. One of the first problems encountered in the early attempts was the effect of pressure. External gaseous pressure not only increases the physical exertion necessary for movement underwater but also increases the rate of absorption of gases from the lungs into the tissues. When the atmospheric pressure is doubled, not only does the body receive more oxygen due to the increased P_{O_2}, but the amount of nitrogen in the tissues is also increased. From this increase of nitrogen two distinct conditions result. *Nitrogen narcosis* occurs when excessive nitrogen enters the nervous system, producing strong psychological reactions often expressed as a feeling of euphoria. In addition, a diver who has absorbed excessive amounts of atmospheric gases has a totally different problem when a rapid ascent is attempted. When the diver ascends toward the surface, decreased pressures cause gases in solution in the tissues to become less soluble. Since gases come out of solution faster than they can be carried to the lungs, bubbles form in the tissues. This is particularly noticeable for nitrogen: since it is not used in metabolism, it tends to build up in the tissues when a human dives for extended periods of time. Bubbles from the dissolved nitrogen form in the nervous system and become quite painful and debilitating. Bubbles which form in the circulatory system result in air embolism and can have a disastrous effect. This collection of conditions associated with the formation of gas bubbles in the tissues is referred to as the *bends, Caisson disease, diver's disease,* and *aroembolism.*

Diving in a *caisson* or with *scuba* gear (i.e., self-contained underwater breathing apparatus) imposes the pressure of the surrounding water on the diver's breathing system. In the caisson the diver utilizes the oxygen in a bubble which surrounds him. As oxygen is consumed from the bubble, the percent of nitrogen increases while the pressure remains constant. In this way the quantity of nitrogen absorbed is tremendous because of the increased partial pressure imposed as oxygen is removed. Because the air is of a constant mixture when supplied by the scuba gear, the diver does not experience the problem encountered with the caisson.

How then can these problems of nitrogen be avoided? Some years ago the only method available was for the diver to ascend slowly, allowing time for the nitrogen to diffuse from the body tissues without forming bubbles. Another method, more recently developed, is to supply the diver with pure oxygen. But oxygen in its pure state is quite toxic, and the amount of time that it can be safely breathed is reduced with increased pressure. A possible remedy for this quandary is to replace the nitrogen and part of the oxygen with more mobile gas such as helium. There are several advantages to the use of helium in place of nitrogen. Helium is less than one-half as soluble in the tissues as nitrogen; and because of its smaller molecular size, it has much greater mobility in solution than nitrogen, so it passes back into the lungs more rapidly than nitrogen does. The decreased solubility and increased mobility reduces the amount of inert gas which goes into solution and allows it to move back into the lungs at a faster rate. Because it does not accumulate and form bubbles readily, helium is much

safer than nitrogen for use in underwater breathing devices. A mixture of 10 percent oxygen and 90 percent helium would mean that a person working at 40 meters below the surface would be receiving 0.5 atmospheres of oxygen (P_{O_2} is equal to 152 mm Hg). This would allow the diver to work for longer periods of time and not show the problem of nitrogen narcosis or embolism normally observed upon ascent. But some problems are known to be caused by helium: after diving to depths greater than are possible with a nitrogen mixture, a diver experiences problems that bear strong resemblance to nitrogen narcosis. An obvious replacement for helium would be hydrogen, which is even more mobile; but it would be a poor choice because of its explosive qualities if accidentally ignited.

HIBERNATION

A number of mammalian species which are unable to compete for food and thus survive in inclement seasons are able to employ an effective means of avoidance. These species reduce to a minimum the metabolic demand on food stores by becoming inactive and allowing body temperatures to approach the ambient. This is characterized by a physiological condition which can occur in winter, whereby the mammal becomes *torpid* for extended periods of time, discards its thermoregulatory ability, and allows metabolism to fall to a maintenance level. This physiological condition, called *hibernation*, is essentially duplicated in some species during summer months, when it is usually termed *estivation.* These torpid conditions allow mammals to reduce the metabolic demand of the body for external food sources and ensures that activity is at a maximum when food sources are available. This process involves a physiological mechanism which is quite profound but which is in general poorly understood. Both hibernation and estivation are responses triggered by environmental changes such as food availability, temperature, and perhaps photoperiod.

In hibernation, which occurs during the winter and fall seasons, the mammal may remain in the torpid condition for several months, only interrupted by short periods of arousal. This process is seen in a number of mammalian orders, and a great many variations are manifested in nature. In some groups, particularly in bats, a short torpid period is sometimes a daily occurrence. The length of torpor is expanded until the bats exhibit the prolonged condition characteristic of hibernation.

Hibernation is an adaptation to inclement, cold conditions. It is usually not observed in larger mammals or flying mammals which can migrate to habitats less demanding on food resources. But such small mammals as red squirrels, lemmings, and pikas do not hibernate. Carnivores sometimes show a response called *carnivoran lethargy* that resembles hibernation and is, indeed, considered to be true hibernation by some authors. Carnivores in the lethargic condition usually maintain body temperature closer to normothermic temperatures found in the active animal. The higher body temperatures of these animals in the torpid state is believed by some to provide the basic difference between carnivoran lethargy and true hibernation.

Advantages of Hibernation

Mammals that hibernate avoid temperature minimums when food availability is limited and when a large expenditure of energy is necessary to maintain an internal homeo-thermic condition. These animals are able to store large quantities of fat in the adipose tissues that sustain them through the time of limited food supply. Body temperature regulation is usually inconsequential during this time, because the *hibernaculum* (i.e., the shelter) is isolated from temperature extremes by being subterranean. Here, the animal essentially allows its body temperature to become equal to environmental temperature or at least fall below the optimum activity temperature of 37° C. The consequent decrease in body temperature during hibernation reduces the demand on the body food stores. The reduction of body temperature effectively lowers the temperature differential between the body and the surrounding environment and decreases the demand for energy production essential to maintaining the normal body temperature of 37° C. As a result of the need for a secure hibernaculum, hibernation is usually restricted to burrowing animals.

Mammals Which Hibernate

Hibernation is probably not a product of recent evolution since it occurs in prototherians as well as eutherians. Hibernation is found in the orders Chiroptera and Rodentia and, according to some authors, also occurs in the order Carnivora. But, again, the situation in carnivores is frequently referred to as lethargy rather than true hibernation. Among the chiropterans true hibernation occurs in the Vespertilionidae. Various species of bats within this family hibernate for only short periods, whereas others in this family are known to hibernate throughout the winter. Bats usually utilize abandoned mine shafts, attics, and hollow trees as hibernacula. In temperate regions, many species have used specific caves for hibernation for hundreds, if not thousands, of years. One species, the red bat *(Lasiurus borealis)*, remains in cold regions throughout the year. It hibernates for short periods of time but becomes active on warm days even in winter. It would appear that the degree of torpor achieved in this species, and in bats generally, is less intense than that found in other groups of hibernators such as rodents.

Among the rodents several degrees of hibernations are achieved. In the cactus mouse *(Peromyscus eremicus)* torpor may be achieved daily when ambient temperatures fall below 30° C. This is definitely a case of torpor in response to decreased temperature as well as food availability. Both hibernators and nonhibernators are found among the hamster group. Some cases are known in which certain genetic strains within a particular species hibernate while others do not. In many cases within the hamster group environmental conditions are extremely critical in evoking the hibernation response. Hibernation can be induced in the laboratory sometimes with relatively minor environmental changes while control groups maintained under different environmental conditions show no signs of hibernation.

The family Sciuridae includes some of the most notable hibernators as well as some obvious exceptions active the year round. Many species within this family are fossorial and thus have a habitat which readily lends itself to hibernation. The sciurids include marmots, many species of ground squirrels, prairie dogs, flying squirrels, chipmunks, and tree squirrels. All of these groups undergo winter hibernation except the tree squirrel *(Tamiascuirus)*, which is active the year round as far south as Arizona and as far north as Alaska.

The exclusively Old World family Gliridae includes the dormouse, which is perhaps the most notable of the hibernators. The glirids include seven genera and twenty-three species. Hibernation is typical in this group

Within the order Carnivora, two families, Ursidae and Mustelidae, undergo winter torpor. In North America the black bear *(Ursula americanus)* becomes torpid and remains in the *den* (hibernaculum) throughout much of the winter. These animals exhibit most of the traits of true hibernators, though they do not typically allow the core temperature to fall to the level observed in hibernating rodents. The mustelids are usually not hibernators, though some members become torpid during the winter months. The North American badger *(Taxidea taxus)* is notable in this group for its ability to undergo winter torpor.

Environmental Factors Which Induce Hibernation

Although environmental situations which control entrance into hibernation are sometimes difficult to achieve in the laboratory, certain basic principles governing the onset of hibernation in the wild have been observed. These include *day length* (i.e., photoperiod), *temperature*, and the *availability of food*. Ambient *humidity* may also be a factor in some cases. The importance of these factors varies with the species, but in most cases a combination of factors is believed to be necessary to induce hibernation.

The dormouse provides an excellent example of a species which responds to photoperiod and prepares itself for hibernation accordingly. In this species reduced periods of light from 19 to 9 hours per day is sufficient to induce hibernation. In contrast, the ground squirrels *(Citellus tridecemlineatus* and *Citellus lateralis)* are not directly affected by photoperiod as a single stimulating factor. But when reduced photoperiods are combined with cooler temperatures, the golden-mantled ground squirrel *(Citellus lateralis)* is induced to hibernate. In some cases, ground squirrels have been maintained for years in the laboratory without going into hibernation and yet begin to hibernate almost immediately after being exposed to an atmospheric temperature a few degrees above freezing. Here, the onset of hibernation culminates in a period of weight gain which results from storage of body fat. If food is removed from these animals prior to the end of the period of fat deposition, hibernation is sometimes prevented. When food is made available to them *ab lib*, hibernation proceeds without interruption.

Environmental factors alone are probably not responsible for the onset of hibernation. It is probable that annual rhythms are essential to the initiation as well as termination of hibernation, and environmental cues such as photoperiod and food availability act only as zeitgebers which modify the time of beginning and ending of hibernation. Consequently, when the annual rhythm is at the point when hibernation would be expected, a reduction in photoperiod or change in some other zeitgeber causes a rapid onset of hibernation. Likewise, when these environmental cues are given at inappropriate times with respect to the annual rhythm, many of the physiological changes associated with winter torpor are evoked without the actual onset of hibernation.

Physiological Changes During Hibernation

When animals go into hibernation a number of changes occur in metabolism as well as behavior. During hibernation there are a number of physiological characteristics that distinguish the process from other situations of dormancy. During the preparation for hibernation, the animal usually stores large quantities of fat. This is associated with a change in metabolism which allows for greater fat deposition. During this time food consumption is at a maximum. With the onset of hibernation, activity decreases and the normal dormant periods become increasingly long. This is usually a process which requires several days or even weeks, but investigators have reported that the onset of hibernation ensues in a very short time in species that are physiologically prepared. The thirteen-lined ground squirrel has been reported to enter hibernation within 12 hours and undergoes a body temperature drop to 4.0° C within 8 hours. Generally, hibernation involves a series of *test bouts* in which the mammal undergoes torpor and decrease of body temperature rather spasmodically over a period lasting for several days. During this time body temperature becomes continuously lower until it is finally equal to the ambient temperature of the hibernaculum. Hibernation after the process reaches its maximum is not continuous, and the hibernator arouses at intervals during the winter for short periods of time.

During hibernation, activity in many of the endocrine glands is reduced to correspond to the minimum level of metabolism. In similar fashion, body temperature decreases to a level comensurate with metabolism, and the animal is consequently able to survive for long periods of time on stored body fats. Breathing rate slows, and heart rate decreases to a few beats per minute. The change in heart rate is extremely profound in small mammals, whose hearts beat under normal circumstances at a rate of 100 to 300 beats per minute. In the hibernators, particularly the hibernating ground squirrel, the heart continues to beat even when body temperature is only a few degrees above freezing. The heart of hibernators will beat *in vitro* at a variety of temperatures without an elaborate experimental setup to distribute oxygen to the cardiac muscle, a phenomenon uncharacteristic of nonhibernators. One of the characteristics frequently associated with true hibernation is the ability of the heart of hibernators to beat at temperatures below 21° C. In most nonhibernators the heart fibrillates at 15° to 21° C and will not beat at lower temperatures. If the heart of a hibernator is removed during the active season, it does not follow the typical pattern seen in the hearts of hibernating mammals but follows the pattern of nonhibernators. Thus, it is impossible to maintain the heart of an active hibernator *in vitro* without the same elaborate laboratory preparations used in maintaining hearts of nonhibernators.

Muscle and bone physiology are also of interest in hibernating mammals. When the nonhibernator goes for long periods of time without activity, the skeletal muscles tend to atrophy and calcium is reabsorbed from skeletal tissue. Neither situation occurs in the hibernator. Even when motor nerves are cut, atrophy of skeletal muscle does not occur until normal activity is resumed.

Brown fat Hibernators have large quantities of *brown fat*, which is in greatest abundance in the interscapular region. Brown fat is well supplied with blood vessels and has a high density of mitochondria and consequently high concentrations of cytochrome enzymes. It is distinguishable in the living mammal by its reddish or brownish coloration and is not strictly limited to hibernators. The red squirrel *(Tamiascuirus)*, which is a nonhibernator and active the year round, has an abundance of this substance. The Norway rat, another nonhibernator, also possesses a small amount of brown fat in the interscapular region.

Brown fat exhibits a very high metabolic rate and is thought to provide much of the heat necessary to bring the body to normothermic temperature during arousal. At times of arousal, the temperature of brown fat may be as much as 5.0° C above the temperature of the body core. It is usually strategically located near the larger veins, apparently to warm the blood returning to the heart.

Carnivoran lethargy Most hibernating mammals assume a poikilothermic condition during torpor which allows their body temperature to drop precipitously with the temperature of the hibernaculum. As a built-in protective mechanism these animals usually awaken before body temperatures reach the point of tissue freezing. Carnivores, on the other hand, do not reach this state of poikilothermy, and core temperatures usually fall by about 5.0° to 10° C below normal. During this time metabolic rate is maintained at 50 to 60 percent of the rate seen in the active animal. Also, these animals exhibit a decrease in heart rate from about 40 to 70 beats per minute in the active mammal to 10 to 20 beats per minute. Folk and others at the University of Iowa report a minimum of 8 beats per minute in lethargic black bears during winter. When subjected to artificial cooling, the hearts of bears continue to beat until a core temperature of 17° to 20° C has been reached. In badgers subjected to the same treatment, heartbeat persisted until core temperature reached 13° C.

Most of the data on carnivores is inconclusive. But an obvious answer to the question of carnivore hibernation is that a degree of lethargy occurs and these animals may indeed be "intermediate" in the process of hibernation as proposed by the late Ray Hock.

A Chemical Model of Hibernation Induction

For several decades scientists have searched for a means of inducing hibernation by some chemical or hormonal means. The brown fat so frequently present in hibernators was at one time thought to be glandular, perhaps secreting a hormone capable of maintaining the torpid condition. If a substance were to occur that controls hibernation, it would be expected to be found in the blood since all of the tissues of the hibernator's body reflect changes in metabolism and activity during hibernation. Many attempts were made to isolate a hibernation substance, but none was found, probably because of minor and seemingly insignificant errors of technique. Dawe and coworkers were finally able to isolate a substance called the *hibernation inducing trigger (HIT)* in the early 1970s. This substance, which is maintained in the plasma, can be stored for long periods of time *in vitro* at low temperatures and will induce hibernation in active individuals which are capable of the hibernation response. This substance does not seem to be species specific, as long as the species normally shows the hibernation response. In other words, the HIT from ground squirrel has been used to induce hibernation in marmots and other hibernating species. The substance appears to be protein and of a fairly high molecular weight, and it can be denatured at high temperatures characteristic of other animal proteins. The substance was found through dialysis to have a molecular weight smaller than 10,000 daltons. The HIT is absent from the blood of active hibernators and from individuals arousing from hibernation.

A substance larger than 10,000 daltons seems to be present in "summer" animals that negates the effect of the HIT and is therefore called the *anti-trigger*. This substance, when injected into animals in the late summer or fall, impedes the onset of hibernation. Dawe and Spurrier collected evidence suggesting that a balance is maintained between the HIT and the anti-trigger. When an animal is hibernating the HIT predominates in plasma concentration and maintains the hibernation state. Likewise, when the animal is active the anti-trigger predominates in both concentration and function.

Arousal from Hibernation

Hibernating mammals are frequently isolated within the hibernaculum and receive very few stimuli from the external environment. In the contiguous United States, the hibernaculum is usually below the frost line, where its temperature does not fall below 2.0° to 5.0° C during the winter months. Even in spring, when *Citellus* emerges from the hibernaculum, the temperature of the burrow is essentially the same as it is in winter. In other words, the hibernaculum provides a very constant environment, one that is quite uniform in temperature and moisture content.

What then are the cues which trigger arousal? Perhaps the hibernator's annual cycle controls the arousal "trigger" and is therefore the primary motivating force. The arousal process is usually accompanied by increased heart rate, shivering, and rapid metabolism, which brings about an equally rapid elevation in body temperature. Arousal to the active state requires varying lengths of time in the mammals. Arousal is reported to take approximately 30 minutes in bats and is apparently quite rapid in other small mammals. In the largest hibernating rodent, the marmot, arousal requires 2 hours for normothermic temperatures to be reached. In the echidna arousal may take as many as 20 hours. Complete arousal occurs in a gradual fashion, very much the same as the onset of hibernation. The dormant periods disappear and the animal is awake for extended periods of time.

SUMMARY

Air pressure at altitudes above 3,000 meters is sufficiently low to make oxygen delivery to the tissues difficult for mammals adapted to altitudes near sea level. When low altitude species are subjected to alpine conditions, acclimatization must occur in order for them to function normally. Physiological changes which occur include increased hematocrit, decreased affinity of hemoglobin for oxygen, and increased respiratory rate. Where lowland species are raised at high altitudes additional changes, such as increased heart size and lung volume, also occur.

Some species are genetically adapted to high altitudes and show very definite physiological differences from lowland species. Several members of the family Camelidae are well-adapted to alpine existence. These species, which include the llama and vicuña, have lower hematocrits than lowland species, but the hemoglobin content per erythrocytes is high enough to offset this apparent problem. Also, the hemoglobin of these species has a high affinity for oxygen, which allows blood saturation at reduced pressures. Other alpine species which are less well known also show these effects. The characteristics of adaptation to alpine existence are not lost when individuals belonging to these species are raised at low elevations.

Diving mammals show very distinct physiological modifications which allow them to survive for long periods and at great depths underwater. These adaptations include greater blood volume, greater muscle myoglobin content and an autonomic reflex which induces a variety of physiological changes. The autonomic reflex imposed in the diving mammal results in constriction of the arteries to peripheral organs, leaving normal blood flow to critical organs such as the heart, lungs, and brain. This diving reflex also causes a reduction in heart rate and perhaps a decrease in metabolic rate. The organs of some mammals also have an abundance of enzymes which are necessary in order to convert pyruvate to lactate, thus enabling them to endure ischemia for longer periods of time through the production of energy from anaerobic glycolysis and the buildup of oxygen debt. The whales, which represent the best of the diving groups, are able to collapse their lungs, thus reducing the accumulation of nitrogen in the blood.

Humans show a relatively poor but noticeable diving response. In order to maintain themselves underwater for long periods of time, humans have developed a number of mechanical devices which supply oxygen to the diver during submergence. Most of these devices harbor certain hazards, which can be overcome by modification of the respiratory gases supplied to the diver. One of the major problems was common early in the development of underwater breathing devices, which employed air as the respiratory gas. Such use led to elevated concentrations of blood nitrogen, which resulted in narcosis and other problems associated with nitrogen embolism. More recently, helium (which has greater mobility and lower solubility than nitrogen) and oxygen have been used in mixtures of respiratory gases with notable success.

Hibernation is a specialized torpor which allows mammals to avoid the coldest portion of winter by reducing metabolism and assuming a poikilothermic condition as a means of energy conservation. It occurs in several groups of mammals, which are usually fossorial and are frequently unable to migrate long distances to areas of more clement weather.

Several environmental factors, such as photoperiod, temperature, and food availability, induce hibernation in species which have evolved the ability to undergo this type of torpor. In addition, an annual rhythm is probably essential for effective hibernation to occur.

Animals enter hibernation by following an ever-increasing pattern of torpor, which culminates with intermittent bouts of quiescence lasting from one to two months. Arousal from hibernation also follows a pat-

tern of decreasing periods of torpor with longer periods of activity. Because of the almost constant environment of the hibernaculum, arousal is probably more dependent upon an animal's intrinsic rhythm than it is upon environmental cues.

A hibernation inducing trigger (HIT) was discovered in the blood of rodents. Hibernation is induced when blood from hibernating rodents is transfused into active hibernators. The hibernation inducing trigger acts in conjunction with a second blood-borne factor, the anti-trigger, which induces arousal. It is believed that the entire hibernation process from induction to arousal depends upon the interaction of these two substances.

SELECTED BIBLIOGRAPHY

CHAPTER 1

Brooks, C. M., and P. F. Cranefield. 1959. *The Historical Development of Physiological Thought.* New York: Hafner.

Bylebyl, J. J., ed. 1979. *William Harvey and His Age: The Professional and Social Context of the Discovery of the Circulation.* Baltimore, MD: Johns Hopkins University Press.

Fulton, J. F. 1983. *Selected Readings in the History of Physiology.* Darby Books.

Leake, C. D. 1956. *Some Founders of Physiology.* Bethesda, MD: International Union of Physiol. Sci. and the Amer. Physiol. Soc.

Rothschuh, K. E. 1973. *History of Physiology.* New York: Krieger.

Sourkes, T. L. 1967. *Nobel Prize Winners in Medicine and Physiology 1901–1965.* Abelard-Schumman Ltd.

CHAPTER 2

Beck, J. S. 1980. *Biomembranes: Fundamentals in Relation to Human Biology.* New York: McGraw-Hill.

Bittar, E. E. 1980. *Membrane Structure and Function.* Vol. 1. New York: Wiley.

Bronner, F., and A. Kleinzeller. 1983. *Current Topics in Membranes and Transport.* Vol. 19, *Structure, Mechanism, and Function of the Na/K Pump.* New York: Academic Press.

DeRobertis, E. D. P., and E. M. DeRobertis, Jr. 1981. *Essentials of Cell and Molecular Biology.* New York: Holt, Rinehart and Winston.

Giese, A. C. 1979. *Cell Physiology.* 5th ed. Philadelphia: Saunders.

Harrison, R., and G. C. Lunt. 1980. *Biological Membranes: Their Structure and Function.* 2nd ed. Bath, England: University of Bath.

Kleinzeller, A. 1983. *Current Topics in Membranes and Transport.* Vol. 18, *Membrane Receptors.* New York: Academic Press.

Kleinzeller, A., et al., eds. 1984. *Current Topics in Membranes and Transport.* Vol. 20, *Molecular Approaches to Epithelial Transport.* New York: Academic Press.

Starzak, M. E. 1984. *The Physical Chemistry of Membranes.* New York: Academic Press.

CHAPTER 3

Aidley, D. J. 1971. *The Physiology of Excitable Cells.* New York: Cambridge University Press.

SELECTED BIBLIOGRAPHY

Bacq, M. 1974. *Chemical Transmission of Nerve Impulses: A Historical Sketch.* Elmsford, NY: Pergamon.

Cooke, I., and M. Lipkin, Jr. 1972. *Cellular Neurophysiology: A Source Book.* New York: Holt.

De Robertis, E., and M. Dekker. 1975. *Synaptic Receptors: Isolation and Molecular Biology.* Philadelphia: Saunders.

Kuffler, S. W., and J. G. Nicholls. 1976. *From Neuron to Brain: A Cellular Approach to the Function of the Nervous System.* Sunderland, MD: Sinauer.

Tasaki, I. 1982. *Physiology and Electrochemistry of Nerve Fibers.* New York: Academic Press.

Triggle, D. J., and C. R. Triggle. 1976. *Chemical Pharmacology of the Synapse.* New York: Academic Press.

CHAPTER 4

de Lahanta, A. 1977. *Veterinary Neuroanatomy and Clinical Neurology.* Philadelphia: Saunders.

Ehrlich, Y. H., ed. 1979. *Modulators, Mediators and Specifiers in Brain Function: Interactions of Neuropeptides, Cyclic Nucleotides and Phosphoproteins in Mechanisms Underlying Neuronal Activity, Behavior and Neuropsychiatric Disorders.* New York: Plenum.

Eyzaguirre, C. 1983. *Physiology of the Nervous System.* Chicago: Year Book.

Hackman, C. H., and D. Bieger. 1976. *Chemical Transmission in the Mammalian Central Nervous System.* Baltimore, MD: University Park Press.

Herman, R. M., ed. 1976. *Neural Control of Locomotion.* New York: Plenum.

Jenkins, T. W. 1978. *Functional Mammalian Neuroanatomy with Emphasis on Dog and Cat.* New York: Lea and Febiger.

Ottoson, D. 1983. *Physiology of the Nervous System.* New York: Oxford University Press.

Pearson, R., and P. Lindsey. 1976. *The Vertebrate Brain.* New York: Academic Press.

Pinsker, H. M., and W. D. Willis, Jr., eds. 1980. *Information Processing in the Nervous System.* New York: Raven Press.

Poliakov, G. I. 1972. *Neuron Structure of the Brain.* T. Pridon (ed.). Cambridge, MA: Harvard University Press.

Schmidt, R. F. 1978. *Fundamentals of Neurophysiology.* New York: Springer-Verlag.

Shepard, G. M. 1979. *The Synaptic Organization of the Brain.* New York: Oxford University Press.

Stephenson, W. K. 1980. *Concepts in Neurophysiology.* New York: Wiley.

Stratton, D. B. 1981. *Neurophysiology.* New York: McGraw-Hill.

CHAPTER 5

Eyzaguirre, C. 1983. *Physiology of the Nervous System.* Chicago: Year Book.

Landsberg, L., and J. B. Young. 1978. Fasting, feeding and regulation of the sympathetic nervous system. *New Engl. J. Med.* 298:1295.

Moore, R. Y., and F. Bloom. 1978. Central catecholamine neuronal systems: Anatomy and physiology of dopaminergic systems. *Ann. Rev. Neurosci.* 1:129.

Ottoson, D. 1983. *Physiology of the Nervous System.* New York: Oxford University Press.

CHAPTER 6

Bouting, S. L., ed. 1976. *Transmitters in the Visual Process.* Elmsford, NY: Pergamon.

Cone, R. A., et al. 1971. *Principles of Receptor Physiology.* New York: Springer-Verlag.

Keidel, W. D. 1983. *Physiological Basis of Hearing.* New York: Thieme-Stratton.

Moller, A. R., ed. 1973. *Basic Mechanisms in Hearing.* New York: Academic Press.

Papper, A. N., and R. R. Fay. 1980. *Comparative Studies of Hearing in Vertebrates.* New York: Springer-Verlag.

Polyak, S. 1957. *The Vertebrate Visual System.* Chicago: University of Chicago Press.

Shichi, H. 1983. *Biochemistry of Vision.* New York: Academic Press.

Smythe, R. H. 1961. *Animal Vision.* London: Purnell.

———. 1975. *Vision in the Animal World.* New York: St. Martin's Press.

Wilson, V. J. 1979. *Mammalian Vestibular Physiology.* New York: Plenum.

Woolridge, D. E. 1979. *Sensory Processing in the Brain: An Exercise in Neuroconnective Modeling.* New York: Wiley.

Zettler, F., and R. Weiler, eds. 1976. *Neural Principles in Vision.* New York: Springer-Verlag.

CHAPTER 7

Alexander, R. M. 1968. *Animal Mechanics.* London: Sedgewick and Jackson.

Bullbring, E., et al. 1970. *Smooth Muscle.* London: Arnold.

Carlson, F. D., and D. R. Wilkie. 1974. *Muscle Physiology.* Englewood Cliffs, NJ: Prentice-Hall.

Close, R. I. 1972. Dynamic properties of mammalian skeletal muscles. *Physiol. Rev.* 52:129.

Cold Springs Harbor Laboratory. 1973. The mechanism of muscle contraction. *Cold Springs Harbor Symp. Quant. Biol.* 37.

Crass, M. F., III, and C. D. Barnes. 1982. *Vascular Smooth Muscle: Metabolic, Ionic and Contractile Mechanisms.* New York: Academic Press.

Hubbard, J. I. 1973. Microphysiology of vertebrate neuromuscular transmission. *Physiol. Rev.* 53:674.

Karpovitch, P. V., and W. E. Sinning. 1965. *Physiology of Muscular Activity.* Philadelphia: Saunders.

Margaria, R. 1976. *Biomechanics and Energetics of Muscular Exercise.* New York: Oxford University Press.

CHAPTER 8

Frost, H. M. 1972. *The Physiology of Cartilagenous, Fibrous and Bony Tissue.* Springfield, IL: Thomas.

Hall, B. K. 1978. *Developmental and Cellular Skeletal Biology.* New York: Academic Press.

Hancox, N. M. 1972. *Biology of Bone.* New York: Cambridge University Press.

Vaughn, J. M. 1970. *The Physiology of Bone.* Oxford: Clarendon Press.

CHAPTER 9

Altman, P. L., and D. S. Dittmer, eds. 1971. *Biological Handbooks: Blood and Other Body Fluids.* Bethesda, MD: Federation of American Societies for Experimental Biology.

Groer, M. W. 1981. *Physiology and Pathophysiology of the Body Fluids.* St. Louis, MO: Mosby.

Weiss, L. 1977. *The Blood Cells and Hemopoietic Tissues.* New York: McGraw-Hill.

CHAPTER 10

Abramson, D. I., and P. B. Dobrin. 1984. *Blood Vessels and Lymphatics in Organ Systems.* New York: Academic Press.

Altman, P. L., and D. S. Dittmer, eds. 1971. *Biological Handbooks: Respiration and Circulation.* Bethesda, MD: Federation of American Societies for Experimental Biology.

Bain, W. H., and A. M. Harper. 1967. *Blood Flow Through Arteries and Tissues.* Baltimore, MD: William and Wilkins.

Burton, A. C. 1972. *Physiology and Biophysics of the Circulation: An Introductory Text.* 2nd ed. Chicago: Year Book.

Carv, C. G., et al. 1978. *The Mechanics of Circulation.* New York: Oxford University Press.

Chien, S., S. Usami, R. J. Dellenback, and C. A. Bryant. 1971. Comparative hemorheology: Hematological implications of species differences in blood viscosity. *Biorheology,* 8:35.

Falkow, B., and E. Neil. 1971. *Circulation.* New York: Oxford University Press.

Hudlicka, O. 1973. *Muscle Blood Flow: Its Relation to Muscle Metabolism and Function.* Amsterdam: Swets and Zeitlinger.

Jarrot, B., and M. McCullock. 1975. *Physiological and Pharmacological Control of Blood Pressure.* Boston: Blackwell.

McFarlane, R. G., ed. 1970. *The Haemostatic Mechanism in Man and Other Animals.* Symposium of the Zoological Society of London, Number 27. London: Academic Press.

Onesti, G., et al. 1975. *Regulation of Blood Pressure by the Central Nervous System.* New York: Grune and Stratton.

Pedley, T. J. 1980. *The Fluid Mechanics of Large Blood Vessels.* New York: Cambridge University Press.

Stebbens, W. E., ed. 1979. *Hemodynamics and the Blood Vessel Wall.* Springfield, IL: Thomas.

Taylor, M. 1973. Hemodynamics. *Ann. Rev. Physiol.* 35:87.

CHAPTER 11

Altman, P. L., and D. S. Dittmer, eds. 1971. *Biological Handbooks: Respiration and Circulation.* Bethesda, MD: Federation of American Societies for Experimental Biology.

Katz, A. M. 1977. *Physiology of the Heart.* New York: Raven Press.

Little, R. C. 1980. *Physiology of Atrial Pacemakers and Conductive Tissue.* Mt. Kisco, NY: Futura.

Opie, L. H. 1984. *The Heart: Physiology, Metabolism, Pharmacology, and Therapy.* New York: Academic Press.

CHAPTER 12

Davenport, H. W., 1982. *Physiology of the Digestive Tract.* 5th ed. Chicago: Year Book.

Jacobson, E. D., and L. L. Shanbour. 1974. *Gastrointestinal Physiology.* Baltimore, MD: University Park Press.

Kidder, D. E., and M. J. Manners. 1978. *Digestion in the Pig.* Scientechnica.

Vonk, H. J., and J. R. H. Western. 1984. *Comparative Biochemistry and Physiology of Enzymatic Digestion.* New York: Academic Press.

CHAPTER 13

Atkinson, D. E. 1977. *Cellular Energy Metabolism and Its Regulation.* New York: Academic Press.

Brady, S. 1964. *Bioenergetics and Growth: With Special References to the Efficiency Complex in Domestic Animals.* New York: Hafner.

Herman, R. H., et al., eds. 1980. *Principles of Metabolic Control in Mammalian Systems.* New York: Plenum.

Hock, F. L. 1971. *Energy Transformation in Mammals.* Philadelphia: Saunders.

Kleiber, M. 1961. *The Fire of Life: An Introduction to Animal Energetics.* New York: Wiley.

Margaria, R. 1976. *Biomechanics and Energetics of Muscular Exercise.* Oxford: Clarendon Press.

Schmidt-Nielsen, K. 1975. Scaling in biology: The consequence of size. *J. Exp. Zool.* 194:287.

Shepherd, R. J. 1982. *Physiology and Biochemistry of Exercise.* New York: Praeger.

Sinclair, J. C., ed. 1978. *Temperature Regulation and Energy Metabolism in the Newborn.* New York: Grune and Stratton.

Sink, J. D., ed. 1974. *The Control of Metabolism.* University Park, PA: Pennsylvania State University Press.

Vonk, H. J., and J. R. H. Western. 1984. *Comparative Biochemistry and Physiology of Enzymatic Digestion.* New York: Academic Press.

CHAPTER 14

Barman, J. M. 1975. *Renal Function: Physiological and Medical Aspects.* St. Louis, MO: Mosby.

Deetjen, P., et al. 1975. *Physiology of the Kidney and of Water Balance.* New York: Springer-Verlag.

Dicker, S. E. 1970. *Mechanisms of Urine Concentration and Dilution in Mammals.* London: Arnold.

Gilmore, J. P. 1972. *Renal Physiology.* Baltimore, MD: William and Wilkins.

Hamburger, J., et al. 1971. *Structure and Function of the Kidney.* Philadelphia: Saunders.

Koushanpour, E. 1976. *Renal Physiology: Principles and Functions.* Philadelphia: Saunders.

Moffat, D. B. 1975. *The Mammalian Kidney.* New York: Cambridge University Press.

Riegel, J. A. 1972. *Comparative Physiology of Renal Excretion.* New York: Hafner.

Smith, H. W. 1961. *From Fish to Philosopher.* New York: Doubleday.

Sullivan, L. P., and J. J. Grantham. 1982. *Physiology of the Kidney.* 2nd ed. New York: Lea and Febiger.

Windhager, E. E. 1968. *Micropuncture Technique and Nephron Function.* New York: Appleton-Century-Crofts.

CHAPTER 15

Altman, P. L., and D. S. Dittmer, eds. 1971. *Biological Handbooks: Respiration and Circulation.* Bethesda, MD: Federation of American Societies for Experimental Biology.

Balfour, N. 1981. *Respiratory Physiology.* St. Louis, MO: Mosby.

Braun, H. A., et al. 1980. *Introduction to Respiratory Physiology.* Boston: Little, Brown.

Comroe, J. H., Jr. 1965. *Physiology of Respiration: An Introductory Text.* Chicago: Year Book.

Davis, D. G., and C. D. Barnes, eds. 1978. *Regulation of Ventilation and Gas Exchange.* New York: Academic Press.

De Jours, P. 1975. *Principles of Comparative Respiratory Physiology.* New York: American Elsivier.

Hughes, G. A. 1963. *Comparative Physiology of Vertebrate Respiration.* Cambridge, MA: Harvard University Press.

Jones, J. D. 1972. *Comparative Physiology of Respiration.* London: Arnold.

Lim, T. P. 1983. *Physiology of the Lung.* Springfield, IL: Thomas.

Pieper, J., and P. Scheid. 1977. Comparative physiology of respiration: Functional analysis of gas exchange organs in vertebrates. *Int. Rev. Physiol.* 14:219.

Stein, J. B. 1971. *Comparative Physiology of Respiratory Mechanics.* New York: Academic Press.

Weibel, E. R. 1973. Morphological basis of alveolar capillary gas exchange. *Physiol. Rev.* 53:419.

Widdicombe, J., and A. Davies. 1984. *Respiratory Physiology.* Baltimore, MD: University Park Press.

CHAPTER 16

Hardy, J. D., et al., eds. 1970. *Physiological and Behavioral Temperature Regulation.* Springfield, IL: Thomas.

Hensel, H. 1973. Neural processes in thermoregulation. *Physiol. Rev.* 53:948.

Kluger, M. J. 1979. *Fever.* Princeton, NJ: Princeton University Press.

Larcher, W. 1973. *Temperature and Life.* New York: Springer-Verlag.

Mount, L. M. 1979. *Adaptation to Thermal Environment: Man and His Productive Animals.* Baltimore, MD: University Park Press.

Newburgh, L. H., ed. 1968. *Physiology of Heat Regulation and the Science of Clothing.* New York: Hafner.

Satinoff, E. 1980. *Thermoregulation.* Stroudsburg, PA: Dowden, Hutchinson, & Ross.

Schmidt-Nielsen, K. 1964. *Desert Animals: Physiological Problems of Heat and Water.* New York: Oxford University Press.

Shinji, I., et al. 1972. *Advances in Climatic Physiology.* New York: Springer-Verlag.

Sinclair, J. C., ed. 1974. *Thermoregulation and Bioenergetics: Patterns of Vertebrate Survival.* New York: American Elsivier.

Whittow, G. C., ed. 1971. *Comparative Physiology of Thermoregulation.* Vol. 2, *Mammals.* New York: Academic Press.

————. 1973. *Comparative Physiology of Thermoregulation.* Vol. 3, *Special Aspects of Thermoregulation.* New York: Academic Press.

CHAPTER 17

Barrington, E. J. W. 1979. *Hormones and Evolution.* New York: Academic Press.

Buth, W. R. 1976. *Hormone Chemistry.* New York: Halsted Press.

Clegg, C. C., and A. G. Clegg. 1969. *Hormones, Cells and Organisms: The Role of Hormones in Mammals.* Stanford, CA: Stanford University Press.

Frieden, E. H. 1976. *Chemical Endocrinology.* New York: Academic Press.

Ganong, W. F., and L. Martini, eds. 1982. *Frontiers in Neuroendocrinology.* Vol. 7. New York: Raven Press.

Goldsworth, G. J., et al. 1981. *Endocrinology.* New York: Wiley.

Rickenberg, H. V., ed. 1978. *Biochemistry and Mode of Action of Hormones, II.* Baltimore, MD: University Park Press.

Suzuki, T. 1983. *Physiology of Adrenocortical Secretion.* Karger.

Turner, C. D., and J. T. Bagnara. 1976. *General Endocrinology.* 6th ed. Philadelphia: Saunders.

CHAPTER 18

Asdell, S. A. 1964. *Patterns of Mammalian Reproduction.* Comstock.

Cole, H. H., and P. T. Cupps, eds. 1977. *Reproduction in Domestic Animals.* New York: Academic Press.

Hafez, E. S. E. 1971. *Comparative Reproduction of Nonhuman Primates.* Springfield, IL: Thomas.

Rawlands, I. W., ed. 1966. *Comparative Biology of Reproduction in Mammals.* New York: Academic Press.

Sadlier, R. M. F. S. 1969. *The Ecology of Reproduction in Wild and Domestic Mammals.* London: Methuen & Co. Ltd.

CHAPTER 19

Dawe, A. R., and W. A. Spurrier. 1969. Hibernation induced in ground squirrels by blood transfusion. *Science* 163:298.

————. 1972. The blood-borne "trigger" for natural mammalian hibernation in the 13-lined ground squirrel and the woodchuck. *Cryobiology* 9:163.

Fischer, K. C., and F. E. South, eds. 1966. *Mammalian Hibernation.* Edinburgh, Scotland: Oliver and Boyd.

Fischer, K. C., A. R. Dawe, C. P. Lyman, E. Schönbaum, and F. E. South, Jr. eds. 1967. *Mammalian Hibernation III.* Edinburgh, Scotland: Oliver and Boyd.

Frisancho, A. R. 1975. Functional adaptation to high altitude hypoxia. *Science* 187:313.

Harrison, R. J., and S. H. Ridgway. 1976. *Deep Diving in Mammals.* Meadowfield Press.

Heath, D., and D. R. Williams. 1979. *Life at High Altitude.* Baltimore, MD: University Park Press.

Hock, R. 1957. *Hibernation.* New York: 5th Conf. on Cold Injury, J. Macy Found, 61–135.

Kooyman, G. L. 1972. Deep diving behavior and effects of pressure in reptiles, birds and mammals. *Symp. Soc. Exp. Biol.* 26:295.

Lyman, C. P., and P. O. Chatfield. 1955. Physiology of hibernation in mammals. *Physiol. Rev.* 35:403.

Schmidt-Nielsen, K. 1983. *Animal Physiology: Adaptation and Environment.* New York: Cambridge University Press.

Soumaleinen, P., ed. 1964. *Mammalian Hibernation II.* Finland: American Academy of Science.

GLOSSARY

Acclimation The process of physiological modification resulting from a single environmental variable or stimulus which enhances adjustment

Acclimatization The physiological modification of an organism resulting from several environmental variables or stimuli which permit better adjustment

Accommodation Adjustment, especially of the eye, for seeing objects at various distances; most frequently involves a change in the shape of the lens

Acetylcholine An acetic acid ester of choline secreted by certain nerve terminals; a *neurotransmitter*

Acetylcholinesterase An enzyme present in nervous tissue and muscle and red blood cells which catalyzes the *hydrolysis* of acetylcholine to choline and acetic acid

Acini Follicles or pouchlike structures; as in the acini of the thyroid or pancreas

Acquired immunity The acquisition of the ability to produce *antibodies* against newly introduced *antigens*; as opposed to *natural immunity*, which is inherent

Acromegaly Abnormal enlargement of the extremities of the skeleton (nose, jaws, fingers, and toes) caused by hypersecretion of the pituitary growth hormone after maturity

Action potential A moving *potential* propagated along a nerve membrane

Active tension Tension developed by contraction within the muscle, as opposed to tension developed as the result of stretching

Adaptation Genetic change in a population which makes it more suitable to exist in a particular habitat

Adaptation (of nerves) The internal adjustment of the receptor which results in a reduced response to the stimulus

Adipose tissue Fat tissue

Adrenergic Capable of releasing *norepinephrin (noradrenalin)* at nerve terminals

Adrenocorticoids (adrenocorticosteroids) One of the steroid *hormones* produced by the adrenal cortex

Aerobic glycolysis The breakdown of carbohydrates in the presence of oxygen; chiefly that part of the glycolytic cycle between citric acid and oxaloacetic acid

---

Italicized terms also appear in the glossary.

Afferent Carrying toward a center; afferent *neurons* carry impulses toward the central nervous system, and afferent arterioles carry blood toward the *glomerulus* of the kidney

After potential A potential developed as part of the *action potential* that follows the peak potential; sometimes called an after depolarization

Agglutination The clumping of particles in blood; usually red blood cells

Agglutinins Specific substances or *antibodies* capable of causing the *agglutination* of bacteria, red blood cells, or other particles

Agglutinogens Genetically determined *antigens* located on the surface of the erythrocyte

Allen's rule Observed reduction in appendage lengths in mammals within the same species or family as the northernmost limits of the range or distribution is approached

Allocortex Cortex of primitive vertebrates which remains as the basal portion of the cortex in mammals, particularly in higher groups of primates and cetaceans

Allometric growth Unequal or disproportionate growth among different portions of the body

All or none law Description of an *action potential* which is not graded; i.e., action potential occurs if *threshold* is reached by the stimulus, but greater stimuli do not result in more intense *potentials*

Alpha receptors Membrane sites which bind to *catecholamines* to mediate vasoconstriction

Altricial Undeveloped; incapable of following the adult; confined to the den or lair

Amphiarthrosis A form of articulation midway between *diarthrosis* and *synarthrosis,* in which the articulating bony surfaces are separated by an elastic substance to which both are attached; mobility is slight but may be exerted in all directions

Anabolism The buildup or assimilation of cellular compounds

Anaerobic glycolysis The breakdown of sugars into simpler compounds, usually beginning with glucose and terminating with pyruvate or lactate

Anamnestic response The rapid reappearance of large quantities of *antibodies* in the blood following entrance of an *antigen* to which an animal has previously developed an immunity

Anastomsis The joining of two or more hollow organs such as blood vessels

Androgens Substances producing or stimulating male characteristics; such as testosterone

Anemia Reduction below normal of the number of erythrocytes, quantity of *hemoglobin*, or the volume of packed red blood cells in the blood

Annulospiral ending Stretch receptor located in *intrafusal* muscle fiber

Anoxia Deficiency of oxygen

Antibody A specific substance which interacts with *antigens* to produce immunity

Antigen A foreign substance in the blood which induces the formation of *antibodies* or reacts with them

Apneustic center A group of nerve cell bodies located in the *pons* which prolongs inspiration when stimulated

Appendicular skeleton Portion of the skeleton consisting of the appendages and related bones of the sacral and pectoral girdles

Arachnoid The membrane interposed between the *dura mater* and the *pia mater* and having a weblike appearance; one of the *meninges*

Arteriosclerosis A disease associated with extensive deposits of calcium in the middle layer of the artery; sometimes called Mönckeberg's arteriosclerosis

Artiodactyla Order of hoofed mammals containing the pigs, peccaries, hippopotami, camels, deer, cattle, sheep, goats, and antelope, whose most diagnostic trait is the presence of a paraxonic hoof

Astigmatism Ametropia caused by differences in curvature in different meridians of the refractive surface of the eye so that light rays are not sharply focused on the retina

Atheroschlerosis A disease primarily associated with the accumulation of fatty deposits called plaques within the lumen of the large arteries

Atresia Abnormal closing of a passage, or the absence of a normal body opening

Auditory bulla The bony structure enclosing the middle ear

Auerbach's plexus (myenteric plexus) A network of nerve fibers located between the muscle layers of the intestine

Auscultatory method The measurement of blood pressure by listening for sounds of blood flow through an artery which has been collapsed by means of external pressure

A-V node Atrioventricular node

Axial skeleton Part of the skeleton consisting of the vertebral column and skull

Axolemma The surface membrane of the *axon*

Axon That process of a nerve cell by which impulses travel away from the *nerve cell body*

Axoplasm Cytoplasm of an *axon*

Bainbridge reflex A rise in heart rate induced by increased pressure in the right atrium

Baroreceptor A receptor stimulated by pressure change in the circulatory system

Basal metabolic rate *Metabolism* determined in a rested individual approximately 12 to 14 hours after the last meal

Bergmann's rule Characteristic increase in size observed in individuals of the same species or family as the northernmost limit of its range is approached

Beta receptors *Catecholamine receptors* which mediate increase in rate and strength of cardiac muscle contraction, dilation of arterial and bronchial smooth muscle and which enhance *glycogenolysis*, lipolysis, and insulin, glucagon, and renin secretion.

Bile Secretion of the liver which is collected in the gall bladder and consists chiefly of *bile salts* and waste products from *catabolism* of *hemoglobin*

Bile salts Sodium and potassium salts of *bile* acids conjugated to glycine and taurine

Bilirubin The orange or yellow pigment in *bile*

Biliverdin A greenish pigment in *bile* formed in the *oxidation* of *bilirubin*

Binocular vision Having sight in which the visual fields of both eyes overlap

Bipolar neuron Nerve cell having a single *dendrite* and a single *axon*

Blastocyst A stage in the development of the mammalian embryo consisting of the trophoblast and an inner cell mass

Blood-brain barrier A selective mechanism which prohibits the entry of many blood-borne substances into the *cerebrospinal fluid*

Bohr effect Decrease in affinity of *hemoglobin* for oxygen in the presence of carbon dioxide and hydrogen ion

Bolus A lump or mass of injested food in the digestive tract

Bowman's capsule The expanded blind end of the *nephron* which encloses the *glomerulus*

Bradycardia Slow heart rate

Bursa A sac or pouch of synovial fluid located at friction points, especially joints

Calcitonin *Hormone* secreted by the parafollicular cells of the thyroid gland

Calorie Standard amount of heat necessary to raise one gram of water one degree Centigrade; 0.239 Joules

Calorimetry A measurement of heat; in thermal physiology, the measurement of the heat transfer between a tissue, an organ, or an organism and its environment

Calorimetry, direct The direct physical measurement of heat, usually the rate of transfer of heat between a tissue, an organ, or an organism and its environment

Calorimetry, indirect The measurement of the rate of transfer of a material involved in the transformation of chemical energy into heat between a tissue, an organ, or an organism and its environment; the process requires the calculation of the heat transfer from an empirically established relation between the material transfer and the heat transfer

Calyx   A cuplike division of the kidney pelvis

Canaliculus   A small channel or canal, as in bones, where they connect the *lacunae*

Cancellous bone   Skeletal portions having a reticular or latticework structure as in *spongy tissue* of bone

Cardiac output   The total volume of blood pumped from the heart in a unit of time

Carnivoran lethargy   Winter sleep seen in members of the order Carnivora which resembles *hibernation*

Carnivore   An animal whose diet is exclusively or largely meat

Catabolism   The breakdown of molecules into smaller units with the release of energy

Catecholamines   Any of a group of sympathomimetic amines (including dopamine, *epinephrine*, and *norepinephrine*), the aromatic portion of whose molecule is catechol

Categorical hemisphere   Portion of the brain devoted to language functions and sequential, analytical processes; dominant hemisphere

Cecant   An animal whose digestive process is dependent upon digestion and fermentation in the intestinal diverticulum known as the *cecum*

Cecum   A blind pouch at the proximal end of the large intestine to which the ileum is attached

Cellulose   A fibrous carbohydrate composed of glucose molecules which are interconnected by means of β-1,4-linkage

Central nervous system (CNS)   Primarily, the brain and spinal cord

Cerebrospinal fluid   Liquid found in the ventricles of the brain, spinal cord, and subarachnoid space

Chloride shift   A series of reactions involving oxygen and carbon dioxide exchange in the blood, signified by the movement of chloride ions into and out of the cell

Cholinergic   A term applied to nerve endings which release *acetylcholine* at a *synapse*

Cholinesterase   see *acetylcholinesterase*

Chondroblast   An immature cartilage-producing cell

Chondrocyte   A cartilage cell

Chronotropic   Affecting the time or rate

Chyme   The semifluid mixture of partly digested food and digestive secretions found in the stomach and small intestine during digestion of a meal

Circadian   About a day; occurring in a 24-hour cycle

Citric acid cycle   see *tricarboxylic acid cycle*

Clo   A unit to express the relative thermal insulation values of various clothing assemblies: 1 clo = $0.18°C \cdot m^2 \cdot h \cdot kcal^{-1}$ = $0.155°C \cdot m^2 \cdot W^{-1}$

Coagulation   Formation of a clot

Cochlea   A winding, cone-shaped tube forming a portion of the inner ear and containing the *organ of Corti*

Collecting duct   Tubule which empties into the pelvis of the kidney

Colloidal osmotic pressure   The pressure generated by the colloids retained in the plasma after filtration of plasma through the endothelial membrane of the capillary

Colostrum   First "milk," usually high in *antibody* concentration

Concentration gradient   A change in concentration over a particular distance

Cone   Retinal cells from which color vision is derived

Copraphagy   To consume feces

Cordal reflex   Neural reflex which can be completed with peripheral nerves and the nerves of the spinal cord

Cornification   Conversion of epithelium to the stratified squamous type

Corpora nigra   Dark pigmented bodies extending inwardly from the rim of the pupil in certain ungulates

Corpus albicans White fibrous tissue that replaces the regressing *corpus luteum* in the ovary during the latter half of pregnancy or soon after *ovulation,* when pregnancy does not supervene

Corpus callosum Arched mass of white matter composed of transverse fibers connecting the cerebral hemispheres

Corpus hemorragicum Ovarian follicle containing blood which is formed immediately after *ovulation*

Corpus luteum Yellow glandular mass in the ovary formed from an ovarian follicle that has matured and discharged its ovum

Cortex The outer layer of an organ or structure

Critical temperature, lower The ambient temperature below which the rate of metabolic heat production of a resting *thermoregulating* animal increases by shivering and/or nonshivering thermogenic processes to maintain thermal balance

Critical temperature, upper The ambient temperature above which *thermoregulatory* evaporative heat loss processes of a resting thermoregulating animal are recruited

Crossed extensor reflex Cordal response involving retraction of a limb on the ipsilateral side and extension of a contralateral limb

Cytochrome system Enzyme system in the mitochondrion which is involved with electron transport and *oxidative phosphorylation*

Cytogenic Forming or producing cells

Cytopempsis Vesicular transport through endothelial cells of capillary walls

Cytopenia Reduction or lack of cellular elements in the circulating blood

Dead air space Portion of inhaled air which does not come in contact with respiratory membranes where gas exchange is possible

Deamination Removal of an amino group ($-NH_2$) from a compound

Decibel A unit for measuring the volume of sound, equal to the logarithm of the ratio of the intensity of the sound to the intensity of an arbitrarily chosen standard sound

Deciduous Anything which is cast off at maturity

Decussation A crossing over, as between corresponding anatomical parts forming an X shape

Delayed implantation The process whereby embryonic development is arrested and the time between fertilization and implantation is prolonged

Dendrite Threadlike processes composing most of the receptive surfaces of a *neuron*

Depolarization The process of neutralizing polarity

Dermatome The cutaneous area developed from one embryonic spinal cord segment and receiving most of its innervation from one spinal nerve

Diabetogenic Capable of producing diabetes

Diapedesis The passage of white blood cells through intact blood vessel walls

Diaphysis The shaft of a long bone

Diarthrosis An articulation in which opposing bones move freely; as in a hinge joint

Diastole Period of relaxation of the heart muscles

Diencephalon The posterior part of the forebrain consisting of the *hypothalamus, thalamus,* epithalamus, and metathalamus

Digestion The act of converting food materials into particles which can be absorbed through the intestinal mucosa

Diuretic An agent which increases the flow of urine

Diurnal Occurring during the day, as distinct from the night; also, occurring daily

Dorsal Pertaining to the back or top

Dura mater The outer, tough covering of the brain; one of the *meninges*

Dyne The metric unit of force, being that amount which would, during each second, produce an acceleration of one centimeter per second in a particle of one gram mass

Ectopic   Out of the normal location

Ectotherm   An animal which depends upon an external source of heat for control of body temperature

Ectothermy   The pattern of *thermoregulation* in which the body temperature depends on the behaviorally and autonomically regulated uptake of heat from the environment

Edema   An abnormal accumulation of fluid in the tissues

Efferent   To carry away from a center; efferent *neurons* carry impulses away from the central nervous system, and efferent arterioles carry blood away from the *glomerulus* of the kidney

Electrocardiogram (EKG)   Record produced by measuring electrical changes of the heart

Embden-Myerhoff pathway   *Anaerobic glycolysis*, generally beginning with glucose and terminating with pyruvic acid

Embolism   The sudden blocking of an artery by a clot or other foreign material

Emiocytosis   Cell regurgitation, *exocytosis*

Emmetropic   An ideal optical condition in which parallel rays focus on the retina of the eye

Emulsion   A colloidal system in which both the dispersed phase and the dispersion medium are liquids

Encephalization   Assumption of greater control by the brain

Endochondral ossification   The formation of bone within cartilage

Endocrine gland   A ductless gland

Endocytosis   The uptake by a cell of particles that are too large to diffuse through the cell membrane; it includes both phagocytosis and *pinocytosis*

Endometrium   Lining of the uterus

Endopeptidase   An enzyme which *hydrolyzes* peptide bonds within an amino-acid chain

Endothelium   The layer of epithelial cells which forms the inner lining of blood and lymph vessels and various cavities of the body

Enzyme   A biological catalyst, usually a protein

Epimysium   The fibrous sheath around the entire skeletal muscle

Epinephrine   A *catecholamine* produced by the adrenal medulla and the sympathetic nervous system

Epiphyseal closure   Termination of linear bone growth which occurs when the shaft of a bone unites with the epiphyses

Epiphyseal plate   The cartilagenous plate separating the primary and secondary *ossification* centers of bone

Epiphysis   The end of a long bone which is usually larger in diameter than the shaft (the diaphysis)

Epithelium   The cells composing the skin and lining the passages of the hollow organs of the digestive, respiratory, and urinary systems

Eructation   The volitional expulsion of gas or solid material from the stomach

Erythrocyte   Red blood cell (rbc)

Estivation   A state of summer lethargy with a reduction in body temperature and *metabolism* demonstrated by some animals which are temperature regulators when active

Excitatory postsynaptic potential   A *potential*, developed on the *dendrite* of a postsynaptic *neuron*, capable of inducing an *action potential*

Exocrine gland   One of the glands whose products are transferred to their site of action by means of ducts or vessels

Exocytosis   The discharge of particles from the cell which are too large to diffuse through the membrane

Exogenous   Originating outside an organ or part

Exopeptidase   An enzyme which *hydrolyzes* a terminal amino acid of a protein molecule

Experimental design   Description of an experiment indicating techniques used and probable data derived

Expiratory reserve   A volume of air which can be exhaled in addition to the *tidal volume*

Exteroceptor   A sense organ adapted for the reception of stimuli from outside the body

Extrafusal fibers Muscle fibers capable of performing the work of contraction in skeletal muscle

Facilitation The increased excitability of a *neuron* after stimulation by a presynaptic impulse below *threshold*

Feces Excrement discharged from the bowels

Feedback regulation The return of some of the output of a system as input, which exerts some control in the rate at which a process proceeds

Fever A pathological condition in which there is an abnormal rise in core temperature; the extent of the rise is variable

Fibrin An insoluble protein essential to the clotting of blood

Filtration pressure The net pressure resulting from *hydrostatic*, colloidal-osmotic, and tissue pressures; responsible for the exchange of fluid between the capillaries and the tissues

Flatus Gas or air in the digestive tract; commonly used to denote the passage of gas rectally

Fontanel A soft area in the skull of an undeveloped animal

Foramen A passage or opening; a communication between two cavities of an organ or a hole in a bone for the passage of vessels or nerves

Fossa A furrow or shallow depression

Fovea centralis A small pit in the center of the *macula lutea* where the retinal layers are spread aside and light falls directly on the *cones*

Funiculus The white substance of the spinal cord lying on either side between the dorsal and ventral roots

Gamete A reproductive cell; spermatozoa or ovum

Gametogenesis Formation of *gametes* in the gonads

Ganglion A group of nerve cell bodies outside the *central nervous system*

Gastrointestinal tract Stomach and intestinal (digestive) tract

G-cells Flask-shaped cells of the gastric (stomach) mucosa which produce and secrete gastrin

General Adaptation Syndrome A series of debilitating responses to nonspecific stress; usually involves the adrenal glands

Generator potential A local *potential* developed on a receptor membrane which is capable of evoking an *action potential*

Gestation The period of intrauterine fetal development

Glial cells (neuroglia) The supporting cells of nervous tissue; consisting of astrocytes, *oligodendrocytes*, and microglia in the central nervous system

Glomerulus A rounded mass of nerves or blood vessels, especially the microscopic tuft of capillaries that is surrounded by the expanded part of each kidney tubule

Glucocorticoids *Adrenocorticoids* which enhance glucose utilization and lipid mobilization

Gluconeogenesis Formation of glucose or glucose intermediates from lipids or proteins

Glycogenesis The formation of glycogen from glucose

Glycogenolysis *Hydrolysis* of glycogen to form glucose

Glycolysis The *catabolism* of glucose

Golgi bottle neuron A cell responsible for postsynaptic inhibition

Graafian follicle Maturing ovarian follicle

Gradient A difference in concentration or intensity over a given distance

Gray matter Portions of the *central nervous system* which are largely unmyelinated and therefore having a gray appearance

Gray ramus communicans Structures of the nervous system which contain the postganglionic fibers that connect the ganglia of the sympathetic trunk to the spinal nerves.

Gut The intestine or bowel

Haldane effect The shift in the carbon dioxide equilibrium curve with deoxygenation and oxygenation of *hemoglobin*

Hematocrit The volume percentage of erythrocytes in whole blood

Hemoconcentration A decrease in fluid content of the blood with resulting increase in concentration of its formed elements

Hemocytoblasts The free stem cells from which blood cells are formed

Hemoglobin Oxygen carrying pigment of the red blood cell

Hemopoietic tissue Blood cell forming tissue

Herbivore An animal which consumes chiefly plant material

Hering-Breuer reflex A method of breathing regulation based upon stimulation of stretch receptors when the lungs are inflated, which results in forced exhalation

Heterothermy A condition of exhibiting widely differing temperatures throughout the body at a given time

Heterotopic skeletal elements Bony units not being directly part of the *axial* or *appendicular skeletons*

Hibernation The state of winter lethargy with a reduction in body temperature and *metabolism* of some animals that are temperature regulators when active

High energy phosphates Compounds containing chemical bond energy for release and utilization by the cell

Homeostasis Steady state, or tendency to stability in the normal physiological state of an organism

Homeotherm An animal capable of maintaining a relatively constant body temperature despite fluctuations in environmental temperature

Hormone A specific regulating or activating substance produced in the body, usually by one of the *endocrine glands*

Humor Any fluid of the body

Hydrolysis The addition of water or water molecules to a substrate in the process of *catabolism*

Hydrostatic Pertaining to the pressure caused by the weight of liquids or force developed by liquids

Hypercapnia An abnormal amount of carbon dioxide in the blood

Hyperemia An excess of blood in an area or part of the body

Hyperglycemia An excess of glucose in the blood

Hyperplasia An abnormal increase in the number of normal cells in a tissue or organ, thus increasing its size

Hyperpolarization Greater than normal polarity developed across a nerve membrane, usually leading to a less excitable state

Hypertrophy An excessive enlargement or overgrowth of an organ or part, normally due to an increase in cell volume with no change in cell number

Hypophyseal portal system One of the two portal systems found in mammals, connecting the hypothalamus with the anterior pituitary

Hypophysis The pituitary gland

Hypothalamus The part of the *diencephalon* forming the floor and part of the lateral wall of the third ventricle of the brain

Hypoxia Lack of adequate oxygen; also *anoxia*

Immunity The condition of being resistant to a disease or foreign substance

Immunodeficiency Incapable of producing sufficient *antibodies*

Immunoglobulin Plasma proteins which combine with *antigens; antibodies*

Implantation (nidation) The fixing or attachment of the *blastocyst* to the *endometrium*

Inhibitory postsynaptic potential Hyperpolarized state of the postsynaptic membrane in which excitation is difficult

Inotropic   Increase in the force of contraction

Inspiratory reserve   The quantity of air which can be inhaled in addition to the *tidal volume*

Integument   Skin; the covering of an organ

Intercalated discs   Disclike appearance of inter-digitated membranes of adjacent cardiac muscle cells

Internal (intrinsic) clotting mechanism   Clotting caused by factors within the bloodstream, not necessarily involving physical trauma

Internal milieu   Internal environment; particularly the blood and lymph in which cells are bathed

Interneuron   *Internuncial cell; neurons* which transmit impulses between different parts of the spinal cord

Internuncial cell   *interneuron*

Interoceptors   Sensory receptors located in the internal organs

Interstitial fluid   Fluid located in the gaps or spaces between cells, tissues, or structures

Intrafusal fiber   Fibers which do not generate force through contraction, but compose the nuclear bag cells and nuclear chain cells

Intramembranous ossification   Bone formation within connective tissue membranes, as opposed to *ossification* of cartilage *(endochondral ossification)*

Ischemia   A deficiency of blood in a cell or tissue

Juxtaglomerular apparatus   Specifically arranged renal arterioles and renal tubules which are responsible for the production of renin

Kinins   A group of endogenous peptides that act on blood vessels, smooth muscles, and nociceptive nerve endings

Krebs cycle   see *tricarboxylic acid cycle*

Lactation   Giving milk; usually expressed as "period of lactation" or that time when the animal is producing milk

Lacteals   Intestinal lymph vessels that absorb fat from digested food

Lactogenesis   The formation of milk in the *mammary glands*

Lacuna   A small cavity, such as that found in bones, which encloses an *osteoblast*

Lamellae   A thin leaf, plate, or disk

Latent period   The period elapsing between the application of a stimulus and the response

Lateral   To the side

Law of specific nerve energies   The concept that for every stimulus there is a specific receptor which is best adapted to receive it

Leukocyte   White blood cell

Leukopenia   A decrease in the number of white blood cells below the normal count for the species

Leutinization   The changes in ovarian follicular tissue brought about by the presence of leutinizing hormone (LH)

Libido   Sex drive

Limbic system   Part of the *allocortex* and composed of several nuclei that control the emotions and basic drives

Lipase   An enzyme which *hydrolyzes* esters of fatty acids

Local circuit theory   The hypothesis that action potentials are propagated by means of local circuits, which bring areas of the cell membrane adjacent to the *action potential* to *threshold*

Lumen   The passageway (interior) or opening of a hollow organ such as a blood vessel

Macula densa   A zone of heavily nucleated cells in the distal *renal* tubule; usually a part of the *juxtaglomerular apparatus*

Macula lutea   A yellowish depression on the retina which has a high density of *cones*

Mammary gland   Milk producing gland of mammals

Marey reflex Also known as the carotid sinus reflex; a change in heart rate as a result of the response of *baroreceptors* to the blood pressure in the carotid sinus

Mastication Chewing

Meatus A passage or opening; especially the external portion of a canal

Medial Pertaining to the midline

Meissner's plexus A nerve net found in the intestine beneath the inner muscle layer

Melatonin A hormone produced by the pineal gland which apparently has a blanching effect in the skin of some species

Meninges Membranes or coverings of the central nervous system, consisting of the *pia mater*, *dura mater*, and *arachnoid*

Mesencephalon The midbrain

Metabolism The chemical changes which occur within an organism; includes *anabolism* and *catabolism*

Metanephros Embryonic kidney which gives rise to the adult mammalian kidney

Microflora Microscopic organisms such as bacteria and protozoans found in various parts of the body, especially the gastrointestinal tract

Micturition Urination

Milliosmole One thousandth of an osmole (standard unit of osmotic pressure)

Mineralocorticoids *Steroid hormones* which have as their primary function the regulation of minerals of the body, usually by means of their effect on the kidney

Miniature end-plate potential A nonpropagated local *potential* caused by continuous release of small amounts of *acetylcholine* from the presynaptic *neuron* during the resting phase

Modality A particular environmental change or factor which gives rise to a specific sensation

Monogastric Possessing a single stomach

Monophasic action potential A moving *potential* recorded by one internal and one external electrode so that a single *spike* is produced as the potential passes over them

Monopolar neuron A nerve cell having only one extension from the *nerve cell body*; not found in adult mammals

Monosynaptic reflex A reflex involving only two *neurons* and therefore a single neuronal *synapse*

Monotocous Giving birth to only one offspring per *gestational* period

Motor end plate The thickened portion of the muscle membrane which forms part of the *myoneural junction*

Motor neuron A nerve cell which excites another nerve cell or such receptive tissue as skeletal muscle

Mucosa Mucous membrane

Multiparous Having given birth to more than one offspring

Multiple fiber summation Recruitment of motor units within a muscle so that more and more fibers are added to the contraction

Multipolar neuron A nerve cell with several extensions from the *nerve cell body*, usually having several *axons*

Muscle twitch A single muscle contraction

Myelin The lipid substance surrounding the *axons* of myelinated nerve fibers

Myeloid (marrow) tissue Pertaining to the cells of bone marrow

Myoepithelium Tissue made up of contractile epithelial cells

Myofibril One of the slender threads of a muscle fiber, composed of numerous *myofilaments*

Myofilament Ultramicroscopic threadlike components of *myofibrils*; thick ones contain myosin, thin ones actin

Myoglobin A ferrous protoporphyrin globin complex resembling *hemoglobin* present in *sarcoplasm* of muscle, which acts as a store of oxygen

Myometrium The muscular wall of the uterus

Myoneural junction   A synapse formed by motor nerve and muscle cells

Myopia   Defect in vision so that objects can only be seen distinctly when very close to the eyes; nearsightedness

Natural immunity   The inherent ability to produce *antibodies* against newly introduced *antigens*; as opposed to *acquired immunity*

Neocortex   The recently evolved cortex found in greatest abundance in higher primates and cetaceans; believed to be directly associated with conscious responses

Nephron   The functional unit of the kidney consisting of Bowman's capsule, convoluted tubules, and loop of Henle.

Nernst Equation   Mathematical analysis of electromotive force based upon diffusion *gradients* of a single ionic species

Nerve cell body   A portion of the *neuron* which contains the nucleus

Nerve center (nucleus)   A group of *nerve cell bodies* in the *central nervous system* which has a specific function or affects a specific part of the organism

Neurolemma (neurilemma)   The thin membrane spirally enwrapping the *myelin* layers of myelinated nerve fibers and the *axons* of unmyelinated nerve cells

Neuron   A nerve cell

Neurotransmitter   A substance produced by a nerve cell to excite or inhibit other nerves or tissues

Newton's law of cooling   Explanation that the rate of cooling is directly proportional to the difference between the temperature of the body in question (the heat source) and the environment (the heat sink)

Nidation   Implantation of the *blastocyst*

Node of Ranvier   Spaces between successive *Schwann cells*

Nonprotein respiratory quotient   The ratio of carbon dioxide produced to oxygen consumed, less the carbon dioxide and oxygen associated with protein *catabolism*

Norepinephrine (noradrenalin)   *Neurotransmitter* produced by the sympathetic nervous system and the adrenal medulla

Nuclear bag cell   *Intrafusal* muscle cells which contain stretch receptors called *annulospiral endings* and have contractile portions at either end of the cell

Nuclear chain cell   *Intrafusal* muscle cell which is similar to nuclear bag cells but contains no contractile portions

Occlusion   A less-than-expected postsynaptic response after presynaptic stimulation; result of spatial summation of stimuli from two or more presynaptic *neurons* on one postsynaptic neuron

Oil-water solubility coefficient   *Partition coefficient*

Oligodendrocytes   The nonneural cells of ectodermal origin forming part of the adventitial structure of the *central nervous system*

Omnivore   Organism which consumes both plants and animals

Oogenesis   The formation and development of the ovum

Opsonization   The rendering of bacterial and other cells subject to phagocytosis

Organ of Corti   Portion of the inner ear believed to be primarily responsible for conversion of mechanical vibrations into neural impulses. This structure consists of hair cells, basilar membrane, and tectorial membrane

Orifice   An aperture or opening

Osmoreceptors   *Neurons* which respond to changing osmotic concentrations in the body fluids

Ossicles   Bones of the middle ear: incus, stapes, and malleus

Ossification   The formation of bone substance

Osteoblast   A cell capable of bone production

Osteoclast A large multinuclear cell associated with absorption and removal of bone

Osteocyte An *osteoblast* that has become embedded within the bone matrix, occupying a flat oval cavity and sending, through openings in its walls, cytoplasmic processes that connect with other osteocytes in developing bone

Ostium Any small opening; especially an entrance into a hollow organ or canal

Ovulation Expulsion of the egg from the mature Graafian follicle

Oxidation The process by which electrons are removed from atoms or ions

Oxidative phosphorylation The production of high-energy phosphate from energy released during oxidation of cytochrome enzymes, inorganic phosphate, and ADP

Oxygen-carrying capacity The total volume of oxygen that can be maintained by a specific unit of blood

Oxygen debt The deficiency of oxygen which may occur during exercise; usually associated with the buildup of lactic acid

P$_{50}$ The partial pressure of a gas, usually oxygen, at which 50 percent saturation of the blood is reached

Papilla A small projection or elevation

Parasympathetic nervous system A branch of the autonomic nervous system associated with ruminating, quiescent activities; produces *acetylcholine* as a *neurotransmitter*

Parenchyma The essential parts of any organ, concerned with its function

Parenteral Situated or occurring outside the intestines

Parous Having borne at least one offspring

Partial pressure The fraction of the total pressure contributed by any particular gas in a mixture of gases

Partition coefficient (oil-water solubility coefficient) The ratio of the concentration of a substance dissolved in oil to its concentration dissolved in water in an oil-water mixture

Parturition Expulsion of the fetus from the womb

Passive tension Any muscle tension not developed through contraction

Pectoral Pertaining to the chest

Perimysium Connective tissue demarcating a fascicle of skeletal muscle fibers; an extension of the *epimysium*

Perineum The pelvic floor; the space between the anus and scrotum in males and between the anus and vulva in females

Perissodactyla One of the hoofed mammals in which only one of the toes of the ancestor remains as the hoof (e.g., zebra)

Peristalsis The rhythmic movement of the gastrointestinal tract resulting in the flow of food toward the anus

Permease An enzyme which transports substances across a membrane

Phagocytosis Literally "cell eating"; the process by which a cell engulfs another cell or particle

Phasic muscle Muscle fibers which contract for short periods of time and do not maintain prolonged tension; fast-twitch muscle fibers

Phenylketonuria An inherent error of *metabolism* in which ketone derivatives of phenylalanine build up in the blood

Pheromones A substance secreted to the outside of the body which elicits specific behavior and physiological patterns when received by other members of the same species

Phosphorylation The addition of a phosphate group to a compound

Physiology The study of function in the living organism

Pia mater The innermost of the *meninges*; adheres tightly to the brain and spinal cord

Pigment A coloration of the body or body part

Pinna The projecting part of the external ear

Pinocytosis Cell drinking, absorption of droplets of fluids by cells

Pitch   Sound frequency; tone

Placenta   The organ formed from maternal and fetal tissues whose primary function is nourishment of the fetus

Plasma   The fluid portion of blood

Platelets   Small granulated bodies in blood formed from bits of cytoplasm broken off from megakaryocytes in the bone marrow; chiefly known for their role in blood clotting

Pleura   The serous membrane that enfolds the lungs and lines the walls of the chest and diaphragm

Plexus   A network of nerves, veins, or lymphatic vessels

Pneumotaxic center   *Central-nervous-system* nucleus located in the *pons* which regulates breathing rate

Poikilothermy   The pattern of *thermoregulation* of a species exhibiting a large variability of core temperature as a proportional function of ambient temperature

Poiseuille's law   Relationship expressing interaction of pressure, flow, and resistance in a liquid system

Polygastric   Possessing more than one stomach

Polysynaptic reflex   A cordal response to a stimulus involving several *neurons*

Polytocous   Usually litter-bearing

Pons   A bridge; the portion of the brainstem between the medulla and the midbrain

Porphyrin   An iron- (or magnesium-) containing cyclic tetrapyrole derivative occurring universally in protoplasm; the iron-containing compound is essential to mammalian respiratory pigments

Portal system   System of veins leading into a specific organ (i.e. hepatic or renal portal systems)

Postpartum   After parturition

Potential (transmembrane potential)   An electrical *gradient* which exists across a membrane

Precapillary sphincter   A valve which controls the release of blood from a metarteriole into a capillary bed

Precocial   Developed to an advanced stage at birth; a mammalian offspring which can follow its mother and is not restricted to a nest at birth

Preload (muscle)   The weight applied to muscle prior to the beginning of active contraction

Prepotential   A *potential* which precedes the discharge of a membrane potential, such as the gradually declining potential which leads to the discharge of the S-A node of the heart

Pressor effects   Factors altering blood pressure

Primordial   Existing first; especially primordial egg cells in the ovary

Principal focus   The point in front of the retina where the maximum number of light rays converge

Pronephros   The first embryonic kidney

Proprioceptors   Any of the sensory nerve endings that give information concerning movements and position of the body; they occur chiefly in muscles, tendons, and the labyrinth

Prosencephalon   The forebrain

Prostaglandins   A group of fatty acids found in semen, menstrual fluid, and various tissues of many species; these chemicals stimulate contractility of smooth muscle and have the ability to lower blood pressure

Protease   An enzyme which *hydrolyzes* proteins

Proteolysis   The hydrolytic breakdown of proteins into smaller peptides

Protuberance   A part that is prominent beyond a surface, such as a knob

Proximal   Near the point of origin; near the center

Pseudomonopolar neuron   A nerve cell which appears to have only one cytoplasmic extension from the *nerve cell body*, but which in fact, is two extensions capable of serving as an *axon* and a *dendrite* (e.g., sensory neurons of the dorsal horn of the spinal cord)

Pseudopregnancy   False pregnancy

Pulmonary circulation (lesser circulation)
The flow of blood from the heart to lungs and
back to the heart

Pulmonary compliance   The ability of the lungs
to assume the shape of the thorax during exhalation and inhalation

Pupillary adaptation   Change in the pupil diameter to control the amount of light entering
the eye

Pyramidal system   Motor tracts in the ventral
portion of the medulla, most prominent in primates

Pyrogen   The generic term for any substance,
whether exogenous or endogenous, which
causes a *fever* when introduced into or released in the body

Q$_{10}$ Effective temperature on biological reactions
in which the reaction rate doubles for every ten
degree rise in temperature

QRS complex   A portion of the electrocardiogram caused by ventricular depolarization
and auricular repolarization

Ramp retina   A retina whose distance from the
center of the lens changes at different locations
within the eye; forms a ramp in which focal
distance can be changed by changing the angle
of incidence of light

Ramus   A branch; especially a nerve or blood
vessel

Receptor   A nerve ending capable of receiving a
stimulus

Reduction   The addition or acceptance of electrons by an ion or molecule so as to reduce its
positive valence

Referred pain   Pain which is apparently mis-
placed from its true site of origin

Refraction   The bending of light rays as they
pass through different media

Refractory period, absolute   The time at which
the cell cannot be stimulated

Refractory period, relative   The time at which
it is more difficult than normal to stimulate the
cell

Renal   Pertaining to the kidney

Renshaw cell   An inhibitory *neuron* located in
the spinal cord

Representational hemisphere   The portion of
the brain thought to be responsible for visual-
spatial relationships; nondominant hemisphere

Residual volume   That volume of air which remains in the lungs after maximum expiration

Respiration, external   The exchange of gases
between the cell and the external environment

Respiration, internal   The utilization of oxygen
in the metabolic process

Respiration rate   The rate at which oxygen is
consumed

Respiratory center   A nerve center in the medulla which controls breathing rate

Respiratory minute volume   The total quantity
of air drawn into the lungs each minute;
breathing rate per minute times tidal volume

Respiratory quotient (RQ)   The volume of carbon dioxide liberated divided by the volume of
oxygen consumed in unit time

Resting membrane potential   The *potential*
which exists across the membrane during the
quiescent period

Resting metabolic rate   The oxygen consumption rate in the inactive animal at normothermic temperatures

Rete   A net

Reticulo-endothelial system   The tissue macro-
phage system; this includes Kupffer cells of the
liver and alveolar macrophages and all of the
cells derived from the circulating monocytes

Reticulospinal tract   A motor tract in the spinal
cord associated with the reticular activating
system of the brain

Reticulum   A network

Reversal potential   Part of the *action potential* in
which the internal charge is reversed (i.e., positive) from its normal negative state

Rhodopsin The visual pigment of the *rods*

Rhogam Rh-positive *antibodies* which are administered into the bloodstream of an Rh-negative mother after parturition of a Rh-positive fetus in order to bind any possible Rh-positive *antigens* which may have crossed the placental barrier

Rhombencephalon The hindbrain

Rickets A disease of the bones associated with vitamin-D deficiency

Rods The light sensitive cells of the retina which are specialized for vision in dim light

Ruminant An animal which harbors gastric microorganisms in a symbiotic relationship; usually a polygastric ungulate

S-A node Sinoatrial node

Saltatory conduction The conduction of an impulse along a nerve, characterized by jumps from one *node of Ranvier* to the next

Sarcolemma The muscle membrane

Sarcomere Repeating contractile units of muscle which exist between two Z lines and consisting of numerous *myofilaments*

Sarcoplasm The cytoplasm of a muscle cell

Sarcoplasmic reticulum A system of channels which surround the *sarcomere* of muscle and is essential for calcium ion exchange

Schwann cell *Myelin*-containing cell which encircles some peripheral nerve fibers

Scotopic vision Vision associated with the *rods* of the retina; night vision

Secretory vesicle A saclike body within the cell capable of releasing the contents to the outside

Segmentation The spontaneous formation of contractile rings in the intestine which tend to divide it into units and results in a sloshing action of the intestinal contents

Sella turcica A saddlelike depression on the upper surface of the sphenoid bone, enclosing the pituitary gland

Sensitization The initial exposure of an individual to a specific *antigen*, which results in an immune response; subsequent exposure usually results in a heightened response

Sensory neuron A nerve cell which detects environmental changes and relays these to the *central nervous system*

Septum A wall dividing two cavities

Serosa Any serous membrane

Serum Blood plasma minus the clotting elements

Set-point theory of thermoregulation The mechanism by which body temperature is regulated after comparing internal temperature or input from peripheral skin receptors with a hypothetical temperature (the set point) located within the hypothalamus

Sigmoid Shaped like the Greek letter sigma

Sliding-filament theory of muscle contraction The theory that thick and thin filaments of the sarcomere slide past each other during contraction

Sodium pump An *active transport* mechanism of sodium and potassium; especially located in the cell membrane of nerve and muscle cells

Somite One of the segmentally arranged, paired masses of mesoderm found alongside the neural tube of the embryo, forming the vertebral column and segmental musculature

Spatial summation The accumulative effects of several presynaptic *neurons* on one postsynaptic neuron

Specific dynamic action Heat generated during the process of *catabolism* which is not derived from the substrate

Specific gravity The weight of a substance compared with an equal volume of water

Spermatogenesis The formation and development of spermatozoa

Spermiation The process by which spermatozoa are released from the Sertoli cells

Spermiogenesis The second stage in the formation of spermatozoa, in which spermatids are transformed into spermatozoa

Sphincter A circular muscle surrounding an orifice

Sphygmomanometer An instrument for measuring arterial blood pressure

Spike An *action potential*

Spinal shock Paralytic period which immediately follows spinal trauma in some higher mammals

Spirometer An apparatus used to measure air capacity of the lungs

Spongy bone Bone usually located at the ends of the long bones, containing numerous vacuoles or spaces in the dried state that give the appearance of a sponge; important in blood cell synthesis; cancellous bone.

Squamous Scalelike

Starling's hypothesis The exchange of fluid between the tissues and the circulatory system is a function of colloidal-osmotic pressure, *hydrostatic pressure*, and tissue pressure

Starling's law of the heart The force of contraction of cardiac muscle is a function of applied tension

Stasis A stoppage or diminution of flow, as of blood or other body fluids; a state of equilibrium among opposing forces

Steroids Lipid soluble compounds containing four carbon rings interlocked to form a cyclopentophenanthrene nucleus; includes many *hormones* and *bile* acids

Stroke volume The quantity of blood pumped from the heart with one complete *systole*

Stroma The tissue that forms the ground substance or framework of an organ

Subliminal area Postsynaptic *neurons* which are affected by presynaptic neurons but are not aroused to action

Substrate phosphorylation Direct transfer of high-energy phosphate between a substrate molecule and ADP

Sulcus A groove or depression between parts, especially a fissure between the convolutions of the brain

Surfactant A substance which lowers the surface tension of membranes lining the inside of the lungs

Suture A type of joint, especially in the skull, where bone surfaces are closely united

Symphysis A line of union; a cartilagenous joint such as that between the bodies of the pubic bone

Synapse The junction between two *neurons*

Synarthrosis A fibrous joint

Synchondrosis A cartilagenous joint in which the cartilage is usually converted to bone before adult life

Syncytium A multinucleate mass of protoplasm produced by the merging of cells

Syndesmosis A joint in which the bones are united by fibrous connective tissue forming an interosseous membrane or ligament

Synostosis A joint between bones formed by osseous material

Synovial joint A union between two bones by means of a fluid-filled sac

Systemic circulation (greater circulation) That part of the vascular system carrying blood to all parts of the body except the lungs

Systole Heart muscle contraction, especially that of the ventricles

Systolic pressure The maximum pressure in the arteries produced by ventricular contraction

Tachycardia Rapid heart beat

Tactile Pertaining to the sense of touch

Tapetum lucidum The iridescent epithelium of the choroid of animals which gives their eyes the property of shining in dim light

Telencephalon The paired brain vesicles which are the anterolateral outpocketings of the forebrain, together with the median unpaired portion, the terminal lamina of the hypothalamus

Temporal summation Recruitment of the effects of a single presynaptic *axon* through rapid stimulation

Terminal buttons Projections from *axons* which terminate on the *dendrites* of postsynaptic *neurons;* responsible for release of *neurotransmitter*

Tetany Maximum contraction developed in a muscle during rapid stimulation in which insufficient time for relaxation is allowed

Thalamus Part of the lateral wall of the third ventricle lying between the *hypothalamus* and epithalamus; primarily a relay center for sensory impulses to the cerebral cortex

Thermogenesis The production of heat

Thermoneutral zone (TNZ) The range of ambient temperature within which metabolic rate is at a minimum, and within which temperature regulation is achieved by nonevaporative physical processes alone

Thermoregulation The regulation of body temperature within narrow limits

Threshold The level of stimulus which must be reached before an effect is produced

Thrombus A clot which is fixed in position

Tidal volume The quantity of air breathed with each breath

Tissue pressure The force developed by the weight of tissue on the circulatory system

Tonic muscles Muscles capable of prolonged contraction

Torpor A state of inactivity and reduced responsiveness to stimuli associated with a reduction in *metabolism* and body temperature

Total tension The summation of *active* and *passive tension* in a muscle

Trabecula A fibrous cord of connective tissue serving as a supporting fiber by forming a septum extending into its wall or capsule

Transcytosis The passage of a vesicle completely through a cell; involves both *endocytosis* and *exocytosis*; also known as cytopempsis

Transport maximum The enzymatic limit of a substance which can be pumped from the kidney tubules by active transport; tubular maximum

Trauma An injury or wound that may be produced by external force or shock

Treppe The staircase phenomenon associated with increased force of contraction following repeated stimuli

Tricarboxylic acid cycle (citric acid or Krebs cycle) The carbon cycle originating with citrate and ending with oxaloacetic acid

Triglycerides Esters of three fatty acids and glycerol

Upper critical temperature The ambient temperature above which body temperature can no longer be regulated by means of physical *thermoregulatory* mechanisms

Vas A vessel or duct

Vasoconstrictor A compound which causes blood vessels to constrict

Vasodilator A compound which causes blood vessels to dilate

Ventilation rate The rate of breathing

Ventral Pertaining to the lower portion of the body

Vesicle A small bladder or sac containing liquid

Vestibular apparatus Part of the inner ear associated with the sensation of balance and motion

Vestibule A small space or cavity at the beginning of a canal, especially the inner ear, larynx, mouth, nose, or vagina

Vestibulospinal tract Motor pathways in the spinal cord which relay impulses from the vestibular nuclei (and hence the *vestibular apparatus*) to the spinal cord

Villus One of the short, vascular, hairlike projections found on certain membranous surfaces, especially the intestinal mucosa

Viscera Organs of the chest or abdominal area

Viscosity The resistance of a liquid to flow

Visual cycle A series of reactions for the replacement of visual pigments in the retinal cells

Visual spectrum That part of the electromagnetic spectrum to which the eye responds

Vital capacity The maximum amount of air which can be exhaled from the lungs after complete filling

Viviparous Giving birth to living young, which develop within the maternal body

Wave summation The summation of contractile responses when stimuli are rapid enough to prevent complete relaxation

Weber-Fechner law An expression of the logarithmic relationship between strength of stimulus and sensation received

White matter Myelinated nerve tissue

White ramus communicans Area of passage of axons of the sympathetic preganglionic neurons which leave the spinal cord and travel to the paravertebral sympathetic ganglion chain

Zeitgeber Environmental cue; usually associated with modification or control of *circadian* rhythms

INDEX